SYMPOSIA OF THE
SOCIETY FOR EXPERIMENTAL BIOLOGY

NUMBER XLIX

PROCEEDINGS OF A
MEETING HELD AT
THE UNIVERSITY OF LEEDS, UK
4–8 JULY 1994

SYMPOSIA OF THE
SOCIETY FOR EXPERIMENTAL BIOLOGY

I Nucleic Acid
II Growth, Differentiation and Morphogenesis
III Selective Toxicity and Antibiotics
IV Physiological Mechanisms in Animal Behaviour
V Fixation of Carbon Dioxide
VI Structural Aspects of Cell Physiology
VII Evolution
VIII Active Transport and Secretion
IX Fibrous Proteins and their Biological Significance
X Mitochondria and other Cytoplasmic Inclusions
XI Biological Action of Growth Substances
XII The Biological Replication of Macromolecules
XIII Utilization of Nitrogen and its Compounds by Plants
XIV Models and Analogues in Biology
XV Mechanisms in Biological Competition
XVI Biological Receptor Mechanisms
XVII Cell Differentiation
XVIII Homeostasis and Feedback Mechanisms
XIX The State and Movement of Water in Living Organisms
XX Nervous and Hormonal Mechanisms of Integration
XXI Aspects of the Biology of Ageing
XXII Aspects of Cell Motility
XXIII Dormancy and Survival
XXIV Control of Organelle Development
XXV Control Mechanisms of Growth and Differentiation
XXVI The Effects of Pressure on Organisms
XXVII Rate Control of Biological Processes
XXVIII Transport at the Cellular Level
XXIX Symbiosis
XXX Calcium in Biological Systems
XXXI Integration of Activity in the Higher Plant
XXXII Cell–Cell Recognition
XXXIII Secretory Mechanisms
XXXIV The Mechanical Properties of Biological Materials
XXXV Prokaryotic and Eukaryotic Flagella
XXXVI The Biology of Photoreceptors
XXXVII Neural Origin of Rhythmic Movements
XXXVIII Controlling Events in Meiosis
XXXIX Physiological Adaptations of Marine Animals
XL Plasticity in Plants
XLI Temperature and Animals Cells
XLII Plants and Temperature
XLIII Mucus and Related Topics
XLIV Hormone Perception and Signal Transduction in Animals and Plants
XLV Molecular Biology of Plant Development
XLVI Molecular Biology of Muscle
XLVII Cell Behaviour: Adhesion and Motility
XLVIII Membrane Transport in Plants and Fungi: Molecular Mechanisms and Control

SYMPOSIA OF THE
SOCIETY FOR EXPERIMENTAL BIOLOGY

NUMBER XLIX

BIOLOGICAL FLUID DYNAMICS

EDITED BY
C. P. ELLINGTON AND T. J. PEDLEY

SOCIETY FOR EXPERIMENTAL BIOLOGY SYMPOSIA

SEB Symposia form a long-standing series of volumes first published in 1947. The series is annual and each publication is a collection of authoritative articles on an aspect of modern experimental Biology. The contributors are all invited and speak on specific topics within the chosen field. Meetings are held annually over a period of two or three days.

The aims of the Symposium series are to stimulate discussion and communication between scientists of all nationalities, to foster the development of, and research on, modern aspects of plant, animal and cell biology.

Published for the Society for Experimental Biology
by The Company of Biologists Limited
Bidder Building, 140 Cowley Road, Cambridge CB4 4DL, UK

Typeset, Printed and Published by The Company of Biologists Limited,
Bidder Building, 140 Cowley Road, Cambridge CB4 4DL, UK

ISBN 0 948601 50 7
ISSN 0081–1386

A CIP Catalogue record for this book is available from The British Library

CONTENTS

PREFACE

This book has arisen out of the SEB Symposium on "Biological Fluid Dynamics", which was held at the University of Leeds on 4-8 July 1994 with about 120 participants. A major aim of the Symposium was the promotion of increased contact and interaction between different groups of scientists within the general area of Biomechanics. We sought to bring together zoologists (and botanists) with their emphasis on comparative aspects and on external biological fluid dynamics (swimming, flying, feeding etc.), and medical scientists, physiologists and bioengineers with their emphasis on man and on internal fluid dynamics (blood flow, breathing etc.). The principles of fluid dynamics are the same for external and internal flows, and the biological principles of adaptation and optimisation apply to all aspects of an organism's response to physical constraints. The scientists invited to the Symposium included both biologists and theoretical and experimental fluid dynamicists.

The Symposium was organised in seven half-day sessions. Each session covered a particular area and each (with one exception) contained two major invited lectures and four shorter ones selected from offered contributions. The seven sessions were entitled (in order of occurrence): Swimming; Flight; Large vessel blood flow; Microcirculation and tissue transport; Micro-organisms, filter feeding, etc.; Invertebrates and intermediate Reynolds number; and Respiration. There was a poster room in which posters were displayed all week, and in which a convivial poster and video session was centred on one evening. There were no parallel sessions.

The presenters of the major lectures were invited to write authoritative surveys of their fields for this volume. Shorter articles were also solicited from some of the other contributors in order to fill gaps in the coverage. It is gratifying that almost everyone invited has responded positively, and we therefore believe that this volume will prove to be of lasting value as a comprehensive survey of Biological Fluid Dynamics.

It is a great pleasure for us, as Chairman and co-Chairman of the Symposium as well as editors of this book, to record our gratitude to the Society for Experimental Biology, the Wellcome Trust and the Company of Biologists for their generous financial support. We would also like to thank the University of Leeds, in particular the School of Mathematics, for their help and support. Much of the organisational burden was borne by the other members of the organising committee: Neill Alexander, John Altringham, Chris Bridges, Jeremy Rayner, Tony Stead and especially Nick Hill, who ensured that all last-minute logistical problems within Leeds were solved effectively. We are grateful to those Leeds research students in Applied Mathematics (Fatma Ayaz, Bindi Brook, Munir Chaudhary, Andy Edwards, David Lynch, Louise Matthews, Jon Pitchford and Richard Vincent) who organised the audio-visual equipment and made sure that the refreshments flowed freely during the poster evening.

Sandra Koura and Victoria Wragg from the SEB Office provided administrative support with their usual efficiency. Final thanks must go to Dr Sandra Ray of the Company of Biologists, who has enabled this volume to be produced with splendid despatch.

C.P.E.
T.J.P.

BODY SURFACE ADAPTATIONS TO BOUNDARY-LAYER DYNAMICS

J. J. VIDELER

Department of Marine Biology, Groningen University, PO Box 14, NL-9750, The Netherlands

Summary

Evolutionary processes have adapted nektonic animals to interact efficiently with the water that surrounds them. Not all these adaptations serve the same purpose. This paper concentrates on reduction of drag due to friction in the boundary layer close to the body surface. Mucus, compliant skins, scales, riblets and roughness may influence the flow velocity gradient, the type of flow and the thickness of the boundary layer around animals, and may seriously affect their drag in a positive or negative way.

The long-chain polymers found in mucus decrease the pressure gradient and considerably reduce drag due to friction. The effect is probably due to channelling of the flow particles in the direction of the main flow, resulting in a reduction of turbulence.

Compliant surfaces could probably reduce drag by equalising and distributing pressure pulses. However, the existing evidence that drag reduction actually occurs is not convincing. There is no indication that instantaneous heating, reducing the viscosity in the boundary layer, is used by animals as a drag-reducing technique.

Small longitudinal ridges on rows of scales on fish can reduce shear stress in the boundary by a maximum of 10 % compared with the shear stress of a smooth surface. The mechanism is based on the impedance of cross flow under well-defined conditions. The effect has been visualized with the use of particle image velocimetry techniques.

The function of the swords and spears of several fast, pelagic, predatory fish species is still enigmatic. The surface structure of the sword of a swordfish is shown to be both rough and porous. The height of the roughness elements on the tip of the sword is close to the critical value for the induction of a laminar-to-turbulent flow transition at moderate cruising speeds.

A flow tank is described that is designed to visualize the effects of surface imperfections on flow in the boundary layer in direct comparison with a smooth flat wall. The flow in a 1 m long, 10 cm high and 1 cm wide channel is visualized by illuminating the particles in a thin laser light sheet. The first results show that a rough surface increases the shear stress in the boundary layer and makes it thinner. The function of the roughness on the sword of a swordfish is probably to reduce the total drag by generating premature turbulence and by boundary layer thinning, despite an increased friction over the surface of the sword.

The function of the porous surface structures on the sword, and of the porous skins of sharks and of the castor oil fish, will probably be discovered soon using new particle

Key words: boundary layer, mucopolysaccharides, mucus, skin, scales, ridges, swordfish, roughness, compliance, drag reduction.

image velocimetry techniques applied under strong magnification to visualize the local behaviour of the flow.

Introduction

This paper deals with a very limited selection of biological adaptations. Body surfaces of animals serve many functions, and virtually every structural feature has developed as a compromise with the demands of other functions in response to evolutionary pressures. Adaptations resulting from pressures with high survival values can be expected to show fewer concessions and might be close to optimal solutions for particular functions. Hydrodynamic drag reduction increases the survival value of animals that rely heavily on their swimming performance to obtain food, to find mates and to escape from predators. Total hydrodynamic drag may be divided artificially into drag due to velocity (and hence pressure) changes around the body and drag due to friction in a layer of fluid close to the animal. In the context of this division, adaptations are either related to the shape of the body or to surface structures. Here, we restrict ourselves mainly to relationships between skin features and the behaviour of the fluid very close to the animals.

Adaptations of the skin

Knowledge of biological relationships between form and function is often based on intuition and common sense. The Dutch functional morphologist J. W. M. Osse (personal communication) calls this the 'Little Red Riding-hood' approach: 'My, grandmother what big eyes you have! All the better to see you with. My, what big teeth you have! All the better to eat you with!' It would be very difficult to prove scientifically that bigger teeth improve the consumption of little girls; however, the assumed connection between the size of the eyes and improved vision is a useful *ad hoc* hypothesis. This approach has been and still is widespread practice in functional morphology, and there is nothing wrong with it as long as the hypotheses are not treated as proven facts.

The surfaces of the bodies of aquatic animals provide a wide range of interesting features that have been considered as adaptations to decrease hydrodynamic drag. These considerations are, however, mainly based on Little Red Riding-hood thinking. In order to turn these hypotheses into factual knowledge, we need to prove that the drag-reducing effect really exists and to find out to what extent it applies. Ultimately, we are interested in the process causing the effect.

Potentially drag-reducing surfaces on the bodies of aquatic animals can be arbitrarily classified into five categories: (1) surfaces excreting long-chain polymers; (2) compliant skins; (3) heat-generating surfaces; (4) skins with longitudinal grooves, hair, ridges or riblets; and (5) surfaces covered with random roughness. A critical overview of the existing measurements and hypotheses should encourage further work in this field and possibly point out the most promising directions to choose.

The boundary layer concept

Prandtl (1904) divided the flow near a solid surface into two regions. Close to the surface, the relative velocity varies from zero right at the surface to the free-stream velocity at some distance away. This region is called the *boundary layer*. The steep velocity gradient normal to the surface is due to the viscosity of the fluid. In the second region, outside the boundary layer, viscosity can be neglected and only inertial forces are taken into consideration (i.e. incompressible frictionless flow, or potential flow). Velocity and hence pressure gradients are relatively uniform there. In both regions, the flow can be either laminar or turbulent. In a laminar flow, individual fluid particles move steadily and follow smooth tracks or streamlines. If particles start to move in a more chaotic way, the flow has become turbulent. The instant of transition from laminar to turbulent flow depends on the size of the solid surface, on the speed of the flow relative to that surface, and on the ratio of inertial to viscous forces expressed dimensionlessly as the *Reynolds number*:

$$Re = UL\nu^{-1}, \tag{1}$$

where ν is the kinematic viscosity or diffusivity of the fluid, U is the velocity of the fluid and L is a typical length. The diffusivity is the ratio of the viscosity (momentum per unit surface area) to the fluid density ρ. Lighthill (1990) shows how a physical quantity, e.g. velocity, diffuses in time t over a surface area proportional to νt; along one direction, the diffusion distance d is therefore proportional to $(\nu t)^{1/2}$.

A simplified two-dimensional description of the flow in the boundary layer over a very thin flat plate, moved in the direction of the plane of the plate, is given in Fig. 1. The plate moves to the left at speed U_∞. Where the sharp leading edge of the plate meets still water, the velocity gradient between the plate moving at U_∞ and the stationary water mass has zero thickness. As the flow then convects along the plate, the velocity diffuses outwards and the thickness $\delta(x)$ of the velocity gradient grows in proportion to $(\nu t)^{1/2}$, or:

$$\delta(x) = (\nu x U_\infty{}^{-1})^{1/2}, \tag{2}$$

where x is the distance along the plate and $xU_\infty{}^{-1}$ denotes the time taken to cover distance x. Equation 2 can be expressed in terms of a local Re, based on length x:

$$\delta(x) = x(xU_\infty \nu^{-1})^{-1/2} = xRe^{-1/2}. \tag{3}$$

Fig. 1 shows how the boundary layer is thin and laminar just beyond the leading edge. The velocity gradient across the boundary layer is relatively steep. Re increases with distance x along the plate up to a critical value. Beyond that point, instability increases, starting with waves and ending in completely chaotic movements beyond the transition zone. The thickness of the boundary layer is everywhere small compared with the length L of the plate. Calculations based on empirical values by Blasius (1908) give:

$$\delta(x) = 3.4xRe^{-1/2} \tag{4}$$

for laminar flow, and:

$$\delta(x) = 0.37xRe^{-1/5} \tag{5}$$

for turbulent flow.

For a flat plate of length 1 m moving in water at 20 °C (ν=$10^{-6}\,m^2\,s^{-1}$) at a velocity of 5 $m\,s^{-1}$, Re at 1 cm from the leading edge is about 5×10^4. The thickness of the boundary layer there is about 0.15 mm. Beyond the transition zone near the end of the plate, Re is 5×10^6 and the maximum value of $\delta(x)$ is 1.7 cm.

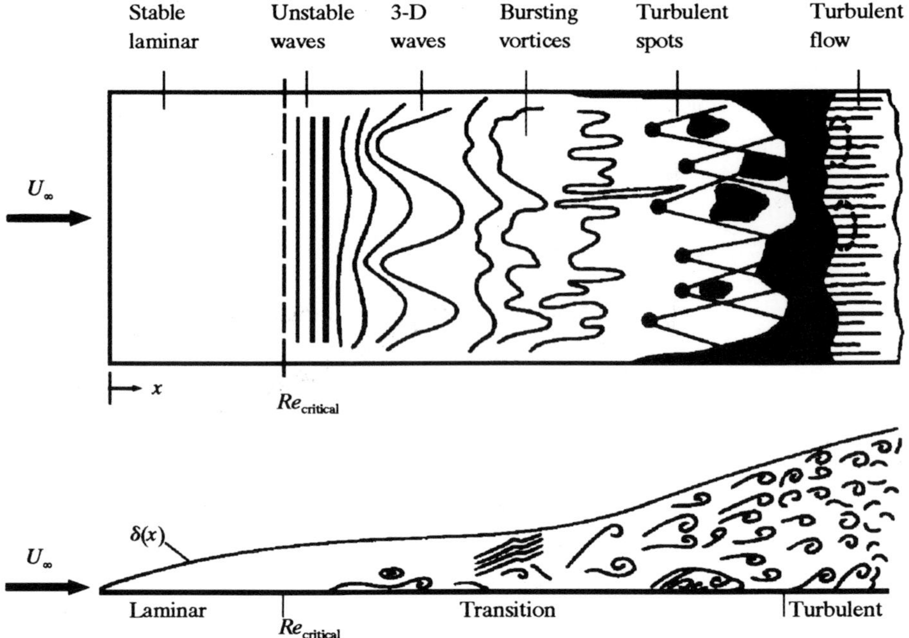

Fig. 1. Schematic summary of the development of the boundary layer over a very thin flat plate. The plate is moving to the left at speed U_∞ in the direction of its plane. The upper part of the diagram provides a top view and describes six stages in the flow pattern from left to right. The lower diagram displays the growth of the boundary layer thickness $\delta(x)$ with a change of character of the flow from laminar to fully turbulent under flow regimes with increasing *Re*. From Schlichting (1979, Fig. 16.23 after White, 1974).

Frictional drag *D*, which is the main drag on a very thin flat plate (with surface area *A*) moving in its own plane, changes with the conditions of the flow. The drag coefficient C_f is defined as:

$$C_f = D(0.5\rho U_\infty{}^2 A)^{-1}. \tag{6}$$

For our smooth flat plate under laminar conditions, C_f is, according to Blasius (1908):

$$C_f = 1.328 Re^{-1/2}. \tag{7}$$

There are several semi-empirical equations describing the drag coefficient for a smooth flat plate under turbulent conditions. Fig. 2, modified from Hoerner (1965), gives a large number of C_f values for smooth flat plates in parallel flow. The data points under laminar conditions follow the Blasius model nicely up to the transitional range of *Re*. The C_f values measured under natural and prematurely forced turbulent conditions are also well described by most models. The coefficient increases during the transition 1.5-fold, from 0.002 under laminar conditions at $Re=3\times10^5$ to approximately 0.003 when the flow is turbulent at $Re=3\times10^6$. If the flow remained laminar at this higher *Re*, the Blasius curve would predict a C_f value of about 0.0008, which would be a reduction of 3.75-fold compared with the turbulent value. Such a delay in the occurrence of turbulence would be

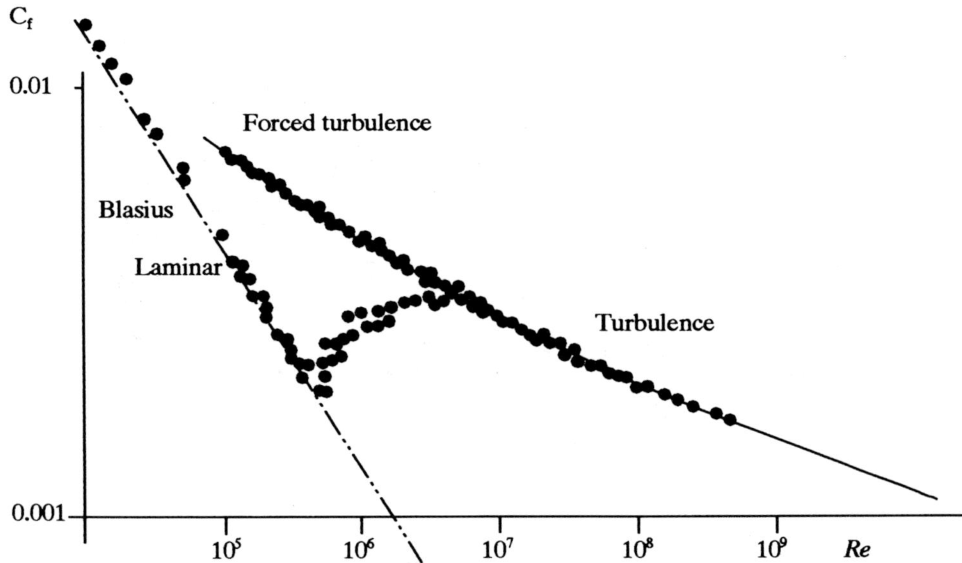

Fig. 2. Measurements and calculations of the frictional drag coefficient C_f as a function of *Re*. Data points are from various measurements, lines are model calculations. See text for further details. Based on Hoerner (1965).

an effective drag-reducing mechanism. It is conceivable that some surface structures are adaptations serving that goal. However, delayed turbulence can also stimulate sudden separation of the flow away from the solid surface, which would strongly increase the drag coefficient. Separation usually occurs as a result of negative pressure gradients in the boundary layer, and it starts when the flow is reversed very close to the surface. This, of course, happens more easily near the end of a blunt body than along a flat plate. Separation of a laminar boundary layer can be delayed by a premature transition to turbulence, where a more uniform distribution of velocities provides a more stable situation. This could be achieved by roughness of the right size and in a place where the flow would be laminar under normal conditions. If such an adaptation exists, it would be expected to occur on the anteriormost part on the body of a fast-swimming animal.

In a fully developed turbulent flow, there are more possibilities for favourable interference with the flow. In the velocity gradient of the boundary layer, water particles rotate and deform each other. Under turbulent conditions, there are movements in all directions superimposed on the average mean path of the flow. In fact, every adaptation reducing the erratic movements of water particles in turbulence or large-scale eddies potentially has a drag-reducing effect.

Polymer drag reduction through mucus, tears and cell shedding

The epidermis of fish usually contains mucoid cells. These cells secrete fibrous mucopolysaccharides, which swell in water to form mucus. The mucus layer may serve a variety of functions. For example, it protects against infections and parasites, reduces the danger of damage, helps the fish to escape from predators, and may prevent the exchange of ions.

Mucus is also assumed to reduce frictional drag during swimming through a mechanism known by physicists as the Toms effect. Toms (1948) found that small amounts of polymers added to turbulent high-*Re* flow in a pipe reduced the pressure drop substantially below that of the fluid alone at the same flow rate (Lumley, 1969). Rosen and Cornford (1971) and Bernadsky *et al.* (1993) investigated the Toms effect of the mucus of a number of fish species from different ecological niches and of two species of marine molluscs. Comparison of the drag-reducing properties of mucus shown in both studies does not provide a consistent picture. A 5 % solution of mucus from the Pacific barracuda *Sphyraena argentata* in sea water gave the highest drag reduction of almost 66 %. The mucus of the Red Sea chevron barracuda *Sphyraena putnamiae* gave maximally less than 10 % drag reduction. The morphology and feeding habits of both species are very similar. No consistent relationship between speed and style of locomotion and the drag-reducing effectiveness of mucus could be found for the species investigated so far.

The mucus produced by two molluscs, the Red Sea sea hare *Aplysia oculifera* and the Pacific nut brown cowrie *Cyprea spadicea*, had excellent drag-reducing properties, providing more than 60 % reduction compared with pure sea water. Both species are very slow crawling organisms. The biomechanical properties of the mucus of molluscs changed from highly elastic under stationary conditions to viscous whenever sliding movements were applied (Denny, 1980). It is quite possible that the large molecules causing this peculiar mechanical behaviour also happen to decrease frictional drag.

The effect of fish mucus on the flow in the boundary layer has been analyzed by Daniel (1981), who compared velocity profiles over the surface of a freshly killed rainbow trout *Oncorhynchus mykiss* with those over smooth wax models of the same fish. Stroboscopic flash photography was used to measure the velocity of 100–300 μm diameter particles in the flow. Fig. 3 shows that the boundary layer velocity profile over the surface of the fish slopes more gradually than that over the model. These slopes were used to approximate the shear stress τ_0 (N m^{-2}) acting on the surface of the fish and the model using Newton's law of viscosity:

$$\tau_0 = \mu \delta U_x / \delta y \,, \tag{8}$$

where $\delta U_x/\delta y$ is the velocity gradient near the surface. Fig. 3 shows that the thickness of the boundary layer over the model is about half as high as that over the fish. The shear forces over the model without mucus are therefore about twice as high as those over the fish. Little can be said about the total drag because a thicker boundary layer displaces and compresses the streamlines of the potential flow around the body, and this will increase velocities and enhance the total drag.

The cells in the skin of the bottle-nosed dolphin *Tursiops truncatus* divide 250–290 times faster than those in the human epidermis (Palmer and Weddel, 1964). These cells are released during swimming and have been thought to have a drag-reducing effect similar to that of the long-chain molecules in fish mucus. Sokolov *et al.* (1969), however, could not detect drag-reducing properties of dolphin cell suspensions when tested against

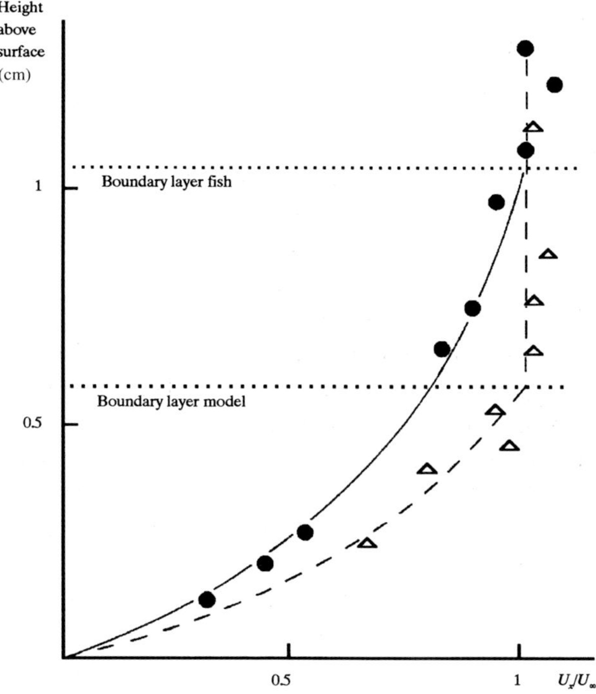

Fig. 3. Flow velocity measurements at different heights above the mucus covering the skin of a trout (filled circles) and a wax model without mucus (open triangles). The speed is normalised with respect to the freestream velocity U_∞. The approximate boundary layer thickness is indicated by horizontal dotted lines. Based on Daniel (1981).

sea water in a Toms effect experiment. They also failed to show any significant effect of dolphin eye secretions on pressure differences in flow tubes.

The causes of the friction-reducing effect of long-chain polymers are still under investigation. There are currently two opposing opinions. The first assumes that the drag-reducing effect is caused by the polymers acting as viscoelastic threads, steering water particles in the main stream direction and thus reducing the turbulence. According to the second opinion, the drag reduction is due to small pieces of the polymer chains which are released from the threads, mix with the fluid and reduce turbulence. Gyr *et al.* (1993) provide experimental evidence showing that at least part of the effect is caused by small fractions of polymer mixed into the fluid.

Hoyt (1975) assumes that a delay in laminar-to-turbulent transition in the boundary layer could be largely responsible for the Toms effect. Polymers may double or triple the *Re* at which this transition occurs. Hoyt also reviews the evidence showing that the friction in a pulsating flow can be reduced by 24% at certain long-chain polymer concentrations. The main feature, however, seems to be a reduction in the shear stresses under turbulent conditions, which agrees well with Daniel's measurements of the decreased average velocity gradient along a slimy fish skin. It is tempting to envisage how the long molecules, orientated in the streamwise direction, limit crossflow and hence the shear stress due to that motion in the fluid. Quantitative support for this picture must await detailed flow visualization.

Compliant and heat-generating surfaces

During the onset of the transition from laminar to turbulent flow over a flat plate, waves develop in the fluid. In an idealized case, these waves start as two-dimensional, so-called Tollmien–Schlichting waves, turning into three-dimensional ones before vortices are formed (stages 2 and 3 of Fig. 1). Waves are an indication of oscillating velocity and pressure changes. Kramer (1960) suggested that compliant natural surfaces such as the dolphin skin could minimize pressure pulsations by elastic deformation processes. The laminar flow pattern would be maintained beyond the critical *Re* through this mechanism, offering reduced drag at high speeds.

The skin of dolphins seems to be adapted for this type of hydrodynamically advantageous behaviour. The outer part of mammalian skin has two layers: an epidermis on the outside and a dermis underneath. Both layers are exceptionally thin in cetaceans. The epidermis of dolphins is only about 0.5 mm thick. The dermis of the common porpoise *Phocaena phocaena* is only 0.34 mm thick (Slijper, 1958). This is the reason why the dermis covering most parts of the body of cetaceans cannot be used for leather production (the penis skin being the main exception). Dermal ridges are another unique feature of cetacean skin. The outer part of the dermis forms papillae arranged on longitudinal ridges, penetrating into the epidermis, firmly connecting the epidermis with the dermis. The ridges supposedly follow the direction of the flow obliquely over the body (Purves, 1963).

Kramer (1960) mounted a thin rubber diaphragm over rubber stubs in a fluid-filled space as an imitation of the dolphin skin structure. Rather crude tests, using models towed by a speed boat, showed a maximum drag reduction of 59 % at $Re = 15 \times 10^6$. Experiments verifying the large drag reductions, however, have failed so far (Gad-El-Hak, 1987; Carpenter, 1990; see Fish and Hui, 1991, for a review of drag minimization in dolphin swimming).

Essapian (1955) recorded skin deformations appearing as transversal folds on fast-swimming and accelerating dolphins. Aleyev (1977) tried to demonstrate that this was a passive drag-enhancing phenomenon by towing naked women through the water at about twice the speed of the world record freestyle for men. Women and dolphins have a subcutaneous fatty layer and virtually hairless bodies in common, which makes them, according to Aleyev, physically analogous. The hydrodynamic resistance of the same women dressed in a tight suit was noticeably lower than that of the nude subjects.

Increased temperature of a fluid decreases viscous effects and could conceivably reduce drag to some extent. Marine mammals and warm-bodied fish are potentially capable of performing such a trick. Drag reduction due to decreased viscosity could, however, only occur if the water in the boundary layer could be heated instantaneously. That requires a very effective heat exchanger in the skin. The blood supply to the epidermis of whales is poorly developed compared with that of other mammals. The small arteries running into the dermal papillae are surrounded by veins forming a heat-preserving system (Slijper, 1958; Parry, 1949). This is the opposite of what one would expect from a system promoting heat loss into the environment. Walters (1962) showed that this mechanism is not likely to work in tunas either.

Ridges, scales and riblets

Drag reduction studies in aircraft research showed that small longitudinal ridges of a particular geometry could reduce drag under turbulent conditions (Walsh, 1980; Walsh and Lindemann, 1984). The maximum drag reduction was found to be dependent on the height h and on the spacing s of the riblets in relation to the local Reynolds number s^+, defined as:

$$s^+ = s(\tau_0 \rho^{-1})^{1/2} \nu^{-1}, \quad (9)$$

where τ_0 is the shear stress of an equivalent flat plate as defined in equation 8. Note that $(\tau_0 \rho^{-1})^{1/2}$ has units of $\mathrm{m\,s^{-1}}$. Maximum drag reductions of 7–8 % were measured by Walsh and Lindemann (1984) in windtunnel tests for s^+ values around 15, using plates with and without riblets mounted on a drag balance. Bechert *et al.* (1985), inspired by naturally occurring riblets on large sharks, tested a variety of riblet configurations as well as the drag-reducing properties of hair. The use of a flow channel filled with 4500 kg of baby oil allowed them to magnify the tiny riblets 100 times. *Re* reached by the channel was between 5000 and 33 000. Test plates with different riblets milled in Plexiglas were compared with flat plates.

The large pelagic predatory sharks swim at speeds up to $20\,\mathrm{m\,s^{-1}}$ (*Re* up to 10^7). They are covered with a variety of small scales varying in diameter between 0.2 and 0.5 mm (Bechert *et al.* 1985). Fig. 4 shows how the shape of the scales depends on the position on the body with respect to the passing flow on a 2.55 m Galapagos shark *Carcharhinus galapagensis*. The pattern on the trunk is repeated across the pectoral fins. The frontal scales have a rounded and smooth front, and bear ridges on the rear end. There are very regular continuous ridges on the scales in the middle section of the body and fins. The rearmost scales bear similar ridges that are somewhat extended at the trailing ends. The implantation of the rearmost scales is flexible, and the scales may bend backwards under pressure. The spacing of the ridges varies among the large sharks between 35 and 105 μm. The scales are firmly attached to the shark skin, which is up to 3 mm thick. The pattern of implantation ensures that the ridges are continuous along the body. Fig. 5A,B shows scanning electron micrographs of the scale configuration of the middle section of the Galapagos shark. Fig. 5C shows a close up of scales on the silky shark *Carcharhinus falciformes*. The base of the scale is smaller than the surface part, leaving a fluid-filled space underneath the outer surface.

Fig. 6 compiles the best results obtained so far with different longitudinal ridges tested against smooth flat plates (Bruse *et al.* 1993). The y-axis gives the difference in shear stress as a percentage of the shear stress measured for the flat plate. Walsh's V-shaped riblets in optimal configuration, with a ratio of protrusion height h over the distance s between the ridges of 0.9, caused a decrease in shear stress of about 6 %. Simple straight ridges, based on the configuration found in the great white shark, provided about 9 % drag reduction.

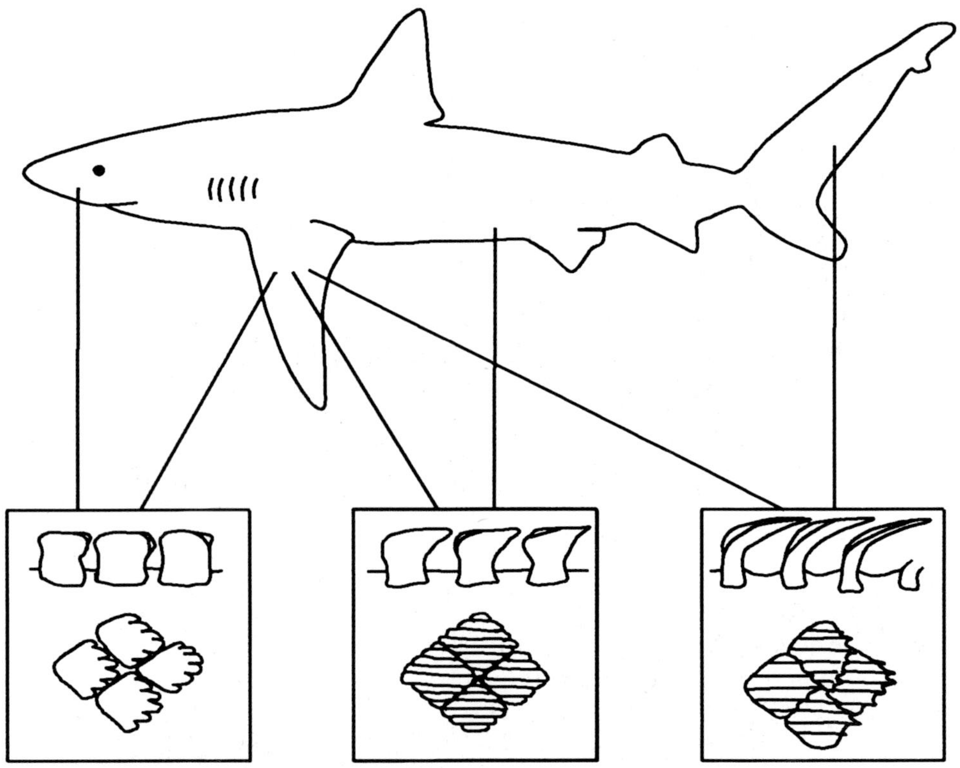

Fig. 4. Repeating patterns of scales with different surface riblets on the body and pectoral fins of a 2.55 m Galapagos shark. From Bechert *et al.* (1986).

Ridges that are scalloped in cross section gave intermediate values. The best spacing found for hair, with h/s=0.1, gave only about 2 % reduction in shear stress. Schneider and Dinkelacker (1993) tested V-grooved riblet films against a smooth surface for a streamlined body of revolution in a water tunnel. They obtained drag reductions of up to 10 % at *Re* of the order of 2×10^6, using spacings between the saw teeth of 62 and 86 μm.

The mechanism behind these drag reductions was probably well devised by Bechert *et al.* (1986). They supposed that longitudinal ribs would straighten the turbulent flow into the mean flow direction by hampering the cross flow components. Quantitative support for the suggestion that rib structures impede cross flow comes from Suzuki and Kasagi (1993), who used three-dimensional particle tracking velocimetry to visualise the effect. At s^+ values of 15, the cross flow very close to the valleys between the ribs was impeded. This s^+ value corresponds well with the range where maximum drag reductions were

Fig. 5. Scanning electron micrographs taken by W.-E. Reif (Tübingen University) of surface structures on the middle section of large pelagic sharks. (A) Overview of the scale configuration of the Galapagos shark of Fig. 4. The flow direction during swimming is from left to right. (B) The scales at approximately the same position viewed from the rear. Note the pit organ, a differential pressure sensor, in the centre of the picture. (C) Single scales of a 2.27 m silky shark. Note the space left by the narrow bases of the scales.

found in Fig. 6. At an s^+ of 31, the drag increase is probably caused by a secondary flow developing near the ribs, enhancing the transport of turbulent movement, which obviously exceeds the drag-reducing effect.

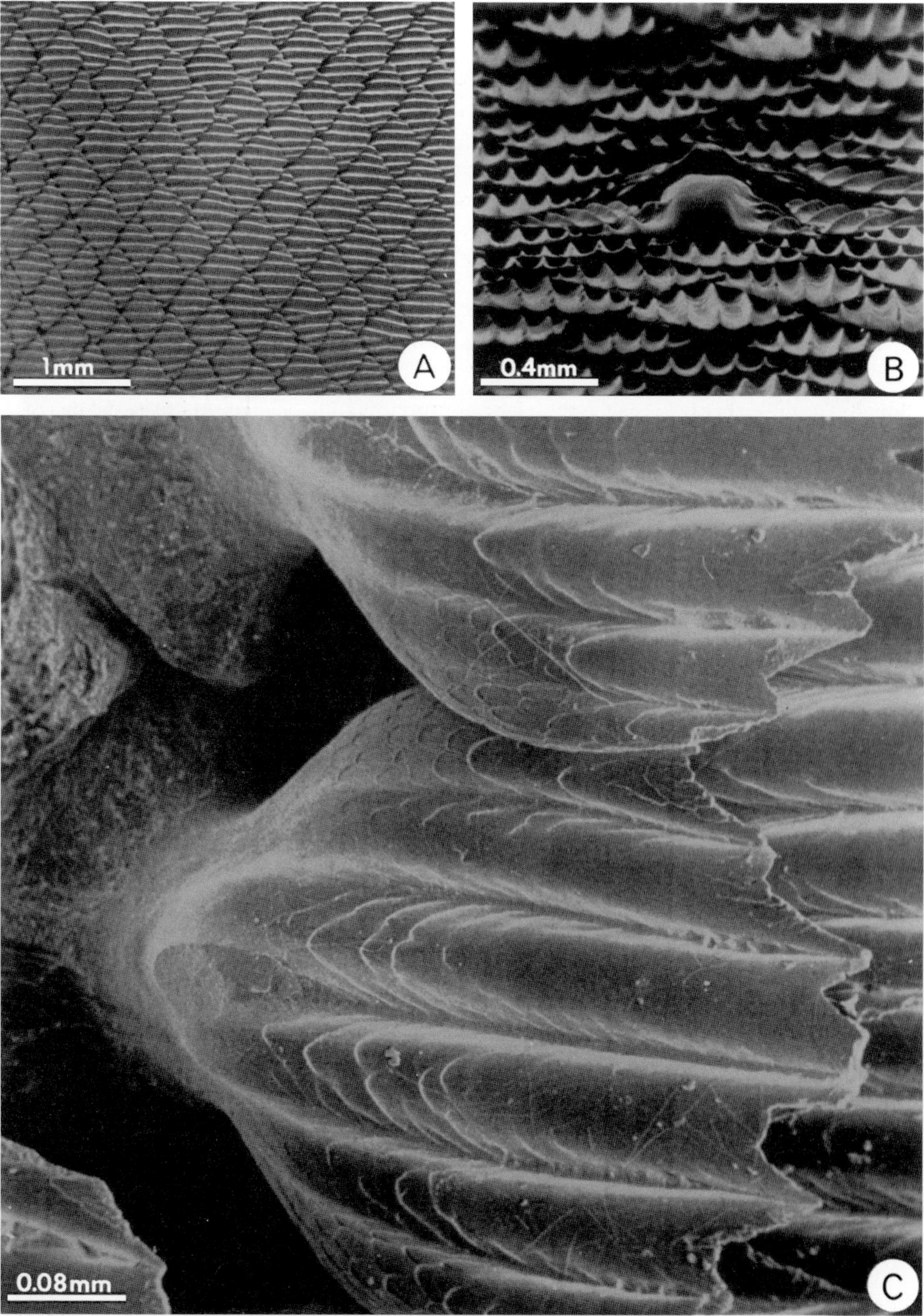

Fig. 5

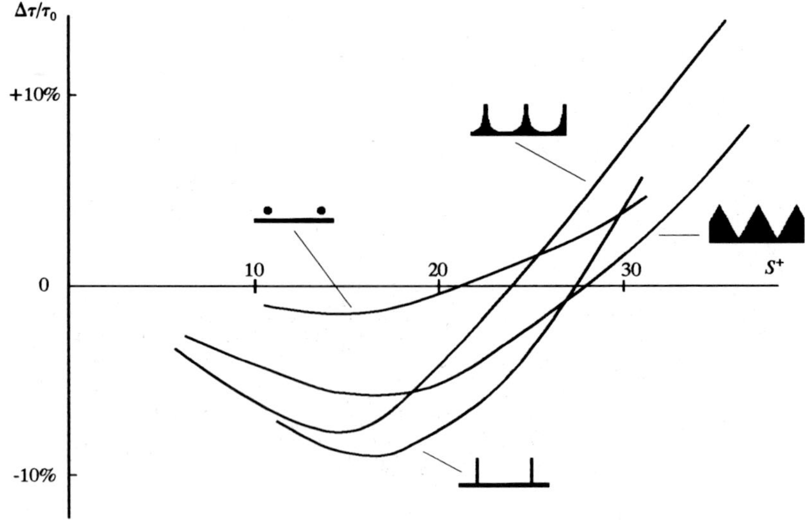

Fig. 6. The difference between the shear stress of surfaces with longitudinal riblets and that of a flat plate, expressed as a percentage of the shear stress of the latter. Positive values indicate a shear stress higher than that of a flat plate. Negative values are found when a test surface has a lower shear stress than that of a smooth flat plate. The horizontal axis is the local *Re*, s^+ (see text). Results obtained with optimal configurations, giving the smallest minimum shear stress, for scalloped, saw-tooth and straight riblets and for hair in the flow direction above the surface are shown. The relative dimensions of the optimal configurations are shown by their transections perpendicular to the flow. Based on Bruse *et al.* (1993) and Walsh (1980).

My, fish what a big sword you have!

The swordfish *Xiphias gladius* can reach a size of up to 4.5 m in length, but adults are usually between 2.5 and 3.5 m long. Scales on the body are functionally absent. The shape of the head beyond the rostrum is concave. The sword, the extended upper jaw, can reach a length of 40–45 % of the body length in adults. It is dorsoventrally flattened and covered with craters and bumps, giving it a rough appearance. The height of the roughness is about 0.1–0.2 mm, with maximum values appearing nearest to the tip. The scanning electron micrograph (Fig. 7A), giving an overview of the surface structure at about 10 % of the length of the sword from the tip, shows some longitudinal orientation in the ridges and grooves. A closer look at the same surface (Fig. 7B) emphasises the presence of many holes with a diameter of about 0.1–0.2 mm. Sections through the sword (Fig. 7C) reveal that the holes are probably interconnected by a system of channels just underneath the rough surface. This figure also shows the size and the spacing of the rough elements.

There are no proper swimming speed measurements for swordfish. Estimates exceed $30\,\mathrm{m\,s^{-1}}$ ($108\,\mathrm{km\,h^{-1}}$). At that speed, a 3 m swordfish would swim at an *Re* of the order of 10^8. The anatomy supports these extreme speed claims. The high lunate caudal fin, the narrow dorsoventrally flattened caudal peduncle fitted with lateral keels and the large muscular streamlined body are all hallmarks of a very fast swimmer (Videler, 1993).

There is a great deal of controversy about the function of the sword. Despite reports on the use of the sword for stabbing enemies, slashing prey and piercing boats (Talbot and

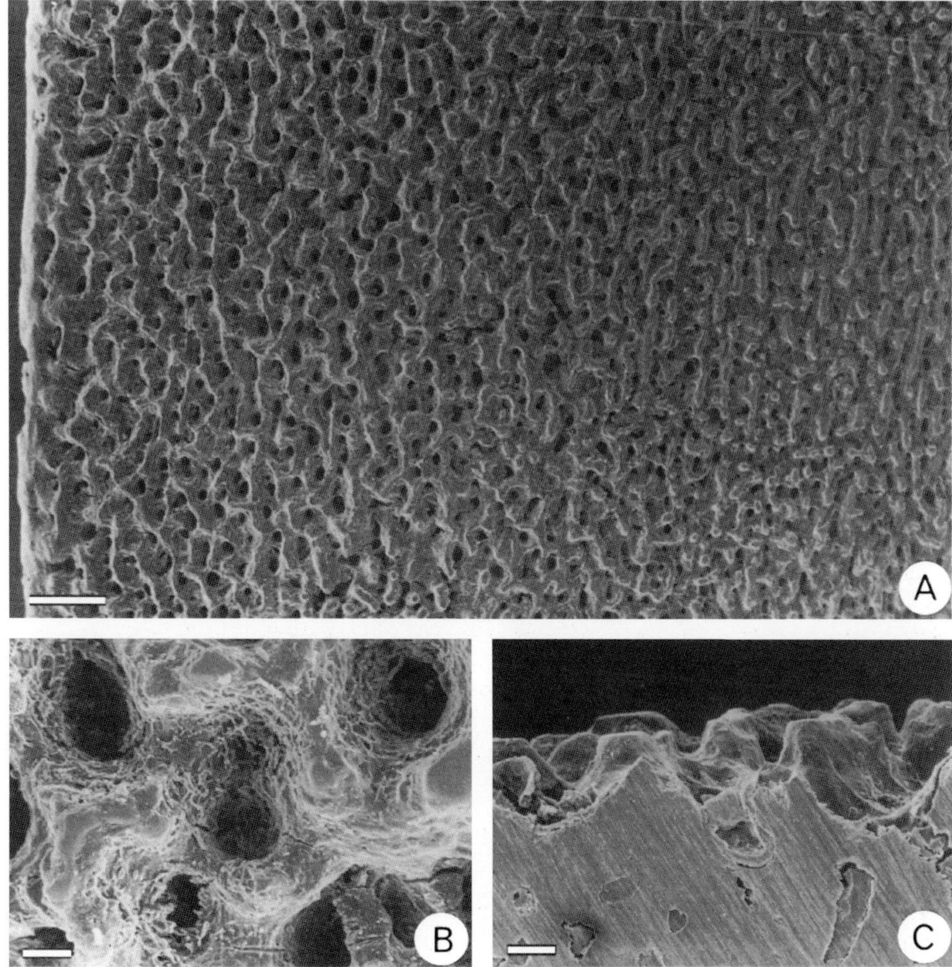

Fig. 7. Scanning electron micrographs of the surface structures on a 76 cm long sword of a swordfish at about 8 cm from the tip. (A) Overview of the upper surface. The local width of the sword is about 2.5 cm. The right edge of the sword is visible on the left, the direction of the tip is to the bottom of the page. Scale bar, 1 mm. (B) Enlarged portion of the same surface showing the size of the holes between the protuberances. Scale bar, 0.1 mm. (C) A cross section showing the size of the rough elements and pores in the bone just underneath the surface, which possibly interconnect the holes. Scale bar, 0.1 mm.

Penrith, 1962), there is little real evidence that this type of use was intentional. Spear- and sword-bearing fish rely on extremely high speeds to overtake and engulf their fast-swimming food items, and the swords presumably serve a hydrodynamic function (Wisner, 1958). Swordfish live pelagically in the open ocean, where they are usually never confronted with solid boundaries. These fast fish cannot swim tight turns, are unable to swim backwards and cannot brake properly. Accidental collisions are to be expected with such bad manoeuvring performance. Another argument against the weapon function is that it would be very difficult for a swordfish to get rid of a stabbed prey item stuck on its sword. Finally, the delicate surface structure of the sword makes it both rough and blunt, properties that are undesirable if it had to be used as a blade.

Aleyev (1977) measured the dynamic pressure coefficient (Fig. 8) over the surface of a smooth model of the swordfish with and without a sword, showing that the presence of the sword prevents extreme pressure values near the onset of the head and at the shoulder. This interesting measurement deals mainly with the pressure drag outside the boundary layer on the basis of the overall shape. However, understanding the function of the sword also requires explanations for aspects of the anatomy of the sword itself, i.e. its roughness and the more complex structural features such as the holes and the porosity.

Studies on the effect of sandpaper roughness by Nikuradse (1933) show (Fig. 9) that roughness of a certain size increases the drag under turbulent conditions; rough surfaces of the order of roughness of the sword of a swordfish do not make much difference under laminar conditions (Schlichting, 1979). These findings predict that a rough sword would increase drag at high speeds and have no effect at low speeds. Despite these discouraging results from well-established early hydrodynamic studies, an attempt was made to examine in more detail the effect of roughness in a direct comparison with a flat surface.

A flow tank for direct comparison of wall structure effects

A flow tank was constructed to investigate the effect of roughness on the flow in the

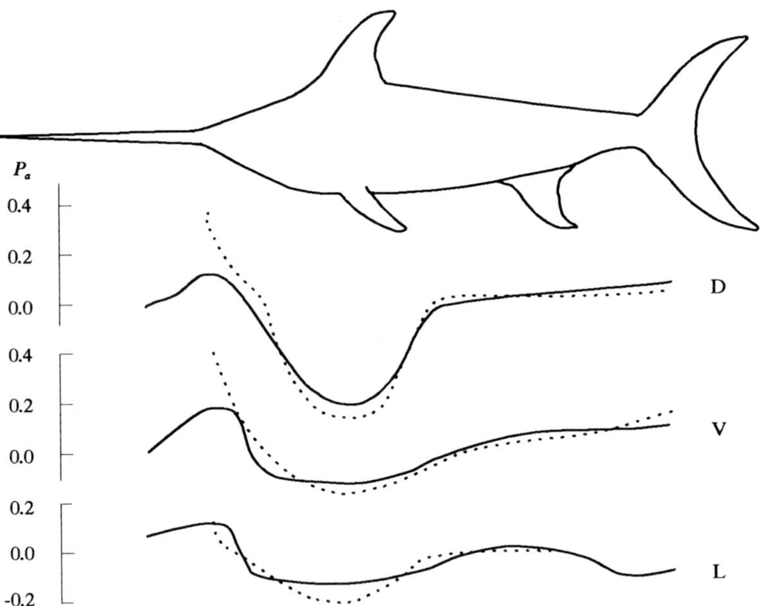

Fig. 8. Distribution of dynamic pressure coefficient P_a over the surface of a model of *Xiphias gladius* along the dorsal (D), ventral (V) and lateral (L) midlines (solid curves). Dotted curves are values for the same model but without the sword. Both models were tested at $6\,m\,s^{-1}$. The length of the complete model is 0.94 m, Re=6.7×10^6; the model without the sword was 0.65 m long, Re=3.9×10^6. Modified from Aleyev (1977). $P_a=2(p-p_0)(\rho U_\infty{}^2)^{-1}$, where p is the pressure at the point of investigation, p_0 is the static pressure in the free stream, ρ is the water density and U_∞ is the velocity of the free stream. Pressures are in Pa=N m^{-1}.

boundary layer, along the same principles used by Reynolds (1883) leading to the discovery of his law of similitude. Fig. 10 shows a schematic drawing of the main 1.5 m high tank and the Perspex 1 cm×10 cm measuring section. Water is directed gradually along smooth walls to the constricted measuring part when the valve at the end of the flow pipe is opened. One wall of the Perspex section can be replaced by a wall with the roughness under investigation. The opposite wall remains smooth and transparent. The water is seeded with 2–5 μm particles. These are visualized in a 0.2–0.5 mm thin, horizontal Krypton laser sheet. Video frames with an electronic exposure time of 200 frames s^{-1} were taken at the normal video rate of 50 Hz. At the highest flow velocities, the particles that remained in the sheet during each single exposure appeared as small stripes with sharp ends. From the length of these stripes, their velocity could be calculated. The velocities of many individual particles collected from a large number of frames were used to compose velocity profiles across the 1 cm wide channel. For further details of the flow visualization techniques and subsequent analyses, see Stamhuis and Videler (1995). The maximum velocity of this system is about 5 m s^{-1}.

Here, I would like to report on the first preliminary results obtained with this apparatus. One Perspex wall was sandblasted until it was uniformly rough. The height of the roughness elements k was about 0.05 mm. The flow in the channel with two smooth walls was compared with that with one smooth and one rough wall.

Average velocity profiles at different positions along the measuring section are shown in Fig. 11. The average velocity of the flow was approximately 3.3 m s^{-1}, giving Re=3×10^4 based on a characteristic length of twice the cross-sectional area divided by

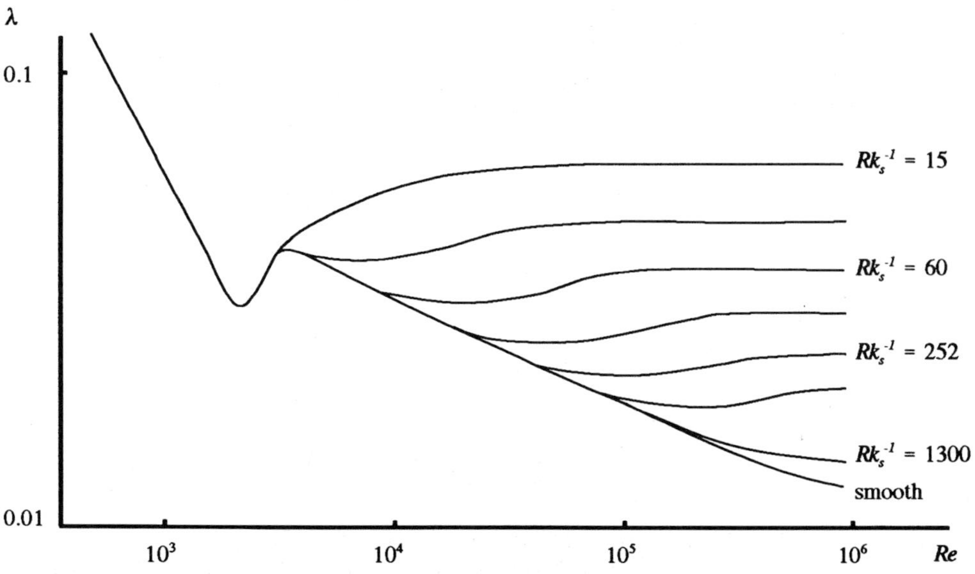

Fig. 9. The resistance of the flow in rough pipes. The resistance coefficient λ is defined as: $\lambda = d\Delta PL^{-1}(0.5\rho U^2)^{-1}$, where d is the diameter of the pipe, ΔP is the pressure difference measured over the length L and U is the flow velocity. The relative roughness is indicated as the ratio of the pipe radius R to the height of the roughness elements, k_S. Re is calculated using d as the length dimension. Based on Sclichting (1979).

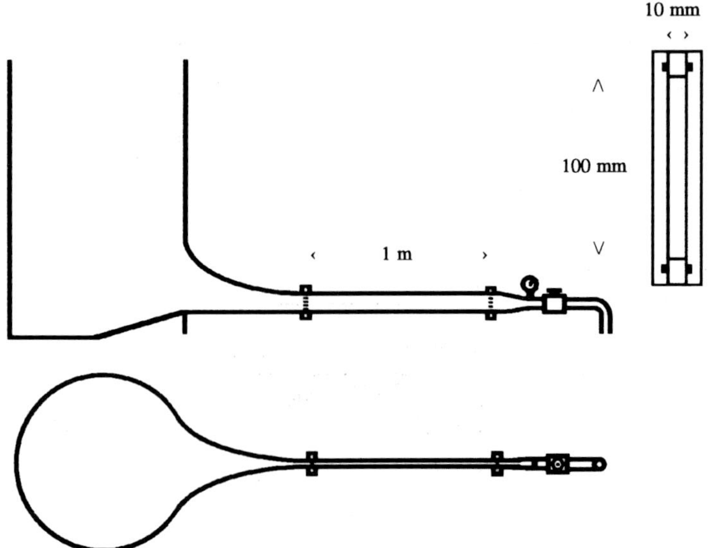

Fig. 10. Schematic side and top views of a 1.1 m^3 polyvinylchloride flow tank with a 1 m long Perspex test section. The internal dimensions of the rectangular test section (inset) are 10 cm×1 cm. The side walls of the test section can be exchanged. The maximum velocity is about 5 m s^{-1}. The water, seeded with particles 2–5 μm in diameter, is collected in a large lower tank and pumped back after the experiments.

the wetted periphery (Prandtl and Tietjens, 1934). The profiles are symmetrical all along the 1 m long channel in the case of the two smooth walls. A clear entrance effect, a uniform velocity over a large part of the cross section at $0.1L$, almost disappeared at $0.5L$ and was no longer visible at $0.9L$. An effect on the velocity profile of the rough wall is clearly visible near the end of the test section, where the velocity profile on the rough side is much steeper. The shear stress (equation 8) in the gradient near the rough wall is 1.7 times that of the smooth side. The boundary layer containing the velocity gradient is thinner at the rough side and almost 56 % of the total amount of water flows through that half of the channel.

The velocity profiles do not increase as steeply as the seventh root of the distance from the wall, as predicted (Prandtl and Tietjens, 1934) for turbulent flow through smooth tubes. However, the observation that the rough side clearly makes a difference near the end of the test section indicates that the flow is turbulent there. This conclusion is also supported by the observation that the trajectories of the particles are not always exactly parallel to the walls. The height of the protuberances on the Perspex wall is less than half that near the tip of the swordfish sword. Nevertheless, it changes the boundary layer structure at speeds well below those that could be achieved by a swordfish.

The critical height k_{crit} of roughness elements causing transition in a laminar boundary layer is (Schlichting, 1979):

$$k_{crit} = 15\nu v_*^{-1}, \qquad (10)$$

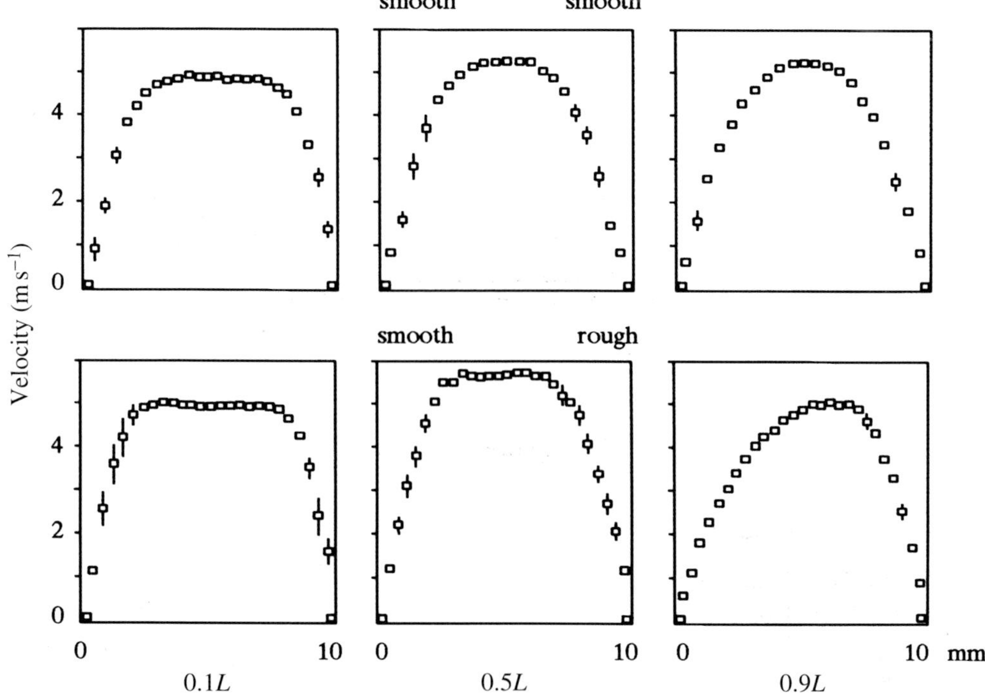

Fig. 11. The average velocity profiles measured at 10, 50 and 90 cm distance from the entrance of the test section of the flow tank shown in Fig. 10. In each diagram, the horizontal axes represent the 10 mm width of the channel. Flow speeds measured across the channel are indicated. The vertical bars are standard deviations, N=18. The three upper diagrams give the velocity profiles in the channel with two smooth walls; in the lower diagram, the right-hand wall is rough. See text for futher details.

where the friction velocity v_*, a measure of the intensity of turbulent eddying, is equal to:

$$v_* = (\tau_0 \rho^{-1})^{1/2}. \tag{11}$$

For a laminar boundary layer, Schlichting's equation 7.32 gives:

$$\tau_0 \rho^{-1} = 0.332 U_\infty{}^2 [\nu (U_\infty x)^{-1}]^{1/2}. \tag{12}$$

These equations can be used to calculate k_{crit} at $0.1L$ on a 1 m long sword of a swordfish swimming at a cruising speed of 5 m s^{-1} in sea water, where ν equals 1.18×10^{-6}. The calculations predict a value of k_{crit} of 0.16 mm. This is exactly the kind of roughness found on the sword. During swimming, *Re* increases from the tip of the sword along the body, and it reaches transitional values prematurely as a result of the roughness over the anterior part. According to our experiments with the roughened Perspex plate, this would give a steeper gradient of shear stress near the surface of the sword, resulting in a thinner boundary layer. The premature turbulence at an advanced position along the sword could decrease the danger of flow separation at the concave part of the head. A thin boundary layer must also tend to reduce the total drag because the streamlines of the potential flow outside the boundary layer would be less compressed.

However, roughness is only one aspect of the intriguingly complex microstructure of the sword of the swordfish shown in Fig. 7. There is still a long way to go before we will fully understand its function and the underlying mechanisms.

Epilogue

There are many more integumental structures on swimming animals that probably have interesting hydrodynamic functions. Webb (1975) provides an overview of these structures, their possible functions and the lack of direct evidence for these functions. This survey shows that the progress made since 1975 has been very limited.

Among the most challenging remaining cases, already described by Bone in 1972, is the skin structure of a teleost up to 3 m long, the castor oil fish *Ruvettus pretiosus*. The adult has a mixture of cycloid and ctenoid scales and a subdermal space communicating with the outside world through caudally directed pores (Fig. 12). This construction is intriguingly complex and so far we may only guess as to its function. Bone suggested that the ctenoid scales might generate turbulence to avoid the large drag penalties caused by separation.

There is one structural feature that the scales of sharks, the sword of the swordfish and the skin of the castor oil fish have in common. Each skin has space underneath the surface in open connection with the water around the animals.

A hint for a possible function comes from the aircraft industry, where two methods are used to prevent separation under adverse pressure conditions. These tricks are called boundary layer suction and injection (Schlichting, 1979). Boundary layer suction is achieved by removing decelerated water particles to the interior of the body. A similar

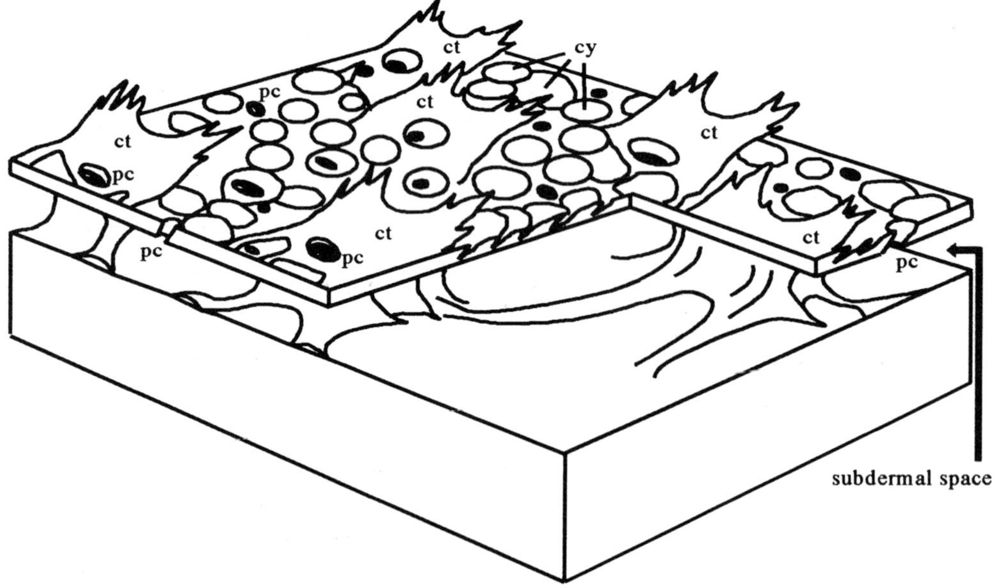

Fig. 12. A schematic drawing of the integument of a castor oil fish. The bases of the ctenoid scales (ct) form pillars supporting a subdermal space. Pore channels (pc) point backwards. Not all the cycloid scales (cy) are shown. Based on Bone (1972).

effect is achieved by injecting water at the right speed and in the right direction into the boundary layer.

The porous walls of the animals and the compliant dolphin skin could probably perform both tricks at once by damping disturbances and equalizing pressure pulses. In the castor oil fish, the holes point backwards, which would not only be the right direction for injection (Bone, 1972) but would also be in the direction of reversed velocities in the case of a danger of flow separation.

New flow visualization and imaging techniques are now within the reach of biologists. These allow direct investigation of flow phenomena on a microscale. Biological fluid dynamics will progress strongly in the next decade through the application of these techniques in combination with increased cooperation among biologists and hydrodynamicists.

The manager of the Biological Centre, Mr G. J. Hartman, kindly provided the extra money needed to employ the technician Mr L. A. Casemier, who cunningly constructed the flow tank shown in Fig. 10. My student Mr M. Stam carried out the pilot experiments and analyzed the data using programs designed by Mr E. J. Stamhuis. I gratefully acknowledge Professor Dr W.-E. Reif (Tübingen University) for the permission to use his scanning electron micrographs of shark skin and Mr J. Zagers (Laboratory for Electron Microscopy of the Department of Biology, Groningen University) for the scanning electron micrographs of sword surface structures. I thank Professor T. J. Pedley and Dr C. P. Ellington for the invitation to present this work and for their organisational and editorial efforts.

References

ALEYEV, Y. G. (1977). *Nekton*. The Hague: Dr W. Junk, 435pp.

BECHERT, D. W., BARTENWERFER, M., HOPPE, G. AND REIF, W.-E. (1986). Drag reduction mechanisms derived from shark skin. AIAA 15th Congress of the international Council of the Aeronautical Sciences. London, pp. 1044–1068.

BECHERT, D. W., HOPPE, G. AND REIF, W.-E. (1985). On the drag reduction of the shark skin. AIAA Shear Flow Control Conference, Boulder, Colorado. p. 18.

BERNADSKY, G., SAR, N. AND ROSENBERG, E. (1993). Drag reduction of fish skin mucus: Relationship to mode of swimming and size. *J. Fish Biol.* **42**, 797–800.

BLASIUS, H. (1908). Grenzschichten in Flüssigkeiten mit kleiner Reibung. *Z. math. Phys.* **56**, 1–37.

BONE, Q. (1972). Buoyancy and hydrodynamic functions of integument in the castor oil fish, *Ruvettus pretiosus* (Pisces: Gempylidae). *Copeia* **1**, 78–87.

BRUSE, M., BECHERT, D. W., VAN DER HOEVEN, J. G. TH., HAGE, W. AND HOPPE, G. (1993). Experiments with conventional and with novel adjustable drag-reducing surfaces. In *Near-Wall Turbulent Flows* (ed. R. M. C. So, C. G. Speziale and B. E. Launder), pp. 717–738. Amsterdam: Elsevier Science Publ.

CARPENTER, P. W. (1990). Status of transition delay using compliant walls. In *Viscous Drag Reduction in Boundary Layers* (ed. D. M. Bushnell and J. N. Heffner), pp. 79–113. Washington DC: AIAA.

DANIEL, T. L. (1981). Fish mucus: *In situ* measurements of polymer drag reduction. *Biol. Bull. mar. biol. Lab., Woods Hole* **160**, 376–382.

DENNY, M. (1980). The role of gastropod pedal mucus in locomotion. *Nature* **285**, 160–161.

ESSAPIAN, F. S. (1955). Speed-induced skin folds in the bottle-nosed porpoise, *Tursiops truncatus*. *Breviora Mus. comp. Zool.* **43**, 1–4.

FISH, F. E. AND HUI, C. A. (1991). Dolphin swimming – a review. *Mammal. Rev.* **21**, 181–195.

GAD-EL-HAK, M. (1987). Compliant coatings research: a guide to the experimentalist. *J. Fluids Structures* **1**, 55–70.

GYR, A., BEWERSDORFF, H.-W., HOYER, K. AND TSINOBER, A. (1993). An investigation of possible mechanisms of heterogeneous drag reduction in pipe and channel flows. In *Near-Wall Turbulent Flows* (ed. R. M. C. So, C. G. Speziale and B. E. Launder), pp. 679–687. Amsterdam: Elsevier Science Publ.

HOERNER, S. F. (1965). *Fluid Dynamic Drag*, 2nd edn. Brick Town, NJ: Hoerner, 452pp.

HOYT, J. W. (1975). Hydrodynamic drag reduction due to fish slimes. In *Swimming and Flying in Nature*, vol. 2 (ed. T. Y.-T. Wu, C. J. Brokaw and C. Brennen), pp. 653–672. New York: Plenum Press.

KRAMER, M. O. (1960). Boundary layer stabilization by distributed damping. *J. Am. Soc. naval Eng.* **F2**, 25–33.

LIGHTHILL, M. J. (1990). *An Informal Introduction to Theoretical Fluid Mechanics.* Oxford: Clarendon Press, 260pp.

LUMLEY, J. L. (1969). Drag reduction by additives. *A. Rev. Fluid Mech.* **3**, 367–384.

NIKURADSE, J. (1933). Strömungsgesetze in rauen Rohren. *Forschg. Arb. Ing.-Wes.* no. 361.

PALMER, E. AND WEDDEL, G. (1964). The relationship between structure, innervation and function of the skin of the bottle nose dolphin (*Tursiops truncatus*). *Proc. zool. Soc. Lond.* **143**, 553–567.

PARRY, D. A. (1949). The structure of whale blubber and a discussion of its thermal properties. *Q. Jl microsc. Sci.* **90**, 13.

PRANDTL, L. (1904). Über Flüssigkeitsbewegung bei sehr kleiner Reibung. *Verhandlungen des dritten internationalen Mathematiker Kongresses, Heidelberg.* Leipzig, pp. 484–491.

PRANDTL, L. AND TIETJENS, O. G. (1934). *Applied Hydro- and Aerodynamics* (translated by J. P. den Hartog) Dover (unabridged republication, 1957), 311pp.

PURVES, P. E. (1963). Locomotion in whales. *Nature* **197**, 334–337.

REYNOLDS, O. (1883). An experimental investigation of the circumstances which determine whether motion of water shall be direct or sinuous, and of the law of resistance in parallel channels. *Phil. Trans. R. Soc. Lond*, **2**, 935–982.

ROSEN, M. W. AND CORNFORD, N. E. (1971). Fluid friction of fish slimes. *Nature* **234**, 49–51.

SCHLICHTING, H. (1979). *Boundary-Layer Theory* (translated by J. Kestin; reissued edition 1987). New York: McGraw-Hill, 814pp.

SCHNEIDER, M. AND DINKELACKER, A. (1993). Drag reduction by means of surface riblets on an inclined body of revolution. In *Near-Wall Turbulent Flows* (ed. R. M. C. So, C. G. Speziale and B. E. Launder), pp. 771–780. Amsterdam: Elsevier Science Publ.

SLIJPER, E. J. (1958). *Walvissen.* Amsterdam: D. B. Centen, 524pp.

SOKOLOV, V., BULINA, I. AND RODIONOV, V. (1969). Interaction of dolphin epidermis with flow boundary layer. *Nature* **222**, 267–268.

STAMHUIS, E. J. AND VIDELER, J. J. (1995). Quantifying and analysing flow around aquatic animals by applying laser sheet particle image velocimetry. *J. exp. Biol.* **198**, 283–294.

SUZUKI, Y. AND KASAGI, N. (1993). Drag reduction mechanism on micro-grooved riblet surface. In *Near-Wall Turbulent Flows* (ed. R. M. C. So, C. G. Speziale and B. E. Launder), pp. 709–718. Amsterdam: Elsevier Science Publ.

TALBOT, F. H. AND PENRITH, J. J. (1962). Spearing behavior in feeding in the black marlin, *Istiompax marlina. Copeia* **2**, 468.

TOMS, B. A. (1948). Some observations on the flow of linear polymer solutions through straight tubes at large Reynolds numbers. *Proceedings of the International Rheological Congress, Scheveningen, The Netherlands* **2**, 135.

VIDELER, J. J. (1993). *Fish Swimming*. London: Chapman & Hall, 260pp.

WALSH, M. J. (1980). Drag characteristics of V-groove and transverse curvature riblets. In *Viscous Flow Drag Reduction* (ed. G. R. Hough). *Prog. Astronaut. Aeronaut.* **72**, New York: AIAA.

WALSH, M. J. AND LINDEMANN, A. M. (1984). Optimization and application of riblets for turbulent drag reduction. AIAA paper 84-0347, 10pp.

WALTERS, V. (1962). Body form and swimming performance in scombroid fishes. *Am. Zool.* **2**, 143–149.

WEBB, P. W. (1975). Hydrodynamics and energetics of fish propulsion. *Bull. Fish. Res. Bd Can.* **190**, 1–159.

WHITE, F. M. (1974). *Viscous Fluid Flow*. New York: McGraw Hill.

WISNER, R. L. (1958). Is the spear of Istiophorid fishes used in feeding? *Pacific Sci.* **12**, 60–70.

SWIMMING OF DOLPHINS: EXPERIMENTS AND MODELLING

E. V. ROMANENKO

Severtsov Institute of Evolutionary Animal Morphology and Ecology, RAS 117071 Leninsky pr. 33, Moscow, Russia

Summary

A critical analysis of the numerous works on dolphin swimming shows that several uncertainties led to incorrect conclusions concerning the estimates of dolphin drag coefficients. Original results on dolphin kinematics and hydrodynamics indicate the existence of a drag-reduction mechanism, caused by the formation of a negative pressure gradient along the body during active swimming. The mathematical model for this mechanism is presented.

Introduction

For many years, researchers have focused attention on dolphin hydrodynamics. They are primarily interested to know whether these animals have special mechanisms for decreasing their resistance during swimming when the critical Reynolds number is exceeded. In 1936, Gray suggested that they do have such a mechanism owing to the favourable (negative) dynamic pressure gradient developing on the body during active swimming. Some other hypotheses for drag reduction were offered later, such as the damping properties of the integument (Kramer, 1960; Babenko *et al.* 1972), reducing resistance by eye and skin secretions (Uskova *et al.* 1975), etc.

The world scientific community has divided on the problem of Gray's paradox. One group of scientists (chiefly from Western Europe and America) believes that Gray's hypothesis is unfounded and that dolphins have no special mechanisms to reduce drag, with the possible exception of their body shape. The other group of scholars (mainly those from Russia and the countries of the former Soviet Union) claims that dolphins do have certain mechanisms to decrease their drag coefficient.

The conclusion that dolphins lack special mechanisms for decreasing their drag coefficient or increasing their critical Reynolds number (Webb, 1975; Yates, 1983; Fish and Hui, 1991; Fish, 1993) is based on indirect estimates and not on direct measurements (Fig. 1). There are flaws in the estimates, however, and the errors may be classified as follows.

(1) In the feathering parameter $\alpha U/(\omega h)$, introduced by Lighthill (1969), the angle α is used by some authors (Webb, 1975; Fish, 1993) as the angle between the wing plane (the plane of the dolphin's caudal lobe) and the tangent to the trajectory of its rotation axis: i.e. what is traditionally called the angle of attack of a wing. The angle α should instead be the inclination of the wing plane to the horizontal axis.

Key words: boundary layer, dolphin, drag, hydrodynamics, kinematics, shearing stress.

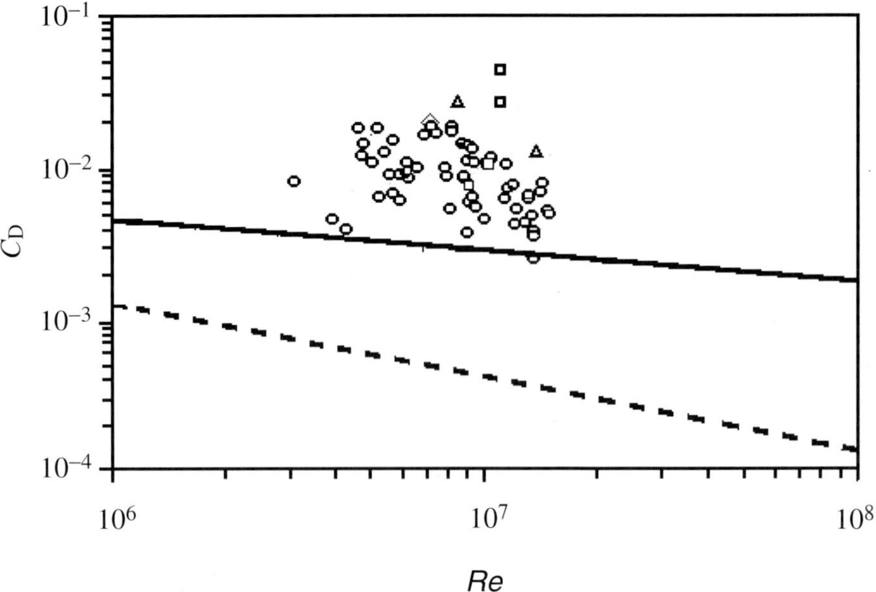

Fig. 1. Comparison of cetacean drag coefficients C_D estimated from hydromechanical models based on kinematics. Drag coefficients are plotted against Reynolds number *Re*. Open circles represent depth-corrected drag coeffficients C_{Dd} for *Tursiops truncatus* from Fish (1993). Other symbols represent *Delphinus bairdi* (◇), *Lagenorhyncus obliquidens* (□), *Phocoenoides dalli* (△). Data are from Lang and Daybell (1963), Webb (1975), Chopra and Kambe (1977) and Yates (1983). The solid line represents the minimum drag coefficient assuming a turbulent boundary layer; the broken line is for the minimum drag coefficient assuming laminar conditions (from Fish, 1993).

(2) Even when the angle α is chosen correctly, its absolute value has been used (Yates, 1983) instead of its tangent, contrary to the warning by Chopra (1976). Furthermore, the one experimental paper (Lang and Daybell, 1963) cited by the above authors does not give an accurate value for the angle, and Yates relied on the suggested value of 0.66 rad.

(3) To estimate the thrust power, Webb (1975) uses the following equation from Parry (1949):

$$E = 0.0175L^2U^3[(0.38Lf/U) - 0.047]\,, \tag{1}$$

where L, U and f are the length of the body, the swimming velocity and the frequency of body oscillations, respectively. However, the numerical coefficients are wrongly specified in this equation, and the error is almost tenfold.

(4) The errors introduced by a number of theoretical assumptions were neglected, although they were specially emphasized by Chopra and Kambe (1977). Other differences between theory and experiments might also have contributed errors: e.g. the elasticity of the caudal lobe, the swimming depth of the dolphin, etc.

In addition to these errors, there are certain practical difficulties which decrease the reliability of the above estimates: it is very difficult to define exactly the spatial position of the rotation axis of the dolphin's lobe, and to differentiate the shape of the lobe from

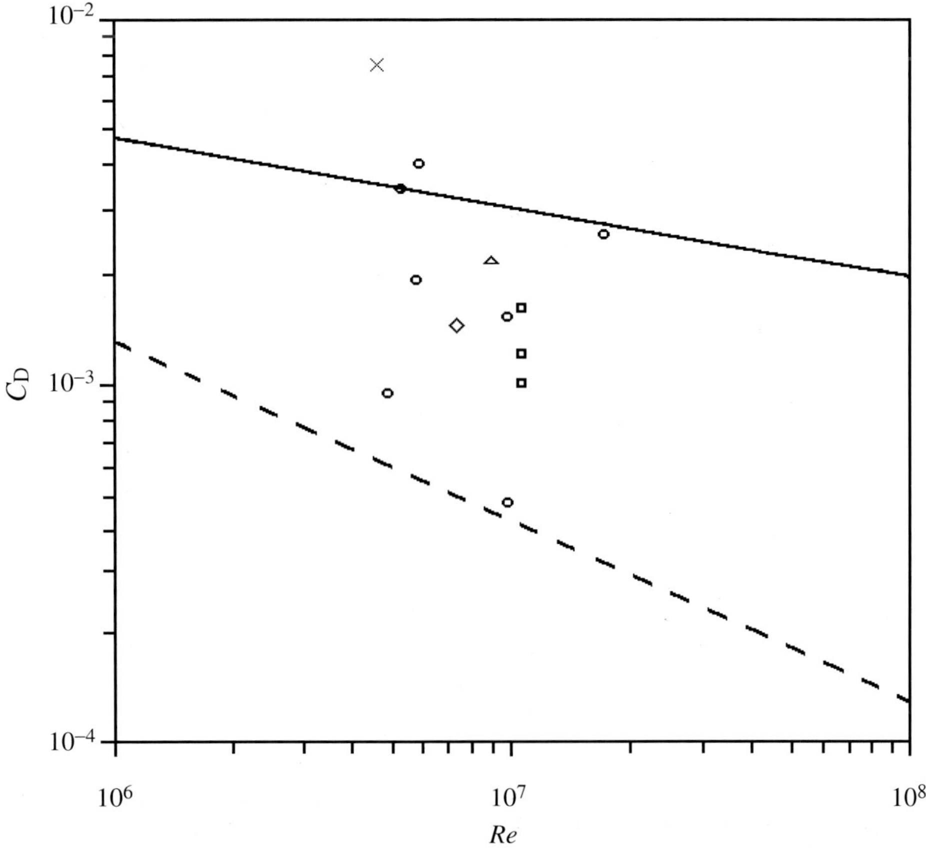

Fig. 2. The corrected values of the frictional drag coefficient. Symbols representing species as in Fig. 1, plus *Sotalia guianensis* (×). Minimum drag coefficients are shown for turbulent (solid line) and laminar (broken line) boundary layers. Data from Webb (1975), Kayan (1979), Yates (1983), Videler and Kamermans (1985), Romanenko (1986) and Fish (1993).

that of theoretical wings. There are also some divergences in the theoretical approach to the problem and, hence, in the conclusions (Ahmadi and Widnall, 1985; Lan, 1979; Chopra and Kambe, 1977). All of this questions the reliability of the estimates and the conclusions drawn from them.

Fig. 2 shows corrected values of frictional drag coefficients, with the data from Fish (1993) presented for selected speeds of 2 and 6 m s^{-1}. It is clear that the dolphin frictional drag coefficients are in good agreement with theoretical values for a turbulent boundary layer on the plate. However, the results cannot be used to conclude whether the dolphin has any special drag-reducing mechanisms. To investigate such mechanisms, it is necessary to measure directly the flow pattern and the fine structure of the boundary layer.

It seems premature to close the problem on dolphin hydrodynamics and to reject Gray's paradox. Moreover, the experiments carried out by scientists from Russia and from the countries of the former Soviet Union testify that dolphins do indeed have special mechanisms to increase the critical Reynolds number and to reduce drag (Kozlov, 1983; Romanenko, 1986; Pershin, 1988).

Flow velocities and pressure gradients

We have been working on Gray's hypothesis for many years, trying to develop it further and to verify it in two ways: experimentally and by mathematical modelling. In our experiments, we measured the flow velocities at three points on the lateral surface of the swimming dolphin. The points were situated 1.2, 1.5 and 1.7 m from the nose tip, the dolphin's body being 2.24 m long. The velocities were measured by microvanes, and the data were recorded by radiotelemetry to the shore; a small radio transmitter was fixed on the dorsal fin. The results are presented in Fig. 3. The vertical axis shows the ratios between the flow velocities measured at the third and first points along the body and at the second and first points. Horizontally, we display the acceleration of the dolphin. It is easy to see that when the dolphin moves at constant velocity, or with positive acceleration, the streamline flow is accelerated to faster velocities downstream on the body. The results were obtained at an average swimming velocity of $4\pm0.5\,\mathrm{m\,s^{-1}}$. Knowing the flow velocities and using Bernoulli's equation, it is not difficult to calculate pressures and

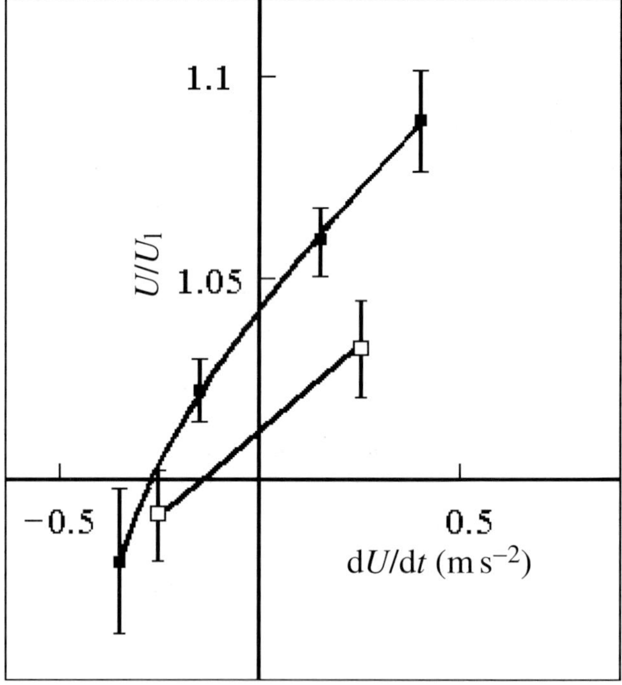

Fig. 3. Relative velocities of flow along the dolphin's body. ■, the ratio of velocities U/U_1 for the third and first points on the body; □, the same ratio for the second and first points. Ratios are plotted against the swimming acceleration dU/dt.

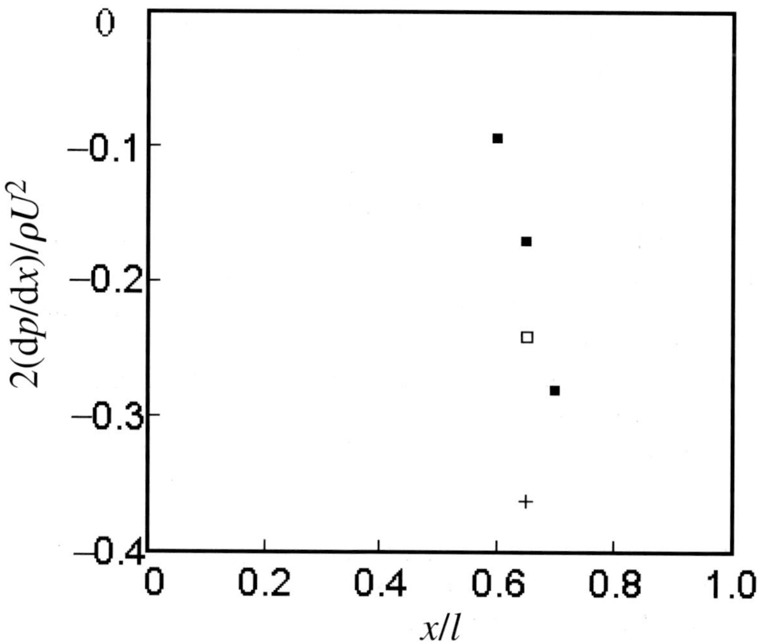

Fig. 4. Normalized pressure gradients along the dolphin's body. ■, at constant velocity; □, at an acceleration of 0.14 m s^{-2}; +, at an acceleration of 0.4 m s^{-2}.

pressure gradients. Fig. 4 presents normalised pressure gradients for swimming at constant velocity and at accelerations of 0.14 m s^{-2} and 0.4 m s^{-2}.

Table 1 shows values of the form parameter of the velocity profile, which is more directly linked with the critical Reynolds number than is the pressure gradient. The expression for the form parameter Λ is:

$$\Lambda = -(\delta^2/\nu\rho U)(\mathrm{d}p/\mathrm{d}x)\,, \tag{2}$$

where δ is the thickness of the boundary layer, ν is the kinematic viscosity of water, ρ is

Table 1. *The form parameter Λ of the velocity profile along the body at different swimming accelerations*

x/l	$\mathrm{d}U/\mathrm{d}t$ (m s^{-1})	$2(\mathrm{d}p/\mathrm{d}x)(\rho U^2)^{-1}$	Λ
0.6	0	−0.093	1.6
0.65	0	−0.168	3.0
0.65	0.14	−0.24	4.35
0.65	0.4	−0.36	6.5
0.71	0	−0.28	5.6

Values for the normalized pressure gradient are taken from Fig. 4.

the water density, U is the velocity of the advancing flow and p is dynamic pressure (Romanenko, 1976). The values of the form parameter are quite sufficient to stabilize the laminar flow or, which is the same, to increase the critical Reynolds number considerably. Indeed, our direct measurements of Reynolds number in the transition from the laminar to the turbulent boundary layer on a freely swimming dolphin, using special devices to register pressure pulsations, revealed the critical Reynolds number to be much higher than on a flat plate and on a rigid model of the dolphin. We also found that the critical Reynolds number depends on the acceleration during swimming.

The favourable (negative) gradient of dynamic pressure along the body is known not only to stabilize the laminar flow but also to damp out turbulent flow, by decreasing the degree of turbulence down to a complete reverse transition. The decreased turbulence in the boundary layer on the dolphin's body, caused by a negative pressure gradient, was determined experimentally by Romanenko (1976, 1986).

The level of pressure pulsations is unambiguously related to the shearing stresses on the body, and these stresses govern the resistance to movement. The decreased level of pressure pulsations during the dolphin's active swimming (either with acceleration or at constant velocity), compared with that during the animal's inert movement, demonstrates that the coefficient of frictional drag should be lower when the dolphin is active than when it is inert. And this is exactly what explains Gray's paradox.

Shearing stresses

This conclusion is so important that we cannot accept it without reservations, even if it seems obvious from the results presented above. For confirmation, it is vital to measure directly the shearing stresses within the boundary layer of a freely swimming dolphin. This was accomplished using a specially designed device to measure shearing stresses, together with a data logger fixed on the dorsal fin. The shearing stress sensor was sequentially placed at different points on the right side of the dolphin: the distances from the nose tip were 0.4, 0.5, 0.67 and 0.78 of the body length l. The sensor was also installed on the caudal lobe of the dolphin. The sensor was situated at 3 mm from the body surface, which equalled about 0.2–0.25 of the boundary layer thickness. According to Schlichting (1974), at this distance from the surface the shearing stresses practically coincide with those at the surface itself.

Fig. 5 displays typical results for points under measurement coinciding with 0.5 of the body length l. The horizontal axis shows time in seconds from the onset of the dolphin's movement; the vertical axis shows the swimming velocity (filled squares) and the local coefficient of resistance (crosses) in relative units. There are sections illustrating swimming with positive acceleration, with constant velocity and with deceleration. During the time interval from 6.4 s and 7.4 s, the dolphin surfaced for inspiration expiration. The swimming velocity decreased slightly before it surfaced, probably because of the termination of thrust. The local coefficient of frictional resistance is lowest during accelerated swimming, and it is highest during decelerations. The difference between the lowest and highest values is very large. It should be noted that the local coefficient of frictional drag reached its highest value twice during the sequence:

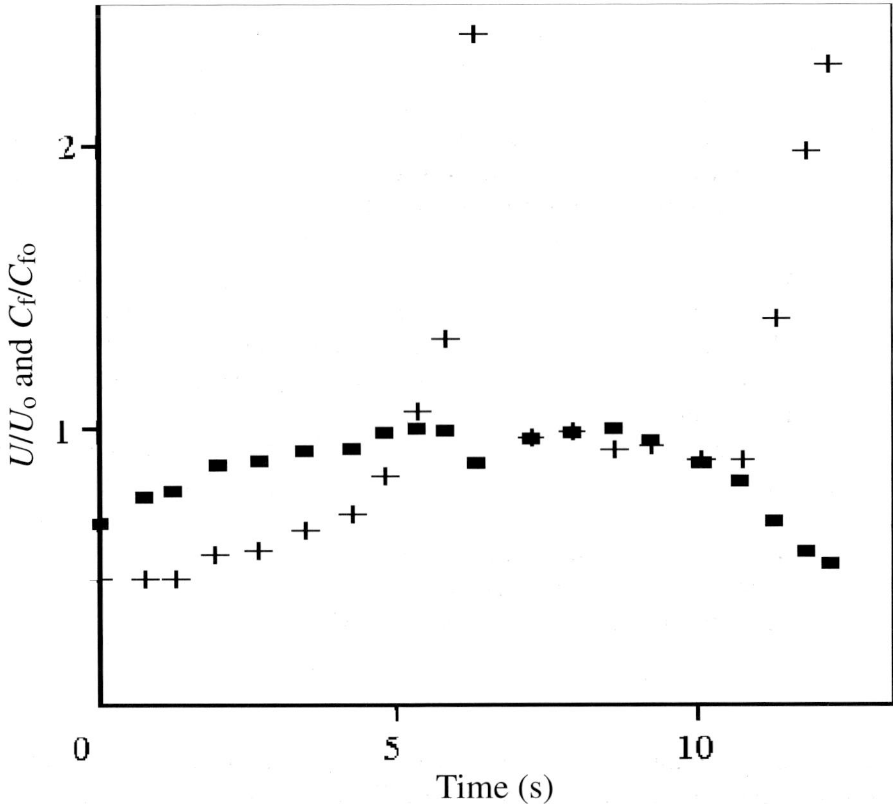

Fig. 5. The swimming velocity (■) and the local drag coefficient (+) on the dolphin's body plotted against swimming time. Velocities are relative to the maximum value, and coefficients are normalized by value corresponding to maximum velocity.

immediately before the dolphin surfaced for inspiration–expiration, and when it decelerated at the end of the run. Other cases of surfacing for inspiration–expiration did not always reveal a deceleration and the accompanying increase in the local coefficient of frictional drag, but these were always observed at the end of swimming.

The results at $0.78l$ show that the local coefficient of frictional drag is 4.7 times lower compared with that at $0.4l$ for a dolphin swimming at constant velocity. When the sensor was placed on the caudal lobe, however, the local coefficient proved to be extremely unstable. This result can be attributed to the unstable pressure gradient on the caudal lobe at different stages of the swimming cycle.

Mathematical modelling

Let us investigate the mechanism underlying the pressure gradient caused by the body oscillations. We shall consider the body as a long cylinder of elliptic or circular profile which makes bending oscillations within one plane. To calculate the dynamic pressure on the body surface, we may use the expression for a circular cylinder in transverse motion (Logvinovich, 1969):

$$p - p_\infty = (\rho v_o^2/2)(1 - 4\sin^2\theta) + (\rho\cos\theta/R)[\mathrm{d}(R^2 v_n)/\mathrm{d}t] , \quad (3)$$

where R and θ are cylindrical coordinates, t is time, and v_n is the transverse velocity of the body given by:

$$v_n = (\partial h/\partial t) + U(\partial h/\partial x) , \quad (4)$$

where h is the transverse displacement and U is the swimming velocity along the x axis (Fig. 6).

Transverse oscillations of the dolphin's body during active swimming can be well described by the following expression (Romanenko, 1986; Yanov, 1990):

$$h(x,t) = h_l[h_o/h_l + a(X) + c(X)^2 + d(X)^8]\sin\{\omega t + (k_o/b)\ln[1 + lb(X)]\} . \quad (5)$$

where $X{=}x/l$, h_o and h_l are the oscillation amplitudes at the head and tail, k_o is the number of wavelengths in the head, b is a parameter for the increase in the phase velocity of the locomotor wave, $\omega{=}2\pi f$ (f is the frequency of oscillations) and a, c and d are constants. This equation incorporates the main features of the locomotor wave spread along the dolphin's body: i.e. the variation in wave amplitude and phase from head to tail. We shall calculate the dynamic pressure distribution on a dolphin's body (*Tursiops truncatus*) for two regimes of swimming, their parameters being presented in Table 2.

Fig. 7 presents the minimum and maximum values of the dynamic pressure gradient for the lateral side of the dolphin's body ($\theta{=}\pi/2$). These values were reached twice during each oscillation. The magnitude of the positive gradient is obviously small, while that of the negative gradient is considerably higher and depends on the swimming regime. In the front part of the body, the gradient permanently remains negative and of large magnitude, being determined by the shape of the body. Fig. 7 also includes the experimental data of Fig. 4 for comparison. The experimental data are in good agreement with the calculated results for the second swimming regime of Table 2.

Some important conclusions can be drawn from the shape of the calculated curves in Fig. 7. The negative pressure gradient is considerable in the head and tail parts of the

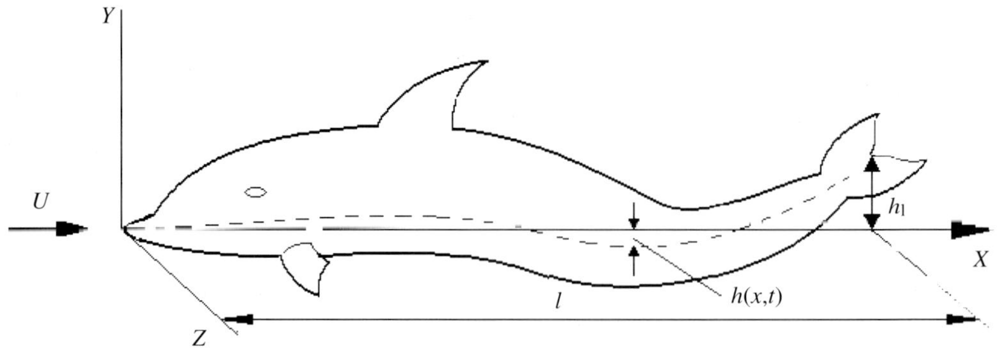

Fig. 6. Definition of the coordinate system for mathematical modelling. See text for details.

Table 2. *The parameters of dolphin swimming under two different regimes*

Parameters	First regime	Second regime
U (m s^{-1})	1.5	4.3
h_1/l	0.18	0.123
f (Hz)	1.46	2.22
b (m^{-1})	0.55	0.23
dU/dt (m s^{-2})	2.6	0
h_o/h_1	0.27	0.21
C_o/U	1.24	0.97
a	−0.58	−0.66
c	1.0	1.1
d	0.31	0.35

C_o is the phase velocity of the locomotor wave in the region of animal's head and other variables are defined in the text.

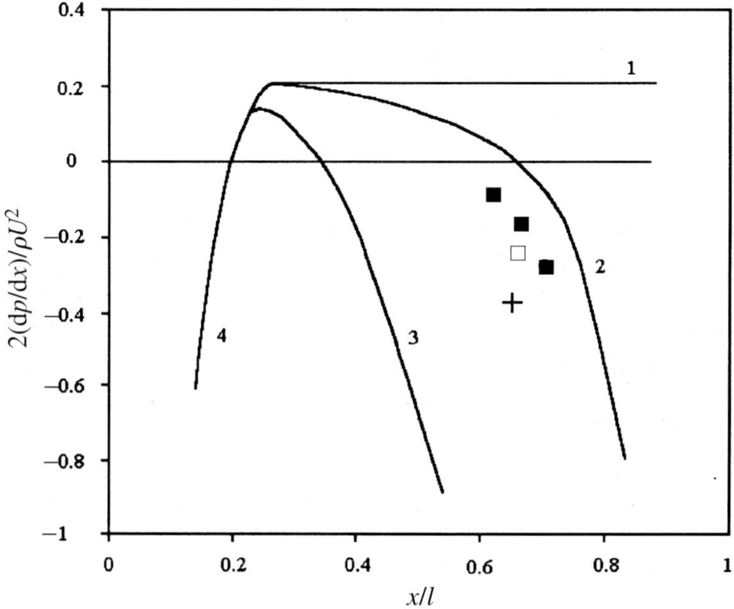

Fig. 7. Comparison of the calculated and experimental pressure gradients along the dolphin's body. Line 1, maximum values of the pressure gradient; lines 2 and 3, mimimum values of the pressure gradient for the second and first regimes, respectively, of dolphin swimming in Table 2; line 4, pressure gradient resulting from the body shape peculiarities on the anterior part of the dolphin's body; symbols represent experimental data (see Fig. 4).

body, and its favourable effect on the boundary layer should be concentrated in those regions. Turbulence in the boundary layer might begin not in the posterior part of the body, which is the case with flow over rigid streamlined bodies, but in the middle part where the pressure gradient is small and perhaps positive. Thus, there might be turbulent flow over the middle of the body with a laminar, or considerably laminated, flow over the head and tail.

Experimental support

Wood (1979) describes observations of a group of Pacific white-side dolphins swimming in phosphorescent water. Fig. 8 shows their sketches. The light areas on the dolphins' bodies indicate a turbulent boundary layer, which is clearly seen to embrace the middle part of the body; the front part and the tail column reveal dark places corresponding to laminar flow. The upper and lower parts of the body are phosphorescent, identifying narrow sections of turbulence on the back and underside of the animals. This observation also agrees with calculations for the dorsal side of the body (θ=0).

The dynamic pressure gradient on the body of the actively swimming dolphin seems to play the leading role in defining the flow pattern. This conclusion follows from an analysis of the body shape of this animal. There are three main parameters of the body, illustrated in Fig. 9, that affect the flow pattern: (i) relative elongation (l/d_{max}), which is the ratio of the body length to the circle diameter equalling in its area the maximum cross section; (ii) the relative position (l_1/l) of the maximum cross section; and (iii) the descent angle (α) of the body of rotation that best approximates the animal's body. In some species of dolphins and large whales, the body shape cannot be approximated very well by a body of rotation. Nevertheless, it is useful to construct a table of comparative data on the body shape of different species of dolphins and whales.

Table 3 presents values for the morphometric parameters derived from the catalogue and pictures in Leatherwood *et al.* (1972). It is important to note that, because there are no accurate data on the maximum cross-sectional area of whales, we used the maximum

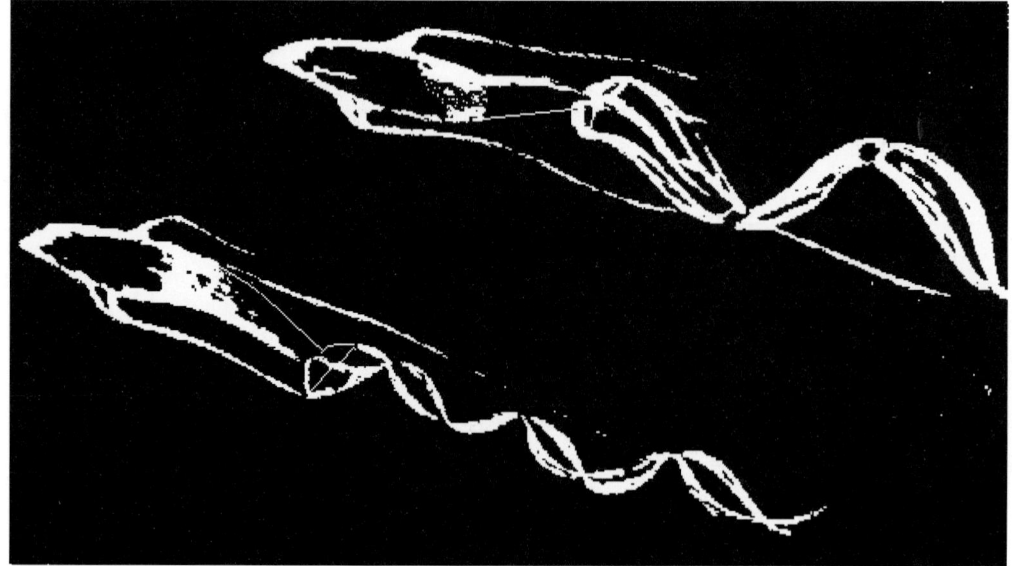

Fig. 8. Illustration from Wood (1979). See text for details.

Table 3. *Morphometric parameters for whale and dolphin*

Species	l/d_{max}	l_1/l	α (degrees)
Tursiops truncatus	5.4	0.35	10
Phocoena phocoena	4.7	0.40	15
Lagenorhynchus obliquidens	6.9	0.36	8
Stenella graffmani	7.1	0.35	7
Stenella longirostris	7.6	0.34	7
Delphinus delphis	6.1	0.36	–
Phocoenoides dalli	4.6	0.33	13
Lissodephis borealis	7.5	0.36	7
Eschrichtius robustus	4.5	0.40	10
Berardius bairdi	6.0	0.39	–
Pseudorca crassioleus	6.9	0.38	–
Physeter catodon	5.1	0.45	–
Kogia breviceps	4.0	0.42	–

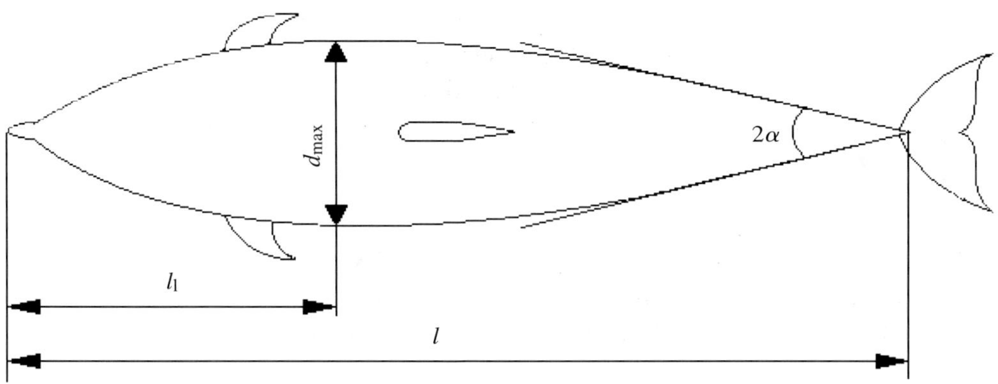

Fig. 9. Illustration of the three main parameters of body shape. Values are given in Table 3.

width of the body as the maximum diameter. For all whales in the table, the relative elongation ranges from 4 to 7.6, the relative position of the cross-section is between 0.33 and 0.45, and the descent angle varies between 7 ° and 15 °.

To assess these data, we turn to the paper of Alekseyeva *et al.* (1968), where the authors calculate parameters of the laminar boundary layer for a series of bodies of rotation which vary in shape. We shall not dwell on their calculation methods but instead cite their main results: (i) when the boundary layer is laminar, flow separation is avoided for $\alpha \leqslant 6.5$; (ii) the minimum resistance in laminar flow with Reynolds numbers of the order of 10^8 is found when the elongation is 9 and the relative position of the maximum cross section equals 0.21; (iii) the minimum resistance in turbulent flow is obtained with an elongation of 5.5–7 and the relative position of the maximum diameter around 0.4.

When the results of Alekseyeva *et al.* (1968) are compared with those in Table 3, the following conclusions can be made.

(1) The descent angle in whales exceeds the maximum angle at which the laminar boundary layer remains attached. Thus, either the laminar boundary layer of dolphins

must separate, or they must somehow be able to prevent this separation. As we saw above, a negative pressure gradient develops on their body when dolphins are swimming actively, and this gradient may prevent separation of the laminar boundary layer.

2. The body of whales is not optimal to minimize resistance in laminar flow, meaning that there is a danger of the boundary layer separation discussed above. However, as we could see for whales, and for dolphins in particular, such a danger does not exist.

3. The body shape in whales approaches the optimum for minimal resistance in turbulent flow.

Thus, given the negative pressure gradient on the dolphin's body (and, most likely, on the body of other whales), their body shape may be considered as optimal both for laminar and for turbulent flow. This is a most important adaptive device created by nature in whales.

References

AHMADI, A. R. AND WIDNALL, S. E. (1985). Unsteady lifting-line theory as a singular-perturbation problem. *J. Fluid Mech.* **153**, 59–81.

ALEKSEYEVA, YE. U., GROMOV, V. P., DMITRIEVA, A. F., KOLOBOV, B. P., KUZNETSOV, B. G., SEMENOV, B. N. AND YANENKO, N. N. (1968). *Characteristics of the Laminar Boundary Flow as Calculated on Rotating Bodies*. Novosibirsk, Nauka, Sibirian Branch. 219pp.

BABENKO, V. B., KOZLOV, L. F. AND PERSHIN, S. V. (1972). On the alternative damping of dolphin's skin at different swimming velocities. *Bionika* **6**, 84–89.

CHOPRA, M. G. (1976). Large amplitude lunate-tail theory of fish locomotion. *J. Fluid Mech.* **74**(1), 161–182.

CHOPRA, M. G. AND KAMBE, T. (1977). Hydromechanics of lunate-tail swimming propulsion. Part 2. *J. Fluid Mech.* **79**(1), 49–69.

FISH, F. E. (1993). Power output and propulsive efficiency of swimming bottlenose dolphins (*Tursiops truncatus*). *J. exp. Biol.* **185**, 179–193.

FISH, F. E. AND HUI, C. A. (1991). Dolphin swimming – a review. *Mammal. Rev.* **21**, 181–195.

GRAY, J. (1936). Studies in animal locomotion. VI. The propulsive powers of the dolphin. *J. exp. Biol.* **13**, 192–199.

KAYAN, V. P. (1979). On hydrodynamic properties of fin propulsion in dolphin. *Bionika* **13**, 9–15.

KOZLOV, L. F. (1983). *Theoretical Biohydrodynamics*. Kiev: Vischa Shkola, 238pp.

KRAMER, M. (1960). The dolphin's secret. *New Scient.* **7**, 1118–1120.

LAN, C. E. (1979). The unsteady quasi-vortex-lattice method with application to animal propulsion. *J. Fluid Mech.* **93**(4), 747–765.

LANG, T. G. AND DAYBELL, D. A. (1963). Porpoise performance tests in a seawater tank. *Nav. Ord. Test Sta. Tech. Rep.* **3063**, 1–50.

LEATHERWOOD, S. W., EVANS, E. AND RICE, D. W. (1972). *The Whales, Dolphins and Porpoises of the North Pacific: a Guide to their Identification in the Water*. Nat. Ocean Atmos Admin. Prop. 343pp.

LIGHTHILL, M. J. (1969). Hydrodynamics of aquatic animal propulsion. *A. Rev. Fluid Mech.* **1**, 413–446.

LOGVINOVICH, G. V. (1969). *Hydrodynamics of a Flow with Free Boundaries*. Kiev: Naukova Dumka. 210pp.

PARRY, D. A. (1949). The swimming of whales and a discussion of Gray's paradox. *J. exp. Biol.* **26**, 24–36.

PERSHIN, S. V. (1988). *Fundamentals of Hydrobionics*. Leningrad: Sudostroenise. 263pp.

ROMANENKO, E. V. (1976). *Fundamentals of Statistic Biohydrodynamics*. M. Nauka. 168pp.

ROMANENKO, E. V. (1986). *A Theory of Swimming of Fishes and Dolphins*. M. Nauka. 152pp.

SCHLICHTING, H. (1974). *Theory of Boundary Layer* (in Russian). M. Nauka, 712pp.

USKOVA, YE. T., RAYEVSKY, V. S., MOMOT, L. N. AND USKOV, I. A. (1975). Comparative studies of hydrodynamic efficiency of polyoxyethylene and cutaneous secretion solutions of marine mammals. *Bionika* **9**, 90–92.

VIDELER, J. AND KAMERMANS, P. (1985). Differences between upstroke and downstroke in swimming dolphins. *J. exp. Biol.* **119**, 265–274.

WEBB, P. W. (1975). Hydrodynamics and energetics of fish propulsion. *Bull. Fish. Res. Bd Can.* **190**, 1–159.

WOOD, F. G. (1979). In *Marine Mammals and Man*. Leningrad: Hidrometeoizdat (in Russian) 267 pp.

YANOV, V. G. (1990). Dolphin's kinematics. New results of experimental studies. *DAN USSR* **315**, 49–52.

YATES, G. T. (1983). Hydrodynamics of body and caudal fin propulsion. In *Fish Biomechanics* (ed. P. W. Webb and D. Weihs), pp. 177–213. New York: Praeger.

THE ROLE OF THE LATERAL LINE IN ACTIVE DRAG REDUCTION BY CLUPEOID FISHES

JAMES LIGHTHILL

Department of Mathematics, University College London, Gower Street, London WC1E 6BT

Summary

The lateral-line canals, confined in clupeoid fishes to the two sides of the head, are centred on the two lateral recesses, where thin membranes separate the sea water in the lateral-line system from another fluid (perilymph) in that subcerebral canal which passes through the head between the two lateral recesses. Any pressure difference between the recesses can accelerate fluid in the subcerebral canal, but it is only the effective acceleration of that fluid (i.e. relative to the lateral acceleration of the head) which can tend to generate motions – sensed by neuromasts – in lateral-line canals near the lateral recesses. Furthermore, it is the same effective lateral acceleration (relative to that of the head) that is experienced by water in the thin boundary layer on the surface of the head, where it tends to generate 'crossflows' that may act to increase hydrodynamic resistance (i.e. drag) to the fish's normal swimming movements.

These regular swimming movements produce oscillatory sideslip of the fish's head which, by itself, would give such substantial values to the effective acceleration that lateral-line sensors near the lateral recesses would be saturated during normal swimming movements. Any such permanent state of saturation seems rather unlikely.

An alternative hypothesis is that the fish actively produces an oscillatory turning of the head, controlled by the sensory output of those same neuromasts in such a way that this output is kept to a minimum. Then that effective pressure difference, which is responsible for the effective lateral acceleration both of perilymph in the subcerebral canal and of sea water in the boundary layer on the head, would be minimised – with advantageous drag-reduction consequences.

In order to test this hypothesis, a detailed hydrodynamic analysis was carried out. It suggested that, in order to minimise the effective pressure difference, the yaw angle (in radians) of the fish's head would need to be kept in phase with the sideslip velocity, their magnitudes being in a ratio of about $0.87U^{-1}$ (where U is the swimming speed). Experiments on a swimming clupeoid fish confirmed these conclusions, both about phases and about magnitudes.

By contrast, a purely passive response of the head to oscillatory sideforce on the caudal fin would be expected to give the yaw angle a substantial lag behind sideslip, along with a ratio of magnitudes much smaller than $0.87U^{-1}$. Thus, the experiments seem to support the hypothesis regarding active control of drag reduction.

Key words: Clupeoidea, herring, lateral line, drag reduction, subcerebral canal, boundary layer, crossflows, fish swimming.

Introduction

The clupeoid fishes, comprising the herring family Clupeidae and the anchovy family Engraulidae, are an interestingly specialised group which moreover represent the leading component – around half by weight – of world fish catches. All of them (see next section) are pelagic plankton-feeders with highly developed schooling tendencies, whose acousticolateralis systems have been shown (Blaxter *et al.* 1981; Denton and Gray, 1983, 1993) to exhibit features that are special to clupeoids and which may facilitate schooling behaviour:

(i) the presence in each ear of a remarkable air-containing organ (the bulla, a spherical cavity half-filled with air); along with

(ii) an exceptional placing of the lateral line, which is confined to the head alone; and

(iii) penetration of the head by a subcerebral canal filled with a fluid (perilymph), motions in which induce seawater motions in the lateral line.

Thus, the entire system – including also, of course, those far commoner anatomical structures (the semicircular canals and otoliths) that sense movement of a fish's own head – is a compact sensory system, entirely located in the head itself (and mainly in its posterior part); a compactness which may tend to minimise delays both in communication between different elements of the system and in the ensuing muscular responses.

In three consecutively paginated papers (Denton and Gray, 1993; Lighthill, 1993; Rowe *et al.* 1993), evidence was presented suggesting that feature iii (above) allows the lateral line to combine its established roles (including that of sensing the movement of nearby fishes in a school, as described in the section on lateral-line responses to movements of nearby fish) with an important contribution to the efficiency of a fish's own swimming movements. The present paper offers a brief overview of those studies.

They began from an attempt to answer the question: how are lateral-line signals affected by a fish's own swimming movements? That question seemed to be important because any movements of the fish itself could be expected to generate a relatively large response which might prejudice the lateral line's role in sensing movements of other fishes.

Actually, the overall sensory output from lateral-line neuromasts may be thought of as being associated with distributions of water pressure comprising a symmetrical component (identical on both sides of the head) and an antisymmetrical component (equal in magnitude but opposite in sign on each side of the head). Denton and Gray (1983) had shown that information about the movement of nearby fishes is mainly derived (see section on lateral-line responses to movements of nearby fish) from the symmetrical component; by contrast, very simple considerations (see section on motions in the subcerebral canal) identify the antisymmetrical component as the one influenced by a fish's own swimming movements.

Motion in the subcerebral canal (see iii above) is driven, of course, only by the antisymmetrical component, comprising equal and opposite pressures at the canal's two ends: the lateral recesses. This motion can generate large flows in parts of the lateral-line system close to the lateral recesses. Indeed, an early estimate of that antisymmetrical component based on a standard assumption of fish hydrodynamics (briefly, that the anterior portion of the fish responds 'in rigid-body fashion' to tail sideforces) suggested that such flows would be so large that the associated sensors – the neuromasts in those parts of the lateral-line system – would be saturated (Denton and Gray, 1993). Clearly, this saturation would rule out their utilisation for extracting information on movements of nearby fishes from responses to the symmetrical component of the pressure distribution. On that early estimate, then, a fish's normal swimming movements would render useless an important part of its sensory system; a conclusion which seemed almost impossible to believe.

Then a fuller analysis (Lighthill 1993), outlined in the section on lateral-line responses to movements of nearby fish, showed that the magnitude of the motions in the subcerebral canal depends essentially on a combination of the head's sideslip velocity and its angle of yaw. Active head turning (relative to the remainder of the fish's body) could in principle be used, then, to keep these motions extremely small.

Such an active system would need, of course, a control input which the system might continually seek to annul; here, this control input could be provided by the sensors themselves (that is, by the neuromasts close to the lateral recesses) – although an additional possibility, that internal sensors contribute to detecting motions in the subcerebral canal, cannot be excluded. Moreover, if active control of head turning kept to a minimum motions in the subcerebral canal driven by an antisymmetrical component in the pressure distribution, the lateral-line system would have no difficulty in detecting that symmetrical component which is associated with movements of nearby fishes.

It remained to consider what advantages, if any, might accrue to clupeoid fishes from a specialised control system which tends to minimise those 'effective' pressure differences (see below) that drive motions in the subcerebral canal. An apparently convincing answer was provided (see section on possibilities for control of boundary-layer crossflow) by drag-reduction considerations. Indeed, because a school of clupeoid fishes tends to keep swimming continually – at least while it moves from one patch of planktonic food to the next available patch – a rather evident advantage of decreased energy expenditure *en route* seemed to be offered by reductions in hydrodynamic drag.

Fishes in general experience minimum drag for a given forward speed whenever they stop swimming and glide forwards with no fin movements, the value of this minimum drag being readily inferred from the rate of deceleration. By contrast, estimates of the thrust generated by tail movements in a steadily swimming fish have tended to exceed that minimum drag by factors of 3 to 4. An obvious interpretation of the excess depends on the fact that these lateral movements of the caudal fin generate not only a steady thrust but also an oscillatory sideforce, to which the anterior part of the fish responds with oscillatory sideslip and yawing motions. These tend to create departures from symmetry, known as crossflows, in the 'boundary layer' of fluid very close to the fish's body. In consequence, the drag on the body is increased rather substantially above its minimum value – which necessitates the augmented thrust.

Now, any crossflows in the boundary layer on the head of a clupeoid fish are driven (see section on possibilities for control of boundary-layer crossflow) by the same 'effective' pressure difference across the head which drives motions in the subcerebral canal; here, that effective pressure difference is defined (in the section on the motions in a fish's subcerebral canal due to its own swimming) as the actual difference in pressure plus an inertial correction for the head's lateral acceleration. (Briefly, this converts the absolute fluid acceleration produced by the actual pressure difference into an acceleration of fluid relative to the moving head.) It follows that any control system which uses active head turning to minimise motions in the subcerebral canal will also minimise boundary-layer crossflows on the head itself.

This can be expected to make a significant contribution to drag reduction, in that the boundary layer on the head will be similar to that on a gliding fish – i.e. essentially free of crossflow. In short, the boundary layer starts off with an effectively symmetrical form all over the head, which must help to reduce drag even if crossflows may begin to appear on posterior parts of the body.

To sum up, feature iii of the clupeoid lateral-line system (see above) provides the sensory input which would be needed by an active control process that used head turning to minimise effective pressure differences between the lateral-line recesses; moreover, such a process would bring a significant drag-reduction advantage. Conversely, the same feature would, in the absence of active head turning, offer a serious disadvantage, in that many lateral-line sensors would be saturated (and therefore useless) during normal swimming movements. A rational hypothesis then is that active head turning is used to maintain an approximately constant ratio between the head's angle of yaw (in radians) and its sideslip velocity; an estimate (see section on motions in a fish's subcerebral canal due to its own swimming) of the ratio necessary to annul the effective pressure difference for the herring *Clupea harengus* swimming at speed U being $0.87U^{-1}$. (By contrast, passive response of the head to sideforces on the tail would produce yaws with substantial lags in phase behind those of sideslip velocities, as well as with amplitudes far smaller than those just indicated.)

Against this background, the suggested hypothesis was subjected to a direct experimental test in herring by Rowe *et al.* (1993), with results that are outlined in the last section. Briefly, the above ratio was found to be rather closely maintained. Their results tend to reinforce views, derived from the earlier arguments, of the lateral line's role in active drag reduction by clupeoid fishes.

Although this paper concentrates exclusively on clupeoid fishes, where a fairly full account of the control system can be pieced together, the possibility that other groups of fishes may – by a process of convergent evolution – have arrived at analogous systems for active control of head turning, is by no means excluded. Rowe *et al.* (1993) provide also some information relevant to this issue.

Clupeoid fishes and their lateral lines

Closely related to the herring, *Clupea harengus*, are members of the clupeoid group of fishes with their interestingly specialised acousticolateralis systems. They include the herring family, Clupeidae, with genus names including *Brevoortia* (the menhaden genus so abundant in the western Atlantic) as well as *Clupea* itself and the self-explanatory *Sprattus*, *Sardina*, *Sardinops* and *Sardinella*; while the genera of the anchovy family Engraulidae include, for example, *Engraulis*, *Cetengraulis* (the main basis of a huge Peruvian fishery) and *Anchoviella*.

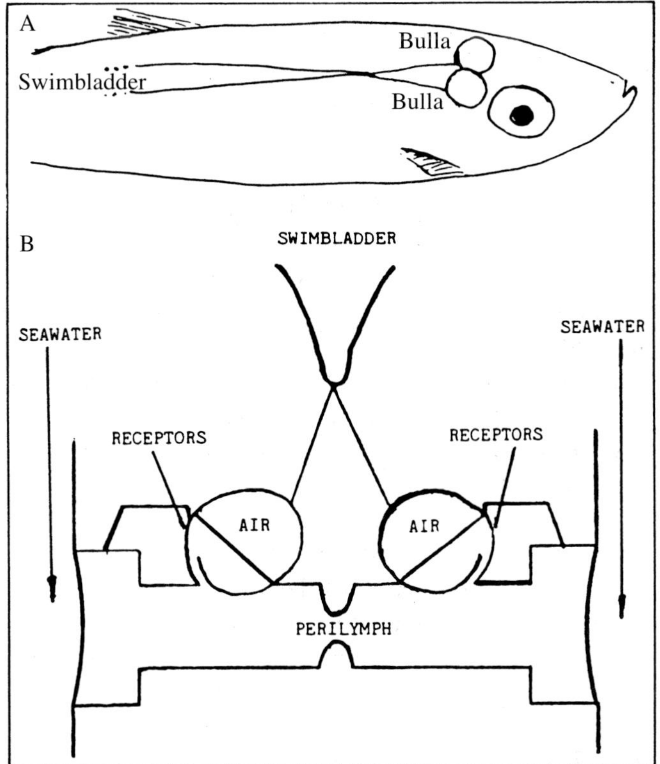

Fig. 1. Each auditory bulla (shown here in a simplified version of a diagrammatic representation after Blaxter *et al.* 1981) includes a roughly hemispherical mass of air. (A) This is renewed from time to time from the swimbladder *via* the associated precoelomic duct. (B) The air mass responds to sudden pressure changes by changes of volume that generate motions of perilymph to which certain hair-cell receptors (in the utricular maculae) are sensitive. Membranes separate the perilymph from the sea water of the lateral-line canals (top view). Note how the subcerebral canal penetrates the head between the two lateral recesses.

Fishes in this group are pelagic (living fairly near the ocean surface) and swim in great schools or shoals as they move between one patch of planktonic food and another. Often, in response to attack by a predator, a school of clupeoid fishes makes a sudden movement, almost like a single organism, so that the predator may become confused. This collective reaction seems to be mediated by the capability of each individual clupeoid fish to respond sensitively to those sudden pressure changes which can be generated by predators in attacks; and the auditory bulla (see i above and Fig. 1), with its optimum frequency response in the range 50–500 Hz, may play an important role in this response. Blaxter *et al.* (1981) explained how the hemispherical air cavity in each bulla is replenished (the swimbladder acting as an air reservoir for this purpose) and showed that the membrane separating air from perilymph moves sensitively – this movement being detected by hair-cell receptors, as shown – in response to sudden pressure changes.

But the important feature of Fig. 1 in the context of the lateral-line system is the

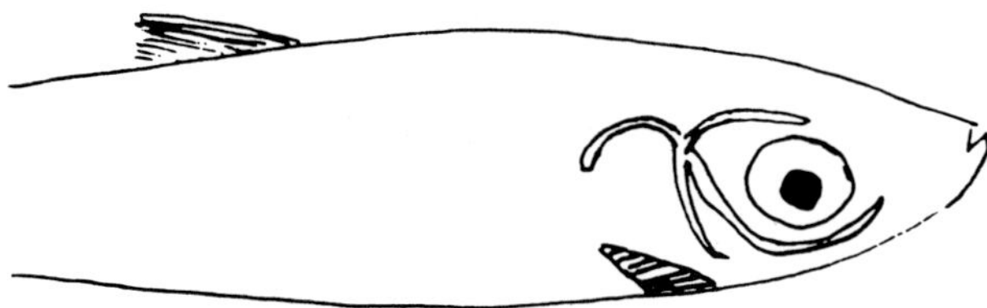

Fig. 2. In clupeoid fishes, the lateral-line system (here shown diagrammatically after Blaxter *et al.* 1981) is confined to the head alone and centred upon the lateral recesses.

presence of the perilymph-filled subcerebral canal which (see iii above) penetrates through the head of a clupeoid fish between the two lateral recesses, where membranes separate it from the sea water of the lateral-line canals. Here we re-emphasize (see ii above and Fig. 2) that these canals are confined to the head alone in clupeoid fishes, and note that the lateral recess on each side of the head acts as a sort of centre for that side's lateral-line canals.

In contrast to the bulla's specialised response to pressure changes produced by sudden movements of a relatively distant predator, the lateral line responds excellently in a lower range of frequencies to movements of nearby fishes in a school. This may be advantageous for the maintenance of schooling behaviour under conditions where visual signals are limited.

Lateral-line responses to movements of nearby fishes

Denton and Gray (1983) made experimental and theoretical studies of how an individual lateral-line canal responds to an externally generated pressure gradient that is varying sinusoidally with radian frequency ω. In the first case investigated, with the fish held stationary in an artificially induced pressure gradient, they were able to verify (see Fig. 3) the theoretically expected dependence of Q, the oscillatory volume flow in the canal, on Δp, the oscillatory difference of pressure between two adjacent openings from the canal into the ambient fluid.

They next investigated cases where the fish is free to move; so that the fish body, with

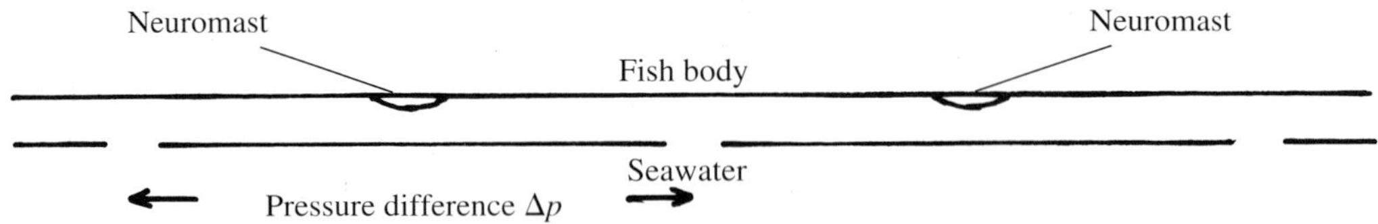

Fig. 3. Diagrammatic representation of an individual lateral-line canal, with the pressure difference Δp generating a capillary-tube flow, which in turn applies strain to the neuromast. The flow Q in the narrow tube is accelerated by the pressure difference and is also subject to viscous resistance; so that, for pressure fluctuations of radian frequency ω, it takes the form $Q=\Delta p/(R+i\omega I)$, where R is the tube's resistance and I its inertance.

its density very close to that of water, can respond to the same external pressure gradient as the water in the lateral-line canals. This raises the possibility that the pressure gradient may be unable to produce any relative motion of water in the canals.

(Parenthetically, we note that this possibility can be described in two alternative ways. The rate of change of relative velocity can be expressed as the acceleration of water in the canals minus the acceleration of the body, which may vanish if both accelerations are produced by the same pressure gradient; no resistive force would then appear since it can act only on the relative velocity itself. Alternatively, the formalism of 'inertial force' can be used to express the forces acting on water in an accelerating container – the lateral-line canal – as a combination of the forces applicable for a container at rest and an inertial force per unit mass equal to minus the acceleration of the container. Needless to say, the two formalisms are equivalent; the first being used for preference in the remainder of this paper.)

Denton and Gray (1983) made, however, an important distinction between the effects of different components of the externally applied pressure gradient. Consider (say) the longitudinal component that acts along the length of a clupeoid fish. Because of the backbone's longitudinal rigidity, all sections of the fish move with the same longitudinal acceleration, determined from a weighted mean of the longitudinal pressure gradients applied to all elements of the body's volume. However, it is only the longitudinal pressure gradient at the head itself which generates longitudinal acceleration of water in the lateral-line canals. Therefore, whenever an external source of oscillatory pressure gradients – such as a nearby fish making swimming movements – produces over the head a much bigger pressure gradient than the average for the body as a whole, the fluid in the lateral-line canals will respond to the difference of those gradients.

Thus, for a fish swimming in a school, any lateral-line canals situated in the head may advantageously provide good sensitivity to swimming movements of the fish immediately in front. Again, however, we stress that this sensitivity is derived from the response of fluid in the canals to longitudinal pressure gradients; depending therefore, in the phraseology of the Introduction, upon elements of the pressure distribution that are symmetrical between the two sides of the head.

By contrast, Denton and Gray (1983) point out that lateral (side-to-side) motions of the head are affected by the same local lateral component of pressure gradient that acts on water in the lateral-line canals. The original argument can be used, then, to rule out the possibility of lateral pressure gradients acting to generate water motions in the canals. They rightly stress, in support of this view, the contrast between the fish's longitudinal rigidity and lateral flexibility (while an additional supporting argument may be that even a completely rigid elongated body with a lateral pressure gradient varying along it would be free to turn in response to such variation, so that the head's acceleration would be closely related to the local pressure gradient). It follows that the lateral-line sensors do not respond to antisymmetrical components of the pressure distribution.

There is, however, some response to vertical pressure gradients, because the head's vertical acceleration depends on an average of such pressure gradients over its depth. This gives lateral-line canals near the top of the head, for example, an advantageous sensitivity to vertical pressure gradients produced by another fish swimming just above it. Once again, however, the sensitivity is to a symmetrical component in the pressure distribution.

Motions in a fish's subcerebral canal due to its own swimming

We now consider the effect of a clupeoid fish's own swimming movements on the flow of perilymph in its subcerebral canal (see Fig. 1). To this end, we define Δp as the pressure difference (left minus right) across the width $2b$ of the head between the two lateral recesses.

If the fish's head were stationary, this pressure difference would tend to produce in the perilymph of the subcerebral canal an acceleration (from right to left) equal to

$$(-\Delta p)/(2b\rho)\,, \tag{1}$$

where ρ is the density of the perilymph; the changing flow being opposed, of course, by any resistance in the canal. If, however, the head were itself moving with lateral acceleration A (from right to left), the relative accelaration of perilymph in the canal would be

$$[(-\Delta p)/(2b\rho)] - A = (-\Delta p)_{\mathrm{eff}}/(2b\rho)\,, \tag{2}$$

where we have written

$$(\Delta p)_{\mathrm{eff}} = \Delta p + 2b\rho A \tag{3}$$

as the effective pressure difference driving motions in the canal.

In the present section, we attempt to calculate the value of this expression (equation 3) which results from a fish's own swimming movements. This is a calculation which takes no account of any effect of the swimming movements of other fishes. But we may note at the outset that any externally induced pressure gradients, such as these movements might generate, would give equation 3 a zero value [because they would produce an acceleration A of the head itself given by expression 1, so that the relative acceleration (equation 2) would be zero]. Therefore, it is logical to ignore them.

In the essentially carangiform swimming of a clupeoid fish, body flexure appears mainly in the fish's posterior region, where large side-to-side movements of the caudal fin generate forward thrust together with oscillatory sideforces. Unavoidably, the fish body as a whole responds in sideslip and yaw to these sideforces (Lighthill, 1970, 1978), since the basic laws of mechanics require that the rate of change of lateral momentum and of angular momentum for the fish as a whole are equal, respectively, to the resultant and to the moment of the lateral forces acting on it. However, the consequential extent to which anterior parts of the fish experience sideslip and yaw is somewhat reduced by 'added-mass' effects (in other words, sideslip of a fish cross-section interacts with neighbouring fluid in a manner which gives the cross-section an effectively increased inertia).

Here, we are not at all concerned with complex problems of estimating values for the sideslip and yaw of the head of a clupeoid fish, but rather with briefly summarising calculations by Lighthill (1993) of equation 3 for arbitrarily assigned values of those quantities. Two principles govern the distribution of pressure p over the head of the swimming fish: (a) outside a very thin boundary layer, potential flow exists – with a

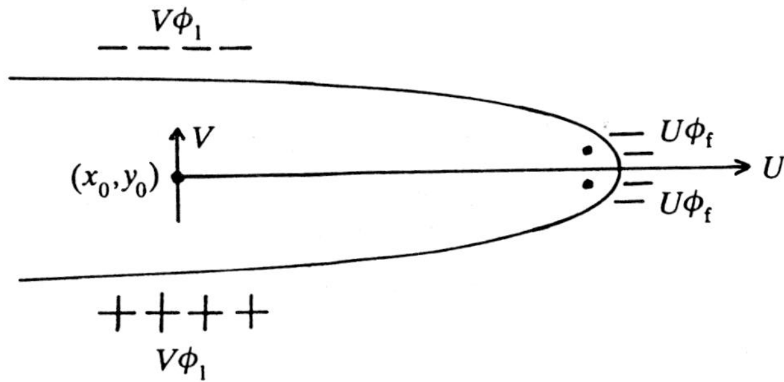

Fig. 4. Movement of a fish's head (in top view) without rotation generates water motions described by a combination of two potentials, as follows. Associated with the forward component, at velocity U, of the head's movement is a symmetrical potential $U\phi_f$, which takes negative values around the snout [giving rise, there, to positive pressures $-\rho(\mathrm{d}U/\mathrm{d}t)\phi_f$ when the velocity U increases]. Also, associated with any lateral component, at velocity V, of the head's movement is an antisymmetrical potential $V\phi_l$ which takes negative values on the side towards which the head is moving and positive values on the opposite side. When V is increasing, these lead to an opposing pressure difference $-\rho(\mathrm{d}V/\mathrm{d}t)\Delta\phi_l$ across the head. This difference is unaffected by the presence of the symmetrical potential $U\phi_f$.

potential ϕ (tending to zero far from the head) whose gradient gradϕ is the flow velocity; while (b) the pressure p on the surface is identical with the pressure just outside the boundary layer, where the unsteady-flow form of Bernoulli's equation determines it as

$$p=-\rho\frac{\partial\phi}{\partial t}-\tfrac{1}{2}\rho\,|\mathrm{grad}\phi|^2\,. \tag{4}$$

On the basis of these principles, Lighthill (1993) approaches the calculation of equation 3 in two stages, beginning with the simple case when the head remains unyawed.

In this case, the head's movement, without any rotation, is a simple combination of a forward movement with velocity U, producing a symmetrical potential $U\phi_f$, and a lateral movement (sideslip) with velocity V, producing an antisymmetrical potential $V\phi_l$ (see Fig. 4). As the head moves, it carries along with it these distributions of potential; thus, if the central point between the two lateral recesses has coordinates (x_0,y_0), satisfying the rules

$$\dot{x}_0=U\,,\quad \dot{y}_0=V\,, \tag{5}$$

then the velocity potential at each instant is

$$\phi=U\phi_f(x-x_0,y-y_0,z)+V\phi_l(x-x_0,y-y_0,z)\,, \tag{6}$$

where equations 5 need to be used in calculating $\partial\phi/\partial t$ for given x and y.

Now, Lighthill (1993), in a thorough analysis using the symmetry of ϕ_f and the antisymmetry of ϕ_l, and taking into account the entire equation 4 for p, demonstrates that the obvious leading term $-\rho(\mathrm{d}V/\mathrm{d}t)\Delta\phi_l$ dominates Δp to very high accuracy. Here the letter Δ refers to a value at one lateral recess (x_0,y_0+b) minus a value at the other (x_0,y_0-b). Also, ϕ_l is the potential for lateral motion of the head with unit velocity so that

$$\Delta\phi_l = -2bk, \tag{7}$$

where the positive number k depends just on the shape (but not on the size) of the fish's head. Equation 3 is now given as

$$\Delta p = 2bk\rho \frac{dV}{dt} \quad \text{and} \quad (\Delta p)_{eff} = 2b(1+k)\rho A \tag{8}$$

in terms of the lateral acceleration A=dV/dt. Thus, the fish's own movements give the two terms in equation 3 the same sign (even though any other fish's movements, as noted earlier, would give them equal magnitudes and opposite signs). It follows that, with sideslip but no rotation, a large effective pressure difference may drive motions in the subcerebral canal.

When rotation as well as sideslip is allowed for, however, a quite different conclusion becomes possible. Fig. 5 shows the notation used, with the fish's head at a varying angle of yaw α to the swimming direction and Ω as the angular velocity dα/dt. Here, it helps to introduce moving axes, for which the coordinates (X,Y) always have their origin at the central point between the two lateral recesses and the X-axis is in the head's plane of symmetry. Equations

$$X = (x-x_0)+(y-y_0)\alpha, \quad Y = y-y_0-(x-x_0)\alpha, \quad U = \dot{x}_0+\alpha\dot{y}_0, \quad V = \dot{y}_0-\alpha\dot{x}_0 \tag{9}$$

relate the new coordinates X,Y and the head's velocity components U and V in the X- and Y-directions to the coordinates x,y and velocity components (equation 5) used previously.

The velocity potential takes the form:

$$\phi = U\phi_f(X,Y,z) + V\phi_l(X,Y,z) + \Omega\phi_r(X,Y,z), \tag{10}$$

with the symmetrical ϕ_f and the antisymmetrical ϕ_l having their previous meaning, while ϕ_r is another antisymmetrical potential generated this time by rotation of the head about the central point (at unit angular velocity). However, an important difference between ϕ_l

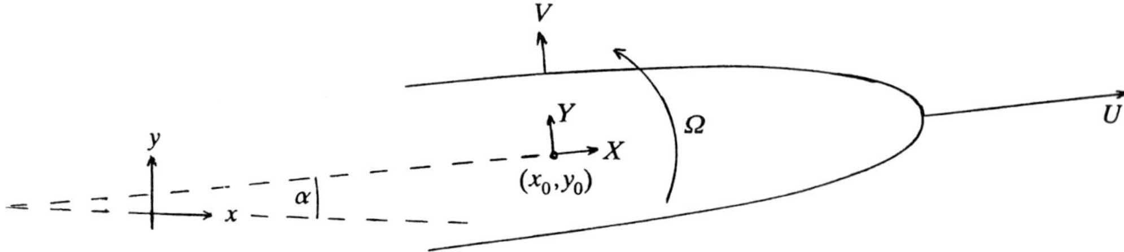

Fig. 5. Horizontal movements of a fish's head are described in two alternative systems of axes: (i) the fixed axes (x,y), in which the central point has coordinates (x_0,y_0) and velocity components (dx_0/dt,dy_0/dt); and (ii) the moving axes (X,Y) with their origin at that central point, and with the X-axis in the head's plane of symmetry, inclined at a variable angle α to the x-axis. Velocity components in the (X,Y) coordinate system are U=dx_0/dt+αdy_0/dt, V=dy_0/d$t$$-$$\alpha$d$x_0$/d$t$, while the angular velocity of the head is Ω=dα/dt. Note that the swimming speed U_0=dx_0/dt differs very little from U; on the oher hand, the sideslip velocity V_0=dy_0/dt differs from V by the large correction $U_0\alpha$.

and ϕ_r is related to their values and those of their X-derivatives at the lateral recesses (where ϕ_l and $\partial\phi_l/\partial X$ but not ϕ_r or $\partial\phi_r/\partial X$ take substantial values).

Now, it is found that

$$\Delta p = -\rho \left[\frac{dV}{dt} \Delta\phi_l - U\Omega\Delta \left(\frac{\partial\phi_r}{\partial X} \right) \right] \quad (11)$$

to high accuracy (with, once again, the entire equation 4 for p taken into account). Here the quantity in square brackets represents two obvious leading terms in $\Delta(\partial\phi/\partial t)$, of which the latter arises because equations 9 give $-U$ as the leading term in $\partial X/\partial t$ for fixed x and y.

Lighthill now introduces the definition

$$\Delta \left(\frac{\partial\phi_r}{\partial X} \right) = -2bk_1 \quad (12)$$

by analogy with equation 7 above, where k_1 like k is a positive constant depending just on the shape (but not on the size) of the fish's head. Then equation 11 becomes

$$\Delta p = 2bk\rho \frac{dV}{dt} - 2bk_1\rho U\Omega ; \quad (13)$$

but care is here required in relating dV/dt to the head's acceleration A in the (lateral) y-direction. A well-known result from the theory of moving axes,

$$A = \frac{dV}{dt} + U\Omega , \quad (14)$$

is in fact evident from Fig. 5, since rotation at angular velocity Ω gives the forward velocity U a lateral component increasing at the rate $U\Omega$. With equations 13 and 14 used to eliminate dV/dt, equation 3 is finally obtained in the form

$$(\Delta p)_{\text{eff}} = 2b(1+k)\rho A - 2b(k+k_1)\rho U\Omega . \quad (15)$$

Another potentially useful form expresses A as dV_0/dt, where $V_0 = dy_0/dt$ is the sideslip velocity in the y-direction (at right angles to the swimming direction), giving

$$(\Delta p)_{\text{eff}} = 2b\rho \frac{d}{dt} [(1+k)V_0 - (k+k_1)\alpha] . \quad (16)$$

Both these equations confirm the suggestion in the Introduction that head turning might always be successful in annulling the effective pressure difference. This could be achieved by giving the ratio Ω/A the value

$$\frac{1+k}{k+k_1} U^{-1} ; \quad (17)$$

or else, as equation 16 shows, by consistently giving the ratio α/V_0 (yaw angle to sideslip velocity) the same value (equation 17), dependent on the swimming velocity U and on the shape (but not the size) of the fish's head.

For the main argument outlined in the Introduction, there is no need to obtain this value (equation 17) in any precise numerical form. This is because the suggested approach which clupeoid fishes may use to annul the effective pressure difference is an active, closed-loop approach which just applies the amount of head turning required for the associated sensory signal to vanish. Also, equation 17 is certain to vary between different clupeoid species and between different individuals within a species.

Nevertheless, Lighthill (1993), in a long Appendix, uses measurements of the head of a particular herring (where measured cross-sections all had a depth-to-width ratio of about 1.8 to 1) to derive the best possible estimate of equation 17 for that head, leading to the value $0.87U^{-1}$ already quoted in the Introduction. Since broad geometrical characteristics of the shapes of different clupeoid fishes' heads are not expected to be highly variable, a roughly similar value (a little less than U^{-1} itself) may apply rather generally.

Possibilities for control of boundary-layer crossflow

From the potential flow outside the boundary layer (see (a) on p. 42), we now turn our attention to the water motions inside the boundary layer itself. This is that very thin layer of fluid which the fish's swimming motion causes to be dragged forward through the action of viscous stresses within the water. Because water has such a low viscosity μ, the layer's thickness tends to remain small; a typical estimate on a head of length a being $(\mu a/\rho U)^{1/2}$, which is considerably less than 1 mm for normal swimming speeds of the order of $1\,\mathrm{m\,s^{-1}}$.

On the other hand, fluid in the boundary layer is subject not only to forces dragging it forward, but also to components of force which act in the plane of a fish cross-section. Such laterally acting forces tend to produce crossflows capable (especially on cross-sections with substantial depth-to-width ratios like those just mentioned) of distorting the entire boundary layer in ways which can substantially increase hydrodynamic resistance.

Lighthill (1993) shows that exactly the same influences are responsible for generating crossflows in the boundary layer over the fish's head and motions of perilymph within the subcerebral canal. The reason is that both these fluid flows are motions relative to the laterally accelerating motion of the head itself. A thorough analysis demonstrates, moreover, that in the boundary-layer crossflow, just as in the subcerebral canal, the Y-component of the fluid acceleration which pressure gradients generate takes the form of expression 1, so that the Y-component of fluid acceleration relative to the moving head takes the value of equation 2 and becomes zero when the effective pressure difference $(\Delta p)_{\mathrm{eff}}$ vanishes.

It follows that a process of oscillatory head turning, actively controlled so as to minimise the sensory output of those lateral-line neuromasts that respond to motions in the subcerebral canal, would also minimise crossflows in the boundary layer over the fish's head. Such minimisation of boundary-layer crossflow is expected to generate substantial reductions in drag that might be particularly advantageous to constantly swimming clupeoid fishes.

Essentially, the boundary layer without any crossflow is similar to that appearing on a fish which is simply gliding forward. The streamlined shape of the fish is then being fully utilised to reduce resistance. Admittedly, the suggested control system for minimising $(\Delta p)_{\rm eff}$ would only be effective for eliminating boundary-layer crossflows on the head of the fish; nevertheless, this effect by itself may be expected to eliminate a significant part of the additional drag resulting from swimming movements. Furthermore, by starting the boundary layer off in a crossflow-free state over the head, it should delay any build-up of substantial boundary-layer crossflows over posterior parts of the fish's body.

The estimate (equation 17) for the required constant ratio of angular velocity Ω to lateral acceleration A (or, alternatively, of yaw angle α to sideslip velocity V_0), which might be effective in minimising crossflows, does not appear to call for any excessively large angles of head turning. It is important to note that such a type of movement differs greatly from any likely passive response of the head to sideforces on the caudal fin. These forces, while generating directly a lateral acceleration A, would be likely rather to produce a rate of change of angular velocity Ω in an essentially passive response, in which case the phase of Ω would lag by about 90° behind that of A. Again, the yaw angle α in a passive response might take a maximum value around $2h/l$, where h is the amplitude of the head's lateral displacement and l is the fish's length, while the amplitude of V_0 for radian frequency ω would be ωh. Thus, the ratio of amplitudes of α and of V_0 would be about $0.2U^{-1}$, far smaller than the value $0.87U^{-1}$ suggested for equation 17, in typical conditions of fish swimming with $\omega l/U$ around 10. All these considerations confirm that head turning, to be effective, must be actively controlled.

An experimental check

In this paper it has been suggested that the lateral-line neuromasts which sense motions in the subcerebral canal of a clupeoid fish could provide effective inputs to an active control process that, by using head turning to minimise those motions, would also minimise boundary-layer crossflows on the head and so produce advantageous drag reduction. This suggestion contrasts with the conclusion by Denton and Gray (1993) that, with head turning limited to the small amounts expected from passive response to sideforces on the caudal fin, motions in the subcerebral canal would be so great that the same neuromasts would be continually saturated under normal swimming conditions. Both arguments conspire to suggest the hypothesis that active head turning is used.

After this point had been reached in the studies described by Lighthill (1993), a decision was taken by Rowe *et al.* (1993) to subject the hypothesis to a classical *experimentum crucis*. If active turning is used, then measurements of the head's yaw angle α and sideslip velocity V_0 for a swimming clupeoid fish should show that the two quantities remain in phase and maintain an approximately constant ratio around $0.87U^{-1}$. (Actually, the cited paper investigates some other matters as well; here, however, reference is made only to the results of this *experimentum crucis*.)

Rowe *et al.* (1993) make several detailed observations on a swimming herring and conclude from all of them that the hypothesis has been verified. Here, we display (Fig. 6)

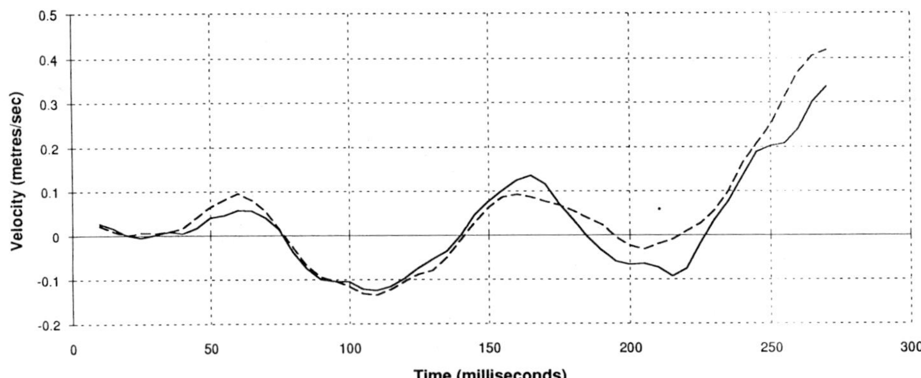

Fig. 6. Measurements of a swimming herring reproduced from Fig. 4 of Rowe *et al.* (1993). The solid line represents $0.87V_0$ (where V_0 is the sideslip velocity), while the broken line represents $U\alpha$ (where α is the angle of yaw of the head and U is the swimming speed).

the data from just one of their experiments; but a particularly interesting one because it represents a case, not of regular, but of accelerating, swimming movements and seems to show that the active control process is able to maintain the relationship between values of yaw angle α and sideslip velocity V_0 for the head even under these conditions. The rather closely coinciding measurements of $U\alpha$ and of $0.87V_0$ throughout the acceleration process may perhaps be viewed as an experimental check on the active-control hypothesis.

References

BLAXTER, J. H. S., DENTON, E. J. AND GRAY, J. A. B. (1981). Acousticolateralis system in clupeoid fishes. In *Hearing and Sound Communication in Fishes* (ed. W. N. Tavolga *et al.*), pp. 39–59. New York: Springer Verlag.

DENTON, E. J. AND GRAY, J. A. B. (1983). Mechanical factors in the excitation of clupeid lateral lines. *Proc. R. Soc. Lond. B* **218**, 1–26.

DENTON, E. J. AND GRAY, J. A. B. (1993). Stimulation of the acousticolateralis of clupeid fish by external sources and their own movements. *Phil. Trans. R. Soc. Lond. B* **341**, 113–127.

LIGHTHILL, J. (1970). Aquatic animal propulsion of high hydromechanical efficiency. *J. Fluid Mech.* **44**, 265–301.

LIGHTHILL, J. (1978). Mathematical theories of fish swimming. In *Fisheries Mathematics* (ed. J. H. Steele), pp. 131–144. London: Academic Press.

LIGHTHILL, J. (1993). Estimates of pressure differences across the head of a swimming clupeid fish. *Phil. Trans. R. Soc. Lond. B* **341**, 129–140.

ROWE, D. M., DENTON, E. J. AND BATTY, R. S. (1993). Head turning in herring and some other fish. *Phil. Trans. R. Soc. Lond. B* **341**, 141–148.

INTERACTIONS BETWEEN MUSCLE ACTIVATION, BODY CURVATURE AND THE WATER IN THE SWIMMING LAMPREY

THELMA L. WILLIAMS[1], *GRAHAM BOWTELL*[2], *JOHN C. CARLING*[1], *KAREN A. SIGVARDT*[3] *and NANCY A. CURTIN*[4]

[1]Physiology Department, St George's Hospital Medical School, University of London, London SW17 0RE, UK, [2]Mathematics Department, City University, Northampton Square, London EC1V 0HB, UK, [3]Department of Neurology, University of California–Davis, Martinez, CA 94553, USA *and* [4]Physiology Department, Charing Cross and Westminster Medical School, University of London, London W6 8RF, UK

Summary

The travelling wave of curvature which propels a fish forward arises from the interaction of the patterns of motoneurone activity generated by the spinal cord with the mechanical properties of (1) the muscle, (2) the skin, bone and connective tissues of the body, and (3) the water in which it is swimming. Furthermore, in the lamprey, a powerful feedback system has been demonstrated which allows local body curvature to influence the timing of the activity pattern generated by the spinal cord. The relative timing between activation and curvature are illustrated for both closed- and open-loop conditions, using data from intact swimming lampreys and from an *in vitro* preparation of lamprey spinal cord and notochord. The mechanical behaviour of a lamprey has been simulated with a mathematical model based on springs, dashpots, light rods, point masses and power units incorporating properties of lamprey muscle. Results are presented which illustrate the behaviour of a lamprey out of water. To anticipate the inclusion of the lamprey body model in the computation of the fluid dynamics, a hydrodynamical model has been developed in which the body motion and the forward swimming have been prescribed by mathematical functions. Results are presented to illustrate the hydrodynamic vortex structure as predicted by a two-dimensional, time-dependent numerical solution of the Navier–Stokes equations, including both viscous and inertial terms.

Introduction

Lampreys are anguilliform (eel-like) swimmers, which develop thrust by passing a lateral wave of curvature down the body. Fig. 1 summarises the problems to be solved in reaching an understanding of such swimming. We need to understand (1) how the pattern-generating circuitry within the nervous system produces the rhythmic patterns of muscle activation, (2) how the physiological properties of muscle interact with the mechanical properties of the system to give rise to a travelling wave of curvature, (3) how this wave of curvature interacts with the water to give forward movement, and (4) what

Key words: fish, locomotion, lamprey, anguilliform, motor control, muscle, mechanics, fluid dynamics.

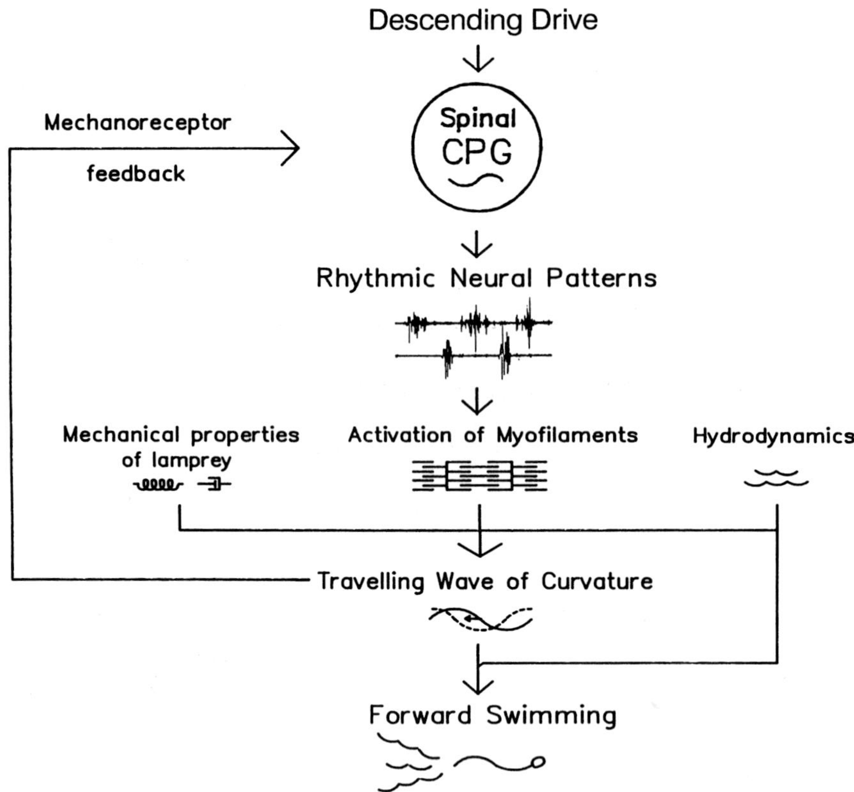

Fig. 1. Control of swimming in the lamprey: descending drive from the brainstem gives rise to forward swimming. CPG, central pattern generator (modified from Sigvardt and Williams, 1992).

role is played by sensory feedback from the resultant body curvature to the rhythm-generating networks.

The mechanisms underlying generation of the locomotor patterns in the lamprey will not be covered in this paper, but a number of recent reviews have appeared (Cohen *et al.* 1992; Grillner *et al.* 1991; Sigvardt, 1993). We will also not discuss the important questions of muscle efficiency and energy flow (Curtin and Woledge, 1993*a*,*b*).

The swimming lamprey

The swimming muscle in the lamprey is arranged in short myomeres parallel to the long axis, corresponding to spinal cord segments (of which there are approximately 100). When a myomere is activated, it develops force tending to shorten the segment and, hence, tending to produce curvature of the body towards the active side. In Fig. 2 are shown the patterns of muscle activation that occur during swimming in an intact lamprey (Wallén and Williams, 1984). Electrodes were placed in the superficial lateral muscle at four positions on the body, as shown in the figure. At any one recording position, muscle

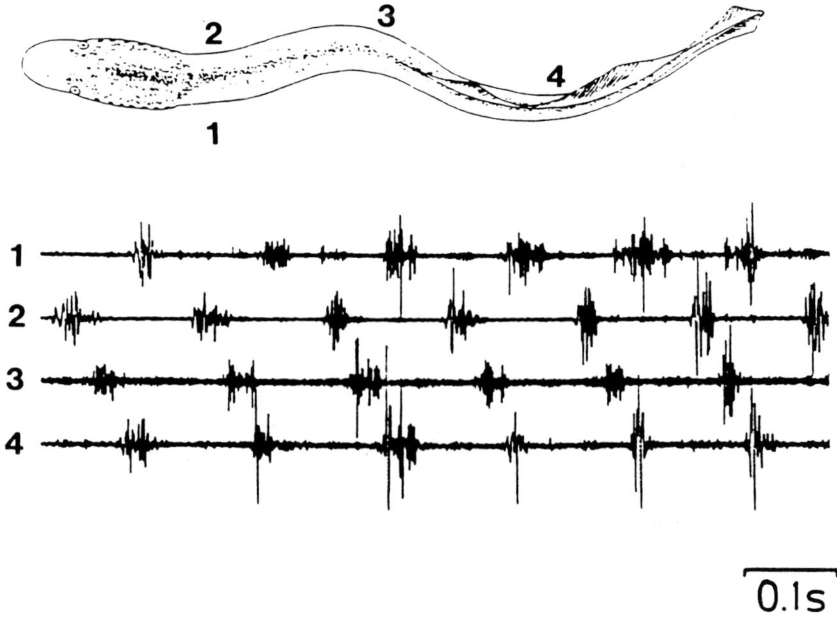

Fig. 2. Patterns of muscle activation in intact lamprey in a swim-mill. Fine-wire electrodes were placed superficially in the lateral musculature at positions 5, 25 and 45 segments behind the last gill slit, as indicated (data from Wallén and Williams, 1984; lamprey drawing by Simon Alford).

activity occurs in bursts, alternating with periods of silence. At any point along the body length, there is a strict left–right alternation of the bursts (e.g. positions 1 and 2 in Fig. 2). Finally, the left–right alternating pattern occurs with a head-to-tail delay. So the activation of the muscle resembles a travelling wave (e.g. positions 2, 3 and 4 in Fig. 2).

From simultaneously recorded elctromyogram (EMG) activity and cine films of the swimming movements, it is possible to deduce where on the body the muscle is active throughout the swimming cycle (Williams *et al.* 1989). This is shown in Fig. 3, which illustrates the simultaneous passage of the wave of activation and the wave of curvature. The lower dashed line indicates the points of maximum curvature and, thus, follows the passage of the mechanical wave. The thick lines show where the muscle is active along one side, and the upper dashed line thus indicates the leading edge of the travelling wave of activation.

The difference in slopes of the dashed lines illustrates that the muscle activity travels faster than the wave of curvature, as first shown by Grillner and Kashin (1976). This difference in wave travel creates a changing phase relationship between activation and curvature along the body length (Williams, 1991). Near the head, the muscle activation begins near the time of maximal body curvature towards the opposite side, and muscle activation occurs during the subsequent shortening of the muscle fibres. By about halfway down, the maximum curvature occurs at about the midpoint of muscle activity, which means that during much of its activity cycle the muscle is being lengthened and is thus

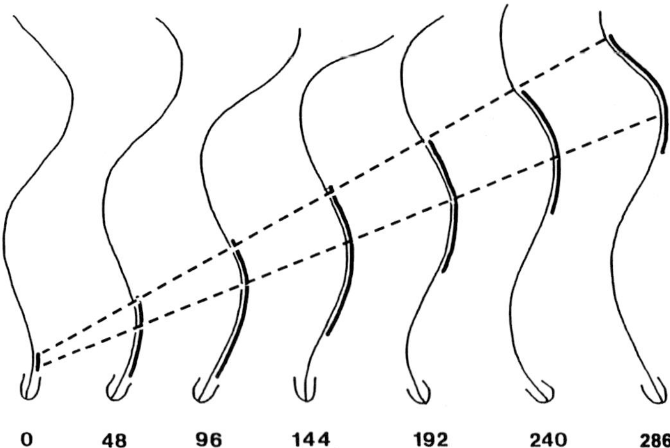

Fig. 3. Muscle activity during swimming in the lamprey. Midline tracings of single cine frames during one cycle of locomotor activity. Solid lines show active regions on one side of the body. Upper dashed line follows the leading edge of the travelling wave of muscle activation; lower dashed line follows maximum curvature to the opposite side; numbers show time (in ms) (modified from Williams, 1986).

absorbing energy (Curtin and Williams, 1990). It is not obvious how this relative timing arises; it must result from all the interactions that take place in the system. It occurs at all swimming speeds, so it is reasonable to assume that this timing is important to the proper working of the system.

Control of neural–mechanical timing

Movement-generated sensory feedback contributes to the control of the phase relationship between activation and movement. As illustrated in Fig. 4, the motor nerves of an isolated preparation of lamprey spinal cord can produce the same patterns of activity as occur during swimming (see Grillner *et al.* 1991). In such a preparation, the muscle has been removed, so the activity does not produce any bending movements. When rhythmic bending is applied by a motor to one end of a preparation, stretch receptor neurones within the spinal cord respond to stretch of the lateral margin (Grillner *et al.* 1982, 1984). These neurones mediate a cycle-by-cycle entrainment of the activity generated by the nervous system (Grillner *et al.* 1981; DiPrisco *et al.* 1990), as shown in Fig. 4.

Fig. 4A shows rectified signals recorded from five motor nerves in an isolated piece of lamprey spinal cord approximately 50 segments long. The bottom trace indicates the rhythmic side-to-side bending which was applied to the upper end of the preparation. This imposed movement entrains the motor nerve activity of the whole preparation, through local mechanoreceptors which feed into the local spinal cord circuits (McClellan and Sigvardt, 1988). The relative timing between the imposed curvature and the entrained activity at the nearest ventral root (vr 9, upper trace) is that which is seen in the caudal half of the body of the intact swimming lamprey (see Fig. 3).

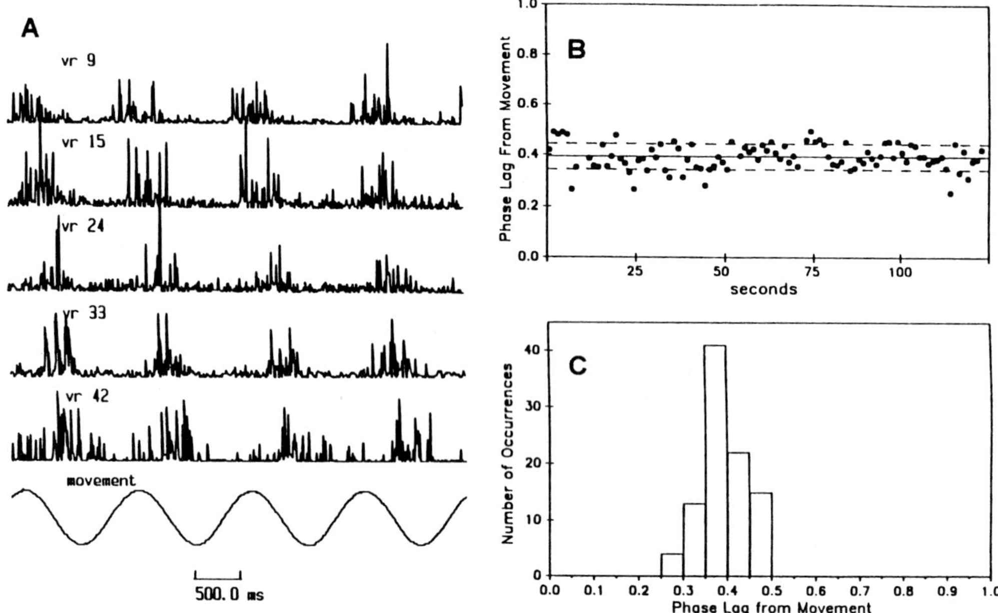

Fig. 4. Phase lag between motor nerve activity and the imposed wave of curvature in an isolated preparation of lamprey cord (still attached to notochord, but with swimming muscles removed). Activity induced by bath application of $0.5\,\mathrm{mmol\,l^{-1}}$ D-glutamate. (A) Upper five traces are rectified electroneurographic activity from ventral roots (vr) at positions 9, 15, 24, 33 and 42 segments behind the gills, as indicated. Lowest trace is signal controlling movement of a servo-controlled pen motor attached to the rostral end of the preparation, imposing curvature at segment 5. (B) Sequential phase lags (as a fraction of cycle duration) from maximal curvature towards recording side to midpoint of motor bursts at position 9. (C) Frequency histogram of data in B (modified from Williams *et al.* 1990).

Fig. 4B shows the phase lags between the imposed movement and the midpoint of the bursts of activity in the nearest motor nerve, cycle by cycle. As with all biological systems, there are apparently random variations around the mean value (see Fig. 4C), but the absence of systematic drift indicates that the activity is truly entrained. If the frequency of the applied movement is increased or decreased somewhat, the spinal cord activity follows, keeping approximately this phase relationship with the nearby motor nerve. When the motor was applied to the opposite end of the preparation, the phasing shifted so that the preferred phase relationship again occurred with the ventral root nearest to the point of imposed bending.

This experiment was performed on pieces of spinal cord taken from several positions along the length of the body (Sigvardt and Williams, 1988). The results are shown by the data points in Fig. 5. When the bending movement was applied at a position more than about seven segments behind the gills, the relative timing of the entrained activity to the movement was such that the midpoint of bursts of activity occurred approximately at the time when the body was maximally bent away from the recording position. Just behind the gills, there were two possible values of phase lag, as shown in Fig. 5. In most

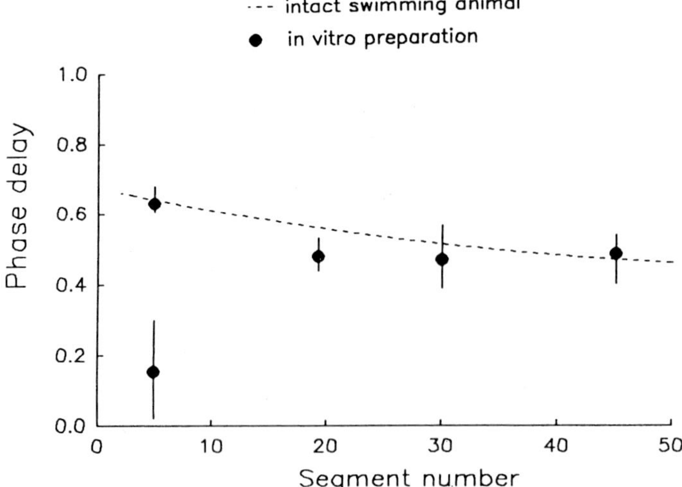

Fig. 5. Phase lag between motor nerve activity and body curvature, closed- and open-loop. Dotted line from intact swimming lampreys (Williams *et al.* 1989) as in Fig. 3. Data points taken from *in vitro* preparations (Sigvardt and Williams, 1988), as in Fig. 4. Segment numbering starts behind the last gill slit (modified from Williams, 1991).

preparations, the phase delay obtained at this most rostral level was stable at one or the other value only, but in some experiments it switched between the two values. These findings indicate that the interactions between the sensory feedback elements and the pattern-generating circuitry are different in the most rostral region from those over the rest of the body. In these experiments the feedback loop has been opened, since the muscle has been removed. For comparison, the dotted line of Fig. 5 shows the phase values obtained in intact swimming lampreys, in which the feedback loop is complete. These results indicate that the sensory feedback system plays a role in maintaining the appropriate phase lag between activation and movement and that, near the head, the mechanical interactions constrain the system to operate within the higher of the two ranges of phase lag which can exist *in vitro.*

Modelling lamprey body mechanics

The lamprey body has been modelled as a chain of pivoted rods, as shown in Fig. 6 (Bowtell and Williams, 1991, 1994). The rods are connected by tissue segments, each of which incorporates an element of stiffness and one of viscosity, which are meant to include the elasticity and viscosity of the muscle itself as well as all the other body tissues. In parallel with these passive elements is a force-generating element, which represents the protein filaments within the muscle. The force developed by this element depends on the velocity of shortening or lengthening, as seen in isolated lamprey muscle (Curtin and Williams, 1990). These force-generating elements are turned on and off sequentially, with a time course representing a travelling wave of activation, such as that

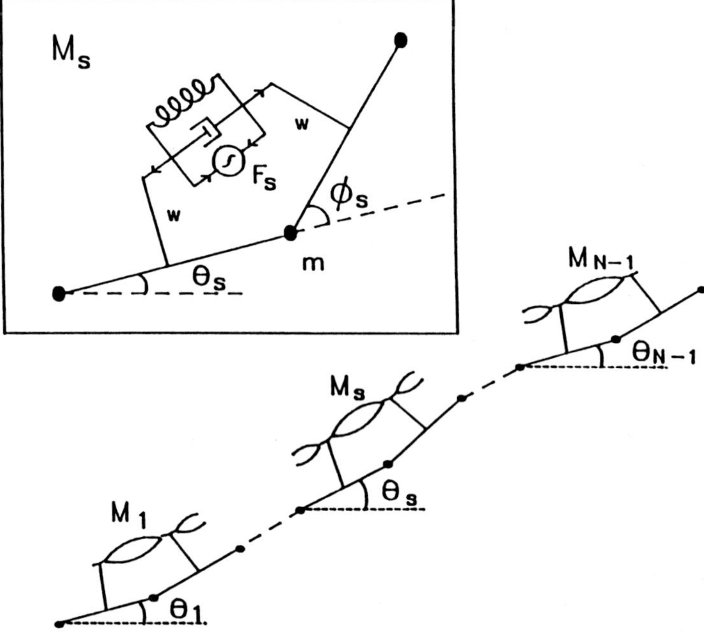

Fig. 6. Model of body mechanics for a lamprey out of water: each tissue segment is composed of a force-generating element (F_S), a viscous element (represented by a dashpot) and an elastic element (represented by a spring). Mass is concentrated at pivot points. Equations of motion are written with angles θ_S as variables. In the real animal, swimming muscles are symmetrical about the midline and activation of muscles on the left and right sides produces turning couples of opposite sign. In the model, each muscle component is capable of producing both positive and negative contractile forces corresponding to the sum of left and right muscle forces. These are mathematically equivalent (modified from Bowtell and Williams, 1991).

generated by the lamprey spinal cord (see Figs 2, 4). This is thus a model of a lamprey out of water.

The equations of motion of the whole system were written in a Lagrangian formulation and solved numerically (Bowtell and Williams, 1991). The system has been solved in two ways, both as a discrete system with some given number of segments (as in Fig. 6) and by taking a continuum limit. If the number of segments was greater than about 10, the results for the discrete model were not significantly different from those for the continuum limit (Bowtell and Williams, 1994).

The behaviour of this model was investigated, using a parameter space covering three orders of magnitude of the constants of elasticity and viscosity. The results are shown in Fig. 7A–C. In each panel, the body shapes at several times during a cycle are superimposed. In qualitative terms, only two kinds of behaviour were obtained, depending on the position in the parameter space. In each case, there is an envelope resembling a standing wave, with either two or three 'nodes'. Within this envelope, there is a travelling wave of curvature. A solution with little attenuation of the envelope at the 'nodes' is shown in Fig. 7A.

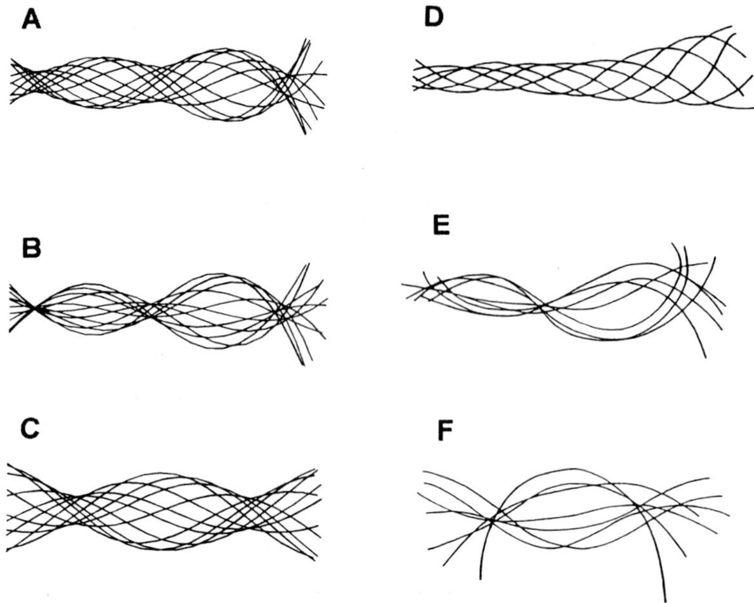

Fig. 7. Calculated profiles compared with body midline drawings of intact lampreys. (A–C) Results (unpublished) of simulations of the model shown in Fig. 6, with muscle force dependent on velocity as in Curtin and Williams (1990). (D) Tracings of body midline from successive cine frames of a swimming lamprey (Williams *et al.* 1989). (E,F) Tracings of the body midline from successive video frames of a lamprey on a slippery bench (Bowtell and Williams, 1991).

Fig. 7D–F shows tracings of the midline of the body of a lamprey. Fig. 7D is from a lamprey swimming in a swim-mill, and the travelling wave nature of the body shape can be clearly seen. This lamprey is in water, however, and the model is of a lamprey out of water. Fig. 7E,F is taken from a lamprey on a slippery bench. As in the model, either a two-node or a three-node pattern was seen. Hence, the model has been successful in predicting the movement of a lamprey out of water.

The next steps to be taken in modelling the body dynamics will be to incorporate the sensory feedback discussed in the previous section and, finally, to model the lamprey immersed in water.

Fluid dynamics of anguilliform swimming

In Fig. 8 are shown contours of instantaneous stream function obtained by numerically solving the two-dimensional Navier–Stokes equations including both viscous and inertial terms. The body shape and movement are prescribed as a backward travelling sine wave whose amplitude increases linearly from head to tail and which moves forward with constant velocity. The swimming animal is thus embedded in the computational grid as a moving time-dependent boundary. (Carling *et al.* 1994, employ a similar technique.)

The values used for the length of the animal, the speed of the backward travelling wave,

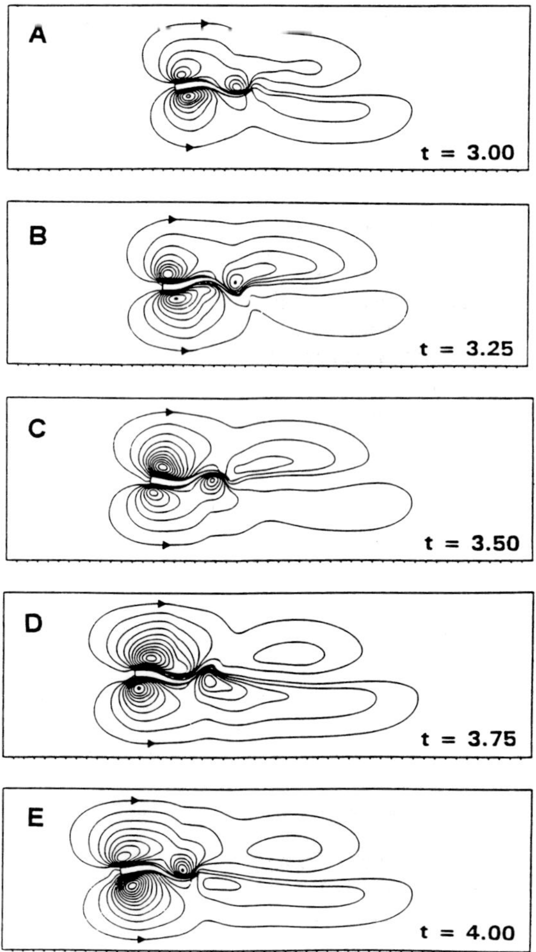

Fig. 8. Hydrodynamics of an eel-like creature: contours of instantaneous stream function during the fourth cycle of motion. Time (t) in A–E is in units of cycle duration (1.2 s). Body length, 8 cm; forward speed, 4 cm s^{-1}; backward travelling wave speed, 6.3 cm s^{-1}. Intervals between contours (representing flow rate) are equal in all cases.

and the speed of forward swimming were obtained from the pictures of a young eel (Gray, 1933). The hypothetical animal in Fig. 8 has been swimming for three cycles, starting from rest in an enclosed tank. The creature moves forwards while the body curvature travels backwards, and the resulting water movement is shown. The contour lines show the directions of water movement at a given instant; the closer together the lines, the faster the velocity of the water. As can be seen in Fig. 8, drag forces near the head set up vortices which remain attached to the body and travel forward with the animal. The vortex near the tail is held back by the travelling wave (Fig. 8A,B) and eventually shed (Fig. 8C,D). Meanwhile, another tail vortex is pinched off (upper half of Fig. 8D,E) as the cycle is completed and the shape of the body returns to that seen in Fig. 8A.

The total force on the body at each time step can be calculated by summing the pressure and drag forces at each point. With the parameters used here, there is a net forward force on the body from the water when summed over a cycle. This is evidence that the chosen ratio of the forward swimming speed to the backward wave speed is not correct for this system, since a net force on the creature would produce acceleration, whereas the imposed swimming speed is constant. An important further step in the modelling process will be to prescribe only the backward travelling wave speed and to allow the forward swimming speed to arise from the solutions of the fluid dynamics equations coupled with equations of force balance on the body.

The calculations giving rise to Fig. 8 were made in two dimensions only, which is equivalent to looking at a horizontal plane through a vertical sheet swimming in an anguilliform manner. So another important step in the modelling will be to go to three dimensions. The picture may look quite different since, in three dimensions, water may travel over the top of the animal, from the leading to the trailing edge of the travelling wave, whereas in two dimensions, water can only move from one side of the creature to the other by circulating around the head or the end of the tail.

The next major step will be to combine the mechanical model of the body with the fluid dynamics. We will then have a model in which the input will be the muscle activation patterns generated by the nervous system and the anticipated output will be forward swimming. The most doubtful part of the whole is the mechanical model of the lamprey body, given that the complex anatomical arrangement of the body tissues is represented by a lumped parameter model of simple geometry. It has worked well for a lamprey on a bench. How will it work for a lamprey in water?

The authors are grateful to the BBSRC, the Wellcome Trust and the NIMH (grant MH47150) for financial support.

References

BOWTELL, G. AND WILLIAMS, T. L. (1991). Anguilliform body dynamics: modelling the interaction between muscle activation and body curvature. *Phil. Trans. R. Soc. B* **234**, 385–390.

BOWTELL, G. AND WILLIAMS, T. L. (1994). Anguilliform body dynamics: a continuum model for the interaction between muscle activation and body curvature. *J. math. Biol.* **32**, 83–91.

CARLING, J. C., BOWTELL, G. AND WILLIAMS, T. L. (1994). Swimming in the lamprey: modelling the neural pattern generation, the body dynamics and the fluid mechanics. In *Mechanics and Physiology of Animal Swimming* (ed. L. Maddock, Q. Bone and J. M. V. Rayner), pp. 119–132. Cambridge: Cambridge University Press.

COHEN, A. H., ERMENTROUT, B. E., KIEMEL, T., KOPELL, N., MELLEN, N., SIGVARDT, K. A. AND WILLIAMS, T. L. (1992). Modelling of intersegmental coordination in the lamprey central pattern generator for locomotion. *Trends Neurosci.* **15**, 434–438.

CURTIN, N. A. AND WILLIAMS, T. L. (1990). Force during shortening and stretch of active muscle fibres isolated from the lamprey, *Ichthyomyzon unicuspis*. *J. Physiol., Lond.* **430**, 67P.

CURTIN, N. A. AND WOLEDGE, R. C. (1993*a*). Efficiency of energy conversion during sinusoidal movement of white muscle fibres from the dogfish *Scyliorhinus canicula*. *J. exp. Biol.* **183**, 137–147.

CURTIN, N. A. AND WOLEDGE, R. C. (1993*b*). Efficiency of energy conversion during sinusoidal movement of red muscle fibres from the dogfish *Scyliorhinus canicula*. *J. exp. Biol.* **185**, 195–206.

DIPRISCO, G. V., WALLÉN, P. AND GRILLNER, S. (1990). Synaptic effects of intraspinal stretch receptor neurons mediating movement-related feedback during locomotion. *Brain Res.* **530**, 161–166.

GRAY, J. (1933). Studies in animal locomotion. I. Movement of the fish with special reference to the eel. *J. exp. Biol.* **10**, 88–104.

GRILLNER, S. AND KASHIN, S. (1976). On the generation and performance of swimming in fish. In *Neural Control of Locomotion* (ed. R. M. Herman, S. Grillner, P. S. G. Stein and D. G. Stuart), pp. 181–201. New York: Plenum.

GRILLNER, S., MCCLELLAN, A. D. AND PERRET, C. (1981). Entrainment of the spinal central pattern generators for swimming by mechanosensitive elements in the lamprey spinal cord *in vitro*. *Brain Res.* **217**, 380–386.

GRILLNER, S., MCCLELLAN, A. AND SIGVARDT, K. (1982). Mechanosensitive neurons in the spinal cord of the lamprey. *Brain Res.* **235**, 169–173.

GRILLNER, S., WALLÉN, P., BRODIN, L. AND LANSNER, A. (1991). Neuronal network generating locomotor behavior in lamprey: circuitry, transmitters, membrane properties and simulation. *A. Rev. Neurosci.* **14**, 169–199.

GRILLNER, S., WILLIAMS, T. L. AND LAGERBÄCK, P-Å. (1984). The edge cell, a possible intraspinal mechanoreceptor. *Science* **223**, 500–503.

MCCLELLAN, A. D. AND SIGVARDT, K. A. (1988). Features of entrainment of spinal pattern generators for locomotor activity in the lamprey spinal cord. *J. Neurosci.* **8**, 133–145.

SIGVARDT, K. A. (1993). Intersegmental coordination in the lamprey central pattern generator for locomotion. *Sem. Neurosci.* **5**, 3–15.

SIGVARDT, K. A. AND WILLIAMS, T. L. (1988). Phase coupling during entrainment of fictive locomotion in the lamprey spinal cord. *Neurosci. Abstr.* **14**, 258.

SIGVARDT, K. A. AND WILLIAMS, T. L. (1992). Models of central pattern generators as oscillators: mathematical analysis and simulations of the lamprey locomotor CPG. In *Seminars in the Neurosciences* **4**, 37–46.

WALLÉN, P. AND WILLIAMS, T. L. (1984). Fictive locomotion in the lamprey spinal cord *in vitro* compared with swimming in the intact and spinal animal. *J. Physiol., Lond.* **347**, 225–239.

WILLIAMS, T. L. (1986). Mechanical and neural patterns underlying swimming by lateral undulations: a review of studies on fish, Amphibia and lamprey. In *Neurobiology of Vertebrate Locomotion* (ed. S. Grillner, P. S. G. Stein, D. Stuart, H. Forssberg and R. Herman), pp. 141–155. London: Macmillan.

WILLIAMS, T. L. (1991). The neural–mechanical link in lamprey locomotion. In *Locomotor Neural Mechanisms in Arthropods and Vertebrates* (ed. D. M. Armstrong and B. M. H. Bush), pp. 227–244. Manchester: Manchester University Press.

WILLIAMS, T. L., GRILLNER, S., SMOLJANINOV, V., WALLÉN, P., KASHIN, S. AND ROSSIGNOL, S. (1989). Locomotion in lamprey and trout: the relative timing of activation and movement. *J. exp. Biol.* **143**, 559–566.

WILLIAMS, T. L., SIGVARDT, K. A., KOPELL, N. AND ERMENTROUT, G. B. (1990). Forcing of coupled non-linear oscillators: studies of intersegmental coordination in the lamprey locomotor central pattern generator. *J. Neurophysiol.* **64**, 862–871.

INVERTEBRATE SWIMMING: INTEGRATING INTERNAL AND EXTERNAL MECHANICS

T. L. DANIEL

Department of Zoology, NJ-15, University of Washington, Seattle, WA 98195, USA

Summary

Challenges in understanding design for locomotion in any swimming animal revolve around the complex interactions between the mechanics of fluid motions around an animal and the mechanics of internal force production. The former is governed by force–velocity relationships that arise from fluid motion, whereas the latter is governed by force–velocity relationships of both active (e.g. muscle) and passive tissues. In reality, all such relationships must be satisfied simultaneously in any swimming creature. Towards this end, I combine traditional analyses of muscle contractility, soft tissue mechanics and hydrodynamic models to examine how organism morphology, muscle physiology and mode of propulsion interact to affect swimming performance. This combination involves a solution to a set of equations that describe the relevant internal and external mechanics. The solution has the unique benefit of providing predictions for both body and propulsor kinematics. Such predictions are examined for a variety swimming animals and are compared with existing kinematic data. Armed with such an approach, I re-examine traditional scaling arguments to show that classical approaches that neglect internal mechanics predict swimming performance relationships that may not be physiologically feasible.

Introduction

Research on aquatic locomotion has enjoyed a rather rich and impressive history of important contributions whose goals have been to understand the mechanics, energetics and control of movement in water. Historically, much of the work in this field has fallen into four rather disparate research areas: hydrodynamic analyses of thrust and energy requirements, analyses of the geometry and contractility of the muscles driving locomotor movements, analyses of the mechanics of passive tissues that are deformed during locomotion, and analyses of the neural control and feedback in regulating locomotor movements. Recently, however, there have been a number of new studies that are merging these areas for vertebrate (Johnston, 1991; van Leeuwen, 1992; Rome *et al.* 1993; Bowtell and Williams, 1991) and invertebrate swimming (Marsh *et al.* 1992). These studies seek to relate the control and dynamics of contracting muscles to the movements observed in swimming animals. All of these studies recognize that there is a complex interaction between the hydrodynamic forces generated by a swimming animal

Key words: hydrodynamics, swimming, models, invertebrates, muscle contraction, locomotion, scaling.

and those forces associated with the motions of internal structures. There is, however, no clear example in which the hydrodynamics and internal mechanics have been examined simultaneously for a swimming animal.

This paper explores ways in which these traditionally separate areas of research may be combined to predict the motions of swimming animals. I draw on invertebrate examples in developing this approach. In some sense, I seek to combine three different force–velocity relationships: one for the hydrodynamics, one for the mechanics of contracting muscle and one for the mechanics of passive soft tissues. While there is not as much known about the dynamics of invertebrate muscle, their relatively simple anatomy and the relatively simple hydrodynamics associated with propulsion by these animals makes the problem more tractable than vertebrate (fish) locomotion driven by muscles in a complex myotomal arrangement. I use, however, many of the ideas developed for vertebrate locomotion, along with the more integrative approaches of Full (1993) for invertebrate terrestrial locomotion to examine two case studies in invertebrates, which combine hydrodynamics, soft tissue mechanics and active muscle mechanics: jet propulsion and swimming with oars.

Diversity and hydrodynamic background

The thrust generated by any swimming animal depends upon the rate and direction in which it changes the momentum of the surrounding fluid. The trick is to elaborate on the precise mechanism that the animal uses in affecting such momentum changes. Armed with some description of the relevant movements of a propulsive surface, we can rely on a host of physical relationships that describe the resultant changes in fluid momentum and thus the resultant thrust generated by the animal. In a general sense, the Navier–Stokes equations provide such a description. But, because these equations are often intractable or cumbersome to solve, we rely instead on the wisdom of hydrodynamicists who have solved these equations for a variety of situations. Below, I indicate a few examples to show how thrust is related to the speeds and amplitudes of moving propulsive surfaces.

Among the invertebrates, we find a myriad of mechanisms for producing thrust, including body undulations, rowing, jet propulsion and lift-based mechanisms (DeMont, 1992; Daniel *et al.* 1992). There are even combinations of propulsive schemes, such as the rowing motions of polychaete parapodia, that result from body undulations (Sleigh and Barlow, 1980). For many examples, we have available a host of quantitative approaches that provide estimates of the instantaneous thrust force or energy requirements for locomotion. For example, the classic works of Taylor (1951) on flagellar locomotion and Lighthill's (1971, 1975) slender body theories provide useful tools for analysing sectional thrust forces associated with body undulations. While these are directed towards extremes in Reynolds number (very low for flagella and very high for anguilliform swimmers), some studies merge the two to examine the mechanics of undulations at intermediate Reynolds numbers (Vlymen, 1974; Jordan, 1992).

Wu (1971) provides the hydrodynamic groundwork for analyses of lift-based locomotion by aquatic animals. His work, along with the contributions from research on insect and vertebrate flight (Weis-Fogh, 1973; Lighthill, 1975; Ellington, 1984; Rayner,

1979), have guided analyses for a variety of aquatic vertebrates (e.g. Blake, 1981). Underwater 'flight' by invertebrates, however, is rather poorly understood, with only a few examples explored in any detail (pteropods: Satterlie *et al.* 1985; portunid crabs: Plotnick, 1985; lobsters: Jacklyn and Ritz, 1986).

Rather than expanding on each possible propulsion mechanism, I focus instead on two examples in some detail: jet propulsion and rowing. The goal of the following is to establish simple expressions that relate the motion of propulsive surfaces to the forces that arise from such motion. Armed with these, we may then proceed to examine the physical and physiological rules that govern force generation by the muscles that drive such motions.

Jet propulsion

Animals such as jellyfish, nautiloids, squid, salps, siphonophores and scallops propel themselves by forcibly expelling fluid from some internal cavity (for a review, see DeMont, 1992). The thrust (T) generated by this mechanism is equal to the rate at which momentum is ejected from the animal:

$$T = \mathrm{d}(mu_\mathrm{e})/\mathrm{d}t\,, \tag{1}$$

where m is the mass of the animal and water within it, t is time and u_e is the velocity of ejected water.

With a quasi-steady approximation and conservation of mass, the thrust can be expressed as a function of the rate of volume change of the animal (Daniel, 1983, 1985):

$$T = (\rho/A_\mathrm{e})(\mathrm{d}V/\mathrm{d}t)^2\,, \tag{2}$$

where ρ is the density of water, A_e is the area through which fluid is ejected and V is the volume of the animal.

Hence, if we prescribe the volume change in time, we can evaluate the instantaneous thrust. The velocity of the animal that results from this thrust is determined from the drag, inertial and added-mass forces that resist the forward motion of the animal. Thus, an instantaneous force balance can be used to determine the translation of the body that arises from some prescribed deformation:

$$T = 0.5\rho SC_\mathrm{D}U^2 + \alpha\rho\mathrm{d}U/\mathrm{d}t + m\mathrm{d}U/\mathrm{d}t\,, \tag{3}$$

where S is the projected area of the animal, C_D is its drag coefficient, U is its velocity and α is its added-mass coefficient.

Daniel (1983) naively solved these equations for swimming jellyfish of a variety of body sizes and shapes in developing scaling arguments for constraints on morphology and swimming motions. A fundamental dilemma with such an approach was the requirement that the volume change of the body must be prescribed. Yet, in scaling arguments of this sort, the hydrodynamics gives no clear clue about what motions are physiologically feasible. Some sizes and shapes would require muscle forces that far exceed those available from the unique myoepithelium that characterizes the motors of these creatures.

It becomes crucial, therefore, to understand the relationships that exist between the hydrodynamic forces and those generated by swimming muscles. One approach for establishing such a relationship can be seen from an analysis of the stresses generated during swimming. As fluid is forcibly ejected from some internal cavity, a pressure stress (P_{hydro}) is generated that is approximately equal to the thrust divided by the area through which fluid is ejected ($P_{hydro}=T/A_e$). Jellyfish generate this pressure with muscles that are arranged circumferentially around the inner surface of the bell. The tensile stress in the wall resulting from the circumferential component of the pressure stress corresponds to the active muscle stress. In their analysis of jellyfish swimming, DeMont and Gosline (1988*a*,*b*,*c*) follow precisely this idea in using measured subumbrellar pressures to calculate an active muscle stress of about 0.1 MPa, a value that falls within the range of previously measured active muscle stresses. Similar analyses of various cephalopods relate pressures to both the energy requirements for locomotion and the stresses within the animal (O'Dor and Wells, 1990; O'Dor and Webber, 1986). The analysis of scallop swimming by Marsh *et al.* (1992) brings us even closer to a realistic accounting of hydrodynamic and muscle forces.

Propulsion by oars

From the rowing motions of aquatic beetles and the myriad of planktonic and nektonic crustaceans (Morris *et al.* 1985; Daniel and Meyhofer, 1989) to the ciliary oars of ctenophores, there is an immense and diverse range of animals that propel themselves with some sort of oar-like appendage. Some, such as shrimp and naupliar forms of many crustaceans, use only one 'oar', their abdomen, in generating thrust (Daniel and Meyhofer, 1989). Others use paired oars, such as hindlimbs in aquatic insects (Nachtigall, 1980, 1985) or antennae in some crustaceans (Morris *et al.* 1985). Yet others swim with metachronal motions of a suite of oars (pleopodal swimming in shrimp or isopods: D. Alexander, 1988; compound cilia in ctenophores: Sleigh and Barlow, 1980). Thrust generated by such creatures arises from at least two (possibly three) physical mechanisms. First, as appendages sweep through the fluid, they generate drag forces which can be resolved into instantaneous thrust and lateral forces. Similarly, because such appendages oscillate in their relative speed, their acceleration relative to the fluid about them yields added-mass forces which may contribute to thrust (Daniel, 1984). The relative contribution of these two forces depends upon the Reynolds number (*Re*) of the appendage: drag forces dominate at very low *Re* and at high *Re* added-mass forces dominate. For any section of the appendage, one may employ a 'blade-element' approach (*sensu* Blake, 1981; Gal and Blake, 1988*a*,*b*) to compute the instantaneous thrust from the appropriate resolution of the hydrodynamic reactions to appendage motion:

$$T = \sin\theta[\int(1/2)\rho C_D h(\omega l - U_b)\,|\omega l - U_b|dl + \int\rho\alpha A d(\omega l - U_b)/dt dl]\ , \qquad (4)$$

= Thrust from sectional drag force + Thrust from sectional added-mass force

where θ is the angle of the appendage relative to the body (see Fig. 8), ρ is the fluid density, C_D and α are the sectional drag and added-mass coefficients of the oar, ω is the angular velocity of the oar, l is the distal position along an oar, U_b is the velocity of the body, h is the thickness of the oar and A is its cross-sectional area.

Note that the sectional force depends upon the velocity of the appendage relative to the surrounding fluid. As the appendage is attached to some moving body, the relative velocity must be resolved from the contributions of the motion of the appendage relative to the body and the motion of the body relative to the fluid.

As with the example of jet propulsion above, we realize that there is another set of equations that tells us how the body moves in response to that thrust. Thus, the thrust generated by appendage motion is equal to the total force resisting the motion of the body which, for simplicity, consists of drag and added-mass forces acting on the body and the inertial force associated with body accelerations:

$$T = (1/2)\rho S_b C_{Db} U_b |U_b| + \alpha_b \rho V_b \mathrm{d}U_b/\mathrm{d}t + m\mathrm{d}U_b/\mathrm{d}t\,, \qquad (5)$$

where C_{Db} and α_b are the drag and added-mass coefficients of the body, S_b is its projected area, V_b is the body volume and m is its mass.

Analyses of this sort have been carried out for a variety of applications, including a number of vertebrate examples (fish and frogs: Blake, 1981; Gal and Blake, 1988*a*,*b*) as well as the selected invertebrate examples mentioned above. As with the example for jet propulsion, all of the analyses require that, at the very least, the motion of the appendage with respect to the body must be prescribed in order to estimate thrust and energy requirements.

During recovery strokes, some feathering of the 'oar' is necessary for generating effective thrust. As was shown by Nachtigall (1980, 1985), this feathering results in a dramatically reduced reaction to appendages during recovery strokes. Lift may also be generated during recovery strokes for certain oar shapes and motions (Plotnik, 1985).

More recent attention has been given to how the setate nature of invertebrate oars affects the pattern of water flow past them and, potentially, the hydrodynamic forces they generate. Cheer and Koehl (1988), for example, developed computational schemes by which they could examine the flows associated with the setate appendages of copepods. The spirit of their approach is to examine the hydrodynamic interactions between closely spaced structures. In a similar manner, we are also concerned with hydrodynamic interactions between propulsive surfaces and the body to which they are attached. Additionally, since many rowing creatures have oars that move quite near each other (end of power strokes for rowing insects, pleopods in crustaceans), we should also be concerned about the effects of such hydrodynamic interactions on instantaneous forces. One example of such a thrust-generating interaction is the force generated by the abdomen of a shrimp as it flexes against the animal's thorax (Daniel and Meyhofer, 1989). Forces arising from such interactions may be quite pronounced.

A general issue

To use any of the analyses that have been developed for the hydrodynamics of aquatic locomotion, we require some description of how the animal moves its propulsive surface in order to calculate thrust, power, efficiency or other locomotor measures of performance. This requirement is problematic for scaling arguments where the hydrodynamics does not provide any direct way to prescribe the motion. It is entirely possible to generate combinations of propulsor motions and body sizes that may violate physiological limits to animal locomotion. For example, the speeds of muscle movements, the stresses that would have to be generated or the times over which muscle may be activated may, in certain scaling limits, go beyond the appropriate physiological range of these parameters. Some attempts to get around this issue examine scaling of aquatic locomotion with the constraint that muscle stress may not exceed its maximum isometric value (Daniel and Meyhofer, 1989; Jordan, 1992). Such arguments, however, may violate the physiological constraint that the force and power output of the muscles must follow, instantaneously, those required to drive the swimming motion. Our dilemma, therefore, is one of relating the instantaneous hydrodynamic reactions to the forces generated by those muscles.

Muscle function in locomotion

A great deal of attention has focused on how muscle is designed to deliver the force and mechanical output seen during locomotion. While studies of vertebrate systems dominate the literature (for general reviews, see Johnston, 1991; Johnston and Altringham, 1991; van Leeuwen, 1992; Rome *et al.* 1993), much of that work follows from the analyses of invertebrate muscles by Josephson (1985), who developed the experimental paradigm for measuring work loops. Below I provide a framework that is parallel, yet separate, from those relationships governed by the fluid dynamics, by which we can develop relationships between the force generated by some propulsor and its motion. Several fundamental concepts about muscle have guided our thinking about this issue. First, as shown in the classic work of Gordon *et al.* (1966), the force generated by active muscle depends upon its instantaneous length, with maximal force occurring when the thick and thin filaments (myosin and actin) are near 100 % overlap. With either a greater or lesser degree of filament overlap, the force declines as the number of potential cross-bridge interactions declines. Second, as Hill (1938) showed, the force (F) generated by active muscle declines as its shortening velocity increases. Moreover, as muscle is actively lengthened at ever greater speeds, the force initially rises above its isometric value and then declines. This force–velocity relationship (known also as Hill's equation) has been formalized with a simple expression:

$$F = (bT_o - av)/(v + b)\,, \tag{6}$$

where a and b are measured constants that are specific to any particular muscle, T_o is the maximum isometric tension and v is the shortening velocity. The tension falls to zero at some maximum velocity (v_{max}=bT_o/a). The ratios a/T_o and b/v_{max} are approximately equal to a constant (about 1/5, McMahon, 1984) for many muscles. Moreover, since the isometric tension depends upon the size (cross-sectional area) of the muscle preparation at hand, it is often more convenient to express Hill's equation in terms of isometric stress (σ_o). With these two modifications, a convenient description of the force–velocity relationship can be written as:

$$F = A_m\sigma_o(v_{max} - v)/(v_{max} + 5v)\,, \tag{7}$$

where A_m is the cross-sectional area of muscle.

A third concept is that the force generated by a muscle depends also upon its activation characteristics. Beginning with the signal from a motor end plate, there are several temporal lags that mediate force production (synaptic delays, diffusion of neurotransmitters and diffusion of Ca^{2+} from intra- or extracellular stores; Almers, 1989). These delays, often quite pronounced, greatly modulate the temporal characteristics of force production. In addition, after motor neurons cease firing, there are pronounced lags in the decline of force with time. These lags arise from the rather longer time it takes actively to sequester Ca^{2+} in intracellular stores.

We see, therefore, five important modulators of internal force production by muscle: (1) its instantaneous length and velocity, (2) its maximum isometric stress, (3) its maximum shortening velocity, (4) its activation time, and (5) its deactivation time. For any particular choice of v_{max}, σ_o and activation/deactivation times, van Leeuwen (1992) provides a useful way to summarize the relationships between the force generated by a muscle and its length and velocity, which is recreated in Fig. 1.

The idea that relationships such as the ones above can be used to estimate *in vivo* mechanical power output was examined in a series of papers by van Leeuwen (1991, 1992), who used measured or assumed temporal patterns of muscle strains to predict the time course of force development and power output by swimming muscles. Thus, knowing how a muscle strains within an organism and when it is activated, one can, in theory, calculate its instantaneous force, work and power output, provided we know v_{max}, σ_o and the various time lags as well as the lengths at which tension declines to zero (length of no myofilament overlap and length at which thin filaments collide). Such calculations were used to estimate the power output from the red axial muscles of swimming carp (van Leeuwen *et al.* 1990).

Some caution should be exercised in using traditional force–velocity and force-length relationships because both are measured under rather non-physiological loading conditions; the former are measured for isotonic loads and the latter for isometric loads. That neither condition really occurs in swimming animals was recognized Josephson (1985), Altringham and Johnston (1990*a*,*b*), Marsh *et al.* (1992), and many others cited above, who developed a combination of *in vitro* and *in vivo* approaches to examine muscle function *in vivo* and to develop scaling arguments. Here, rather than using the more traditional metrics of muscle contractility, a three-pronged approach is used. First, both the time course of *in vivo* strains and the pattern of muscle activation are measured simultaneously for locomotor muscles. Then, muscles are removed and exposed to experimental recreations of both these motions and patterns of excitation while force and deformation are simultaneously measured. From such experiments, one can calculate the work and mechanical power output of those muscles directly without worrying about artifacts introduced by the assumptions from either isometric or isotonic experiments.

It is clear that such 'oscillatory work loops' (*sensu* Josephson, 1985) provide direct estimates of the mechanical work done by muscle *in vivo*. Moreover, such ideas have been carried still further to examine variation in mechanical power output (Rome *et al.* 1993; Johnston and Altringham, 1991) as well as other physiological determinants of muscle activity (Altringham and Johnston, 1990*b*). Importantly, the approach used by van Leeuwen *et al.* (1990) and van Leeuwen (1991), which emphasizes the use of

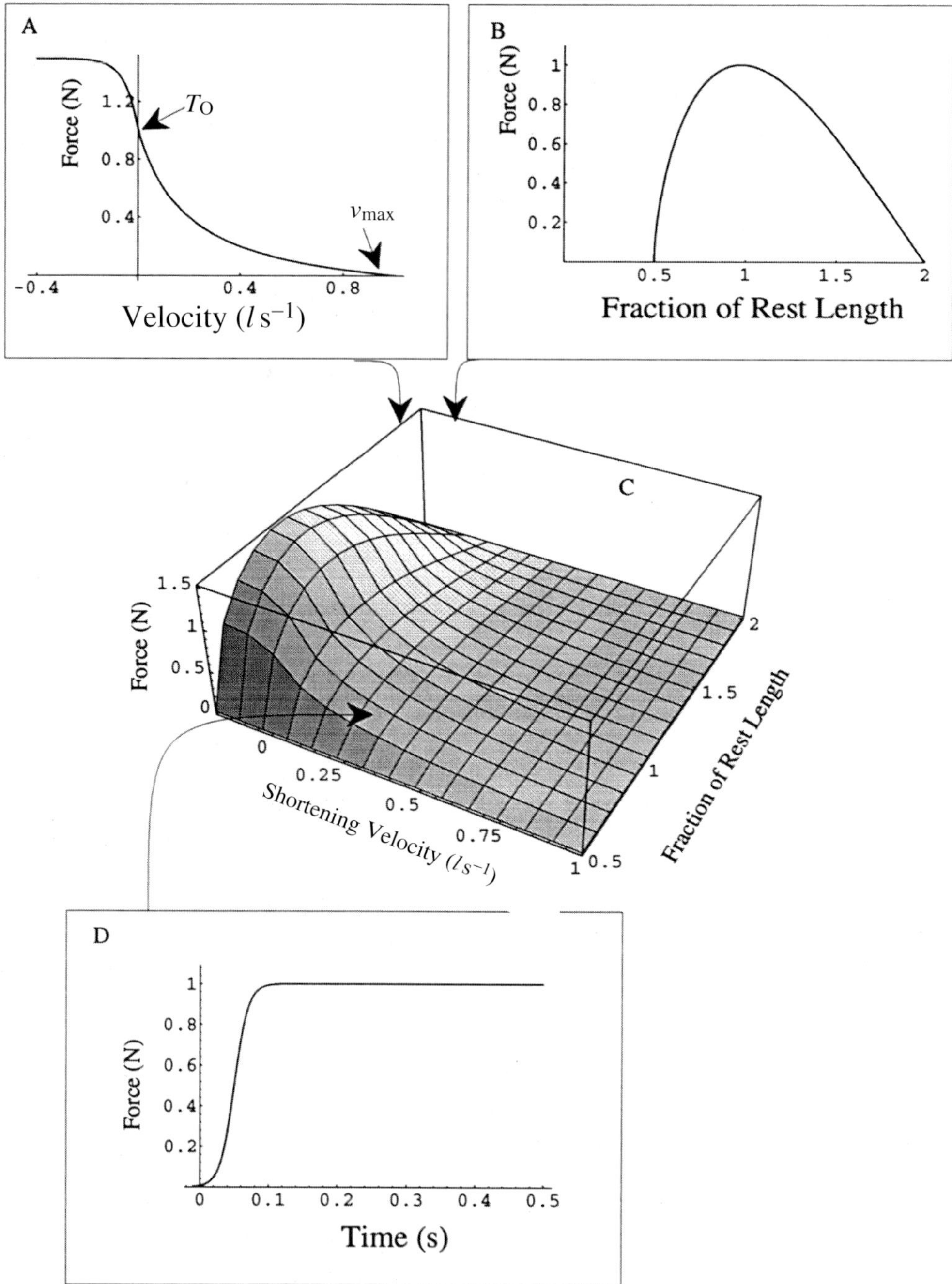

Fig. 1. The major factors that govern force production for muscle are shown diagrammatically. (A) The force–velocity relationship; (B) the force–length curve; (C) the combined effects of muscle length and shortening velocity on force. The local height of the surface is also determined by the time following activation or deactivation of a muscle (D). *l*, resting muscle length.

force–velocity and length–tension relationships, captures many of the details of work loops that have been measured independently (e.g. Altringham and Johnston, 1990*a*). Among swimming invertebrates, Marsh *et al.* (1992) provide the only data and analysis that are analogous to the vertebrate studies.

In addition to these physiological determinants of muscle force production, we must also account for the geometric arrangement of muscle fibers within an animal. For example, Alexander's (1969) study of myomeric arrangement in teleosts and elasmobranchs points out the crucial role of fiber geometry as an important determinant of force or speed output. Accordingly, the mechanical advantage or speed ratio of muscle fibers (Alexander, 1983) must be considered in developing models of force production by swimming animals.

One central issue still remains problematic. Both the work-loop analyses (Josephson, 1985) and the more mathematically inclined approaches of van Leeuwen (1992) require a knowledge of the temporal patterns of muscle strain and activation during locomotion. Just as with the hydrodynamic models that have been developed so far, the motion must be specified in order to calculate the relevant forces. There is, however, the exciting possibility that we could, armed with appropriate physical relationships, predict these motions provided we solve all of the relevant force–velocity relationships simultaneously.

The role of passive tissue mechanics in locomotion

Just as muscles must do work to develop some level of instantaneous thrust, so too must they do work to deform and move portions of an animal's body in generating appropriate swimming motions. Some of this work must be devoted to accelerating and decelerating portions of a swimming animal. For example, in a rowing creature, muscles must periodically accelerate and decelerate the oar and we must account for these inertial forces in addition to the hydrodynamic drag and added-mass forces. Moreover, swimming muscles must also do work to deform passive structures as the animal generates its swimming motions. Antagonistic muscles that may be either active or relaxed must be extended (Josephson, 1985; Daniel and Meyhofer, 1989; Meyhofer, 1993); passive elastic structures such as the bell of jellyfish (Alexander, 1988; DeMont and Gosline, 1988*a,b,c*) or the hinge ligaments in scallops (Marsh *et al.* 1992; DeMont, 1990) are deformed as fluid is ejected from the animal. Skeletal elements of rowing creatures, collagenous connective tissues in squid mantles (Gosline and Shadwick, 1983) or cuticles of cheatognaths (Jordan, 1992) also deform when these animals swim. Accordingly, we must account for any elastic and viscous behaviors of such structures in accounting for the total force developed by swimming muscles. In general, we can assert that there is a third set of force–displacement or force–velocity relationships that must be satisfied. These relationships follow from three ingredients: an elastic component, a viscous component and an inertial component. The inertial component is simply the force associated with periodic accelerations and decelerations of body portions during swimming, whereas the elastic and viscous components depend, respectively, on the deformation and rate of deformation of propulsive structures. These components can be summarized with a simplified equation that relates motions of passive structures to the force:

$$F_{\text{passive}} = kx + \eta \mathrm{d}x/\mathrm{d}t + m\mathrm{d}^2x/\mathrm{d}t^2\,, \tag{8}$$

where x is the displacement of some structure from its rest position, k is a spring constant for a particular structure, η is its damping coefficient and m is its effective mass. While DeMont and Gosline (1988*a*,*b*,*c*) successfully used such an approach in their analysis of jellyfish swimming, one cannot often assume a linear behavior for passive tissues. Indeed, many studies of invertebrate and vertebrate soft tissues show strong non-linearities in their mechanical behavior (see, for example, Wainwright *et al.* 1982). As Gosline and Shadwick (1983) point out, the non-linear stress–strain relationship for the collagen in squid mantle is an important determinant of how strain energy may be used in refilling the mantle. Additionally, equation 8 pertains to a simple material that could be represented by a parallel arrangement of an elastic and a viscous component. For many biological materials, however, more complicated formulations may be required to account for their dynamic behavior (Fung, 1990).

The idea that elastic strain energy, stored either in passive tissues or in activated antagonistic muscles, plays an important role in the energetics of locomotion has been a central theme in studies of vertebrate locomotion (Alexander and Bennet-Clark, 1977; Alexander, 1988; Cavagna *et al.* 1977; Biewener *et al.* 1981; Tidball and Daniel, 1986). Aquatic invertebrate examples, while less commonly reported, are likely to follow the same principles. Examples such as mantle refilling in squid (Gosline and Shadwick, 1983), jellyfish swimming (Daniel, 1983; DeMont and Gosline, 1988*c*), scallop swimming (DeMont, 1990) and shrimp swimming (Meyhofer and Daniel, 1990) all show that the storage of elastic strain energy may greatly modulate both the kinematics and energetics of locomotion.

The energy dissipated by some viscous component of the materials that make up a swimming animal is commonly viewed as a necessary evil: biological materials are inherently viscoelastic and any viscous energy dissipation is simply a factor that is unavoidable. This energy loss may, however, afford some advantage. In particular, Meyhofer and Daniel (1990) and Meyhofer (1993) suggest that energy dissipation may confer dynamic stability to invertebrate muscular systems subject to rapid force transients or continued periodic loading. The idea that some energy dissipation is needed for dynamic stability has not been examined in detail for any locomotor system and deserves additional attention.

Combining approaches

Over the past several years, significant inroads have been made in understanding how the hydrodynamics of locomotion may be integrated with analyses of the active and passive mechanics of internal and skeletal structures. The recent computational development by Fauci (1993), which integrates hydrodynamics at low Reynolds number with elastic mechanics to explore propulsion by flagellated algal cells, shows an exciting method by which we can solve these simultaneous problems. But such 'immersed elastic boundary problems' (Fauci and Peskin, 1988) often miss many features that are characteristics of contracting muscle. In contrast, the recent studies that have been developed for vertebrates (van Leeuwen, 1992; Johnston, 1991; Bowtell and Williams, 1991) and invertebrates (Marsh *et al.* 1992; Full, 1993) nicely combine internal force estimates or predictions with body motions. These, however, differ from Fauci's approach in that the fluid dynamics associated with locomotion is not explicitly incorporated.

Armed only with activation paradigms for the muscles that drive swimming motions, our goal, therefore, is to use the information we have garnered above for the mechanics of active and passive tissues as well as the hydrodynamics of propulsion to predict both the body motions and the fluid forces. I modify the conceptual framework established by van Leeuwen *et al.* (1992) and Johnston and Altringham (1991) to account simultaneously for both internal and external dynamics (Fig. 2). Here, propulsor motions are not specified; rather, they are predicted from the combined set of equations that describe both internal and external mechanics. I, unfortunately, avoid the computational finesse of Fauci (1993) and use, instead, rather simplified views of the relevant hydrodynamics in the two case studies below.

Case study 1: jellyfish

As mentioned above, jellyfish swim by periodically expelling water from an internal cavity (the subumbrellar cavity). This motion is generated by a set of muscles that are circumferentially arranged around the subumbrellar surface (Fig. 3). As these muscles contract, the radius of the bell decreases and water is expelled through an aperture subtended by a ring of tissue called the velum. In addition to developing the force required to expel water, the subumbrellar muscles also deform the bell, overcoming the inertial, viscous and elastic forces required for that deformation. The goal of the analysis that follows is to merge the three mechanical components of locomotion described above: the fluid dynamics, the passive tissue mechanics and the active muscle mechanics. The result of this approach is that we predict both the motions of the bell and the displacements of the body from a suite of morphological and physiological parameters. More importantly, we are armed with an approach that permits the development of scaling arguments which do not violate either physical (fluid dynamic) or physiological (muscle contractility) constraints.

Balance of forces

The thrust generated by a jet reaction mechanism is manifest as a rise in the pressure within the subumbrellar cavity. This pressure, in turn, is a result of the circumferential stress produced by subumbrellar muscles. Using the equations above and assuming that the subumbrellar cavity is approximately cylindrical, we can relate hydrodynamic thrust to muscle force (or stress) production:

$$T = \rho(\mathrm{d}V/\mathrm{d}t)^2/A_\mathrm{e}\,, \tag{9a}$$

$$P = T/A_\mathrm{e}\,, \tag{9b}$$

$$F_{\mathrm{c,h}} = 2Prh = 2\rho rh(\mathrm{d}V/\mathrm{d}t)^2/A_\mathrm{e}^2\,, \tag{9c}$$

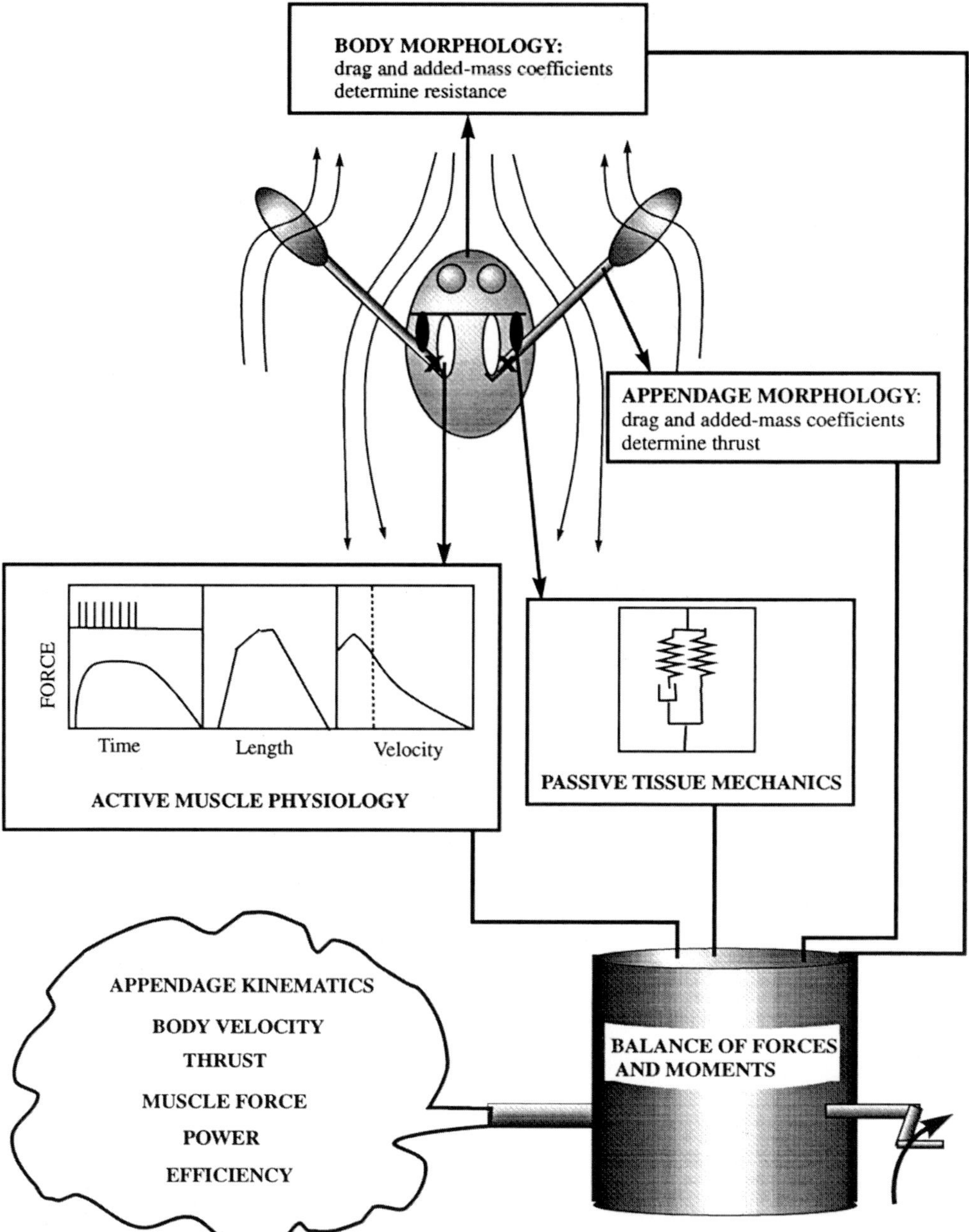

Fig. 2. The various components of a locomotor system are shown diagrammatically for a hypothetical creature that moves with some oar-like device. The flows about the body and appendages determine resistance to motion and thrust and depend upon the external morphology of the animal. Active muscles (white ovals inside the creature) follow the behaviors outlined in Fig. 1. Passive muscles (black ovals inside the creature) are assumed to be viscoelastic. All of these components determine thrust, body velocity and appendage kinematics.

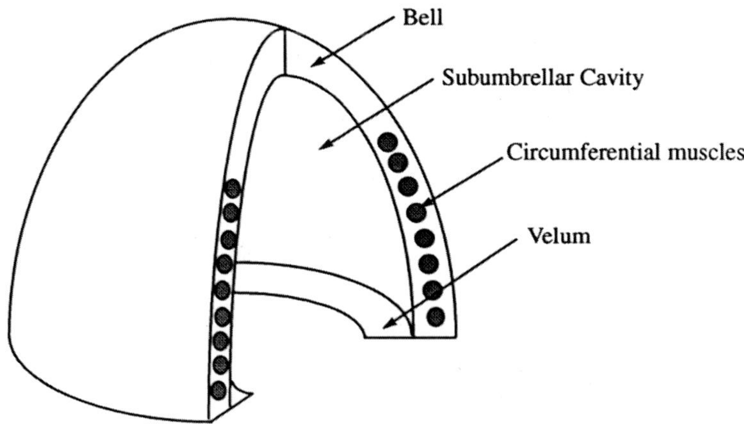

Fig. 3. This schematic diagram of a jellyfish shows the arrangement of circumferentially oriented swimming muscles that expel fluid from the subumbrellar cavity through the velar aperture.

where P is the pressure associated with the thrust, $F_{c,h}$ is the circumferential force resulting from that pressure, and r, h and V are the radius, height and volume of the subumbrellar cavity, respectively. We can relate the instantaneous volume change to the instantaneous radius of the animal by assuming that the volume of the bell itself (not including the fluid within it) and its thickness are constant.

Since the circumferential stress is generated by the subumbrellar muscles, we must balance muscle forces (F_m) against hydrodynamic forces and passive mechanical forces (elastic, viscous and inertial components):

$$F_m = \sigma_{c,h}A_m + k(r - r_o) + \eta dr/dt + md^2r/dt^2 , \tag{10}$$

where A_m is the cross-sectional area of swimming muscles and r_o is the radius of an undeformed bell.

Finally, the force generated by subumbrellar muscles (F_m) depends upon their shortening velocity ($-dr/dt$), their length ($r-r_o$) and the time following either activation or deactivation:

$$F_m = f(l)g(t)\{A_m\sigma_o(v_{max} + 2\pi dr/dt)/[v_{max} - 5(2\pi)dr/dt]\} , \tag{11}$$

where $f(l)$ is a function that adjusts the muscle force for the amount of filament overlap and $g(t)$ is a function that adjusts the muscle force for the time following activation or deactivation (see Fig. 1 for graphs of these functions). The sign change in equation 11 arises from the fact that decreases in the circumference of the bell correspond to positive values for shortening velocity. A factor of 2π accounts for changes in circumference rather than radius.

Since the radius of the animal changes over time, instantaneous drag and added-mass forces that resist the motion of the body vary temporally as well. Thus, we cannot determine the velocity of the body without a simultaneous solution to the balance between the instantaneous thrust and the reactions to the body in the surrounding fluid.

Accordingly, one additional set of equations must be solved to determine both the changes in the shape of the animal and its translation. Thus, we set the thrust (T) equal to the drag, added-mass and inertial forces resisting body motion:

$$T = \rho(\mathrm{d}V/\mathrm{d}t)^2/A_e = 0.5\rho SC_D U^2 + \alpha\rho V\mathrm{d}U/\mathrm{d}t + \rho V\mathrm{d}U/\mathrm{d}t\,. \qquad (12)$$

Equations 10 and 11 give a non-linear second-order differential equation for the temporal changes in bell radius. Equation 12 is a non-linear first-order differential equation for velocity. The equations contain expressions that depend upon the instantaneous radius of the animal and, as such, form a coupled system that must be solved simultaneously. Since an analytical solution is not available, I solve these equations numerically (fourth-order Runge–Kutta method with adaptive time stepping).

During recovery strokes, a similar set of equations is developed to describe the instantaneous motions of the body and deformations of the bell. Here, however, bell deformations are driven not by muscles but by the elastic energy stored in the bell. Moreover, the expansion of the bell generates a negative thrust as it refills. During this time, the velar muscles relax, yielding a significantly larger area through which water is drawn and thus the negative thrust is greatly diminished (Gladfelter, 1972). The equations above are modified to account for these issues by setting the active muscle force to zero during recovery strokes and letting the elastic force in the bell drive the resultant motions.

Where are the data?

There are several past studies which, while not all examining similar species, provide some estimates for relevant parameters (Table 1). For example, DeMont and Gosline's (1988*a*,*b*,*c*) analyses of jet propulsion by *Polyorchis penicillatus* provide direct estimates of the modulus of a bell (and of its spring constant), the damping factor and the effective mass. Gladfelter's (1972) data on the same species are used to estimate the dimensions of the bell and of the circumferential muscles (cross-sectional area). Studies of other jellyfish (Daniel, 1983, 1985) provide estimates of drag and added-mass coefficients.

A much more problematic issue relates to the relevant physiological characteristics of subumbrellar muscles. Here, the maximum shortening velocity (v_{max}) and isometric tension (σ_o), as well as the activation and deactivation times, are not known. We can only rely on estimates based on the range of values reported for other invertebrate muscles. Isometric stress values for a variety of invertebrate muscles range from approximately 0.1 to 1.0 MPa, with many (e.g. annelids, bivalves, insects) having values near 0.5 MPa (Schmidt-Nielsen, 1979), a value I use in the equations above.

Much greater variation is seen in the maximum shortening velocity and in the activation and relaxation times of muscle. Shortening velocity for invertebrate muscles shows a rather dramatic range from about $0.1\,l\,\mathrm{s}^{-1}$ (muscle lengths per second) in the byssus retractor muscle of *Mytilus* to about $15\,l\,\mathrm{s}^{-1}$ for direct flight muscle of locusts (Wilson, 1979; Wilkie, 1966). I use $1.0\,l\,\mathrm{s}^{-1}$ as a conservative estimate of the maximum shortening velocity.

Activation times range from a few milliseconds for indirect insect flight muscle to about 30 s for sea anemone tonic muscles (Prosser, 1991). Deactivation times for certain specialized invertebrate muscles can be quite dramatic (many minutes for the byssus

Table 1. *Values used in the analysis of jellyfish swimming*

Parameter	Value	Source
Morphological parameters		
Bell radius at rest	2 cm	DeMont and Gosline (1988*a*)
Bell height at rest	4 cm	DeMont and Gosline (1988*a*)
Bell thickness	0.4 cm	DeMont and Gosline (1988*a*)
Velum radius	1 cm	Gladfelter (1972)
Thickness of muscle	20 μm	Gladfelter (1972)
Physiological parameters		
Isometric stress	0.5 MPa	Estimate
Maximum shortening velocity	1.0 $l\,s^{-1}$	Estimate
Activation time	0.25 s	Estimate
Bell mechanical parameters		
Stiffness	500 Pa	DeMont and Gosline (1988*a*)
Effective mass	0.02 kg	DeMont and Gosline (1988*a*)
Damping coefficient	0.1 N s m^{-1}	DeMont and Gosline (1988*a*)
Hydrodynamic parameters		
Drag coefficient	1.0	Daniel (1985)
Added-mass coefficient	0.5	Daniel (1985)

These values are approximated from published ones or are estimated.
l is muscle length.

retractor muscle of *Mytilus*) but, more commonly, they are slightly longer than activation times. For the jellyfish *Aurelia*, Prosser (1991) reports activation and deactivation times of the order of 0.5 s. In the analyses below, I assume that muscle is maximally activated in 0.25 s and fully deactivates in the same time.

Some predictions

Armed with a suite of parameter estimates, equations 9–12 can be solved to predict both the temporal pattern of bell deformations and body translations (Fig. 4). Thus, for a jellyfish whose dimensions correspond to those of *Polyorchis* (2 cm in radius and 4 cm tall), we note that these parameters give cycle times of about 0.8 s, with the contraction phase lasting about half of that time. During this time, there is a reduction in the bell radius of about 25 %. This motion results in a peak velocity of about 7 cm s^{-1} and an average cycle velocity of about 2.5 cm s^{-1}. For comparison, the cycle times of *Polyorchis* fall well within the range reported by DeMont and Gosline (1988*a*,*b*,*c*) and Gladfelter (1972), as well as those reported by Daniel (1985) for similarly sized jellyfish.

The approach above can also be used to examine instantaneous pressures (Fig. 4D) and muscle stress (Fig. 4E). Here, peak pressures of about 15 Pa are predicted, which are somewhat lower than those reported by DeMont and Gosline and may result from an underestimate of the activation time. Nevertheless, the temporal pattern of pressure is similar to that reported by DeMont and Gosline (1988*b*). The

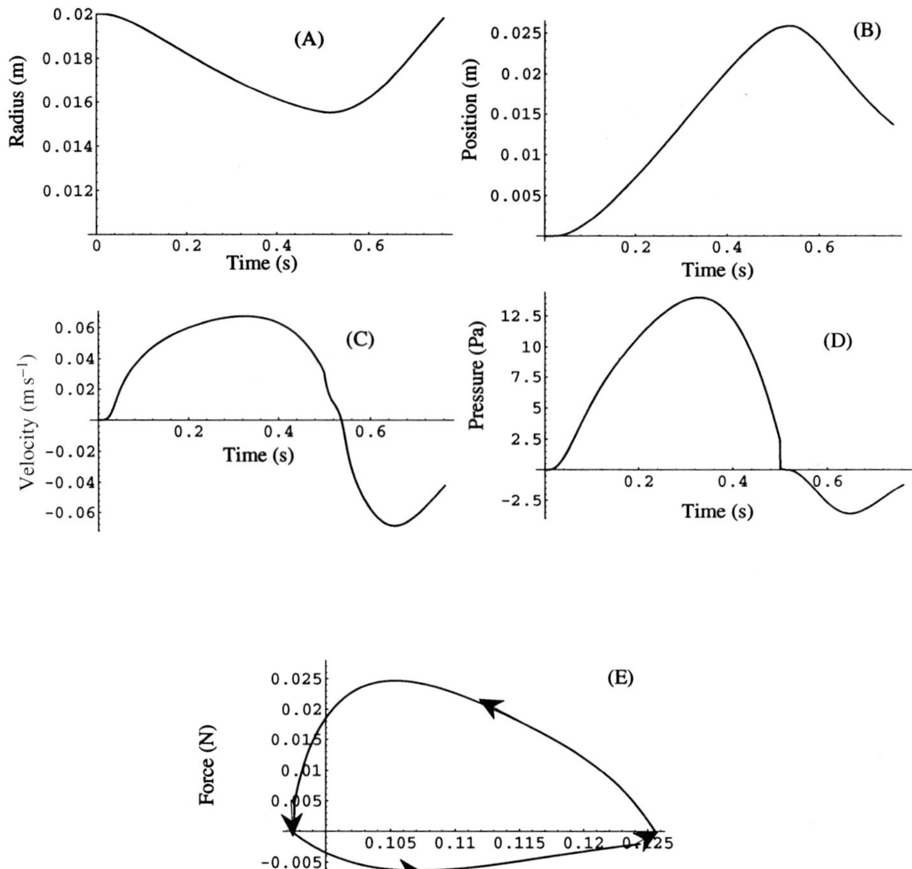

Fig. 4. The instantaneous kinematics and mechanics for a swimming jellyfish. All parameters used in this simulation are shown in Table 1. Instantaneous plots of the radius (A), position (B), body velocity (C) and subumbrellar pressure (D) show motions and forces that correspond to a single cycle of jetting. A work loop (E) is also shown.

circumferential stress corresponding to that pressure plotted against the instantaneous radius of the bell gives a 'work loop' (Fig. 4E) much like those seen in other systems (e.g. Johnston, 1991), with the exception that rather large transients dominate the predicted pattern.

Scale arguments: classic versus *new approaches*

While there are some discrepancies between predicted and measured values for swimming jellyfish, the general results are in good agreement. Integrating muscle mechanics, soft tissue mechanics and hydrodynamics therefore permits us to examine the consequences of variations in morphological and physiological parameters. Classically, we have been interested in the issue of scale. In past approaches, we have naively made

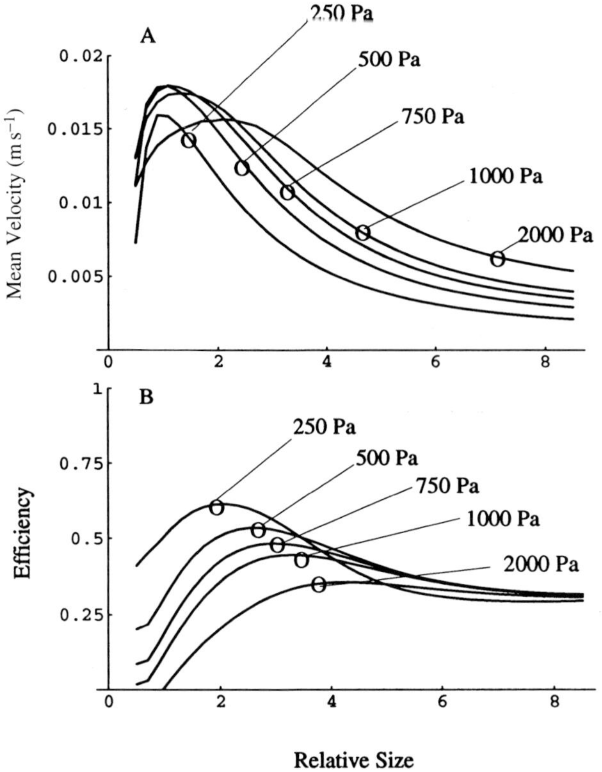

Fig. 5. The consequence of varying both the size of the animal and the stiffness of the bell is shown in a series of plots for the mean cycle velocity (A) and the efficiency (B). All physiological characteristics of the muscles were held constant in these simulations. Note that a bell stiffness of about 500 Pa corresponds to the maximum swimming velocity for an animal whose relative size is 1.0.

assumptions about the kinematics of motion in examining issues of size with hydrodynamic models of aquatic locomotion (for a good example of such naivete, see Daniel, 1983). One conclusion reached by such studies is that, as long as the kinematics remains constant, larger creatures will swim faster. However, larger creatures require greater muscle stress to expel ever larger volumes of fluid in the same time – the constraint imposed by the assumption of constant kinematics. In reality, muscle stress associated with deforming passive tissues and with generating hydrodynamic forces scales in non-intuitive ways. Thus, we can examine the consequences of size variation by assuming (1) that the physiological properties of muscle do not vary and (2) that the material properties that make up an animal remain constant. Under these assumptions, we can examine the consequences of size variation while maintaining results that are both physically and physiologically reasonable.

For the particular choice of bell mechanical properties and muscle contractile properties, we see that either increasing or decreasing the relative size of the animal leads to reductions in both the speed of movement and the efficiency (the curves for the

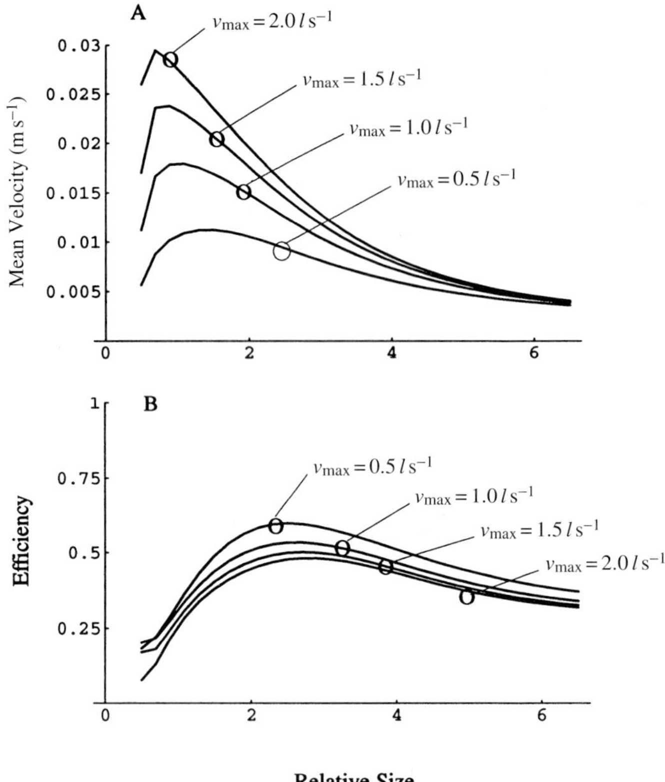

Fig. 6. The consequence of varying both the size of the animal and the maximum shortening velocity (v_{max}) is shown in a series of plots for the mean cycle velocity (A) and the efficiency (B). Increasing v_{max} leads to greater swimming speeds with lower efficiencies. Note, however, that the size at which speed or efficiency is maximal depends upon v_{max}. All other parameters were held constant in these simulations. *l*, resting muscle length.

estimated stiffness of 500 Pa in Fig. 5). This result contrasts to the more classic approach in which the kinematics is assumed to be constant. The latter case leads to predictions of ever greater speed with increasing size, but will yield instantaneous muscle stresses that are not physiologically feasible.

It is likely that the size at which swimming speed or efficiency is maximal may well depend on the particular choice of bell mechanical properties and of muscle contractile properties. Indeed, Fig. 5 shows that increasing the stiffness of the bell changes the size at which speed and efficiency are maximized. Interestingly, a value of 500 Pa – about the average reported by DeMont and Gosline (1988*c*) – leads to the highest overall swimming speed. Increasing either the maximum shortening velocity or the isometric stress increases the swimming speed and decreases efficiency. However, the size at which either speed or efficiency is maximal depends upon the particular choices of these parameters (Fig. 6). For example, the maximal swimming speed occurs at a smaller size as the maximum shortening velocity increases (Fig. 6A). Changing the amount of time

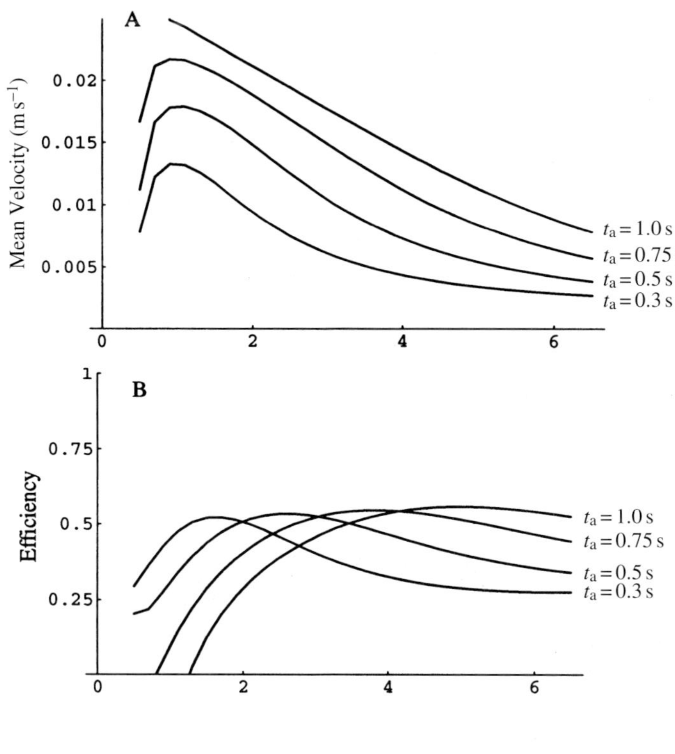

Fig. 7. The consequence of varying both the size of the animal and the activation time (t_a) of the swimming muscles is shown in a series of plots for the mean cycle velocity (A) and the efficiency (B). As with previous figures, the size at which swimming performance is maximal depends upon the value of this parameter.

that muscles are activated also has dramatic effects on swimming performance; efficiency reaches similar maxima for large animals with long contraction times and small ones with short contraction times (Fig. 7).

Each of the figures shows the consequence of varying, at most, two parameters at once (e.g. size and bell stiffness or size and v_{max}). In reality, it is very likely that identical levels of swimming performance (swimming speed or efficiency) can be achieved by varying many of the parameters simultaneously.

Case study 2: notonectids

Notonectids are aquatic bugs that swim by using reciprocating hindlimbs fringed with setae, in a manner quite similar to that reported for other aquatic insects (Nachtigall, 1985). During power strokes, the hindlimbs swing posteriorly with their setae expanded; during recovery strokes, the setae fold and the appendage flexes as it swings anteriorly. The muscle responsible for the power stroke extends from the anterior thoracic antecosta

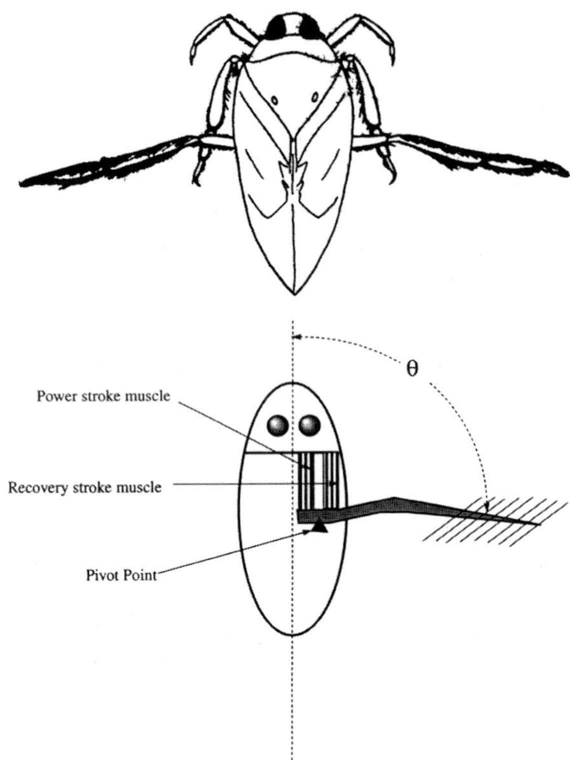

Fig. 8. The geometry of *Notonecta undulata* is reduced to a simple appendage that is driven by two muscles. Power stroke muscles swing the appendage posteriorly about a pivot point. Recovery stroke muscles swing the appendage anteriorly. The angle (θ) subtended by the appendage is also shown.

to the coxo-trochanteral apodeme. The recovery stroke muscle is similarly attached but extends more laterally to a separate apodeme for the coxo-trochanteral joint (Fig. 8; T. L. Daniel, M. Decher and C. E. Jordan, in preparation). Both the power and recovery muscles insert on either side of the joint about which appendage rotation occurs. As with the analysis above, we seek a solution to a set of physical and physiological relationships that describe the mechanics of muscle contraction, the hydrodynamics of thrust production and body motions, and the mechanics of passive tissues.

Balance of forces and moments

The thrust generated during power strokes is given by the integral, along the length of the hindlimb, of the sectional drag and added-mass forces (equation 4). For the purposes of this analysis, thrust is dominated by reactions to the fluid motion normal to the surface of the appendage. Moreover, the integral is approximated as a discrete sum (a more detailed analysis is given by T. L. Daniel, M. Decher and C. E. Jordan, in preparation). This instantaneous thrust, in turn, is balanced by the instantaneous drag, added-mass and inertial forces that resist motion of the body. Accordingly, one equation we must solve is precisely this force balance, which in words and symbols is:

$$\text{Thrust} = \text{Drag Force} + \text{Added Mass} + \text{Inertial Force}\,, \tag{13a}$$

$$2\Sigma F_{\mathrm{n}}\sin\theta = 0.5\rho S C_{\mathrm{Db}} U_{\mathrm{b}}\,|U_{\mathrm{b}}| + \alpha\rho V_{\mathrm{b}}\mathrm{d}U_{\mathrm{b}}/\mathrm{d}t + m\mathrm{d}U_{\mathrm{b}}/\mathrm{d}t\,, \tag{13b}$$

where F_{n} is the sectional force resulting from the hydrodynamic reaction normal to the surface of the appendage and all other symbols are defined in equations 4 and 5. The sectional force is a function of the angular velocity of the appendage, $\omega = \mathrm{d}\theta/\mathrm{d}t$, and the velocity of the body U_{b}:

$$F_{\mathrm{n}} = 0.5\rho C_{\mathrm{Dn}} h u_{\mathrm{n}} |u_{\mathrm{n}}| \mathrm{d}l + \alpha_{\mathrm{l}}\rho A_{\mathrm{l}} \mathrm{d}l \mathrm{d}u_{\mathrm{n}}/\mathrm{d}t\ , \tag{14a}$$

$$u_{\mathrm{n}} = \mathbf{u_r}\cdot\{\cos\theta,\ \sin\theta\}\,, \tag{14b}$$

$$\mathbf{u_r} = \{l\mathrm{d}\theta/\mathrm{d}t\cos\theta,\ l\mathrm{d}\theta/\mathrm{d}t\sin\theta - U_{\mathrm{b}}\}\,, \tag{14c}$$

where C_{Dn} and α_{l} are the sectional drag and added-mass coefficients for the limb, h is the thickness of the limb, A_{l} is the cross-sectional area of the limb, l is the position along the limb and u_{n} is the component of flow normal to the limb.

Power stroke muscles also generate a moment about the pivot point which is balanced, instantaneously, with the moment generated by the hydrodynamic reaction to appendage motions, the moment associated with the inertia of the limb and the moment required to deform the antagonistic muscles:

$$F_{\mathrm{m}} l_{\mathrm{m}} = \Sigma(l F_{\mathrm{n}} + l A_{\mathrm{l}} \mathrm{d}l \mathrm{d}u_{\mathrm{n}}/\mathrm{d}t) + F_{\mathrm{passive}} l_{\mathrm{p}}\,, \tag{15}$$

where F_{m} is the instantaneous force generated by power stroke muscles, l_{m} is the moment arm over which that force acts, F_{passive} is the force required to extend the recovery muscles when they are relaxed and l_{p} is the moment arm over which the recovery muscles act. The quantity within the sum represents the moment required to overcome the hydrodynamic reaction to appendage motion and the appendage inertia. Just as we established with the jellyfish problem, the active force generated by the swimming muscles (F_{m}) is some function of the shortening velocity, length and activation characteristics of the power stroke muscles and follows a paradigm similar to the one established for that problem. As with the case study for jellyfish, we are armed with a system of differential equations that describe the instantaneous position of the limb, the thrust force, muscle force and body velocity.

Where are the data?

Body dimensions, the relevant drag and added-mass coefficients, and the geometry of the muscles and their attachments are summarized in Table 2 for *Notonecta undulata* (T. L. Daniel, M. Decher and C. E. Jordan, in preparation). While details of the appropriate physiological metrics of muscle contractility are not known for this species, there is a good deal of information about insect skeletal muscle that can be used for reasonable estimates of V_{max}, σ_{o} and the temporal characteristics of activation.

It appears that the force required to extend relaxed antagonistic muscles is the dominant

Table 2. *Values used in the analysis of notonectid swimming*

Parameter	Value
Morphological parameters	
Body length	6 mm
Body width	4 mm
Appendage length	12 mm
Setal span	2 mm
Power stroke starting angle	1.0 rad
Physiological parameters	
Isometric stress	0.1 MPa
Maximum shortening velocity	$1.0\,l\,s^{-1}$
Activation time	25 ms
Mechanical parameters for passive muscle	
Stiffness	0.1 MPa
Damping constant	$1.0\,N\,s\,m^{-1}$
Hydrodynamic parameters	
Body drag coefficient	0.4
Body added-mass coefficient	0.5
Appendage sectional drag coefficient	1.0
Appendage sectional added-mass coefficient	1.0

These values are mostly derived from Daniel *et al.* (1994).
l, starting muscle length.

passive force faced by swimming muscles. In the analysis used here, we model this as a non-linear viscoelastic solid whose length-dependent spring constants and damping coefficient were determined from dynamic mechanical data for passive muscles from other arthropods (Meyhofer and Daniel, 1990; Meyhofer, 1993).

In addition to setting values for the various parameters that underlie the analysis above, high-speed cine films of freely swimming notonectids provide data against which any theoretical predictions may be tested (Fig. 9). These provide instantaneous measures of body position and appendage angle which, if the choice of parameters is reasonable, should match predicted values for these data. The basic patterns seen from such kinematics is that the body moves about 3 cm in 0.2 s with an average velocity of $15\,cm\,s^{-1}$. The appendages swing through an arc of about 2 rad in just under 0.1 s and return to their starting position in about 0.15 s. The theoretical predictions for these motions (solid lines in Fig. 9) agree quite nicely, suggesting that our estimates of all of the various parameters are reasonable.

Derived predictions and dilemmas

While it is common to presume that motions of swimming appendages are roughly sinusoidal, both the measured and predicted values for the appendage angle show a pattern that is dramatically different. Here, we see that the hindlimb rapidly reaches a constant angular velocity; the slope of the angle–time curve is constant during most of the power stroke. The mechanism that gives rise to this pattern follows from the

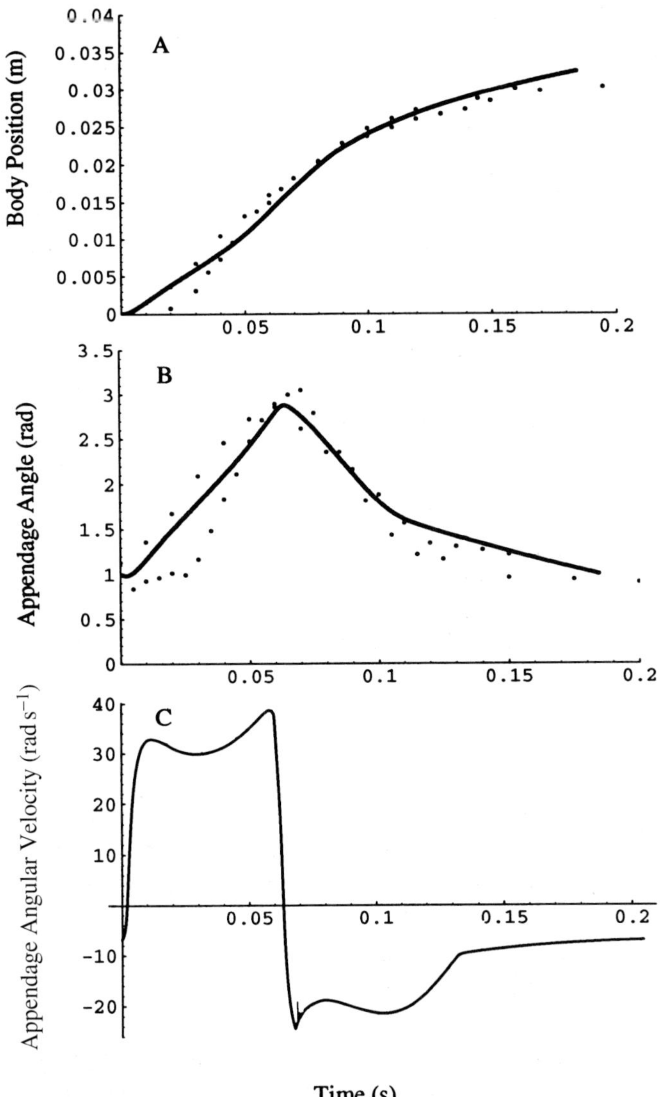

Fig. 9. Instantaneous plots of the body position (A) and appendage angle (B) are shown for both measured (points) and predicted (lines) for *Notonecta undulata*. The angular velocity of the appendage (C) shows very rapid transients, implying that large angular accelerations are present.

force–velocity behavior for contracting muscle. Since the muscle power (the product of force and velocity) has a maximum at one particular shortening velocity, there will be a rapid transient to that maximal power output. Any increase in appendage angular velocity (and thus shortening velocity) beyond the maximal power cannot be accomplished as the hydrodynamic power will only rise.

The rapid transients in angular velocity imply large accelerations at the onset and end

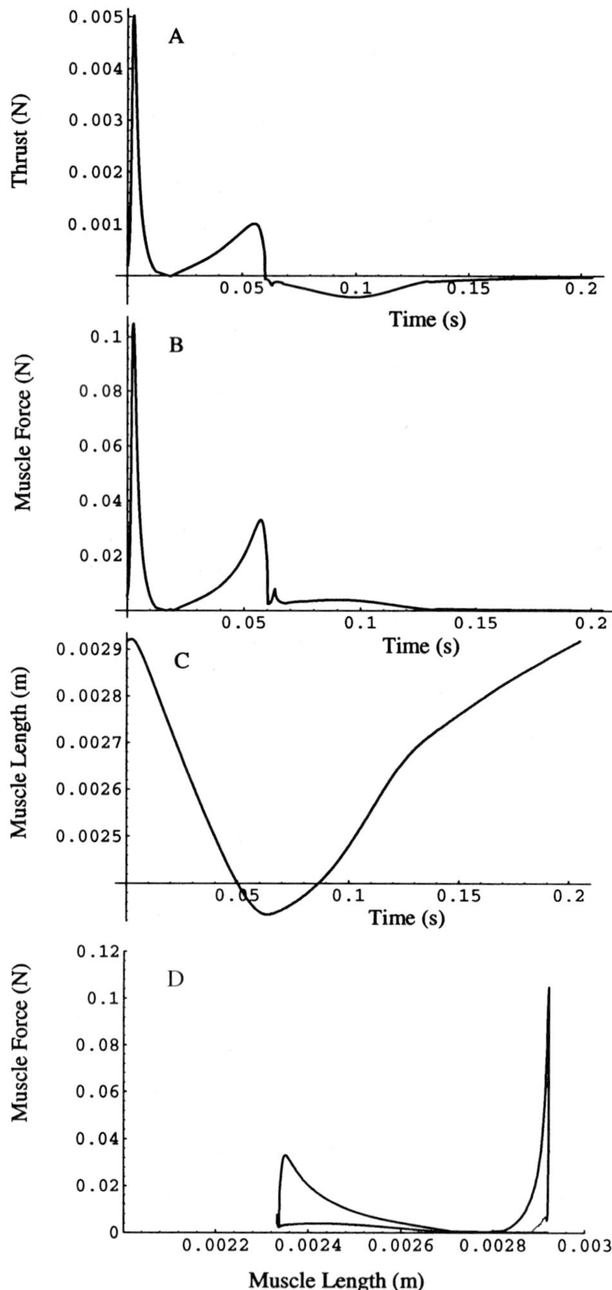

Fig. 10. Predicted instantaneous thrust (A) and muscle force (B) show rapid transients that correspond to the large angular accelerations of the hindlimb. Muscle length (C) and muscle force, when plotted against each other, show a predicted work loop (D) that is quite different from those that have been measured for other swimming animals.

of a power stroke. Such accelerations are likely to be manifest as large hydrodynamic forces. Indeed, the predictions for the instantaneous thrust (Fig. 10) show large peaks at the onset and end of the power stroke, which correspond to changes in body velocity. Since the accelerations of the appendage are quite large, the hydrodynamic reactions to appendage motion will give rise to such peaks. Moreover, during these brief transients, the swimming muscles have not yet achieved the shortening velocity associated with maximal power output. Rather, they are operating at lower speeds. Accordingly, the force–velocity relationship suggests that these muscles are capable of producing instantaneously high forces.

Such rapid transients in propulsor velocity yield a particularly vexing dilemma in any analysis that would require measurements of the appropriate kinematics. These transients, which are quite difficult to measure experimentally, are extremely important determinants of thrust and power output. For example, predictions show that the angular velocity rises from about 0 to 30 rad s^{-1} in about 0.01 s. To capture this acceleration reliably on film would require a frame rate of about 500 frames s^{-1} to get just five points. Thus, studies that analyse hydrodynamic forces from prescribed propulsor motions may miss essential features if the data are smoothed or gathered with insufficient temporal resolution. The same problem would be seen for those studies that use measurements of *in vivo* muscle strain in establishing *in vitro* work loops for locomotor muscles. One example of a predicted work loop (Fig. 10D) shows a pattern quite different from those that have been measured or suggested by previous investigators. This difference arises from the rapid velocity transients and resultant force peaks that are predicted for motions driven by activated muscles.

Scaling arguments

Rather than explore the wide range of parameters that underlie the analysis above, I focus here on variation in just the size of the hindlimb, leaving all other aspects of the internal anatomy, mechanics and physiology unchanged. As with the case study of jellyfish swimming, analyses that hold the kinematics of propulsor motion constant lead to a prediction that creatures with larger 'oars' would swim faster. But, as was suggested above, larger oars require greater muscle power to move them with the same speeds and accelerations. In reality, as the oar gets ever larger, the constraint imposed by the physiology of contracting muscle leads to ever diminishing speeds of oar motion.

By constraining the angles through which bug hindlimbs sweep, we note that there is a fundamental difference between predictions about swimming speed based on assumed kinematics and those based on the muscle physiology (Fig. 11). There is a peak in swimming performance for a hindlimb length of about 1.0 cm – a value quite close to that observed for notonectids. Limbs much shorter than this length may move rapidly but, by virtue of their reduced size, generate little thrust. For longer limbs, reductions in their speeds and accelerations, despite increases in their size, lead to lower average thrust forces.

Directions

The analyses above point out several intriguing issues. First, the condition that

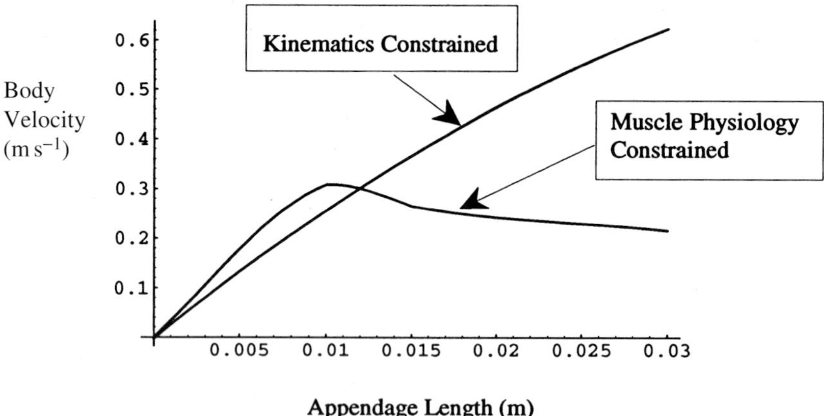

Fig. 11. The consequence of size variation is shown for both classic and new approaches. The former presumes constant appendage kinematics. The latter presumes that the physiology of the muscles remain unchanged.

locomotor motions must be both physically and physiologically feasible gives rise to scaling arguments that are quite different from those based on purely hydrodynamic grounds. Here, we see optimal sizes and shapes for either speed or efficiency. Moreover, the determinants of these optima depend upon a suite of biological and physical parameters that include not only those associated with muscle contractility but also soft tissue mechanical behavior.

A second issue that emerges from these analyses is that predicted motions show transients that are much more rapid than we would anticipate or measure experimentally. In some cases (notonectids) these transients give rise to large peaks in instantaneous thrust forces and in the work loops. The mechanism that facilitates such transients follows from two issues: (1) muscle force may be high when shortening velocity is low (the onset of a transient), and (2) the differential equations predict that shortening velocity will rapidly increase to the value at which power output is maximal. These conditions, combined with activation times of the order of 10–20 ms, yield sharp spikes in thrust and muscle force. It seems that such transients will be important determinants of swimming performance and that motions of animals should be measured with high temporal resolution to assess whether such transients arise.

There are, however, a number of crucial ingredients that are missing from the approach outlined above. In particular, the analyses only implicitly include sensory feedback in modulating the motions of swimming animals. For example, in the simulations of swimming notonectids, the power stroke muscles are turned off at a specific appendage angle. This condition mimics a sensory mechanism that would provide feedback to some central pattern generator that governs swimming motions. In the absence of any details about sensory mechanisms in these animals, however, we cannot draw any firm conclusions about the role of feedback in regulating locomotion. It would be exciting to include sensory feedback in future models of this sort.

This work was supported, in part, by a grant from the National Science Foundation. I thank C. Jordan, E. Stockwell and A. Trimble for many useful comments on the work.

References

ALEXANDER, D. E. (1988). Kinematics of swimming in two species of *Idotea* (Isopod: Valvifera). *J. exp. Biol.* **138**, 37–49.

ALEXANDER, R. McN. (1969). Orientation of muscle fibres in the myomeres of fish. *J. mar. biol. Ass. U.K.* **49**, 263–290.

ALEXANDER, R. McN. (1983). *Animal Mechanics*. 2nd edn. London: Blackwell.

ALEXANDER, R. McN. (1988). *Elastic Mechanisms in Animal Movement*. Cambridge: Cambridge University Press.

ALEXANDER, R. AND BENNET-CLARK, H. C. (1977). Storage of elastic strain energy in muscle and other tissues. *Nature* **265**, 114–117.

ALMERS, W. (1989). Excitation–contraction coupling in skeletal muscle. In *Textbook of Physiology*, vol. 1 (ed. H. D. Patton, A. F. Fuchs, B. H. Hille, A. M. Scher and R. Steiner), pp. 156–170. W. B. Saunders.

ALTRINGHAM, J. D. AND JOHNSTON, I. A. (1990*a*). Modelling muscle power output in a swimming fish. *J. exp. Biol.* **148**, 395–402.

ALTRINGHAM, J. D. AND JOHNSTON, I. A. (1990*b*). Scaling effects on muscle function: power output of isolated fish muscle fibres performing oscillatory work. *J. exp. Biol.* **151**, 453–467.

BIEWENER, A. A., ALEXANDER, R. McN. AND HEGLUND, N. C. (1981). Elastic energy storage in the hopping of kangaroo rates (*Dipodomus spectabilis*). *J. Zool., Lond.* **195**, 369–383.

BLAKE, R. W. (1981). Influence of pectoral fin shape on thrust and drag in labriform locomotion. *J. Zool., Lond.* **194**, 53–66.

BOWTELL, G. AND WILLIAMS, T. L. (1991). Anguilliform body dynamics: modelling the interaction between muscle activation and body curvature. *Phil. Trans. R. Soc. Lond. B* **334**, 385–390.

CAVAGNA, G. A., HEGLUND, N. C. AND TAYLOR, C. R. (1977). Mechanical work in terrestrial locomotion: two basic mechanisms for minimizing energy expenditure. *Am. J. Physiol.* **233**, 398–410.

CHEER, A. Y. AND KOEHL, M. A. R. (1988). Paddles and rakes: fluid flow through bristled appendages of small organisms. *J. theor. Biol.* **129**, 17–39.

DANIEL, T. L. (1983). Mechanics and energetics of medusan jet propulsion. *Can. J. Zool.* **61**, 1406–1420.

DANIEL, T. L. (1984). Unsteady aspects of aquatic locomotion. *Am. Zool.* **24**, 121–134.

DANIEL, T. L. (1985). Cost of locomotion: unsteady medusan swimming. *J. exp. Biol.* **119**, 149–164.

DANIEL, T. L., JORDAN, C. AND GRUNBAUM, D. (1992). Hydromechanics of swimming. In *Advances in Comparative and Environmental Physiology*, vol. 11, *Mechanics of Animal Locomotion* (ed. R. McN. Alexander), pp. 17–49. Springer-Verlag.

DANIEL, T. L. AND MEYHOFER, E. (1989). Size limits in escape locomotion of carridean shrimp. *J. exp. Biol.* **143**, 245–265.

DEMONT, M. E. (1990). Tuned oscillations in the swimming scallop *Pecten maximus*. *Can. J. Zool.* **68**, 786–791.

DEMONT, M. E. (1992). Locomotion of soft bodied animals. In *Advances in Comparative and Environmental Physiology*, vol. 11, *Mechanics of Animal Locomotion* (ed. R. McN. Alexander), pp. 167–190. Springer-Verlag.

DEMONT, M. E. AND GOSLINE, J. M. (1988*a*). Mechanics of jet propulsion in the hydromedusan jellyfish, *Polyorchis penicillatus*. I. Mechanical properties of the locomotor structure. *J. exp. Biol.* **134**, 313–332.

DEMONT, M. E. AND GOSLINE, J. M. (1988*b*). Mechanics of jet propulsion in the hydromedusan jellyfish, *Polyorchis penicillatus*. II. Energetics of the jet cycle. *J. exp. Biol.* **134**, 333–345.

DEMONT, M. E. AND GOSLINE, J. M. (1988*c*). Mechanics of jet propulsion in the hydromedusan jellyfish, *Polyorchis penicillatus*. III. A natural resonating bell and the importance of a resonant phenomenon in the locomotor structure. *J. exp. Biol.* **134**, 347–361.

ELLINGTON, C. P. (1984). The aerodynamics of hovering insect flight. IV. Aerodynamic mechanisms. *Phil. Trans. R. Soc. Lond. B* **305**, 79–113.

FAUCI, L. (1993). Computational modeling of the swimming of biflagellated algal cells. In *Contemporary Mathematics*, vol. 141, *Fluid Dynamics in Biology* (ed. A. Y. Cheer and C. P. van Dam), American Mathematical Society.

FAUCI, L. AND PESKIN, C. S. (1988). A computational model of aquatic animal locomotion. *J. comput. Phys.* **77**, 85–108.

FULL, R. J. (1993). Integration of individual leg dynamics with whole body movement in arthropod locomotion. In *Biological Neural Networks in Invertebrate Neuroethology and Robotics* (ed. R. Beer, R. Ritzmann and T. McKenna), pp. 3–20. New York: Academic Press.

FUNG, Y. C. (1990). *Biomechanics: Motion, Flow, Stress and Growth*. Springer-Verlag.

GAL, J. M. AND BLAKE, R. W. (1988*a*). Biomechanics of frog swimming. I. Estimation of the propulsive force generated by *Hymenochirus boettgeri*. *J. exp. Biol.* **138**, 399–411.

GAL, J. M. AND BLAKE, R. W. (1988*b*). Biomechanics of frog swimming. II. Mechanics of the limb-beat cycle in *Hymenochirus boettgeri*. *J. exp. Biol.* **138**, 413–429.

GLADFELTER, W. B. (1972). Structure and function of the locomotory system of *Polyorchis montereyensis* (Cnidaria, Hydrozoa). *Helgolander wiss. Meeresunters.* **23**, 38–79.

GORDON, A. M., HUXLEY, A. F. AND JULINAN, F. J. (1966). The variation in isometric tension with sarcomere length in vertebrate muscle fibres. *J. Phyiol., Lond.* **84**, 170–192.

GOSLINE, J. M. AND SHADWICK, R. E. (1983). The role of elastic energy storage mechanisms in swimming: an analysis of mantle elasticity in escape jetting in the squid, *Loligo opalescens*. *Can. J. Zool.* **61**, 1421–1431.

HILL, A. V. (1938). The heat of shortening and the dynamic constants of muscle. *Proc. R. Soc. Lond. B* **126**, 136–195.

JACKLYN, P. M. AND RITZ, D. A. (1986). Hydrodynamics of swimming in scyllarid lobsters. *J. exp. mar. Biol. Ecol.* **101**, 85–99.

JOHNSTON, I. A. (1991). Muscle action during locomotion: a comparative perspective. *J. exp. Biol.* **160**, 167–185.

JOHNSTON, I. A. AND ALTRINGHAM, J. D. (1991). Movement in water: constraints and adaptations. In *Biochemistry and Molecular Biology of Fishes*, vol 1 (ed. P. Hochachka and E. Mommsen), pp. 249–268. Amsterdam: Elsevier Science Publishers.

JORDAN, C. E. (1992). A model of rapid-start swimming at intermediate Reynolds number: undulatory locomotion in the chaetognath *Sagitta elegans*. *J. exp. Biol.* **163**, 119–137.

JOSEPHSON, R. K. (1985). Mechanical power output from striated muscle during cyclical contraction. *J. exp. Biol.* **114**, 493–512.

LIGHTHILL, M. J. (1971). Large-amplitude elongated-body theory of fish locomotion. *Proc. R. Soc. Lond.* **179**, 125–138.

LIGHTHILL, M. J. (1975). *Mathematical Biofluiddynamics*. Regional Conference Series in Applied Mathematics, vol. 17. Philadelphia: SIAM.

MARSH, R. L., OLSON, J. M. AND GUZIK, S. K. (1992). Mechanical performance of scallop adductor muscle during swimming. *Nature* **357**, 411–413.

MCMAHON, T. A. (1984).*Muscles, Reflexes, and Locomotion*. Princeton, NJ: Princeton University Press.

MEYHOFER, E. (1993). Dynamic mechanical properties of passive single cardiac fibers from the crab *Cancer magister*. *J. exp. Biol.* **185**, 207–249.

MEYHOFER, E. AND DANIEL, T. L. (1990). Dynamic mechanical properties of extensor muscle cells of the shrimp *Pandalus danae*: cell design for escape locomotion. *J. exp. Biol.* **151**, 435–452.

MORRIS, M. J., GUST, G. AND TORRES, J. J. (1985). Propulsion efficiency and cost of transport for copepods: hydromechanical model of crustacean swimming. *Mar. Biol.* **86**, 283–295.

NACHTIGALL, W. (1980). Mechanics of swimming in water beetles. In *Aspects of Animal Movement* (ed. H. Y. Elder and E. R. Trueman), pp. 107–124. Cambridge: Cambridge University Press.

NACHTIGALL, W. (1985). Swimming in aquatic insects. In *Comprehensive Insect Physiology, Biochemistry and Pharmacology. Nervous System: Structure and Motor Function* (ed. G. A. Kerkut and L. I. Gilbert), pp. 467–490. Pergamon Press.

O'DOR, R. K. AND WEBBER, D. M. (1986). The constraints on cephalopods: why squid aren't fish. *Can. J. Zool.* **64**, 1591–1605.

O'DOR, R. K. AND WELLS, M. J. (1990). Speed, jet pressure and oxygen consumption in free-swimming *Nautilus*. *J. exp. Biol.* **154**, 383–396.

PLOTNIK, R. E. (1985). Lift based mechanisms for swimming in eurypterids and portunid crabs. *Trans. R. Soc. Edinb.* **76**, 325–337.

PROSSER, C. L. (1991). Animal movement. In *Comparative Animal Physiology: Neural and Integrative Animal Physiology* (ed. C. L. Prosser), pp. 67–129. New York: Wiley-Liss.

RAYNER, J. M. V. (1979). A vortex theory of animal flight. II. The forward flight of birds. *J. Fluid Mech.* **91**, 731–763.

ROME, L. C., SWANK, D. AND CORDA, D. (1993). How fish power swimming. *Science* **261**, 340–343.

SATTERLIE, R. A., LABARBERA, M. AND SPENCER, A. N. (1985). Swimming in the pteropod mollusc *Clione limacina*. I. Behaviour and morphology. *J. exp. Biol.* **116**, 189–204.

SCHMIDT-NIELSEN, K. (1979). *Animal Physiology*. Cambridge: Cambridge University Press.

SLEIGH, M. A. AND BARLOW, D. A. (1980). Metachronism and control in animals with many propulsive structures. In *Aspects of Animal Movement* (ed. H. Y. Elder and E. R. Trueman), pp. 49–70. Cambridge: Cambridge University Press.

TAYLOR, G. I. (1951). Analysis of swimming microscopic organisms. *Proc. R. Soc. Lond. B* **209**, 447–461.

TIDBALL, J. G. AND DANIEL, T. L. (1986). Elastic energy storage in rigored skeletal muscle under physiological loading conditions. *Am. J. Physiol.* **250**, R56–R64.

VAN LEEUWEN, J. L. (1991). Optimum power output and structural design of sarcomeres. *J. theor. Biol.* **149**, 229–256.

VAN LEEUWEN, J. L. (1992). Muscle function in locomotion. In *Advances in Comparative and Environmental Physiology,* vol. 11, *Mechanics of Animal Locomotion* (ed. R. McN. Alexander), pp. 191–250. Springer-Verlag.

VAN LEEUWEN, J. L., LANKHEET, M. J. M., AKSTER, H. A. AND OSSE, J. W. M. (1990). Function of red axial muscles of carp (*Cyprinus carpio* L.): recruitments and normalized power output during swimming in different modes. *J. Zool., Lond.* **220**, 123–145.

VLYMEN, W. J. (1974). Swimming energetics of larval anchovy. *Fishery Bull. Fish Wildl. Serv. U.S.* **72**, 885–899.

WAINWRIGHT, S. A., BIGGS, W. D., CURREY, J. D. AND GOSLINE, J. M. (1982). *Mechanical Design in Organisms*. Princeton: Princeton University Press.

WEIS-FOGH, T. (1973). Quick estimates of flight fitness in hovering animals, including novel mechanisms for lift production. *J. exp. Biol.* **59**, 169–230.

WILKIE, D. R. (1966). Muscle. *A. Rev. Physiol.* **28**, 17–38.

WILSON, J. A. (1979). *Principles of Animal Physiology*. 2nd edn. New York: Macmillan Publishing .

WU, T. Y. (1971). Hydromechanics of swimming. I. Swimming of a two-dimensional waving plate at variable forward speeds in an inviscid fluid. *J. Fluid Mech.* **46**, 337–355.

PATHS AND PATTERNS: THE BIOLOGY AND PHYSICS OF SWIMMING BACTERIAL POPULATIONS

J. O. KESSLER[1], *R. P. STRITTMATTER*[1], *D. L. SWARTZ*[1], *D. A. WISELEY*[1] *and M. F. WOJCIECHOWSKI*[2]

[1]Department of Physics *and* [2]Department of Ecology and Evolutionary Biology, University of Arizona, Tucson, AZ 85721, USA

Summary

The velocity distribution of swimming micro-organisms depends on directional cues supplied by the environment. Directional swimming within a bounded space results in the accumulation of organisms near one or more surfaces. Gravity, gradients of chemical concentration and illumination affect the motile behaviour of individual swimmers. Concentrated populations of organisms scatter and absorb light or consume molecules, such as oxygen. When supply is one-sided, consumption creates gradients; the presence of the population alters the intensity and the symmetry of the environmental cues. Patterns of cues interact dynamically with patterns of the consumer population. In suspensions, spatial variations in the concentration of organisms are equivalent to variations of mean mass density of the fluid. When organisms accumulate in one region whilst moving away from another region, the force of gravity causes convection that translocates both organisms and dissolved substances. The geometry of the resulting concentration–convection patterns has features that are remarkably reproducible. Of interest for biology are (1) the long-range organisation achieved by organisms that do not communicate, and (2) that the entire system, consisting of fluid, cells, directional supply of consumables, boundaries and gravity, generates a dynamic that improves the organisms' habitat by enhancing transport and mixing. Velocity distributions of the bacterium *Bacillus subtilis* have been measured within the milieu of the spatially and temporally varying oxygen concentration which they themselves create. These distributions of swimming speed and direction are the fundamental ingredients required for a quantitative mathematical treatment of the patterns. The quantitative measurement of swimming behaviour also contributes to our understanding of aerotaxis of individual cells.

Introduction

Of all the world's living creatures, the most numerous are the smallest. Algal and bacterial cells are significant at all levels of the world's dynamics, from global climate to the gut of insects. This paper is concerned with the self-organization of great populations

Key words: aerotaxis, *Bacillus subtilis*, bacteria, chemotaxis, convection, diffusion, pattern, swimming, hydrodynamics, micro-organisms, respiration.

of micro-organisms and with their swimming paths that are both the cause of and the response to these patterns. The emphasis is on bacteria that consume oxygen. Behaviour and physics jointly cause convection–concentration patterns that mix the fluid, modify transport and improve viability.

The populations of micro-organisms described here live in aqueous suspension. Individual cells may orient their swimming velocity, on average, in a spatio-temporal field that is embedded in the fluid; illumination, chemical concentration, gravity or fluid flow are examples. Cell–cell signalling is not a significant correlating factor. In spite of this 'blindness' *vis-à-vis* each other, great populations of such cells organize themselves into regular, extended (>10^4 cell diameters) patterns of organism concentration and fluid convection (Fig. 1). The ingredients for bioconvection are (1) consumption, by the entire population, of a directionally supplied requirement of life; (2) the response of the individual cell's swimming to environmental gradients, either gravitational or the ones created by consumption; (3) fluid mechanics and conservation of momentum, molecules, photons, mass and organisms; and (4) the gravity force acting on density variations within a fluid.

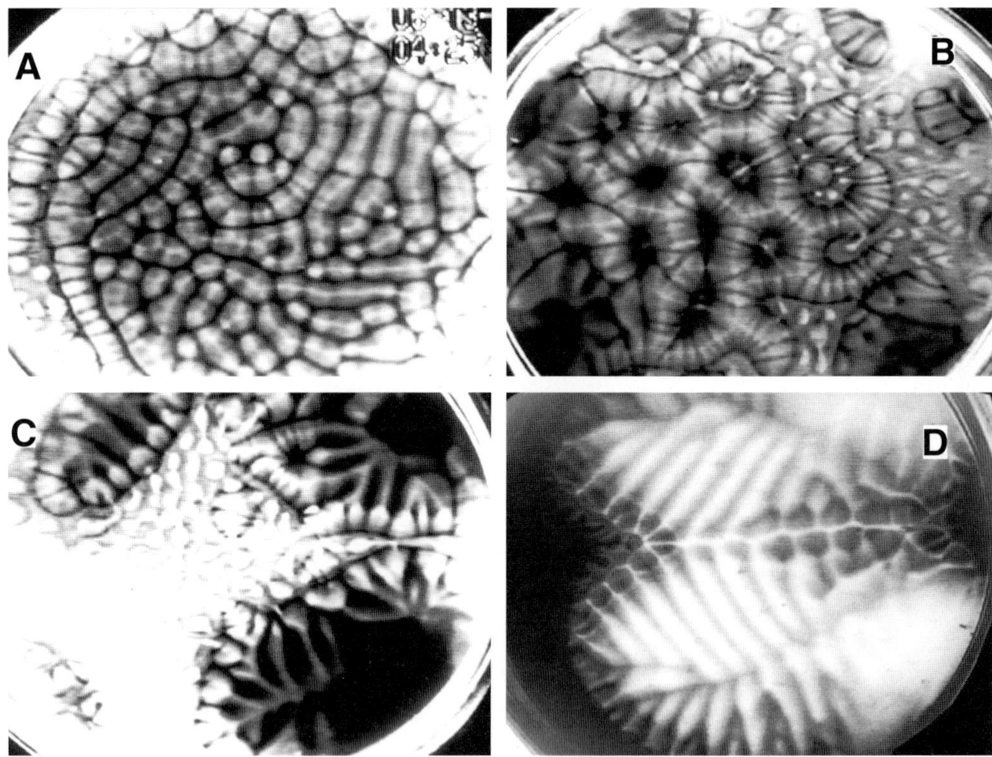

Fig. 1. Bacterial bioconvection in plan view. The photographs are part of a time-lapse video sequence. The depth of fluid was 3 mm, the diameter of the Petri dish was 5.5 cm. Dark-field illumination was provided by an annular high-frequency fluorescent light. The time interval between each of the images A–D is about 4 h. Contrast was reversed in the last image, to improve visibility of details.

The self concentration and convection patterns generated by algae that swim upwards because of their morphology are reasonably well understood and have been previously summarized (Pedley and Kessler, 1992*a*,*b*). Light and gravity jointly affect the swimming velocity distribution of algae, but the details that are required as ingredients of a theory of complex patterns are not yet well known. Some discussion of algal patterns that depend on gravity and self-shading of individual cells by the rest of the population can be found in Kessler and Hill (1994). Bacterial convection patterns, their function and their joint origin in behaviour and fluid mechanics are the chief subject of this paper.

A suspension of swimming aerobic *Bacillus subtilis*, which have multiplied under conditions of good nutrient supply and aeration, typically contains 10^7–10^9 organisms per cm^3; the spacing between them is $\geqslant 10^{-3}$ cm or about 10 cell diameters. The volume fraction of bacteria is then in the range 10^{-4} to 10^{-2}. The hydrodynamic properties of these suspensions, the average density and the viscosity, are virtually the same as those of water. The mass density of the individual cells is about 10% greater than that of water; they consume oxygen at a substantial rate.

Although the bacteria do not directly communicate with one another, they generate macroscopic dynamic patterns that function to transport both themselves and oxygen. The patterns constitute correlations among the concentration of cells, of oxygen and the velocity field of the fluid. Spatial variation of the organisms' concentration n is the most readily observed feature. The patterns' geometry is a function of the average concentration of the organisms and of the response of the distribution of their swimming velocity V to spatial and temporal variations of the oxygen concentration $c(\mathbf{x},t)$ and the fluid's velocity field $\mathbf{u}(\mathbf{x},t)$. The depth of fluid is another parameter that affects the geometry. Measurements of the statistical distributions that occur for various circumstances are reported in the section on experiments.

When the organisms consume dissolved oxygen within the bulk of the fluid, it is replenished by diffusion from the air interface. In this way, consumption and supply generate an oxygen concentration gradient within the fluid. The gradient, pointing towards higher concentrations, is initially directed towards the interface, usually upwards. After convection sets in, the gradient still points generally upwards. In the appropriate locations, it points towards the fluid that descends from the vicinity of the air interface since that fluid contains more dissolved oxygen than the bulk.

During the time when the oxygen concentration decreases, owing to consumption, the mean direction of the cells' velocity distribution points in the direction of the oxygen concentration gradient. As a result of this behaviour, and since the swimming cells cannot penetrate the air interface, they accumulate in its vicinity. The cell concentration diminishes in the portion of the bulk fluid that supports the oxygen gradient. The increase of cell concentration immediately below the air interface, the decrease of concentration to below average in a depletion layer just beneath, and the maintenance of the original average concentration beyond reach of the oxygen gradient complete the first phase of pattern generation (Fig. 2A).

Since the density of the bacteria is greater than that of water, an accumulation of cells in some region of fluid is equivalent to an increase of the mean mass density of that region of fluid, at least in the continuum approximation. Since the effect of gravity is to cause

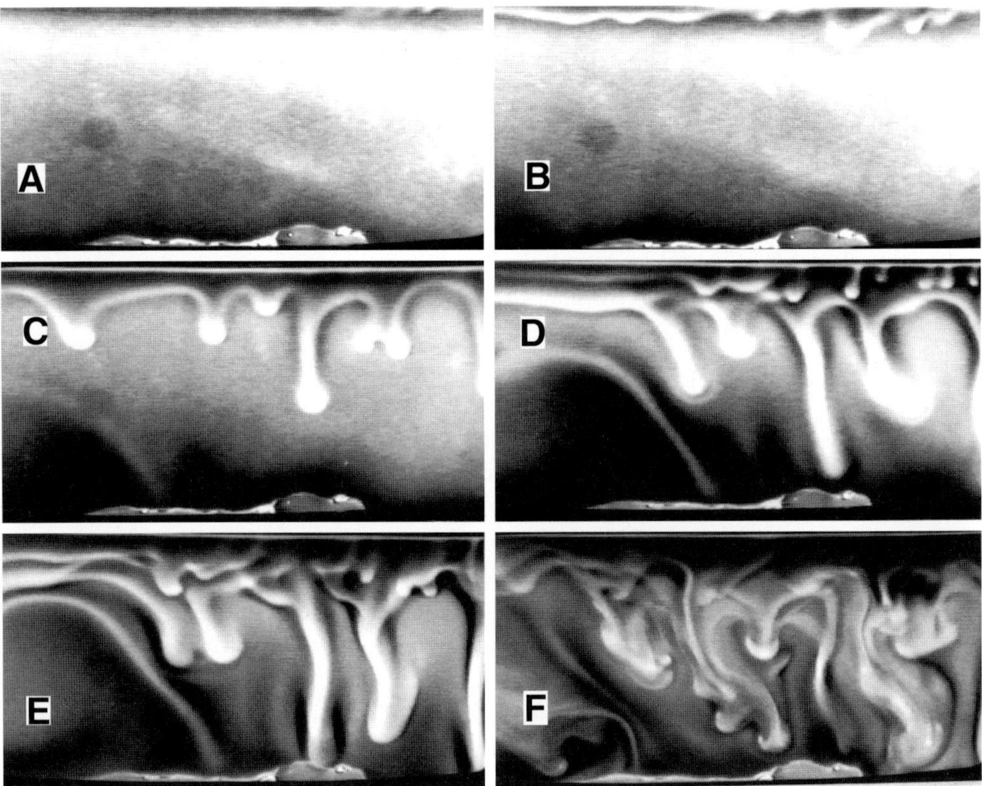

Fig. 2. The development of plumes, from upswimming, to the onset of the gravitational instability, to chaotic mixing. The times in the sequence were (A) t=0, (B) t=39 s, (C) t=103 s, (D) t=170 s, (E) t=213 s, (F) t=253 s. The illumination is dark field; when the image is bright, the cell concentration is high. In A, note the dark band near the top, next to the meniscus. Most of the bacteria have swum from there, upwards to the air interface. The height of fluid is 7 mm. The thickness is 1 mm; gravity is downwards. The dark region that develops near the bottom is due to cells swimming downwards towards the oxygen supplied by the grease seal of the cuvette.

regions that are denser than average to sink, and lighter ones to rise, the local accumulation and depletion of bacteria due to their directional swimming generates gravitational instability. Almost steady convection–concentration patterns are the eventual result. They may consist of plumes (Fig. 2), columns or rolls (Fig. 1), depending on the specifics of the bounding geometry and cell concentration. In any of these cases, the dynamic structural coherence of the patterns persists over distances very much greater than the dimensions of individual bacteria (Fig. 1).

The governing equations

Bioconvection can be mathematically modelled by continuum conservation equations that link the fluid mechanics, the cells' swimming behaviour and the distribution, consumption and supply of some quantity Q that elicits directional swimming. For algal populations, Q is illumination. For bacteria, Q could be a nutrient, an exudate from the cells or various attractants and repellents. The oxygen concentration c is the only Q-factor explicitly recognised in this paper.

Volume is approximately conserved when

$$\nabla \cdot \mathbf{u} = 0 \tag{1}$$

as usual. The expression becomes exact as $(V/u)vn \rightarrow 0$. The ratio of cell swimming speed to the magnitude of fluid velocity is (V/u), the volume fraction of cells is a single cell's volume v times the cell concentration n. The difference between a cell's mass density and the density of water is $\Delta\rho$; the mean density is $\bar{\rho}$.

The fluid momentum conservation is given by:

$$\bar{\rho}\frac{\partial \mathbf{u}}{\partial t} + \mathbf{u} \cdot \nabla \mathbf{u} = \mu \nabla^2 \mathbf{u} - \nabla p + gnv\Delta\rho, \tag{2}$$

the driving body force being supplied by the last term, which is the force of gravity acting on the buoyancy-corrected mass of the swimming cells. The pressure is p and the viscosity is μ.

The conservation, consumption and transport of the oxygen concentration c (molecules cm^{-3}) is given by:

$$\frac{\partial c}{\partial t} = D\nabla^2 c - \nabla \cdot (\mathbf{u}c) - \gamma n. \tag{3}$$

The bacterial consumption of oxygen is γ (molecules $\text{cell}^{-1}\,\text{s}^{-1}$), the diffusion coefficient is D ($\text{cm}^2\,\text{s}^{-1}$). If only the vertical direction is of interest, $\nabla \rightarrow \partial/\partial z$. The fluid, velocity $\mathbf{u}$, transports oxygen; hence, the flux term is $\mathbf{u}c$ (molecules $\text{cm}^{-2}\,\text{s}^{-1}$). The quantity γ may be a function of c and of the time t. The diffusion coefficient can be a function of cell activity and collisions, i.e. of $\mathbf{V}$ and n. The conservation equation for cells is:

$$\frac{\partial n}{\partial t} = -\nabla \cdot [(\mathbf{u} + \mathbf{V})n)]. \tag{4}$$

The swimming velocity $\mathbf{V}(c)$ is a function of c, its derivatives, and possibly a function of the history of c in the cells' reference frame. Both deterministic and stochastic motile behaviours are included in $\mathbf{V}(c)$. When $c<c$(threshold), $\mathbf{V}(c)=0$.

Equation 4 requires a probability density $f(\mathbf{V})$ for the distribution of $\mathbf{V}$. A Fokker–Planck equation may be used (Pedley and Kessler, 1990) to supply f, given suitable experimentally or theoretically derived ingredients. Equation 4 may also be written so that cell swimming is separated into deterministic and stochastic parts (Kessler, 1985, 1986), the latter modelled by a diffusion coefficient D_c for cell swimming. Then:

$$\frac{\partial n}{\partial t} = -\nabla \cdot [(\mathbf{u} + \mathbf{V})n - D_c \nabla n]. \tag{5}$$

In the laboratory reference frame, the distribution of $\mathbf{V}$ depends on $\mathbf{u}$ and its derivatives. For algae, the cells' orientation in the dark is co-determined by gravity, vorticity and rate of strain and by the swimming response to those environmental influences. It is unlikely that bacterial cells are individually oriented by gravitationally supplied torque (Kessler, 1992), but rotational motions of the fluid do affect the orientation of the distribution of $\mathbf{V}$.

The diffusion flux $D_c \nabla n$ that appears in equation 5 is in standard form. A very useful and important discussion of other forms appears in Schnitzer *et al.* (1990). They do not consider collisional effects. When the cell concentration becomes large enough, cell collisions can become an important factor in changing the orientations of trajectories. The diffusion coefficient due solely to collisions, D_b, has the form $A[f(\mathbf{V})]V\lambda$, where A is a number that depends on the local general motion $f(\mathbf{V})$ and λ is a mean free path, proportional to $(nR^2)^{-1}$, where R is an effective collision radius. When cells pass each other at a distance less than $2R$ apart, they disorient each other's trajectories.

The diameters of bacterial bodies are approximately 10^{-4} cm but flagella are much longer, e.g. 5×10^{-4} to 10×10^{-4} cm. When bacteria tumble, they are 'larger' than when they swim smoothly. During smooth swimming, their flagella neatly stream behind in a rotating bundle. Furthermore, when most of the cells swim in the same direction, there will be few collisions but a good possibility of vortical interactions. These are the reasons for the dependence of A on $f(\mathbf{V})$. Under conditions when the cell concentration is high, $D=D_cD_b(D_c+D_b)^{-1}$ is the combined diffusion coefficient (Kessler, 1986).

The plumes of bacteria that develop due to upswimming are reminiscent of those situations in thermal convection where there is a distributed heat source within the fluid. For bioconvection, there is of course no heat source; rather, the density inversion is caused by upswimming of the organism population. Straughan (1993) provides instructive insights into externally energized but otherwise somewhat similar sorts of convection. Bioconvection deviates from the standard variety once the convective nonlinear regime is under way: (1) the fluid's boundaries neither maintain nor extract a density-upsetting flux, and (2) after convective plumes have begun to descend, the (denser than water) organisms swim transversely to gravity, into the plumes, thus reinforcing and sharpening the convection. For algae, the transverse swimming is usually due to gyrotaxis (Kessler, 1985; Pedley and Kessler, 1992*a*,*b*). For bacteria, the attractive gradient due to surface oxygen entrained in the descending plumes causes transverse, i.e. horizontal, oxygen taxis.

The conservation of cell numbers and of energy require some sort of intermittency in bioconvection processes. The potential energy that is viscously dissipated by plumes and mixing processes is generated by upward swimming. Under time-independent conditions, cell conservation requires that the net upward flux of swimmers vanishes. Hence, there would be no generation of potential energy and thus no convection. However, when upswimming and pattern formation are intermittent, there is no problem. Intermittent flushing and accumulation of water in a toilet tank are a suitable analogy. The bacterial patterns discussed here and the bottom-standing plumes that are characteristic of gyrotaxis both exhibit intermittency.

Materials and methods

We have studied swimming behavior in *Bacillus subtilis*, a gram-positive, endospore-forming, aerobic eubacterium commonly found in soils. The strain used in this work is YB886 (*trpC2*, *metB5*, *amyE*, *sigB*, *xin–1*, SPβ−), a derivative of the naturally transformable *B. subtilis* strain 168 (Yasbin *et al.* 1980). Liquid cultures of *B. subtilis* YB886 were grown in GM1/GM2, Spizizen's minimal glucose salts medium (Spizizen, 1958) supplemented with 0.1 % yeast extract, 0.02 % casein hydrolysate, 5 mmol l^{-1} $MgCl_2$, 0.5 mmol l^{-1} $CaCl_2$ (GM2) and the appropriate amino acids at a final concentration of 50 μg ml^{-1}. Cultures were grown in GM1 at 37 °C with vigorous shaking

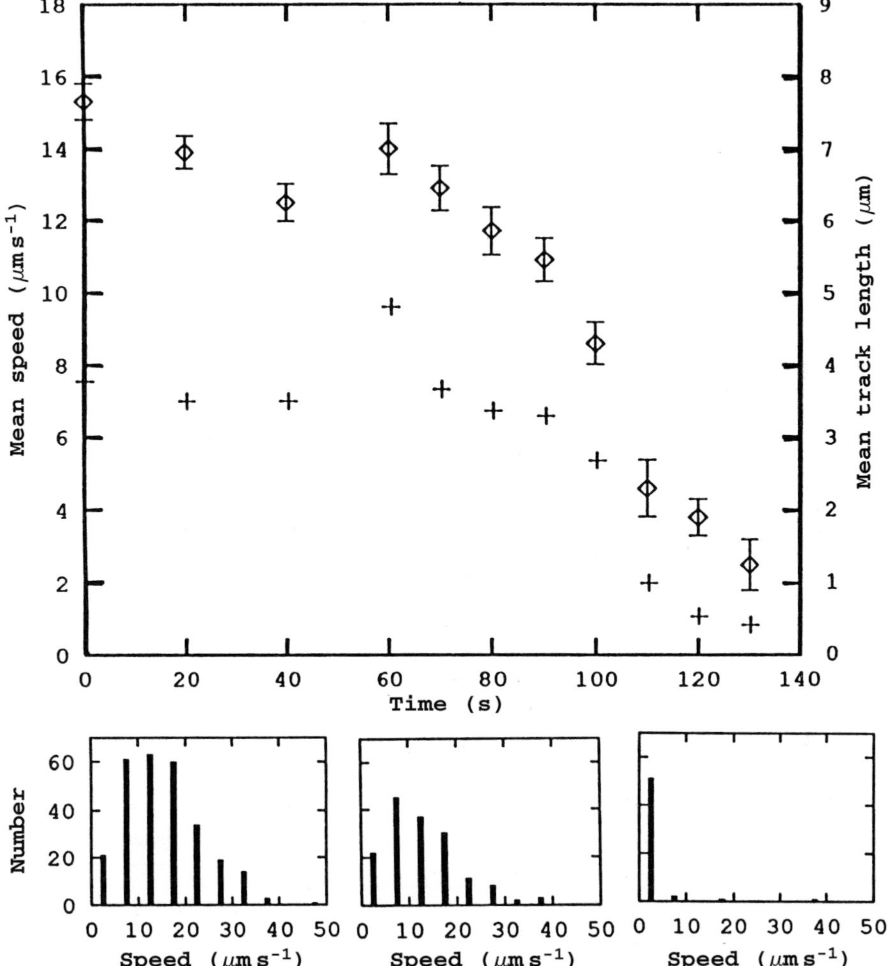

Fig. 3. Choking, the collapse of cell motility as consumption decreases the oxygen concentration. These data were acquired at a location 2985 μm from the air–fluid interface, beyond the range of diffusion of significant amounts of oxygen during the time available. No directionality was observed in the cell trajectories. The diamonds indicate speed; error bars are standard errors of the mean. The crosses are the mean lengths of the observed trajectories. Each point is the mean of a distribution. Histograms for the distribution of swimming speeds are presented below. The first corresponds to t=0, the second to t=70 s and the third to t=130 s. Although the distributions shift to low values of speed as the oxygen runs out, a few fast cells seem to remain.

V+/V-
A
n+/n-
B
d+/d-
C
mean angle (degrees)
D
Rayleigh stat
E
number
F
Time (s)

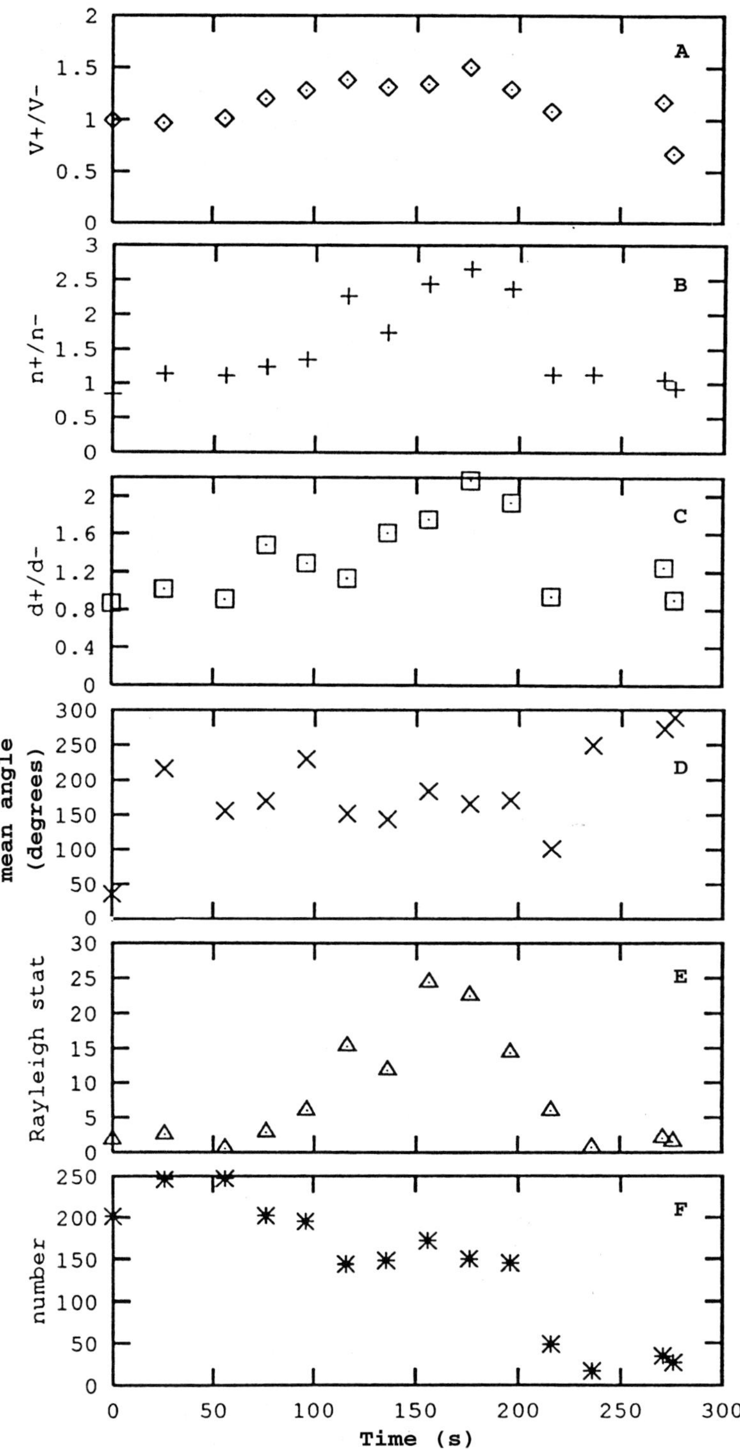

Fig. 4

(250 revs min^{-1}) in a water bath until 90 min following the end of exponential growth (designated as T_0), with growth monitored by measuring turbidity using a Klett–Summerson colorimeter (no. 66 filter). At T_0+90 min the cells were then diluted tenfold into warm GM2 medium and incubated at 37 °C with aeration for a minimum of 60 min before measurements of swimming activity were begun. Cell densities at this time are typically 8×10^7 to 1×10^8 cm^{-3}.

All experiments described here were performed at 20±1 °C. During experimental runs, cultures were maintained at that temperature on a shaker. The cell concentration increased during these experiments, within the range 10^8–10^9 cells ml^{-1}. The 'steady-state' experiments often lasted several days. No nutrients were added during that time. Patterns were observed in plan view using bacterial cultures placed in a covered plastic Petri dish. A water bath below the Petri dish absorbed heat from the illumination. As a control for thermal convection, we showed that dead cells did not produce patterns. Slight thermal gradients could have had a minor effect on pattern symmetry.

To observe plumes, standing cuvettes were made from microscope slides and 1 mm spacers, using Vaseline or stopcock grease as sealants. Patterns and plumes were illuminated with skew light beams, i.e. the dark-field system was used.

For measurements of cell velocities, the bacterial culture was filled half-way into a 'flat microslide' (Vitro Dynamics). The air–fluid meniscus served as a source of oxygen. The ends of the microslide were sealed with silicone vacuum grease (Dow Corning). This preparation was then placed flat on a standard microscope stage. The cell trajectories were recorded on a video recorder for later measurement. The lumen of the microslide was 100 μm. Cell tracks were recorded near the top of the lumen. Thermal convection was absent judged by the fact that small inert particles did not move. The statistical analysis of the cell trajectories was carried out by a computer system and software supplied by the Motion Analysis Corporation, modified and augmented by ourselves.

The data acquired and presented here are two-dimensional projections of three-dimensional activity. The angular and speed distributions have not been modified to remove the projection effect. Further experiments will be required to un-project the

---

Fig. 4. Six measures of motional asymmetry, as a function of the time during which consumption causes an oxygen gradient. The air–fluid interface is located at 180 °, 1300 μm to the left of the location where these data were obtained. The times on the abscissa start at the beginning of measurements; see legend to Fig. 6. (A) Ratio of speeds of cells swimming up-gradient (V+) to speeds down-gradient ($V-$). The plotted points correspond to the sequence in Fig. 5A. (B) Ratio of numbers of cells swimming up/down-gradient. Three corresponding angular distributions of velocity are shown in Fig. 11. (C) Ratio of mean observed track lengths. The track length d is related, in a rather complex way, to the length of a cell's trajectory; it is the projection of the portion of the trajectory within the depth of field onto the plane of observation. (D) The mean direction of cell trajectories. Cells seem to be heading mostly towards 180 °, up-gradient, at all times. However, the statistical confidence for t<100 s and t>200 s is very low; see E and Fig. 11. (E) The Rayleigh Statistic, $\mathbf{r}^2 n$, a measure of the statistical sharpness of directionality. This measure implies that the mean angle (see D) is most meaningful for 100 s<t<200 s. (F) The total sample, i.e. the number of cell trajectories on which the data are based. The decrease is due to the tactic swimming up-gradient, demonstrated by the data in A–E.

distributions. In some of the cases, we present data on left/right, i.e. +/−, asymmetries. These data are not affected by the projection.

Results

Convection patterns

Fig. 1 shows the development of convection patterns, observed in plan view. The duration of the sequence is several hours. Although thermal perturbations cannot be ruled out, the time development and general symmetry are reproducible. Cell division occurs during the course of pattern development. It appears that regions that contain relatively few cells often 'compress' regions with more cells. The mean intensity of scattered light and the pattern morphology are evidence for that inference. A considerable amount of motion occurs, in the form of travelling 'black' bands (few cells), as well as general changes of shape. The narrow black bands are characteristic of bacterial bioconvection. We believe that they are related to horizontal oxygen taxis.

Fig. 2 shows the depletion of cells near the air interface, due to upswimming (inside view). That initial phase is followed by the descent of a single array of bacteria-heavy plumes. The plume array eventually generates a complex mixing flow system. In shallower layers, the mixing flows are in the form of standing waves. Mixing has been traced using dissolved dyes.

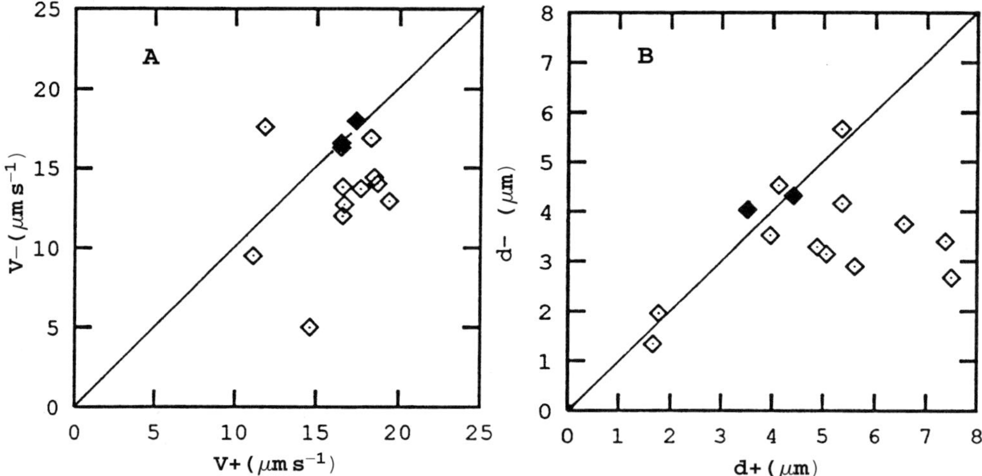

Fig. 5. Asymmetric response to the time-varying gradient of oxygen concentration. Experimental measurements, at a fixed location, of (A) the average magnitudes of speeds V and (B) track length d, up the gradient of oxygen concentration (+) and down the gradient (−). The interface between air and fluid is located 1300 μm to the left, i.e. at 180°. $V(+)$ is the average speed of all cell tracks whose direction of travel θ lies in the interval 90° to 270°; $V(-)$ is the average speed of tracks within $-90° < \theta < 90°$. The two filled points are 'early' in the development of the oxygen gradient; they correspond to the first two points, where t<50 s, on Figs 4 and 6. These diagrams indicate that there is a strong bias, both in track length and in swimming direction, for travel up the oxygen gradient. This bias complements the directional bias in the mean direction of travel θ, plotted in Fig. 4D.

Oxygen taxis and choking

The basis of the pattern formation found in these experiments is the bacterial response to the spatio-temporally varying oxygen concentration created by consumption and supply. Measurements of behaviour that are reported here were made in the actual setting of cell concentration for which the pattern formation occurs. These measurements are some of the ingredients required for a quantitative theory based on equations 1–5.

Consumption and supply create a time-varying dissolved oxygen concentration $c(\mathbf{x},t)$. Bacteria that are an appropriate distance from the interface experience the gradient of c and swim in that direction. When the cells are so far from the interface that they deplete the local dissolved oxygen before the diffusion front arrives, they lose motility. Fig. 3 shows the mean speed, the speed distribution and the mean track length for that case.

The correlation of c with consumption, supply and diffusion are discussed by Kessler *et al.* (1994). Direct measurements of c are in the planning stage. Figs 4–7 show various ways of quantifying oxygen taxis. The length of directional smooth runs, the directional speed and the orientation of tracks all cause accumulation up the gradient. The asymmetry of directional cell trajectories $n(+)/n(-)$ is a projection-independent measure.

Each of the plots in Fig. 4 emphasizes one distinct aspect of the bacterial cell population's behaviour. The time axis is common to all. The time axis is correlated with

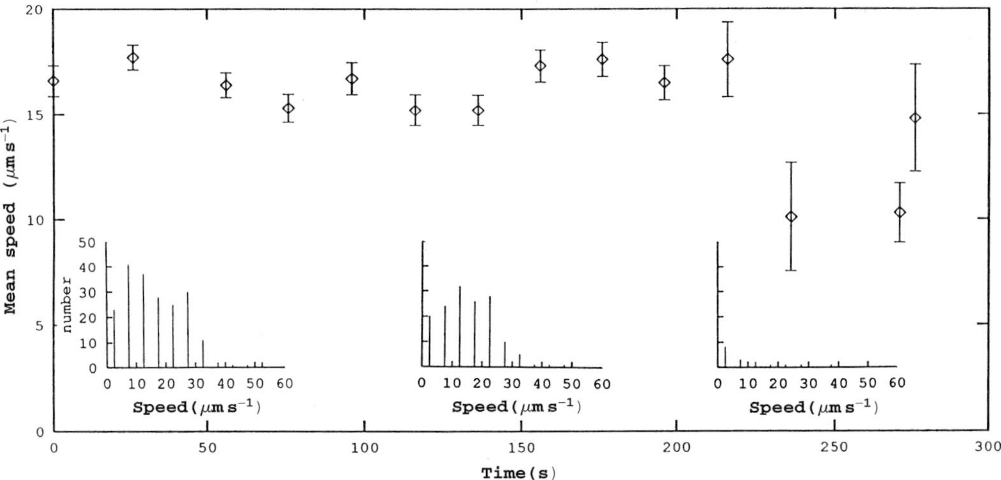

Fig. 6. Swimming speed, averaged over all directions of travel, as a function of the time during which the oxygen concentration decreases and the gradient develops. These data are taken at a fixed location 1300 μm from the air–fluid interface. Averages are over all cells in the field of view. The error bars are the standard error of the mean. The number of cells in the samples decreases with time because of the tactic migration up-gradient (see insets and Fig. 4). This decrease is responsible for the larger error bars at the longer times. The time specified on the abscissa is the time from the beginning of measurements, approximately 2 min after the bacterial culture is filled into the microslide. Oxygen consumption and diffusion have therefore taken place well before t=0. The initial concentration of dissolved oxygen is unknown. The average swimming speeds are derived from distributions of speeds. Three representative histograms of these distributions are shown, located near the associated mean speed data point. The first histogram corresponds to the first point, at t=0, the second to t=130 s and the third to t=230 s.

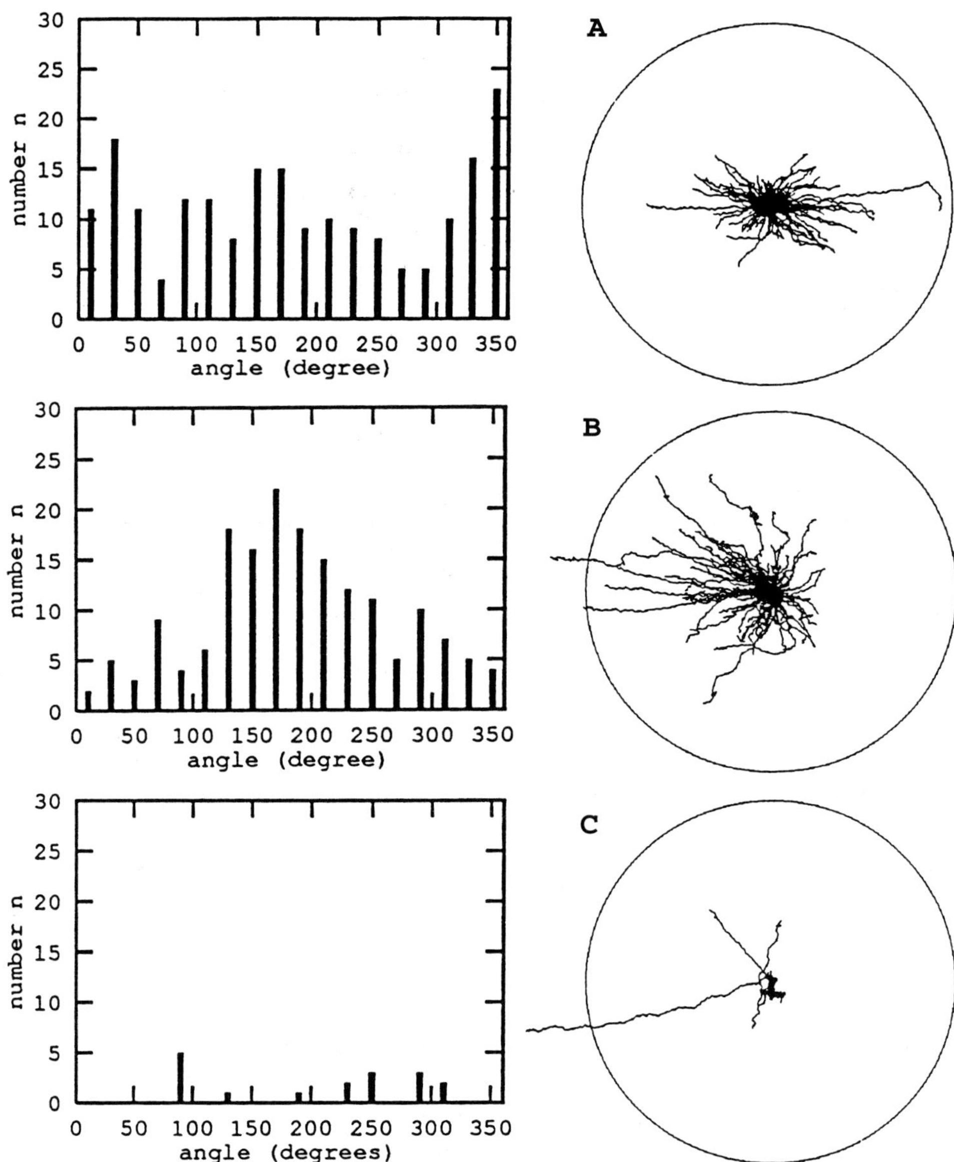

Fig. 7. The angular distribution of trajectory directions. These histograms and corresponding rose-track diagrams are examples of the distributions that yield the average directions shown in Fig. 4D, and the sum-unit vector **r** that is included in the Rayleigh Statistic (Fig. 4E). Histogram A corresponds to t=0 on Fig. 4, (B) to t=156 s and (C) to t=236 s. The height of each of the bars on this histogram represents the number of tracks within its 20° range. Each bar is centred in its range. To construct the rose-track diagrams, the starting points of all the cell trajectories in a sample are translated to the centre of the circle. Because the majority of the tracks are short, they mask one another; only the longer tracks are easily seen. The scale diameter of the circle is 55 μm and the oxygen gradient is oriented towards 180°. These diagrams demonstrate that directional motility develops during the formation of the oxygen concentration gradient. They are the fundamental ingredient of the angular part of the velocity distribution function.

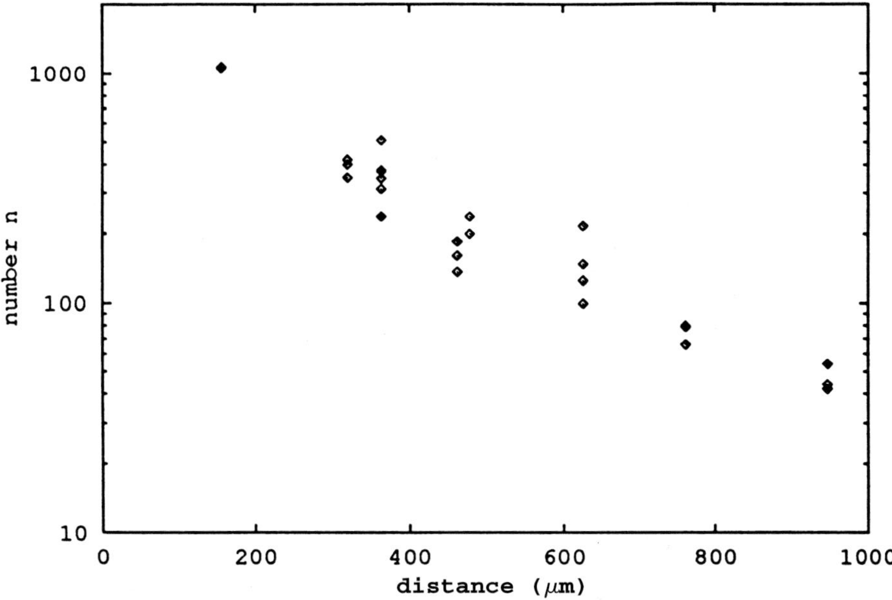

Fig. 8. The spatial distribution of bacterial cells under time-independent conditions. The number of swimming bacterial cells is recorded within an area of fixed size during a measurement interval of 5 s. The abscissa is the distance from the air–fluid interface. These steady-state data were obtained about 20 h after the cuvette was first filled with the bacterial culture; the observed cell numbers include the effects of tactic accumulation, as well as the change in total cell numbers due to cell division and cell decay. Collectively driven roiling and mixing of the fluid occurs for locations $x<100\,\mu m$.

the decline of the local concentration of oxygen, due to consumption, and the appearance of an oxygen concentration gradient, as oxygen diffuses in from the air–fluid interface, approximately 1.3 mm away. The spatial and temporal dependence of the oxygen concentration is a function of the consumption rate of the cells and of their shifting location. The work of Boon and Herpigny (1984) and Hillesdon *et al.* (1994) contains calculations for various cases implied by equations 4 and 5. Experimentally obtained plots of the oxygen concentration, and its gradient, are not yet available.

Figs 4A and 5A show that cells swim more quickly up-gradient than down. That there are more cells that swim up-gradient than down is shown in Fig. 4B–E and, by implication, in Fig. 4F. Figs 4C and 5B show that the mean length d for which tracks remain visible is also skewed towards the oxygen sources. Tracks remain visible if they have no sudden turns and if their orientation is flat, i.e. within the depth of field. The sum over a sample of n directional paths of the unit vectors that point from the beginning to the end of each path specifies θ. The length of that direction vector, divided by n, is called $\mathbf{r}$ (Zar, 1984). For completely randomly oriented directions, $\mathbf{r}=0$. When all unit vectors coincide, $\mathbf{r}=1$. The Rayleigh Statistic $\mathbf{r}^2 n$ is a measure of directionality that takes into account both the distribution of directions and the sample size. Fig. 4D plots θ, and Fig. 4E the Rayleigh Statistic. The latter shows that the data for $100\,s \leqslant t \leqslant 200\,s$ are much more strongly unimodal than the rest. Since the air–fluid meniscus is curved, and since the flat microslide cuvette is much wider than the area within which tracks are observed, exact orientation towards 180° could not be expected, even for completely deterministic swimmers.

Fig. 5 is derived from the same data as Fig. 4A,C. It demonstrates the asymmetry of the cells' response to the oxygen gradient, when it arrives. Fig. 6 shows that the mean swimming speed $<V>$ does not vary significantly during the time $100\,\mathrm{s}<t<200\,\mathrm{s}$ when Fig. 4 demonstrates the most asymmetric response. This observation is surprising; one might think that $<V>$ ought to increase with time since $n(+)V(+)>n(-)V(-)$. To resolve this problem, one may define $n(\pm)=n/2\pm\Delta n$ and $V(\pm)=V^*\pm\Delta V$.

Then:

$$n<V> = (n/2+\Delta n)(V^* + \Delta V) + (n/2-\Delta n)(V^* - \Delta V)\,, \tag{6}$$

or

$$<V> = V^* + 2\,(\Delta n/n)\Delta V\,. \tag{7}$$

The lack of dependence of $<V>$ on time and oxygen concentration, whilst Δn and ΔV are both positive, implies that V^* decreases with time. Fig. 3 shows motility far from the meniscus, beyond the diffusion range of oxygen. As the consumption of oxygen causes a substantial decrease in its concentration, the observed mean speed declines. It can probably be identified with V^*.

The response to the appearance of the oxygen gradient is shown in Fig. 7. These data will yield the angular part of the velocity probability density $f(\mathbf{V})$. The rose-track diagrams will be used to derive estimates of D_c (D. A. Hill, personal communication; Pedley and Kessler, 1990).

Long-term behaviour: steady state and turbulence

The asymmetry of directional swimming nearly vanishes after the initial migration up the oxygen gradient and after the loss of motility of the more remote population. Eventually both n and dn/dx become quite large (Fig. 8).

A new collective behaviour pattern then appears in the microslide preparation. It does not depend on gravity. Close to the meniscus, where oxygen taxis has concentrated the population, the volume fraction of cells approaches unity. Collisions, flagellar interactions and possibly some sort of chemical signalling generate violent turbulent vortical motion

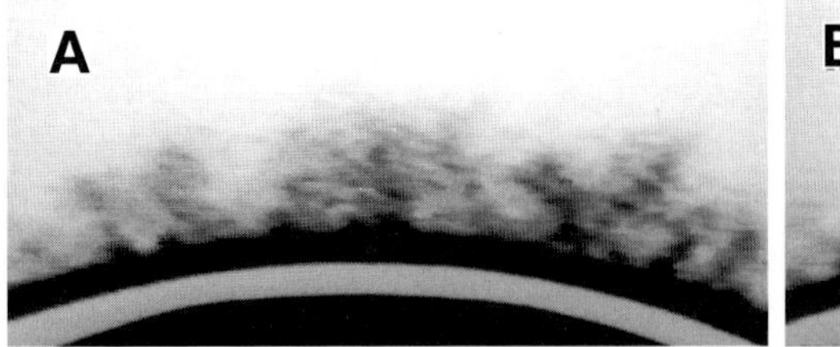

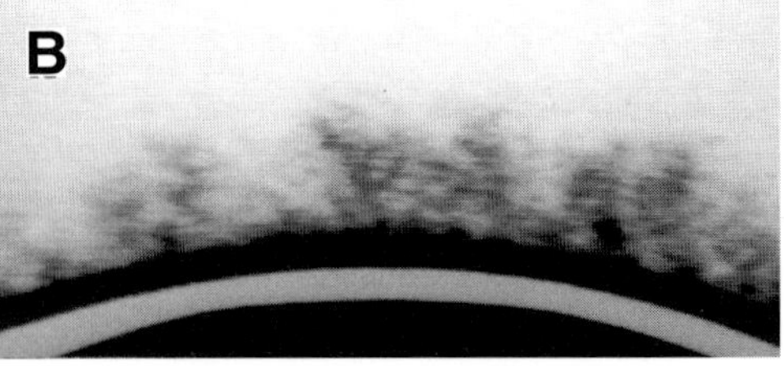

Fig. 9. Roiling at the meniscus. This view of bacteria that have swum to the edge of the meniscus was taken in flat microslide 0.1 mm deep. The distance from the edge of the interface to the top of the plumes is about 100 μm. The two images shown were acquired less than 1 min apart. Both are shown to indicate the frenetic level of activity.

that can be seen as great rotating clouds of cells and intermittent jets that appear near the meniscus (Fig. 9). The overall extent of these collective dynamic interactions is 50–100 μm. A range of smaller scales of collective movements reaches down to a few cell diameters, especially near the triple line, where water, glass and air meet.

The direct contact interactions among the cells appear to be augmented by motions of the meniscus driven by a surface tension gradient, presumably caused by cell exudates. Evidence for this source of motion is provided by the rapid shuttling back and forth of large groups of cells adjacent to the meniscus.

The roiling and mixing action often continues for days. Then, at the distal end of the dynamic cell clouds, one can observe individuals that have inadvertently swum away from the densely populated region suddenly turn and swim back. This behaviour is probably due to a chemotactic attraction of the cells to each other, augmenting the effect of the oxygen gradient. Oxygen, chemical signals and the cell population itself are all transported and mixed by these collective dynamics.

The statistics that govern the 'steady state' in the calm regions more than 50 μm away from the meniscus have so far not yielded a detailed mechanism for the maintenance of the approximately exponential spatial variation of n. For the simple situation where diffusion D due to random swimming balances directional swimming with average velocity V, the solution of equation 5 is:

$$n(x) = n(0)\exp[-(V/D)x] . \tag{8}$$

The more complicated situation where large n causes collisions is discussed in Kessler (1986). The observed length D/V is 2–300 μm.

Fig. 10 shows that for the steady state there is little or no directionality in the individuals' swimming dynamics. Within measurement accuracy, the mean speed V was

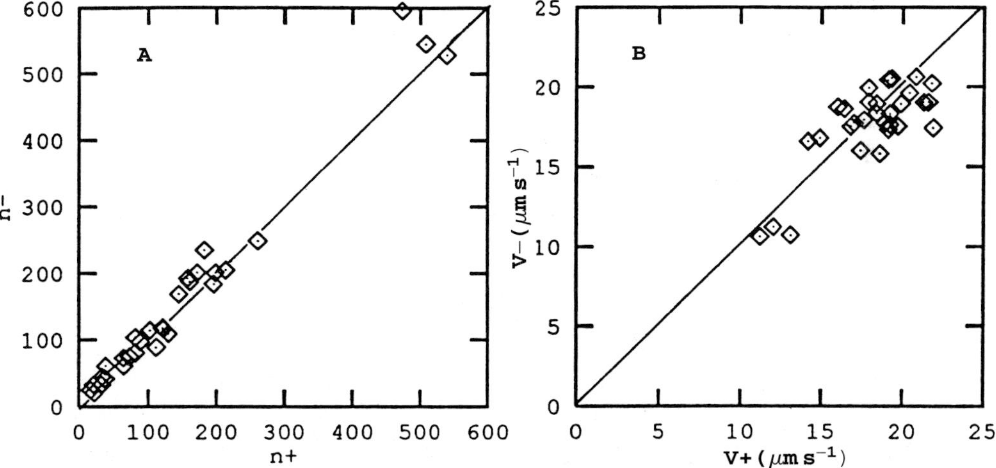

Fig. 10. Lack of asymmetry within the time-independent oxygen gradient. (A) The number of cells $n(-)$ that swim away from the oxygen source and that swim towards it $n(+)$, as detailed in the legend to Fig. 5. The points correspond to eight different distances from the air–fluid interface. (B) $V(+)$ and $V(-)$ are the corresponding speeds. The distribution of swimming directions, not shown, is also flat.

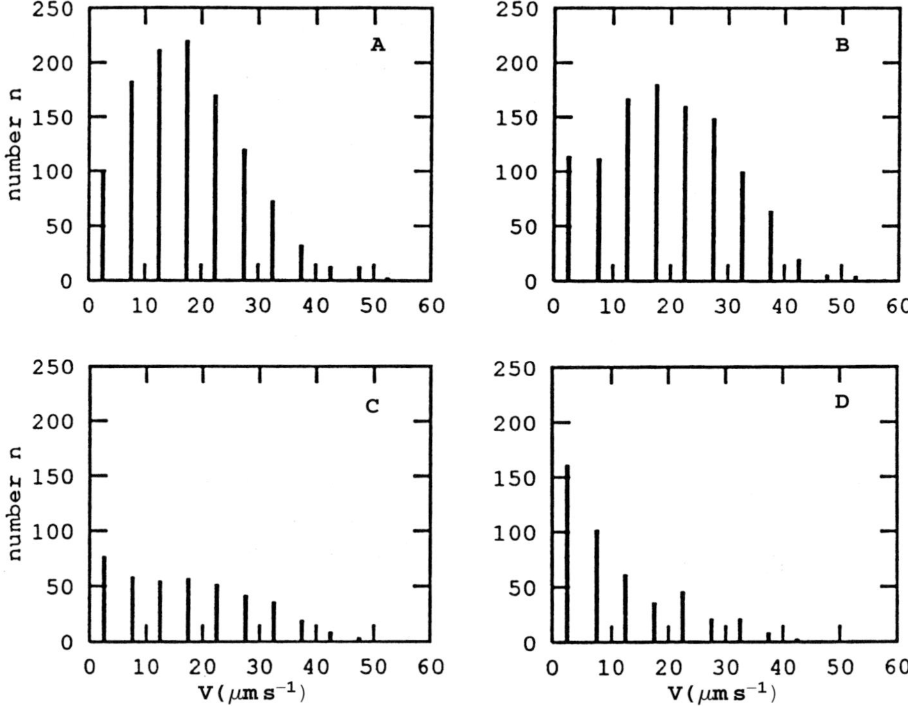

Fig. 11. Four samples of the distribution of swimming speeds under approximately time-independent conditions. The distributions were measured at various distances from the air–fluid interface. The numbers of bacteria per trial at the measuring sites are shown in Fig. 8. Each of the histograms is the sum of three separate trials. Three single points not visible in A are located at V=58, 63 and 78 μm s^{-1}. The distances x from the interface, the mean speeds and the standard deviations S.D., derived from all the trials comprising N tracks, at a particular values of x are: (A) x=156 μm, $\bar{V}$=17.9±0.7 μm s^{-1}, N=1143; (B) x=364 μm, $\bar{V}$=18.7±1.2 μm s^{-1}, N=1079; (C) x=626 μm, $\bar{V}$=18.1±1.7 μm s^{-1}, N=409; (D) x=947 μm, $\bar{V}$=11.3±0.4 μm s^{-1}, N=461. The standard deviations of the *distributions* of V were independent of x, in spite of the changes in shape. They ranged from 10 to 12 μm s^{-1}.

not a function of distance from the meniscus, but the distribution of speeds varied markedly (Fig. 11). These distributions are involved in the shape of $n(x)$.

Discussion

Managed microbial ecosystems have been studied in the past. Some of that work is summarized by Wimpenny (1988). There has also been much illuminating work on bacterial taxes where the attractant or repellent and the organisms are well controlled for maximum insight into some particular aspect of the problem (Armitage, 1992). The research presented here differs from this previous work by using a method that allows the micro-organisms to create their own fluid environment that varies in time and across the space available to the organisms. Physical and biochemical factors come jointly into play. Whatever dependence there may be on the history of the cells' surroundings is automatically accounted for. The experimental results concerning time-dependent and directional motility and the associated population frequency spectra are therefore quite 'natural'. They are appropriate ingredients for an eventual quantitative description of bioconvection patterns that are driven by swimming, oriented by consumption and catalyzed by gravitational symmetry-breaking. For example, one would like to discover the cause of the very unusual (in the sense of convection, generally) cell-depleted migrating 'black' bands seen in Fig. 1.

These patterns can serve as models for a primitive type of biological self-organization. It is primitive because it requires no direct communication between cells. Yet it creates dynamic systems comprising organisms, physical factors and environmental supplies of nutrients. These dynamic systems transport and mix cells and chemicals rapidly and efficiently. They also generate local environments (e.g. anoxic and well-aerated) that may function to select diversity among the initially unspecialised cells.

This work was aided by NASA grant NAG 9442 and by the very generous support of Ralph and Alice Sheets, through the University of Arizona Foundation. We should also like to thank Mitzi de Martino for her help with this manuscript.

References

ARMITAGE, J. P. (1992). Behavioral responses in bacteria. *A. Rev. Physiol.* **54**, 683–714.

BOON, J. P. AND HERPIGNY, B. (1984). Formation and evolution of spatial structures. *Springer Lect. Notes Biomath.* **55**, 13–29.

HILLESDON, A. J., PEDLEY, T. J. AND KESSLER, J. O. (1995). The development of concentration gradients in a suspension of chemotactic bacteria. *Bull. Math. Biol.* **57**, 299–344.

KESSLER, J. O. (1985). Cooperative and concentrative phenomena in swimming micro-organisms. *Contem. Phys.* **26**, 147–166.

KESSLER, J. O. (1986). The external dynamics of swimming micro-organisms. In *Progress in Phycological Research*, vol. 4 (ed. F. E. Round and D. J. Chapman), pp. 257–307. Bristol: Biopress.

KESSLER, J. O. (1992). Theory and experimental results on gravitational effects on monocellular algae. *Adv. Space Res.* **12**, 33–42.

KESSLER, J. O. AND HILL, N. A. (1994). Microbial consumption patterns. In *Spatio-Temporal Patterns* (ed. P. E. Cladis and P. Palffy-Muhoray), pp. 635–648. Reading, MA: Addison-Wesley (in press).

KESSLER, J. O., HOELZER, M. A., PEDLEY, T. J. AND HILL, N. A. (1994). Functional patterns of swimming bacteria. In *Mechanics and Physiology of Animal Swimming* (ed. L. Maddock, Q. Bone and J. M. V. Rayner), pp. 3–12. Cambridge: Cambridge University Press (in press).

PEDLEY, T. J. AND KESSLER, J. O. (1990). A new continuum model for suspensions of gyrotactic micro-organisms. *J. Fluid Mech.* **212**, 155–182.

PEDLEY, T. J. AND KESSLER, J. O. (1992*a*). Hydrodynamic phenomena in suspensions of swimming micro-organisms. *A. Rev. Fluid Mech.* **24**, 313–358.

PEDLEY, T. J. AND KESSLER, J. O. (1992*b*). Bioconvection. *Sci. Prog.* **76**, 105–123.

SCHNITZER, M. J., BLOCK, S. M., BERG, H. C. AND PURCELL, E. M. (1990). Strategies for chemotaxis. In *Biology of the Chemotactic Response* (ed. J. P. Armitage and J. M. Lackie), pp. 15–33. Cambridge: Cambridge University Press.

SPIZIZEN, J. (1958). Transformation of biochemically deficient strains of *Bacillus subtilis* by deoxyribonucleate. *Proc. natn. Acad. Sci. U.S.A.* **44**, 1072–1078.

STRAUGHAN, B. (1993). *Mathematical Aspects of Penetrative Convection*. Harlow: Longman Scientific.

WIMPENNY, J. W. T. (1988). (ed.) *CRC Handbook of Laboratory Model Systems for Microbial Ecosystems*, vols 1 and 2. Boca Raton: CRC Press.

YASBIN, R. E., FIELDS, P. I. AND ANDERSEN, B. J. (1980). Properties of *Bacillus subtilis* 168 derivatives freed of their natural prophages. *Gene* **12**, 155–159.

ZAR, J. H. (1984). *Biostatistical Analysis*, chapters 24 and 25. Englewood Cliffs: Prentice Hall.

UNSTEADY AERODYNAMICS OF INSECT FLIGHT

C. P. ELLINGTON

Department of Zoology, University of Cambridge, Downing Street, Cambridge CB2 3EJ, United Kingdom

Summary

Over the past decade, the importance of unsteady aerodynamic mechanisms for flapping insect flight has become widely recognised. Even at the fastest flight speeds, the old quasi-steady aerodynamic interpretation seems inadequate to explain the extra lift produced by the wings. Recent experiments on rigid model wings have confirmed the effectiveness of several postulated high-lift mechanisms. Delayed stall can produce extra lift for several chords of travel during the translational phases of the wingbeat. Lift can also be enhanced by circulation created during pronation and supination by rotational mechanisms: the fling/peel, the near fling/peel and isolated rotation. These studies have revealed large leading-edge vortices which contribute to the circulation around the wing, augmenting the lift. The mechanisms show distinctive patterns of vortex shedding from leading and trailing edges.

The results of flow visualization experiments on tethered insects are reviewed in an attempt to identify the high-lift mechanisms actually employed. The fling/peel mechanism is clearly used by some insects. The near fling/peel is the wing motion most commonly observed, but evidence for the production of high lift remains indirect. For many insects, lift on the upstroke probably results from delayed stall instead of the flex mechanism of isolated rotation.

The large leading-edge vortices from experiments on rigid model wings are greatly reduced or missing around the real insect wings, often making the identification of aerodynamic mechanisms inconclusive. A substantial spanwise flow component has been detected over the aerodynamic upper wing surface, which should transport leading-edge vorticity towards the wingtip before it has much time to roll up. This spanwise transport, arising from centrifugal acceleration, is probably a general phenomenon for flapping insect flight. It should reduce and stabilise any leading-edge vortices that are present, which is essential for preventing stall and maintaining the circulation of high-lift mechanisms during translation.

Introduction

How do the flapping wings of an insect generate lift? We used to have a simple and comfortable answer to that question: they produce lift according to the same principles as conventional aeroplane wings. It was thought that the instantaneous force on a flapping wing is the same as that which the wing would experience in steady motion at the same

Key words: insect flight, unsteady aerodynamics, insects.

instantaneous velocity and angle of attack. This *quasi-steady assumption* was a logical first step in the aerodynamic analysis of flapping flight and, by ignoring any influence of the past history of the wing motion, it greatly simplified a problem in dynamics to a sequence of independent, static conditions. The assumption is most justifiable for fast forward flight, where the steady flight velocity dominates the flow over the wings and the flapping motion is but a small perturbation of this steady flow. Whether the assumption is valid for large-amplitude flapping at low flight speeds and hovering has been the source of much controversy; unsteady aerodynamic effects may dominate over quasi-steady ones under such conditions.

Nevertheless, the quasi-steady assumption appeared to provide a satisfactory explanation of flapping flight for most animals, from hovering to fast forward flight (e.g. Jensen, 1956; Weis-Fogh, 1956, 1972, 1973; Pennycuick, 1968; U. M. Norberg, 1976*a*). This was a palatable conclusion for most biologists because the quasi-steady interpretation of flight is relatively easy (in as much as any aerodynamics can be easy). Alternative aerodynamic mechanisms had not been discounted, or even investigated very seriously, but there was little incentive to question a plausible quasi-steady explanation that seemed to work. There were a few cases where the quasi-steady explanation failed (Weis-Fogh, 1973; Ellington, 1975; R. Å. Norberg, 1975; U. M. Norberg, 1975, 1976*b*): the required lift was greater than the wings could produce in steady motion. These cases were associated with unusual wing motions, and Weis-Fogh (1973) proposed two novel mechanisms of lift generation that seemed to explain most of the results. The lift produced by these mechanisms depends on events during the rotational phases (pronation and supination) at either end of the wingbeat, when the wing rapidly rotates through about 120° in preparation for the next half-stroke. It is hardly surprising that these mechanisms were new to aerodynamics; conventional wings are never operated in this extreme manner.

Since the 1980s, however, our confidence in the quasi-steady explanation has been eroded almost completely. Cloupeau *et al.* (1979) and Wilkin (1990) succeeded in measuring the fluctuating lift forces on tethered locusts flying in a wind tunnel. The mean lift was comparable to that in the earlier quasi-steady analysis of Jensen (1956), but the peak lift was about twice the quasi-steady value. The discrepancy, both qualitative and quantitative, between the measured instantaneous lift and the quasi-steady calculations indicates important but as yet unexplained unsteady aerodynamic effects. Similarly, serious discrepancies between measured forces and quasi-steady predictions have been found for tethered *Drosophila melanogaster* fruit flies (Zanker and Götz, 1990) and *Manduca sexta* hawkmoths (Wilkin and Williams, 1993).

Other studies invalidated the quasi-steady explanation by showing that the predicted lift force was insufficient to support the body weight. A comprehensive study by Ellington (1984*a–e*), using new data and a new aerodynamic theory, cast doubt on the applicability of the quasi-steady mechanism to hovering flight. The tentative conclusion was that unsteady lift mechanisms are used by *all* hovering animals, and this conclusion has been strengthened by subsequent studies; the quasi-steady explanation has proved inadequate for various Diptera (Ennos, 1989), bumblebees (Dudley and Ellington, 1990*b*) and hummingbirds (Wells, 1993). Studies of bumblebees (Dudley and Ellington,

1990*a*,*b*) and neotropical butterflies (Dudley, 1991) also showed that the quasi-steady explanation fails in free forward flight. There remains some controversy about the significance of unsteady effects in dragonfly flight (R. Å. Norberg, 1975; Newman *et al.* 1977; Savage *et al.* 1979; Somps and Luttges, 1985; Azuma *et al.* 1985; Azuma and Watanabe, 1988), but the weight of modern evidence is clearly against the quasi-steady mechanism in virtually all types of flapping animal flight, except perhaps for birds and bats at fast speeds. Even then, first-order unsteady corrections to the quasi-steady model might be required: see the excellent reviews by Spedding (1992, 1993) and Spedding and DeLaurier (1995).

Definition of the aerodynamic problem

What explanation can be offered in place of the quasi-steady mechanism; how do the flapping wings generate so much lift? Before that question can be addressed properly, some background knowledge of aerodynamics is needed.

Consider a conventional wing, initially at rest with respect to the air, which is suddenly given a constant forward velocity: an 'impulsive start' (Fig. 1). For the wing to experience an upward lift force, the average air pressure must be greater below than above it. The average air velocity must therefore be higher above the wing than below, because of the inverse relationship between pressure and velocity from Bernoulli's principle. This velocity difference can be represented by a vortex 'bound' to the wing; the strength or *circulation* of the bound vortex is a measure of the velocity difference and is directly proportional to the lift force. For a given speed and angle of attack, there is a

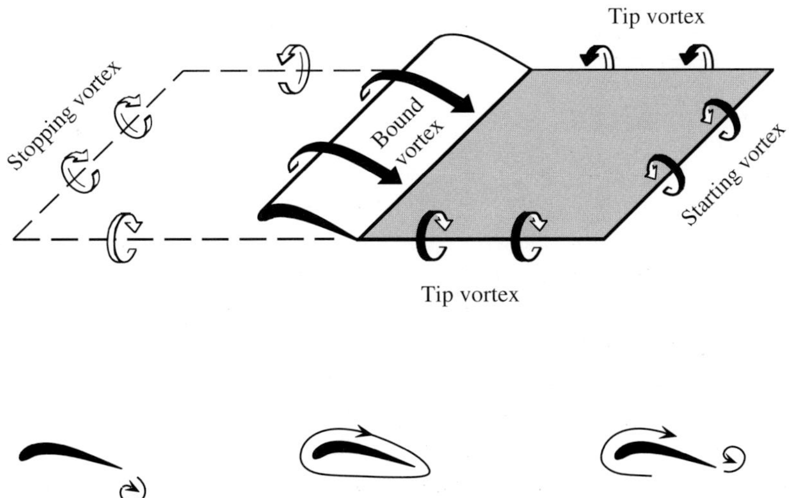

Fig. 1. The 3-D vortex wake created by the impulsive start of a rectangular wing is shown at the top. The stippled area represents air given a downwards impulse. Dashed lines and unshaded vortices indicate future events. Creation of the starting, bound and stopping vortices is shown below in a 2-D view, depicting the vertical plane.

unique value of the circulation, and hence of the lift, for which the air flows smoothly and tangentially from the trailing edge – the Kutta condition.

At the beginning of the motion, air swirls around the trailing edge, shedding vorticity into the wake. This continues until the bound vortex grows to the Kutta value for steady motion and the air flows smoothly from the edge; the gradual build-up of circulation is called the *Wagner effect*, and even after six chord lengths of travel the circulation and lift are only 90 % of the final values. The shed vorticity rolls up into a concentrated 'starting' vortex equal in magnitude but opposite in sense of rotation to the bound vortex. 'Trailing' or 'tip' vortices join up the starting and bound vortices, and they are created as air swirls around the tips from the higher pressure region below the wing to the lower pressure above. Thus, the lifting wing generates a rectangular vortex 'ring', enclosing air that has been blown downwards. When the wing motion stops, there should be no lift or circulation. The circulating flow around the wing then swirls off the trailing edge, shedding the bound vortex as a 'stopping' vortex, and the freed vortex ring moves downwards into the wake. Whether the aerodynamic mechanism is unsteady or quasi-steady, as described here, the reaction force to the lift must impart downward momentum to the air, and the resulting air motion must correspond to a vortex 'ring' structure.

Armed with this description of lift production and vorticity, the aerodynamic problems of flapping insect flight can be illustrated by the bumblebee (Fig. 2), for which the quasi-steady explanation fails at all flight speeds (Dudley and Ellington, 1990*b*). The path of the wing tip through the air at different flight speeds is drawn from the kinematic data presented by Dudley and Ellington (1990*a*). Lift and drag are perpendicular and parallel to the path, respectively, and the resultant force vectors are drawn to scale for each half-stroke. In hovering, only the flapping velocity and the downwash determine the wing path. The downstroke and upstroke are nearly symmetrical, providing weight support but no net horizontal thrust. The wing rotates through about 120° between the half-strokes, so the leading edge always leads, and the morphological lower surface of the wing becomes the aerodynamic upper surface on the upstroke. The circulation changes sense between half-strokes, and must therefore pass through zero at the ends of the wingbeat. Because of the reversal of circulation, a new bound vortex and associated starting and stopping vortices must be created each half-stroke. Stopping vortices will have the same sense as starting vortices on the subsequent half-stroke. They will also be in close proximity and might well coalesce into a single vortex: a 'pronation' vortex at the dorsal end of the wingbeat and a 'supination' vortex at the ventral end. The figure is drawn as if they have coalesced, for clarity.

The pattern of circulation reversal is also seen in forward flight, where the downstroke increasingly dominates the force balance as speed increases; the downstroke path becomes relatively longer, indicating a higher velocity and thus larger forces. At fast speeds, the asymmetry is very pronounced, with the powerful downstroke responsible for weight support, but the direction of the feeble upstroke force is suitable only for thrust.

The required lift is greater than a bumblebee wing can achieve before it stalls in steady motion. Stall places an upper limit on the circulation that can be attained by the quasi-steady mechanism, so *how is an enhanced circulation created to provide the extra lift?* That is the fundamental aerodynamic question. A corollary question is *how is the*

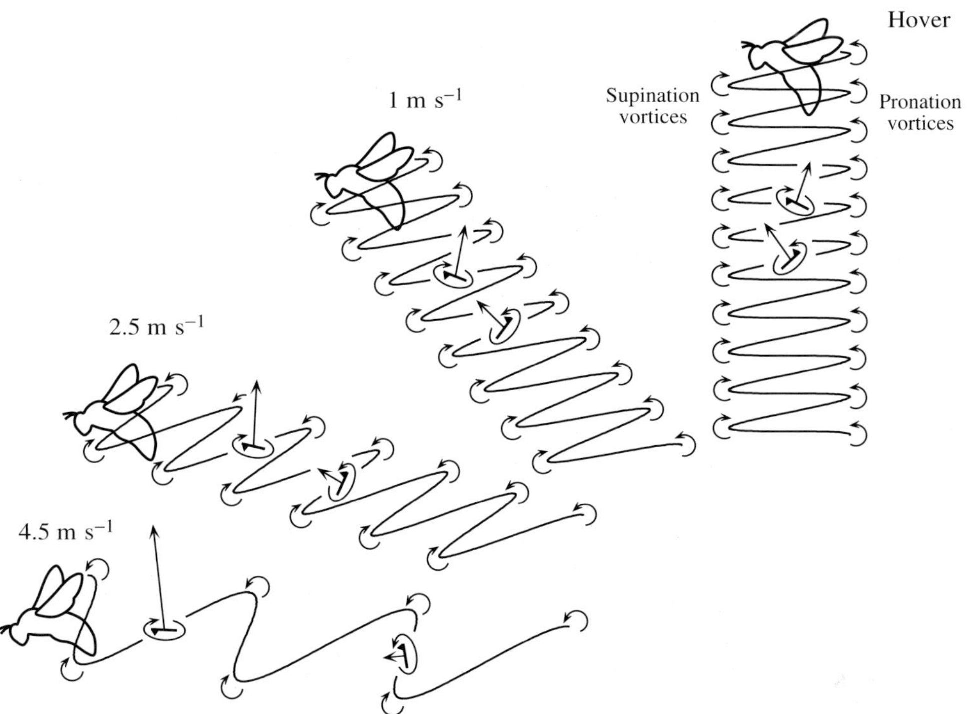

Fig. 2. A 2-D view of the wingtip path for a bumblebee *Bombus terrestris* at different flight speeds. Bound vortices and the resultant aerodynamic forces are shown for representative downstrokes and upstrokes. The morphological lower wing surface is marked by a triangle at the leading edge. Stopping and starting vortices shed during pronation would be in close proximity and of the same sense; they are drawn as if coalesced into a single 'pronation' vortex. Similarly, a single 'supination' vortex represents the stopping and starting vortices shed at the other end of the wingbeat.

enhanced circulation maintained? The wing should stall, shedding the extra bound vorticity and reducing the circulation to that of the Kutta condition for the quasi-steady motion.

In fact, the problem is even worse because the quasi-steady analysis ignores past history and therefore the Wagner effect. Circulation and lift will not grow to final values on each half-stroke because the bumblebee wing moves only 3–4 chord lengths during hovering and about 6 during fast flight. Thus, the quasi-steady estimate of lift is overly optimistic, and even more extra lift will be required in practice.

High-lift mechanisms

As our faith in the quasi-steady explanation came under attack, a number of high-lift mechanisms were proposed as alternatives (Weis-Fogh, 1973; Nachtigall, 1979; Ellington, 1980, 1984*c*). Most of these were conjectural, but the main ones have since been investigated.

High-lift mechanisms can be divided conveniently into those applicable to the *translational* phase of the wingbeat, when the fundamental flapping motion imparts a curvilinear motion to wing elements, and to the *rotational* phase at either end of the wingbeat, when the angle of attack changes quickly in preparation for the next half-stroke.

Translational motion

The translational phase is traditionally the province of the quasi-steady analysis, where wing forces are assumed to be those that the wing would experience in steady motion at the same instantaneous speed and angle of attack. Under high-lift conditions, however, 'stall' can become a very dynamic process, and the lift can briefly exceed the maximum stalled value for steady motion. If the angle of attack is suddenly increased above the stall angle, or if the wing is impulsively started with a high angle of attack, the wing can travel several chord lengths before the separation associated with stall becomes well-developed (Francis and Cohen, 1933): a phenomenon known as *delayed stall* or *dynamic stall*. Stall is also delayed by forward accelerations and decelerations (Maresca *et al.* 1979; Gursul and Ho, 1992) and by rotations that increase the angle of attack (Kramer, 1932; Farren, 1935; Bennett, 1970; Rüppell, 1977). During the brief period before the onset of stall, circulation and lift will exceed the maximum quasi-steady stalled value. The enhanced lift must eventually be lost as the flow separates from the upper wing surface and the steady-state stall is reached, but this does not occur for several chords of travel.

Given the Reynolds numbers and sharp leading edges of insect wings, it is very likely that delayed stall will be accompanied by a *leading-edge vortex*, or leading-edge 'bubble'. At moderate to high angles of attack, the flow separates as it swirls around the sharp leading edge, but it re-attaches to the wing before the trailing edge, enclosing a separation bubble. The circulation of this vortex adds to the circulation around the wing, and thus increases the lift. These leading-edge vortices are common for thin aerofoils with sharp leading edges, and they give a characteristic, gradual 'thin-aerofoil stall' (McCullough and Gault, 1951; Tani, 1964; Ellington, 1984*c*).

Most of the experiments on delayed stall are at a Reynolds number *Re* much higher than is appropriate to insect flight, but Dickinson and Götz (1993) have investigated the impulsive start of model wings at *Re* around 75–230: the aerodynamic realm of the fruit fly. Fig. 3 is traced from their flow visualization records for a flat wing suddenly set in motion at an angle of attack of 45°. After one chord of travel (Fig. 3A), the starting vortex shed from the trailing edge is clearly visible, as is a large counter-rotating leading-edge vortex. The leading-edge vortex grows for 2–3 chords of travel (Fig. 3B,C), and maximum lift is reached during this period; the peak lift is about 2.5 times the maximum value measured under steady conditions at similar *Re* (Thom and Swart, 1940; Vogel, 1967). A new starting vortex forms after 3–4 chords of travel as the leading-edge vortex moves slowly downstream over the wing and gradually breaks away (Fig. 3C,D); there is a corresponding trough in the lift force. The pattern then repeats with the formation of a new leading-edge vortex, and the lift reaches a second but smaller peak after 5–6 chords of travel. The lift oscillations decayed with time but were still present when translation ceased after 7.5 chords of travel.

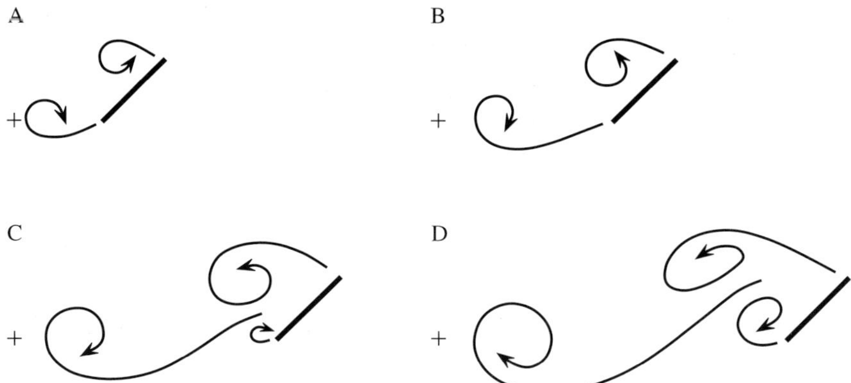

Fig. 3. Leading- and trailing-edge vortex shedding from a flat wing model suddenly set in motion at an angle of attack of 45° and a Reynolds number of 192. Traced from Fig. 3 of Dickinson and Götz (1993). A cross marks the initial position of the trailing edge. (A–D) The vortices after 1–4 chords of travel, respectively. Delayed stall produces maximum lift when the leading-edge vortex is located above the wing (B–C).

Delayed stall is an ideal mechanism for explaining the extra lift of insect wings when they move but a short distance in hovering and slow flight, especially for dragonflies and hoverflies with their low-amplitude wingbeats. For several chords of travel, the limitation of stall is temporarily removed and the wings can operate effectively at higher angles of attack. Large leading-edge vortices enhance the circulatory lift and are likely to feature prominently in the delayed stall of insect wings; indeed, they are commonly observed in model experiments at appropriate *Re* (e.g. Newman *et al.* 1977; Savage *et al.* 1979; Somps and Luttges, 1985; Luttges, 1989; Saharon and Luttges, 1989; Dickinson and Götz, 1993). However, the instability of these vortices would restrict the usefulness of delayed stall as a high-lift mechanism for the greater distances travelled at moderate to fast flight speeds.

The only evidence against the use of the delayed stall mechanism is given by Ellington (1984*e*). From a kinematic and aerodynamic analysis of hovering insects, he suggested that angles of attack were often smaller for insects that required more lift. If true, those results would rule out any mechanism of lift enhancement that is based on the angle of attack during translational phases of the wing motion. Angles of attack were only estimated visually, however, so the results are not conclusive.

Rotational motion

The fling mechanism

The rotational phase of the wingbeat is commonly ignored in a quasi-steady analysis because the wings are translating too slowly to produce significant forces. In his pioneering study of 1973, however, Weis-Fogh excited our interest with a completely new mechanism of lift generation for the tiny wasp *Encarsia formosa*, based on the rotational motion of the wings. The *fling* mechanism creates circulation around the wings

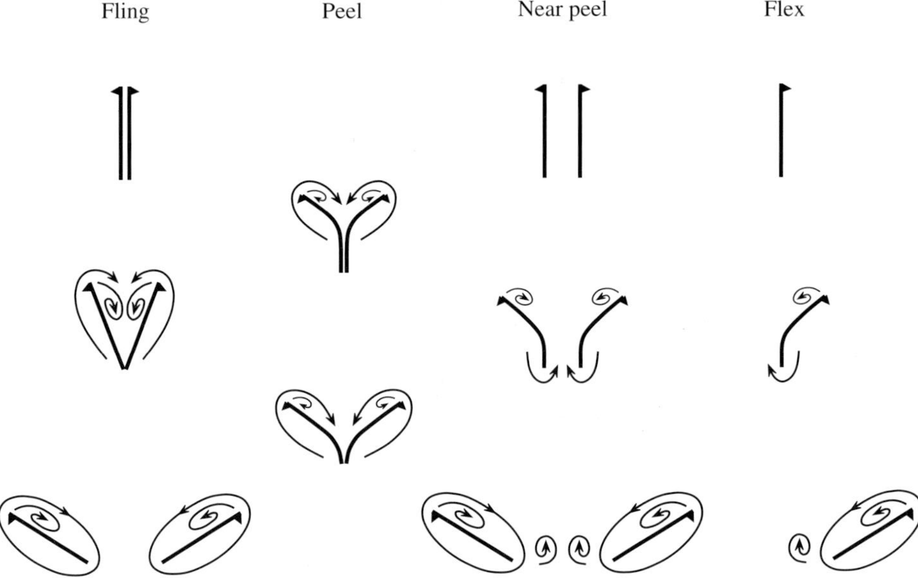

Fig. 4. Rotational mechanisms that create useful circulation prior to translation. A chordwise section of the wings is shown, and triangles mark the lower surface of the leading edges. Vorticity shed from the leading edges during rotation is of the correct sense for lift if recaptured upon subsequent translation.

during the rotational phase, and this circulation then determines the lift during subsequent translation. Prior to the beginning of a downstroke, the wings of *Encarsia* are 'clapped' together dorsally with the longitudinal wing axes horizontal, as shown in vertical section in Fig. 4. The wings then fling open about their trailing edges, and the flow of air into the opening gap creates equal circulations around each wing, but of opposite sense. The circulation is proportional to the angular velocity of rotation and thus can exceed the maximum quasi-steady value for translational motion. When the fling ends, the wings separate and move apart in the downstroke, immediately generating an enhanced lift from the fling circulation. No starting vortices are left behind: the bound vortex of each wing is, in effect, the starting vortex for the other.

The fling mechanism is *the* great success story for insect flight aerodynamics. It has been analysed theoretically (Lighthill, 1973; Edwards and Cheng, 1982; Wu and Hu-chen, 1984), modelled numerically (Haussling, 1979) and verified experimentally (Bennett, 1977; Maxworthy, 1979; Spedding and Maxworthy, 1986). It is a very effective lift mechanism used by certain insects, and even the most casual observer can see the clap and fling motion in commonplace butterflies and moths.

The studies cited above have established that very large leading-edge vortices are produced by the fling of rigid wings with sharp leading edges. The swirl around the leading edge enhances the circulation and lift, but the vortex is unstable during subsequent translation for 2-D motions. The circulation is greater than the quasi-steady maximum and, as in delayed stall, the leading-edge vortex must break away from the wing after a few chords of travel. Using a 3-D mechanical flapping model, Maxworthy (1979) discovered a strong spanwise transport of vorticity towards the wing tip within the leading-edge vortex, somewhat analogous to the conical leading-edge vortices above delta wings. This spanwise removal of vorticity stabilised the vortex more than 2-D considerations would predict, and sustained the fling circulation during the entire downstroke.

Variations on the fling

Ellington (1980, 1984*b*,*c*) noted several kinematic variations on the basic fling motion and discussed the possible aerodynamic consequences. To begin with, few animals perform a rigid fling; the wings 'peel' apart instead, rather like two pieces of paper being pulled apart (Fig. 4). A theoretical analysis of the peel showed that it is very effective in creating circulation, and that stability problems with leading-edge vortices should be much reduced (Ellington, 1984*c*). Vorticity shed from the leading edge should be sucked steadily along the upper wing surface as the peel proceeds, distributing the vorticity more uniformly than in the fling.

Although many insects take advantage of the circulation created by a fling/peel motion, most seem to shun the mechanisms in spite of the aerodynamic benefits. If nothing else, there must be significant mechanical wear and damage to the wings caused by repeated clapping. Much more widespread in occurrence is the *near fling*, or *near peel* (Fig. 4), where most of the wings remain separated by a fraction of the chord length and do not actually touch. For some insects, more proximal, posterior regions of the wings may still touch rather late in pronation, causing a *partial fling* or *partial peel* near the wing bases. A partial peel confined to the very base of the wings with a near peel distally is probably the most ubiquitous pattern I have observed in flying insects.

The separation distance between the wings distinguishes the near, partial and complete fling/peel. The partial fling/peel should be somewhat less effective than a complete fling/peel in creating circulation, and the near fling/peel even less so, because air moving around the trailing edges should reduce the shear past the leading edges. It has been suggested that some insects vary the separation distance between the wings to modulate the aerodynamic force under different conditions (Ellington, 1984*c*).

Isolated rotation

At one end of the spectrum of fling motions, the separation distance becomes so large that the wings are well clear of each other during the rotational phase. Such 'isolated rotation' is commonly observed during supination, and it is also found during pronation for some insects. If the wings simply rotated about their trailing edges as rigid flat plates, then the vortex pattern should be similar to that proposed for the near fling. The rotational motion should produce a leading-edge vortex of the correct sense for lift on subsequent translation, while vorticity of the opposite sense is concentrated at the trailing edge, ready to be shed as a starting vortex for translation.

The only problem is that insects do not rotate their wings about the trailing edge. The rotation axis is instead located near the 1/4 chord axis, which would cause concentrated vortex shedding at the trailing edge; vorticity of the correct sense for translation would therefore be left behind and wasted. However, the wing flexes during the latter half of rotation, as in the peel motions. As shown in Fig. 4, this flexion might cause the trailing edge to become relatively stationary while the leading edge continues rotation, ensuring the correct leading edge shedding. This *flex* mechanism (Ellington, 1984*c*) is probably supplemented by a *delayed rotation* preceding the powerful downstroke of hoverflies (Ellington, 1984*b*,*c*); pronation overlaps the beginning of the downstroke, enhancing the leading edge movement and keeping the trailing edge stationary. Similarly, Dickinson *et al.* (1993) report that the relative timing of supination is actively controlled for turning manoeuvres in *Drosophila*.

Experimental studies of rotational mechanisms

Experimental studies which verified the fling mechanism were cited above. A new study (Sunada *et al.* 1993) has investigated the near fling for rigid wings rotating about their trailing edges; by varying the separation distance between the wings, it covered the spectrum from a complete fling to isolated rotation. Flow visualization results were similar for 2-D and 3-D models, with a large separation vortex shed from the leading edge and a counter-rotating vortex centred at the trailing edge. Vortex shedding from the outside edges joined these vortices for the 3-D model, as expected. There was little qualitative difference between the vortex patterns for isolated rotation and for a complete fling. Force measurements and numerical modelling also revealed remarkably small quantitative differences; the interference effect from the opposite wing is important only during the early stage of rotation, when the opening angle between the wings is small.

Sunada *et al.* (1993) did not investigate the fate of these vortices created during rotation when the wings subsequently began to translate, but Dickinson (1994) extended his 2-D towing tank studies to wing models that rotated and translated. When the rotation axis was close to the trailing edge, the wing indeed recaptured the leading-edge vortex created during rotation, and thus generated more lift upon translation; lift was produced even at an angle of attack of zero. The lift declined dramatically after about 3 chords of travel, showing the same 2-D delayed stall characteristics found in his study of pure translation (Dickinson and Götz, 1993). These results, combined with those of Sunada *et al.* provide stong experimental support for the effectiveness of the postulated rotational mechanisms. From isolated rotation to the complete fling, rotation about the trailing edge does produce a strong leading-edge vortex, and this vortex can be recaptured upon translation, augmenting the circulatory lift of the wings.

Two major questions remain unanswered for the rotational mechanisms. Does the flex mechanism work? The effectiveness of isolated rotation about the trailing edge offers limited support for the flex mechanism, but experimental studies are still needed for flexing wings with an anterior rotation axis. The second question is what kinematic motion best couples rotation and translation to maximize lift enhancement? Dickinson (1994) found that the pattern of vortex shedding, the extent of lift enhancement and the time course of the forces were all affected in a complicated manner by the location of the rotation axis, the speed of rotation and the pattern of any vortices previously shed into the wake.

Coupled translation and rotation

Because of the great interest in fluttering aeroplane wings, flapping flight and swimming, the literature is brimming with theoretical, numerical and experimental studies on pitching (rotating) and heaving (translating, or plunging) aerofoils. However, very few of these studies are applicable to insect flight, where the oscillation amplitudes are large, the mean free-stream velocity is low, and leading-edge shedding greatly complicates theoretical and numerical work. Experimental work is sorely needed to lead the way into this difficult fluid regime, and to identify the best coupling of rotational and translational motions.

The most relevant study is an investigation of 'hovering' by a 2-D model wing in still air executing harmonic translational and rotational motions about the mid-chord axis (Freymuth, 1990). This is broadly similar to the hovering kinematics of most insects. The amplitudes of the two movements were varied in an attempt to identify the conditions for maximum lift production. Lift was estimated at a Reynolds number of 1700 from velocity measurements in the wake using a Pitot tube, but the velocities proved too low for very accurate readings. Some extraordinarily high lifts were reported and need to be verified, but they occurred under conditions that are not too unreasonable for insects such as hoverflies and dragonflies with high-lift, low-amplitude wingbeats: translation distances of 1–2 chord lengths, and angles of attack approaching 65 ° in the middle of translation. Lift was less sensitive to translation amplitude for more moderate angles of attack, and good lift performance was obtained over distances up to about 3 chord lengths, which corresponds to the enhanced lift plateau in Dickinson's experiments.

The hovering wake was a highly structured, staggered array of vortices, with one vortex shed at either end of the cycle. Although details of the shedding are not clear, the stopping vortex of one half-stroke must combine with the starting vortex of the next half-stroke, as proposed in Fig. 2 for the bumblebee. More detail can be seen in Gustafson and Leben (1991), who present preliminary computational flow visualization results using a Navier–Stokes solver for the same hovering motion used by Freymuth. A leading-edge vortex forms about half-way through rotation, grows in strength during the rest of rotation and subsequent translation, and is shed from the trailing edge during the next rotation; as it is shed, it rolls up with a newly created starting vortex from the rotational motion. That such a relatively simple pattern of vortex shedding corresponds to maximum lift production was predicted by Ellington (1984*c*).

Flow visualization around insects

Much more work is needed on details of the high-lift mechanisms, but all of those presented above are indeed capable of generating extra lift. Which ones do insects actually use? Their wing motions are a subtle blend of smoothly coupled 3-D flapping, rotational and cambering movements. Studies on high-lift mechanisms are primarily 2-D with simplified motions that are usually uncoupled. It is difficult to predict how those results might apply to real wings, because vortex shedding is likely to be concentrated at those moments when different motions are coupled at the ends of the half-strokes. The creation and subsequent shedding of vorticity by the wings are direct manifestations of the lift force, and if we could visualize the vortex patterns produced by insects we might be able to identify the associated mechanisms.

The laboratories of Brodsky and Grodnitsky have, over the past decade, produced the most detailed studies using smoke and particle visualization. Most of the early work was published in Russian, but later papers (Brodsky, 1991; Grodnitsky and Morozov 1992, 1993) and a book (Brodsky, 1994) are now in English. Recently, A. L. R. Thomas, A. P. Willmott and I have also studied the airflow around the hawkmoth *Manduca sexta*, a model for the 'normal' wing motion of most insects. A vertical smoke rake was positioned on the windtunnel axis, and different spanwise positions were examined by moving the tethered moth relative to the smoke. Flow patterns were recorded by stereophotography for sharp resolution in 3-D, and by high-speed video for good temporal detail. Final analysis of all the information is not yet complete, but we have reconstructed the flow patterns at an airspeed of $1.5\,\mathrm{m\,s^{-1}}$.

It should be noted that flow visualization around the wings is quite different from visualization of the wake, which is a method that has recently advanced flight studies of birds (Kokshaysky, 1979; Spedding *et al.* 1984; Spedding, 1986, 1987*a*,*b*) and bats (Rayner *et al.* 1986). These wake studies reveal the structure and movement of the air periodically blown downwards by the flapping wings, as modelled in modern vortex theories of flapping flight. However, wake visualization studies cannot unveil the aerodynamic mechanisms employed by the wings; they visualize air that has been blown downwards, but not the manner in which it was blown down. The reader can consult Brodsky (1991, 1994) and Grodnitsky and Morozov (1992, 1993) for discussions of the vortex wakes of insects. My present objective is to focus on the flow around the wings, and on the pattern of vortex shedding from trailing and leading edges, in an attempt to identify aerodynamic mechanisms.

The fling/peel mechanism

The flow created by the fling/peel mechanism has been visualised in studies on two butterflies: the Essex skipper *Thymelicus lineola* (Brodsky and Ivanov; 1984; Brodsky and Grodnitsky, 1985; Brodsky, 1994; Grodnitsky and Morozov, 1993) and the peacock butterfly *Inachis io* (Brodsky, 1991). Fig. 5A–C shows a side view of the clap and fling of *Inachis* with smoke streams illuminated in the sagittal (symmetry) plane; the forewings are starting to clap in Fig. 5A, they peel apart while the hindwings clap in Fig. 5B, and the hindwings peel apart in Fig. 5C. A strong rush of air into the gap between the wings is created by the peel, confirming expectations about the mechanism. This flow is best seen starting with Fig. 5D, when the wings have moved out of the way. A relatively small leading-edge vortex is formed (Fig. 5B), as predicted for the actual peeling motion, instead of the large vortex of an idealised, rigid fling. There is little shedding of starting vorticity from the trailing edges as the downstroke begins (Fig. 5C). The fling/peel is clearly quite effective in creating bound vorticity during the rotational phase of movement, and the bound vortex of either wing pair acts as the starting vortex for the other. The counter-clockwise vortex close to the outer edge of the forewing in Fig. 5C is the tip vortex in sagittal section, and it convects downwards and backwards during the downstroke (Fig. 5C,D). It is joined at the wing tips, out of the plane of smoke, to the

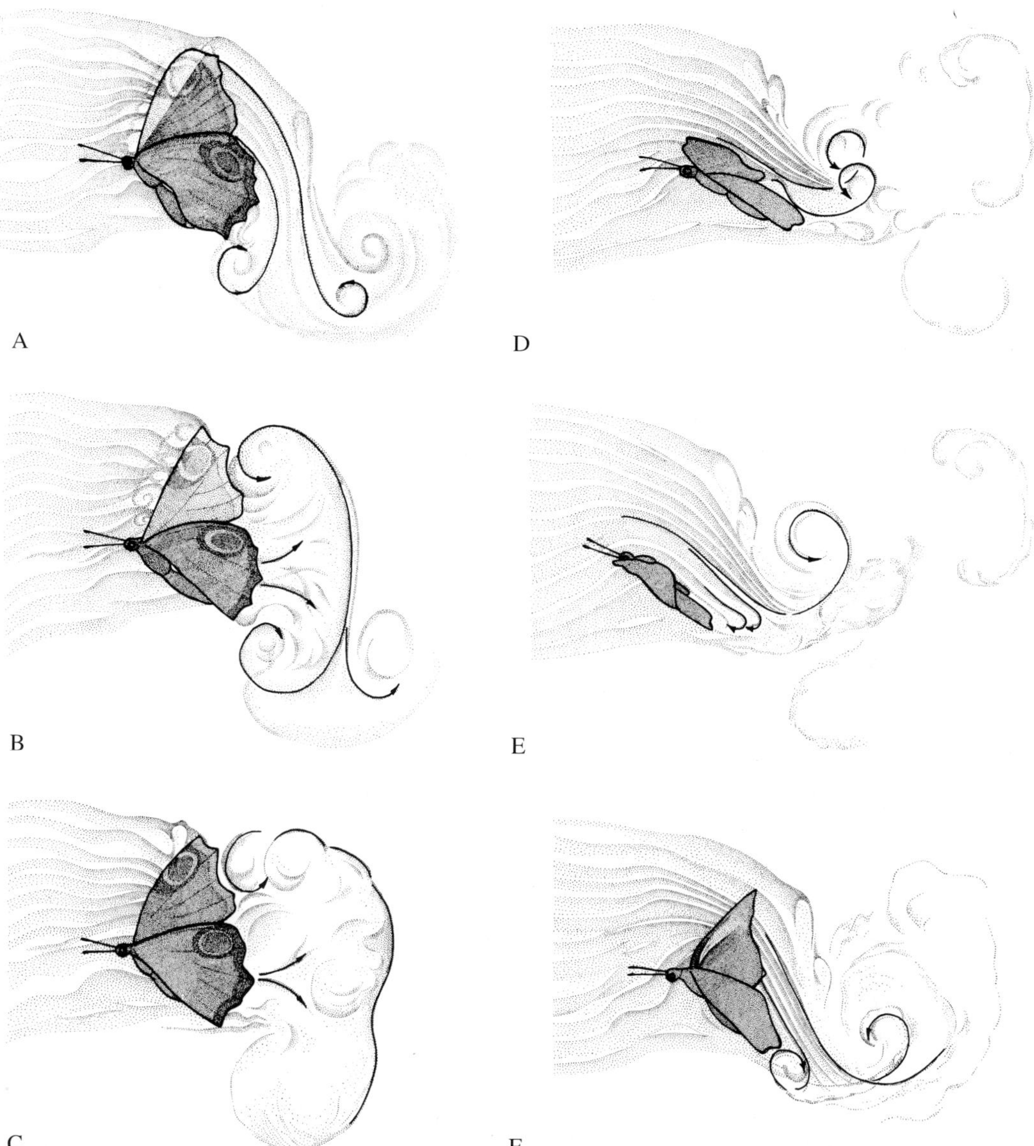

Fig. 5. Drawings from smoke flow visualization in the sagittal plane for a tethered peacock butterfly *Inachis io*. Arrows summarise airflows. Adapted from Brodsky (1991). See text for details.

bound vortex of each wing, forming a vortex loop structure. The leading-edge vortices, if they persist during the downstroke, are also out of the plane of smoke and cannot be seen. The strong downward and backward impulse imparted to the air during the downstroke, providing lift and thrust, is clearly seen by the airflow over the body.

The airflow pattern for the skipper is very similar (Brodsky and Ivanov, 1984; Brodsky and Grodnitsky, 1985; reviewed in English by Brodsky, 1994), except that Grodnitsky

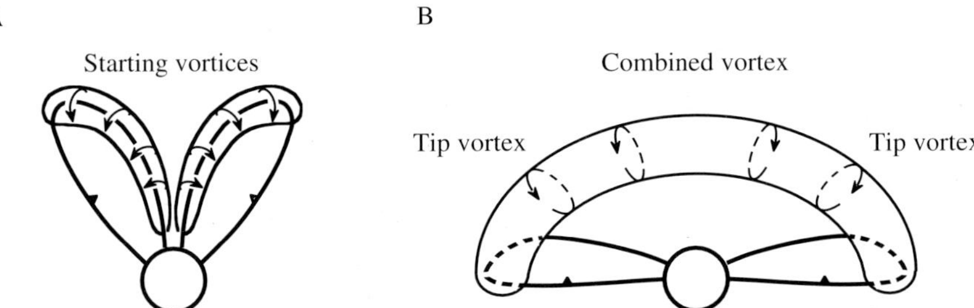

Fig. 6. Formation of the vortex loop structure on the downstroke for insects that perform a near fling, viewed perpendicular to the stroke plane. (A) Starting vortices are shed at the beginning of the downstroke. Their proximal ends join up in the sagittal plane, forming a combined vortex with uniform curvature. The combined vortex is connected to the wings by tip vortices, producing the vortex loop in B. Adapted from Grodnitsky and Morozov (1993).

and Morozov (1993) rarely detected leading-edge vortices. They suggest that leading-edge separation is prevented by the effects of wing surface microstructure or deformation, and tentatively conclude that the vortices are absent. However, they admit that such vortices might be too small for their particle visualization technique to detect.

The near fling/peel

Grodnitsky and Morozov (1993) also studied four species (two bugs, a muscid fly and a crane fly) that perform a near clap and fling during pronation, but the wings do not actually touch. As the wings accelerate at the beginning of the downstroke, transverse starting vortices are shed by each wing (Fig. 6A). Their proximal ends migrate towards the sagittal plane and join up after the wings have moved 45–60 °, resulting in a single, combined starting vortex. This resembles the 'dorsal vortex' in the sagittal plane of the skipper and the peacock butterfly, but it is composed of transverse rather than tip vorticity. The combined vortex connects smoothly to the tip vortices, and therefore to the wings, forming the vortex loop structure of the downstroke (Fig. 6B).

Brodsky (1986) obtained somewhat different results for another crane fly species. He observed that the starting vortices did not join up during the downstroke, but this could be explained if the dorsal extent of the wingbeat was lower than for Grodnitsky's and Morozov's crane fly: tethering can easily introduce such kinematic differences. The starting vortices would then be well separated by the crane fly's stalked wings and the angle between them, and they may not join to form the combined vortex reported by Grodnitsky and Morozov.

Airflow around the green lacewing *Chrysopa dasyptera* was studied by Grodnitsky and Morozov (1992). They do not describe the motion of the uncoupled wings in detail, but their photographs and drawings suggest that it is similar to that of *C. carnea*: a near/partial fling/peel for the forewings during pronation and for the hindwings during pronation and supination (Ellington, 1984*b*). Grodnitsky and Morozov observed that transverse starting vortices are shed from the forewings after their near/partial fling, and these vortices join up in the sagittal plane as described above. A similar pattern is generated by the hindwings, resulting in another common starting vortex. The two common vortices then coalesce into a single large dorsal vortex, which connects to the wings *via* the tip vortices, and this vortex loop dominates the downstroke.

These results provide ambiguous evidence that the near fling/peel creates circulation during the rotational phase, which is exploited upon subsequent translation. The starting vorticity shed at the beginning of translation is consistent with that mechanism, but also with delayed stall. Without clear proof of a leading-edge vortex created during rotation, of correct sense for recapture upon translation, these two mechanisms cannot be distinguished. A leading-edge vortex was not observed in any of the studies, but it might have been too small for the particle visualization techniques. Using the more sensitive smoke visualization method, we searched for a leading-edge vortex during pronation for *Manduca*, but to little avail. However, we obtained indirect support for the near fling/peel using high-speed video recording of the flow in the sagittal plane. There is some natural variation in the separation distance between the pronating wings, and the downwash at the beginning of the downstroke was greater when this distance was smaller. Thus, it appears that *Manduca* produces more powerful downstrokes when the near fling/peel separation is smaller, which is not consistent with the delayed stall mechanism.

Isolated rotation

For most insects, the effects of rotation without interference from the other wing are best studied in supination. Results for the Essex skipper (Brodsky and Ivanov, 1984; Brodsky and Grodnitsky, 1985; reviewed in English by Brodsky, 1994; Grodnitsky and Morozov, 1993) and other insects (Grodnitsky and Morozov, 1993) are very similar. As the flapping slows down and the wing begins to supinate, the air continues to flow smoothly over the upper wing surface but deviates somewhat radially towards the wing tip. Shedding from the trailing edge is observed late in supination (see Fig. 5E for the butterfly). The rolled-up vortex has the sense of a stopping vortex for the downstroke and, perhaps, a starting vortex for the upstroke. The vortices from the left and right wings join together across the midline during the upstroke, forming a combined, clockwise 'ventral vortex'. The point at which they join together varies somewhat between species, and Brodsky (1986) found that they did not connect for the stalked wings of the crane fly.

As with the near fling, these flow visualization results are equivocal. Shedding of the downstroke stopping vortex late in supination is consistent both with the flex mechanism and with the delayed stall of a wing with rapidly increasing angle of attack. A separate starting vortex for the upstroke has not been reported, so if there is upstroke lift then the stopping and starting vortices must roll up as a combined supination vortex. Circulatory lift on the upstroke is verified by upstroke tip vortices for *Manduca* and all of the insects investigated by Brodsky (e.g. 1986, 1991, 1994). Conversely, Grodnitsky and Morozov (1992, 1993) failed to observe upstroke tip vortices for their insects. Their description of a 'fan-like throw-off' during pronation suggests that some stopping vorticity is shed at the end of the upstroke, however, so corresponding bound and tip vortices must be present. The tip vortices would have the same sense of rotation as the downstroke tip vortices, and would be in very close proximity to them; the experiments were performed in still air, which compresses the wake structure compared with windtunnel results and keeps the tip vortices close together. It seems more probable that upstroke tip vortices were indeed shed but quickly rolled up into the stronger downstroke tip vortices. To me, the weight of evidence is certainly in favour of a lifting upstroke with reversed circulation.

Is the upstroke circulation created by the flex mechanism during rotation or by delayed stall during the initial phase of translation? Clear proof of a leading-edge vortex during rotation, of correct sense for recapture upon translation, would support the flex mechanism. Only for the skipper, however, has a small leading-edge vortex been observed near the start of the upstroke (Brodsky, 1994). More commonly reported is that the combined supination vortex grows in strength during the upstroke (e.g. Fig. 5E,F and A), suggesting that starting vorticity is still shed during the translational phase and that the bound vortex increases during the upstroke. If this is the case, then the delayed stall mechanism would be operative.

Our flow visualization of supination for *Manduca* may have resolved the issue. Fig. 7A shows a small leading-edge bubble at the end of the downstroke. The separated flow re-attaches over the posterior wing area and moves radially towards the tip, where it rolls up into the tip vortex of the downstroke. The circulatory flow remains until the very end of supination, when a transverse stopping vortex swirls off the trailing edge (Fig. 7B). This downstroke stopping vortex is separated, temporally and spatially, from the formation of an upstroke starting vortex during translation. Although the separation can be small, it is often quite pronounced, as in Fig. 7C; the figure also shows a tip vortex where the wingtip cuts the smoke in the late upstroke, confirming the presence of an upstroke bound vortex. The stopping and starting vortices coalesce into a rather large, messy supination vortex in which the two vortices may (Fig. 7A,C) or may not (Fig. 7B) be distinguishable after a short time. Shedding of the upstroke starting vortex is similar to that for a wing in pure translation, and there is no indication that the upstroke circulation is created during the preceding rotation.

Concluding remarks

Identification of the high-lift mechanisms employed by insects has proved remarkably difficult. Two-dimensional studies on rigid, model wings have established the effectiveness of several mechanisms and shown distinctive patterns of vortex shedding, particularly for the phasing of leading-edge shedding. However, the large leading-edge vortices of 2-D experiments are missing around the real insect wings, making many flow visualization results inconclusive. The fling/peel mechanism works, but the leading-edge vortex is much smaller than anticipated. The near fling/peel is the most widespread wing motion during pronation, but a leading-edge vortex has not been observed, and evidence that the near fling/peel creates circulation prior to downstroke translation is indirect at best. Judging by *Manduca*, the flex mechanism of producing circulation by isolated rotation is not used in supination; circulation is created instead by delayed stall on the upstroke. Whether circulation is generated by hoverflies and *Drosophila* using a delayed rotation, overlapping the onset of translation, has not been investigated. And finally, the relative importance of translation and rotation remains unclear for the powerful, small-

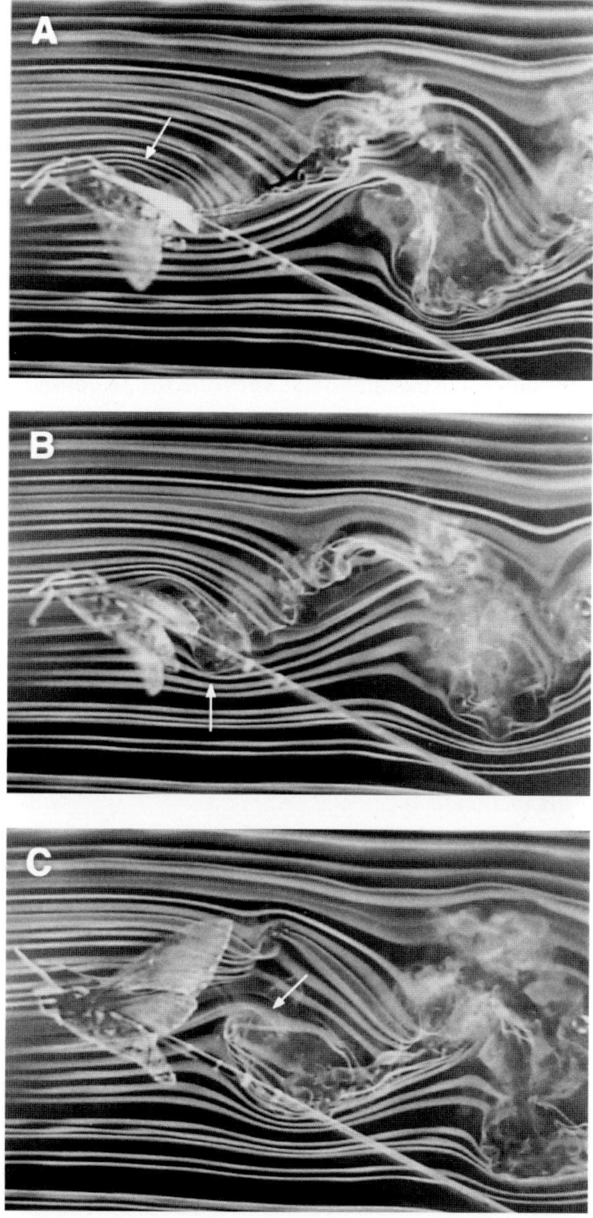

Fig. 7. Flow visualization for the hawkmoth *Manduca sexta* at 1.5 m s^{-1}. (A) A small leading-edge vortex (arrow) is visible at the end of the downstroke. (B) The bound vortex of the downstroke is shed as a stopping vortex (arrow) from the trailing edge at the end of supination. (C) The transverse starting vortex (arrow) for the upstroke is created during early translation and is distinct from the downstroke stopping vortex.

amplitude downstrokes of dragonflies (Brodsky, 1994; Reavis and Luttges, 1988; Luttges, 1989; Saharon and Luttges, 1989).

Why is the leading-edge vortex so elusive? During pronation and supination, the 'peeling' motion is likely to reduce the size of the vortex compared with 2-D expectations from rigid models. But should it virtually disappear? During translation, we see it reasonably clearly for *Manduca* over the outer half of the wing length during the downstroke, but otherwise it is not convincing. When visible, the leading-edge vortex covers about half the chord and does not protrude very far above the wing surface. Seeing it with smoke is difficult enough, and it is probably undetectable with the particle visualization of Grodnitsky and Morozov (1992, 1993).

One possible reason for the small size of leading-edge vortices could be a spanwise flow component over the aerodynamic upper surface, which transports vorticity towards the wingtip before it has much time to roll up. We have observed this spanwise flow in stereophotographs of the downstroke and the upstroke for *Manduca*; it extends from near the wing base all the way out to the tip and can displace smoke filaments radially by up to 1/4 of the wing length as they move from leading to trailing edge. The air motion is similar to the 'fan-like throw-off' described by Grodnitsky and Morozov (1992, 1993) for pronation and supination, but we see it during translation as well.

This radial flow component, probably arising from centrifugal acceleration, is very similar to the spanwise transport of vorticity within the large leading-edge vortex created by a rigid fling in Maxworthy's (1979) 3-D model, as discussed earlier. That vortex was unstable in a 2-D model, and he suggested that the spanwise transport acts to stabilise the fling vortex in natural flight. We now see that spanwise transport is probably a general phenomenon for flapping insect flight. It should reduce and stabilise any leading-edge vortices that are present, which is essential for preventing stall and maintaining the circulation of high-lift mechanisms.

I am grateful to A. P. Willmott for many discussions and for comments on the manuscript. The work on *Manduca sexta* was supported by grants from the Science and Engineering Research Council and from the Hasselblad Foundation.

References

AZUMA, A., AZUMA, S., WATANABE, I. AND FURUTA, T. (1985). Flight mechanics of a dragonfly. *J. exp. Biol.* **116**, 79–107.

AZUMA, A. AND WATANABE, T. (1988). Flight performance of a dragonfly. *J. exp. Biol.* **137**, 221–252.

BENNETT, L. (1970). Insect flight: lift and rate of change of incidence. *Science* **167**, 177–179.

BENNETT, L. (1977). Clap and fling aerodynamics – an experimental evaluation. *J. exp. Biol.* **69**, 261–272.

BRODSKY, A. K. (1986). Flight of insects with high wingbeat frequencies. *Ent. obozr.* **65**, 269–279. (In Russian).

BRODSKY, A. K. (1991). Vortex formation in the tethered flight of the peacock butterfly *Inachis io* L. (Lepidoptera, Nymphalidae) and some aspects of insect flight evolution. *J. exp. Biol.* **161**, 77–95.

BRODSKY, A. K. (1994). *The Evolution of Insect Flight.* Oxford: Oxford University Press.

BRODSKY, A. K. AND GRODNITSKY, D. L. (1985). Aerodynamics of tethered flight of skipper *Thymelicus lineola* Ochs. (Lepidoptera, Hesperiidae). *Ent. obozr.* **64**, 484–492. (In Russian).

BRODSKY, A. K. AND IVANOV, V. D. (1984). The role of vortices in insect flight. *Zool. Zhurn.* **63**, 197–208. (In Russian).

CLOUPEAU, M., DEVILLIERS, J. F. AND DEVEZEAUX, D. (1979). Direct measurements of instantaneous lift in desert locust; comparison with Jensen's experiments on detached wings. *J. exp. Biol.* **180**, 1–15.

DICKINSON, M. H. (1994). The effects of wing rotation on unsteady aerodynamic performance at low Reynolds numbers. *J. exp. Biol.* **192**, 179–206.

DICKINSON, M. H. AND GÖTZ, K. G. (1993). Unsteady aerodynamic performance of model wings at low Reynolds numbers. *J. exp. Biol.* **174**, 45–64.

DICKINSON, M. H., LEHMANN, F.-O. AND GÖTZ, K. G. (1993). The active control of wing rotation by *Drosophila*. *J. exp. Biol.* **182**, 173–189.

DUDLEY, R. (1991). Biomechanics of flight in neotropical butterflies: aerodynamics and mechanical power requirements. *J. exp. Biol.* **159**, 335–357.

DUDLEY, R. AND ELLINGTON, C. P. (1990*a*). Mechanics of forward flight in bumblebees. I. Kinematics and morphology. *J. exp. Biol.* **148**, 19–52.

DUDLEY, R. AND ELLINGTON, C. P. (1990*b*). Mechanics of forward flight in bumblebees. II. Quasi-steady lift and power requirements. *J. exp. Biol.* **148**, 53–88.

EDWARDS, R. H. AND CHENG, H. K. (1982). The separation vortex in the Weis-Fogh circulation-generation mechanism. *J. Fluid Mech.* **120**, 463–473.

ELLINGTON, C. P. (1975). Non-steady-state aerodynamics of the flight of *Encarsia formosa*. In *Swimming and Flying in Nature*, vol. 2 (ed. T. Y. Wu, C. J. Brokaw and C. Brennen), pp. 783–796. New York: Plenum Press.

ELLINGTON, C. P. (1980). Vortices and hovering flight. In *Instationäre Effekte an Schwingenden Tierflügeln* (ed. W. Nachtigall), pp. 64–101. Wiesbaden: Franz Steiner.

ELLINGTON, C. P. (1984*a*). The aerodynamics of hovering insect flight. II. Morphological parameters. *Phil. Trans. R. Soc. Lond. B* **305**, 17–40.

ELLINGTON, C. P. (1984*b*). The aerodynamics of hovering insect flight. III. Kinematics. *Phil. Trans. R. Soc. Lond. B* **305**, 41–78.

ELLINGTON, C. P. (1984*c*). The aerodynamics of hovering insect flight. IV. Aerodynamic mechanisms. *Phil. Trans. R. Soc. Lond. B* **305**, 79–113.

ELLINGTON, C. P. (1984*d*). The aerodynamics of hovering insect flight. V. A vortex theory. *Phil. Trans. R. Soc. Lond. B* **305**, 115–144.

ELLINGTON, C. P. (1984*e*). The aerodynamics of hovering insect flight. VI. Lift and power requirements. *Phil. Trans. R. Soc. Lond. B* **305**, 145–181.

ENNOS, A. R. (1989). The kinematics and aerodynamics of the free flight of some Diptera. *J. exp. Biol.* **142**, 49–85.

FARREN, W. S. (1935). The reaction on a wing whose angle of incidence is changing rapidly. *Rep. Memo. aeronaut. Res. Comm. (Coun.)* no. 1648.

FRANCIS, R. H. AND COHEN, J. (1933). The flow near a wing which starts suddenly from rest and then stalls. *Rep. Memo. aeronaut. Res. Comm. (Coun.)* no. 1561.

FREYMUTH, P. (1990). Thrust generation by an airfoil in hover modes. *Expts Fluids* **9**, 17–24.

GRODNITSKY, D. L. AND MOROZOV, P. P. (1992). Flow visualization experiments on tethered flying green lacewings *Chrysopa dasyptera*. *J. exp. Biol.* **169**, 143–163.

GRODNITSKY, D. L. AND MOROZOV, P. P. (1993). Vortex formation during tethered flight of functionally and morphologically two-winged insects, including evolutionary considerations on insect flight. *J. exp. Biol.* **182**, 11–40.

GURSUL, I. AND HO, C-M. (1992). High aerodynamic loads on an airfoil submerged in an unsteady stream. *AIAA J.* **30(4)**, 1117–1119.

GUSTAFSON, K. AND LEBEN, R. (1991). Computation of dragonfly aerodynamics. *Comp. Phys. Comms* **65**, 121–132.

HAUSSLING, H. J. (1979). Boundary-fitted coordinates for accurate numerical solution of multi-body flow problems. *J. comput. Phys.* **30**, 107–124.

JENSEN, M. (1956). Biology and physics of locust flight. III. The aerodynamics of locust flight. *Phil. Trans. R. Soc. Lond. B* **239**, 511–552.

KOKSHAYSKY, N. V. (1979). Tracing the wake of a flying bird. *Nature* **279**, 146–148.

KRAMER, M. (1932). Die Zunahme des Maximalauftriebes von Tragflügeln bei plötzlicher Anstellwinkelvergrösserung (Böeneffekt). *Z. Flugtech. Motorluftschiff.* **23**, 185–189.

LIGHTHILL, M. J. (1973). On the Weis-Fogh mechanism of lift generation. *J. Fluid Mech.* **60**, 1–17.

LUTTGES, M. W. (1989). Accomplished insect fliers. In *Frontiers in Experimental Fluid Mechanics* (ed. M. Gad-el-Hak). Lecture Notes in Engineering 46. Berlin: Springer.

MARESCA, C., FAVIER, D. AND REBONT, J. (1979). Experiments on an aerofoil at high angle of incidence in longitudinal oscillations. *J. Fluid Mech.* **92**, 671–690.

MAXWORTHY, T. (1979). Experiments on the Weis-Fogh mechanism of lift generation by insects in hovering flight. Part 1. Dynamics of the 'fling'. *J. Fluid Mech.* **93**, 47–63.

McCULLOUGH, G. B. AND GAULT, D. E. (1951). Examples of three representative types of airfoil-section stall at low speed. *Tech. Notes natn. advis. Comm. Aeronaut., Washington* no. 2502.

NACHTIGALL, W. (1979). Rasche Richtungsänderungen und Torsionen schwingender Fliegenflügel und Hypothesen über zugeordnete instationäre Strömungseffekte. *J. comp. Physiol.* **133**, 351–355.

NEWMAN, B. G., SAVAGE, S. B. AND SCHOUELLA, D. (1977). Model tests on a wing section of an *Aeschna* dragonfly. In *Scale Effects in Animal Locomotion* (ed. T. J. Pedley), pp. 445–477. London: Academic Press.

NORBERG, R. Å. (1975). Hovering flight of the dragonfly *Aeschna juncea.* L., kinematics and aerodynamics. In *Swimming and Flying in Nature*, vol. 2 (ed. T. Y. Wu, C. J. Brokaw and C. Brennen), pp. 763–781. New York: Plenum Press.

NORBERG, U. M. (1975). Hovering flight of the pied flycatcher (*Ficedula hypoleuca*). In *Swimming and Flying in Nature*, vol. 2 (ed. T. Y. Wu, C. J. Brokaw and C. Brennen), pp. 869–881. New York: Plenum Press.

NORBERG, U. M. (1976*a*). Kinematics, aerodynamics and energetics of horizontal flapping flight in the long-eared bat *Plecotus auritus. J. exp. Biol.* **65**, 179–212.

NORBERG, U. M. (1976*b*). Aerodynamics of hovering flight in the long-eared bat *Plecotus auritus. J. exp. Biol.* **65**, 459–470.

PENNYCUICK, C. J. (1968). Power requirements for horizontal flight in the pigeon *Columba livia. J. exp. Biol.* **49**, 527–555.

RAYNER, J. M. V., JONES, G. AND THOMAS, A. (1986). Vortex flow visualizations reveal change in upstroke function with flight speed in bats. *Nature* **321**, 162–164.

REAVIS, M. A. AND LUTTGES, M. W. (1988). Aerodynamic forces produced by a dragonfly. *AIAA* Paper no. 80-0330.

RÜPPELL, G. (1977). The course of the upper-side flow on a wing model of the Fulmar (*Fulmaris glacialis*) in slow flight. In *The Physiology of Movement; Biomechanics* (ed. W. Nachtigall), pp. 287–295. Stuttgart: Fischer.

SAHARON, D. AND LUTTGES, M. W. (1989). Dragonfly unsteady aerodynamics: the role of the wing phase relations in controlling the produced flows. *AIAA* Paper no. 89-0832.

SAVAGE, S. B., NEWMAN, B. G. AND WONG, D. T.-M. (1979). The role of vortices and unsteady effects during the hovering flight of dragonflies. *J. exp. Biol.* **83**, 59–77.

SOMPS, C. AND LUTTGES, M. (1985). Dragonfly flight: novel uses of unsteady separated flows. *Science* **228**, 1326–1329.

SPEDDING, G. R. (1986). The wake of a jackdaw (*Corvus monedula*) in slow flight. *J. exp. Biol.* **125**, 287–307.

SPEDDING, G. R. (1987*a*). The wake of a kestrel (*Falco tinnunculus*) in gliding flight. *J. exp. Biol.* **127**, 45–57.

SPEDDING, G. R. (1987*b*). The wake of a kestrel (*Falco tinnunculus*) in flapping flight. *J. exp. Biol.* **127**, 59–78.

SPEDDING, G. R. (1992). The aerodynamics of flight. In *Mechanics of Animal Locomotion* (ed. R. McN. Alexander), *Adv. comp. env. Physiol.* **11**, 51–111. Berlin: Springer-Verlag.

SPEDDING, G. R. (1993). On the significance of unsteady effects in the aerodynamic performance of flying animals. *Contemp. Maths* **141**, 401–419.

SPEDDING, G. R. AND DELAURIER, J. D. (1995). Animal and ornithopter flight. In *Handbook of Fluid Dynamics and Fluid Machinery* (ed. J. A. Schetz and A. E. Fuhs). New York: Wiley (in press).

SPEDDING, G. R. AND MAXWORTHY, T. (1986). The generation of circulation and lift in a rigid two-dimensional fling. *J. Fluid Mech.* **165**, 247–272.

SPEDDING, G. R., RAYNER, J. M. V. AND PENNYCUICK, C. J. (1984). Momentum and energy in the wake of a pigeon (*Columba livia*) in slow flight. *J. exp. Biol.* **111**, 81–102.

SUNADA, S., KAWACHI, K., WATANABE, I. AND AZUMA, A. (1993). Fundamental analysis of three-dimensional 'near fling'. *J. exp. Biol.* **183**, 217–248.

TANI, I. (1964). Low-speed flows involving bubble separations. *Prog. aeronaut. Sci.* **5**, 70–103.

THOM, A. AND SWART, P. (1940). The forces on an aerofoil at very low speeds. *J. R. aeronaut. Soc.* **44**, 761–770.

VOGEL, S. (1967). Flight in *Drosophila*. III. Aerodynamic characteristics of fly wings and wing models. *J. exp. Biol.* **46**, 431–443.

WEIS-FOGH, T. (1956). Biology and physics of locust flight. II. Flight performance of the desert locust (*Schistocerca gregaria*). *Phil. Trans. R. Soc. Lond. B* **239**, 459–510.

WEIS-FOGH, T. (1972). Energetics of hovering flight in hummingbirds and in *Drosophila*. *J. exp. Biol.* **56**, 79–104.

WEIS-FOGH, T. (1973). Quick estimates of flight fitness in hovering animals, including novel mechanisms for lift production. *J. exp. Biol.* **59**, 169–230.

WELLS, D. J. (1993). Muscle performance in hovering hummingbirds. *J. exp. Biol.* **178**, 39–57.

WILKIN, P. J. (1990). The instantaneous force on a desert locust, *Schistocerca gregaria* (Orthoptera: Acrididae), flying in a wind tunnel. *J. Kansas ent. Soc.* **63**, 316–328.

WILKIN, P. J. AND WILLIAMS, M. H. (1993). Comparison of the aerodynamic forces on a flying sphingid moth with those predicted by quasi-steady theory. *Physiol. Zool.* **66**, 1015–1044.

WU, J. AND HU-CHEN, H. (1984). Unsteady aerodynamics of articulate lifting bodies. *AIAA* Paper no. 2184.

ZANKER, J. M. AND GÖTZ, K. G. (1990). The wing beat of *Drosophila melanogaster*. II. Dynamics. *Phil. Trans. R. Soc. Lond. B* **327**, 19–44.

DYNAMICS OF THE VORTEX WAKES OF FLYING AND SWIMMING VERTEBRATES

JEREMY M. V. RAYNER

School of Biological Sciences, University of Bristol, Woodland Road, Bristol BS8 1UG, UK

Summary

The vortex wakes of flying and swimming animals provide evidence of the history of aero- and hydrodynamic force generation during the locomotor cycle. Vortex-induced momentum flux in the wake is the reaction of forces the animal imposes on its environment, which must be in equilibrium with inertial and external forces.

In flying birds and bats, the flapping wings generate lift both to provide thrust and to support the weight. Distinct wingbeat and wake movement patterns can be identified as gaits. In flow visualization experiments, only two wake patterns have been identified: a vortex ring gait with inactive upstroke, and a continuous vortex gait with active upstroke. These gaits may be modelled theoretically by free vortex and lifting line theory to predict mechanical energy consumption, aerodynamic forces and muscle activity. Longer-winged birds undergo a distinct gait change with speed, but shorter-winged species use the vortex ring gait at all speeds.

In swimming fish, the situation is more complex: the wake vortices form a reversed von Kármán vortex street, but little is known about the mechanism of generation of the wake, or about how it varies with speed and acceleration or with body form and swimming mode. An unresolved complicating factor is the interaction between the drag wake of the flapping fish body and the thrusting wake from the tail.

Introduction

'For every action there is an equal and opposite reaction'. As an animal moves in a fluid, it experiences inertial, gravitational and frictional forces, and must impose forces on the fluid so that it is in equilibrium. A flying bird or a swimming fish leaves a momentum flow in its wake as evidence of the propelling and sustaining forces it has generated. At the Reynolds numbers typical of flying vertebrates, and of all but the smallest swimming fish, the wake momentum must be accompanied by vortex structures, because closed-loop vortices are the only mechanism of momentum flux in an inviscid fluid. The vortices induce the fluid movements which are the reaction of the forces generated by the animal, and effectively therefore define the wake.

The wake vortices are an essential component of the locomotion mechanics of any swimming or flying vertebrate. The animal must expend energy to generate the vortices (this is experienced as induced drag), and this has led to a common claim in the literature

Key words: flight, swimming, vortex, wake, bird, bat, fish, aerodynamics, hydrodynamics, wing, tail.

that the vortex wake is detrimental, and should be eliminated. *This is false*. Without the vortices, there could be no momentum flux, and hence no movement. However, the energy invested in the vortices can be considerable, and the vortex wake should be optimized to minimize energy consumption, while maintaining the force (or momentum transport) required for locomotion.

One approach to the mechanical problems of swimming and flying is therefore to consider the problem of generating an efficient vortex wake. How should this be done? Drag-based paddling or rowing gives rise to local, intense drag vortices which are generally inefficient and cannot generate sufficient lift for flying vertebrates; because the paddling limb or fin must travel backwards relative to the water, rowing is restricted to relatively slow swimming. Lifting structures such as the aerofoil or hydrofoil are more effective; the aircraft wing is an obvious and well-studied example, and bird wings and some fish tails operate by the same mechanism. Other force-generating mechanisms used for thrust in swimming and flying, such as propellers and jets, also produce vortex wakes, but for anatomical and morphological reasons have no direct analogue in vertebrates (but see Fish, 1987).

Aerofoil vortices have a number of important properties which make them valuable for the study of locomotion. They are symptomatic of lift generation: a flow in the wake – which may be located and quantified by flow visualization – is indicative of the magnitude and direction of the lift force when that vortex was generated. Vortices interact and deform, and tend to adopt relatively stable structures which can readily be described and interpreted. Experiment and theory indicate that there are a limited number of optimum structures, formed of vortex lines, loops and rings, which are appropriate for flying and swimming. The structure and the degree of organization of the wake are therefore measures of the competence of locomotion. Disorganized or poorly structured wakes are likely to correspond to high induced drag and, therefore, will be inefficient.

In this paper, I review experimental evidence on the wakes of swimming and flying vertebrates, concentrating on lift-based, rather than drag-based, methods of propulsion. Details of the aerodynamic background to these results, and further information on some of the theoretical treatments which may be used, are given by Rayner (1980, 1985*a*, 1993), Vogel (1981), Lugt (1983), Spedding (1992, 1993; Spedding and DeLaurier, 1995) and Azuma (1993).

Flying

Because of the obvious parallels with aircraft, the wakes of birds and bats are the best understood. [I do not discuss the extensive qualitative visualization work on flying insects – see, for example, Brodsky and Ivanov (1984), Brodsky (1988), Luttges (1989), Grodnitsky and Morozov (1993) and Ellington (1995) – except to note that flow patterns in larger insects appear to have much in common with those of smaller birds, although they may differ in structure, and that unsteady aerodynamic factors are significantly more important to flying insects than they are to vertebrates.]

The first experiments on the wakes of animals in flight did little more than demonstrate the presence of localized air currents (e.g. Demoll, 1918). The first published report on wake structures in birds was by Magnan *et al.* (1938), who used tobacco smoke to visualize *Tourbillons* (vortex rings) generated on each downstroke by a slow-flying pigeon. The wake appears the same as that later visualized at Bristol by the helium bubble technique (Spedding *et al.* 1984). In 1979, I published a theoretical model in which the wake was a series of vortex rings each associated with a single downstroke (Rayner, 1979*b*,*c*, 1980), and almost simultaneously Kokshaysky (1979, 1980; Kokshaysky and Pyetrovsky, 1979) reported experiments on finches flying through clouds of small particles. Their results concurred closely with the theoretical predictions and gave the first detailed information on the three-dimensional structure of the wake. Subsequent experiments at Bristol have enabled the wake flows to be quantified, and these are described in the following sections.

The gliding wake

The combination of the vortex ring theory and Kokshaysky's experiments confirmed that weight support and thrust are the reaction of vortex flows in the wake. Evidence that these flows are generated by aerofoil action was provided by visualization of the wake of a kestrel *Falco tinnunculus* in gliding flight (Spedding, 1987*a*). The wake consisted of a vortex sheet which was shed from the trailing edge of the wing and which rolled up within a short distance into a pair of trailing line vortices. The flow is very similar to that behind a low-speed aircraft wing and can be described by the same theoretical models (e.g. lifting-line theory; Katz and Plotkin, 1991). The trailing vortex pair is an important vortex structure since it maximizes vertical momentum while minimizing the energy required to generate the wake, or the induced drag; another wake structure with this property is the circular vortex ring, which is significant for flapping animals.

From the geometry of the wake, Spedding estimated the Munk or span efficiency of the kestrel wing as 0.96. The wing operates close to the theoretical aerodynamic optimum of an elliptically loaded wing. However, this optimum applies to fixed (gliding) wings for which induced drag for given lift is minimal, and is not necessarily appropriate for flapping wings (Rayner, 1986, 1993): alternative constraints, such as maximum thrust for given weight, maximum net thrust less total drag or minimum wing weight, are all potentially important design criteria; each is associated with a different spanwise loading (circulation) distribution and will imply different optimum wing shape. Gliding span efficiency may vary modestly from 1: the optimum thrusting wing (Jones, 1980) has a span efficiency of 8/9; the enhanced thrust offsets the increase in induced drag.

Subsequent experiments by J. M. V. Rayner and A. L. R. Thomas (unpublished) on a wider range of birds demonstrate that Spedding's results with the kestrel are representative, and that all bird wings act in gliding as slow-speed aerofoils. Span efficiencies vary from 0.79 to 1.25; higher values were obtained from the rounded wings of owls, with extensive separated primary feathers, and with substantial spanwise and chordwise camber.

As with fixed aircraft wings, the aerodynamic performance of a gliding wing will depend on wing shape; the rules that relate wing shape to ecological or behavioural factors are relatively well understood (Norberg and Rayner, 1987; Rayner, 1988), but the significance of aerodynamic constraints for wing design is less clear. Wing shape affects the distribution of circulation across the wingspan, and hence the span efficiency, lift and induced drag. Few birds have elliptical wings (these appear to occur only in high-aspect-ratio gliding birds such as larids and procellariids), and some species differ substantially in wing shape. For example, relatively short and pointed triangular wings occur in birds such as ducks (Anatini) and shorebirds (Chardriiformes); these species have high wingbeat frequencies, and it is important for them to minimize inertial forces by reducing distal wing weight and aerodynamic loading (Rayner, 1988). Wingtip shape also has a significant effect on the wake. Tucker (1993) used flow visualization methods to show that the separated primary feathers of a Harris' hawk (*Parabuteo unicinctus*) wing achieved a span efficiency of approximately 1.3 by spreading the vortex cores behind the wingtips; for this mechanism to work effectively, it is essential that the wingtip feathers be splayed vertically. There is as yet no comprehensive theoretical model of how the separate wakes from the individual primary feathers interact.

Forward flight in birds and bats

The purpose of wing flapping in steady forward flight is to generate the thrust necessary to balance drag; the mean lift is inclined forwards so that it provides a horizontal thrust as well as supporting the weight (e.g. Rayner, 1986, 1993). This means that flapping movements should be considered in terms of their contribution to horizontal force rather than vertical force; the vertical force must be present, and is usually an order of magnitude greater than the drag, but it is the presence of the horizontal thrusting component that characterizes flapping geometry. Assuming that the wings continue to generate lift by the aerofoil mechanism (subsequent work described below has confirmed that this is the case), then the vortices shed from the trailing edges of the wings will roll up into small-cored vortex lines. The mean momentum flow induced by these vortices in the wake must have downwards (supporting weight) and backwards (thrusting) components.

The wingbeat pattern is cyclic, and it is impossible to generate constant vector lift throughout. Thrust and weight support therefore vary in magnitude during the wingbeat. The strength and geometry of the vortices in the wake are symptomatic of the lift force on the wings at the time the vortices were shed (provided allowance is made for self-induced deformation of the wake, and, on a longer timescale, for viscous diffusion). Much of our work at Bristol has focused on experiments to visualize the wake flows to determine the vortex structures and to understand the aerodynamic processes involved in flapping vertebrate flight. The vortex patterns are used to develop and test theoretical models of aerodynamic forces, muscle activity and mechanical energetics in flapping flight (e.g. Rayner, 1979*b*,*c*, 1986, 1993); I have applied these models to consider factors determining migration behaviour and energetics (Rayner, 1990, 1995), wing design (Rayner, 1987, 1988), wingbeat kinematics (Rayner, 1993, 1995) and the evolution of flight (Rayner, 1991).

Vortex ring wake

The wake described by Kokshaysky (1979) in small passerines (Fig. 1A), and by Spedding in the pigeon (Spedding, 1982; Spedding *et al.* 1984; Fig. 1B) and Eurasian jackdaw *Corvus monedula* in very slow flight (Spedding, 1982, 1986), consists of a series of small-cored, near-circular vortex rings, each generated by a downstroke. The upstroke is aerodynamically inactive and generates no lift, and wake components from each downstroke remain separate, although they do interact with one another. Each ring is tilted from the horizontal, and the inclination of the ring at the time of generation is equivalent to the thrust:weight ratio. The momentum transport is proportional to the product of the strength (circulation) and the area of the ring; however, ring energy is proportional to strength squared but inversely proportional to ring diameter: a larger ring is a more efficient means of transporting momentum, although the size of the ring is limited by wingspan and the geometry of the wingbeat (Rayner 1979*b*).

Subsequent experiments have shown that this wake pattern is widespread, occurring also in bats (Rayner *et al.* 1986; Rayner, 1987). It appears to be used by all birds and bats in slow, steady flight (Fig. 1). The vortex ring description is a convenient shorthand for this structure, although the vortex distribution may be more complex than is immediately evident from the photographs. Spedding (1986) argued that vorticity may be distributed along the axis (or wake) of each individual ring, as well as in the vortex core, and the rings are sometimes elliptical initially, rather than circular. The vortex loops are frequently asymmetric: there is an intense and concentrated starting vortex, but the 'stopping' vortex formed at the end of the downstroke may be more diffuse (Rayner *et al.* 1986; Rayner and Thomas, 1991).

The measured momentum transported by each of the rings generated by a pigeon or a jackdaw was sufficient to support only about two-thirds of the animal's weight. Spedding (1986) considered that the flow measurement method might not be identifying all vorticity, and hence all momentum, in the wake, and suggested that the complexity of the vortex structure might be responsible. However, it is difficult to see how flows sufficiently intense to explain the discrepancy could fail to register in the images, and the momentum discrepancy is not present in bats. Cine-film and accelerometer measurements of pigeons in repeated experiments have shown that the bird was decelerating vertically at about $0.3g$ (J. M. V. Rayner and A. L. R. Thomas, unpublished; Rayner, 1993). The momentum in the wake is equivalent to the force experienced by the animal, but some birds either choose not to support their weight (the flight path in these experiments was short), or cannot do so at very low speeds. I suspect that the birds are close to an aerodynamic constraint: they cannot increase vortex ring size because they already use a large wingbeat amplitude and cannot increase ring strength because the bound wing circulation is near maximum. These constraints are less significant at faster flight speeds.

Continuous vortex wake

A very different wake pattern was found in long-winged animals such as the common kestrel *Falco tinnunculus* (Spedding, 1982, 1987*b*) and both micro- and megachiropteran bats (*Nyctalus noctula* and *Rousettus aegyptiacus*, Rayner *et al.* 1986; Fig. 2). Now the upstroke is aerodynamically active; air currents in the upstroke wake are downwards but *forwards*, showing that the upstroke supports the weight, but retards the animal by producing a negative thrust. The striking feature of this pattern is that wake circulations in mid-upstroke and mid-downstroke are equal, which strongly implies that the animal somehow maintains bound wing circulation constant. If the animal flew with constant

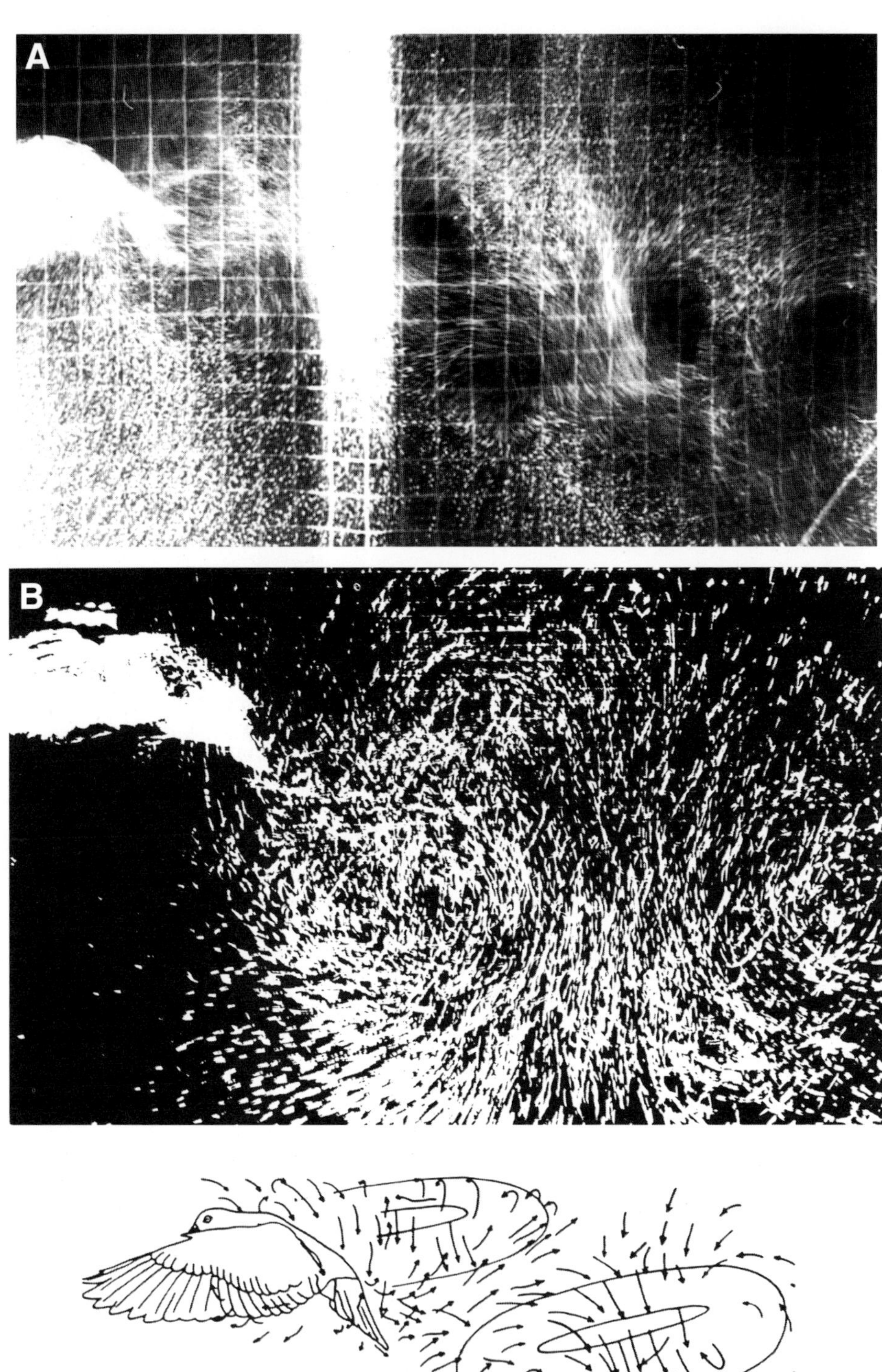
A
B

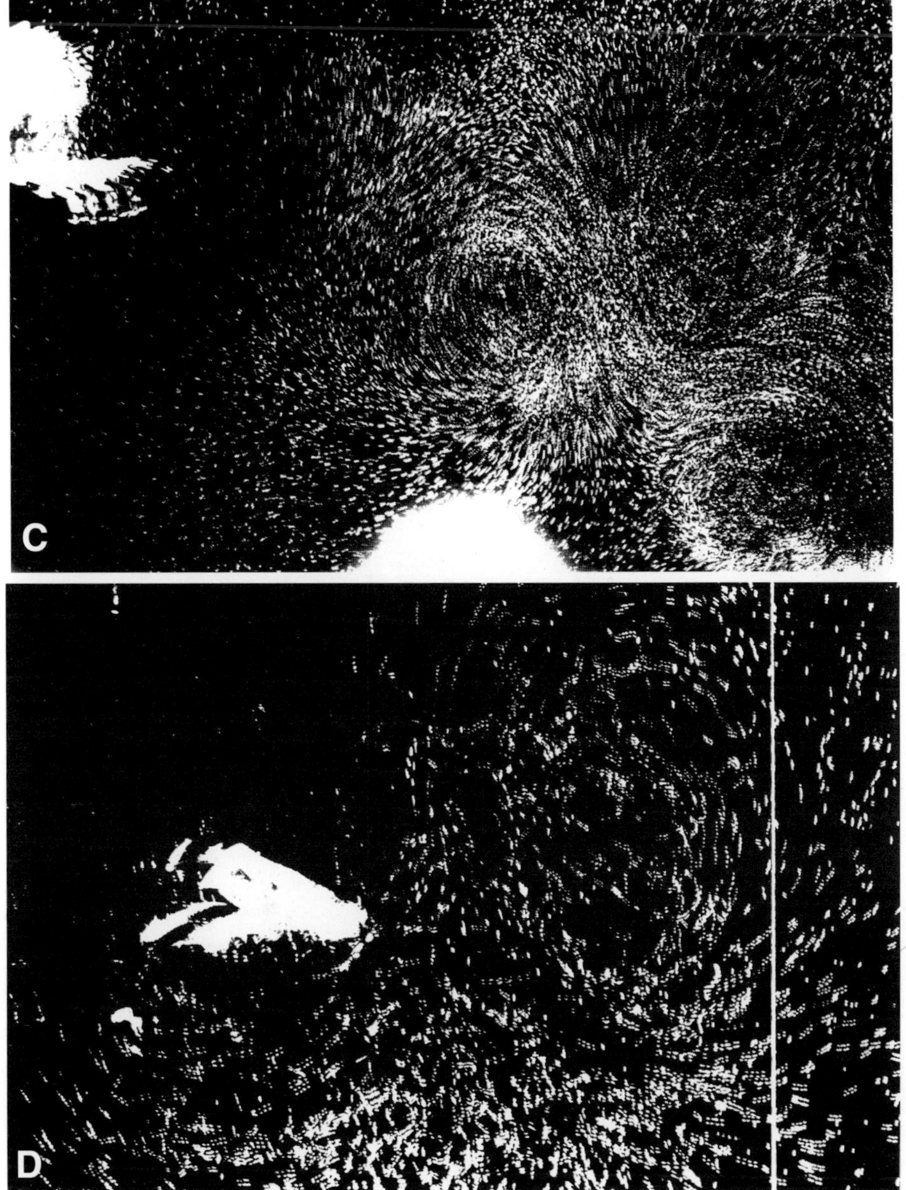

Fig. 1. Flow visualizations of animals using the vortex ring gait. (A) Chaffinch *Fringilla coelebs*, photographed by Kokshaysky flying through a cloud of dust particles. The bird is accelerating, as can be deduced from the steep inclination of the vortex rings, and is probably using bounding flight (from Kokshaysky, 1979). (B) Pigeon *Columba livia* in slow flight at approximately $2\,\mathrm{m\,s^{-1}}$. The flow is visualized by a cloud of helium-filled soap bubbles, which are neutrally buoyant and follow the movements of the air. The photograph is one of a stereo pair; three-dimensional information is used to reconstruct the pattern of the flow and the location of the vortices shown in the sketch (from Spedding, 1982; Spedding *et al.* 1984). (C) Tawny owl *Strix aluco* in steady level flight, showing a wake consisting of a series of ring vortices; note the separated primary feathers in this species. Two rings are visible, in each of which the starting vortex is clearly defined, but the stopping vortex is more diffuse (from Rayner, 1993). (D) Long-eared bat *Plecotus auritus* (Vespertilionidae) in slow flight, showing a single vortex ring part-formed (from Rayner *et al.* 1986); the ring core radius is large, possibly because of the small size of the bat, but possibly because of the structure of the bat wing.

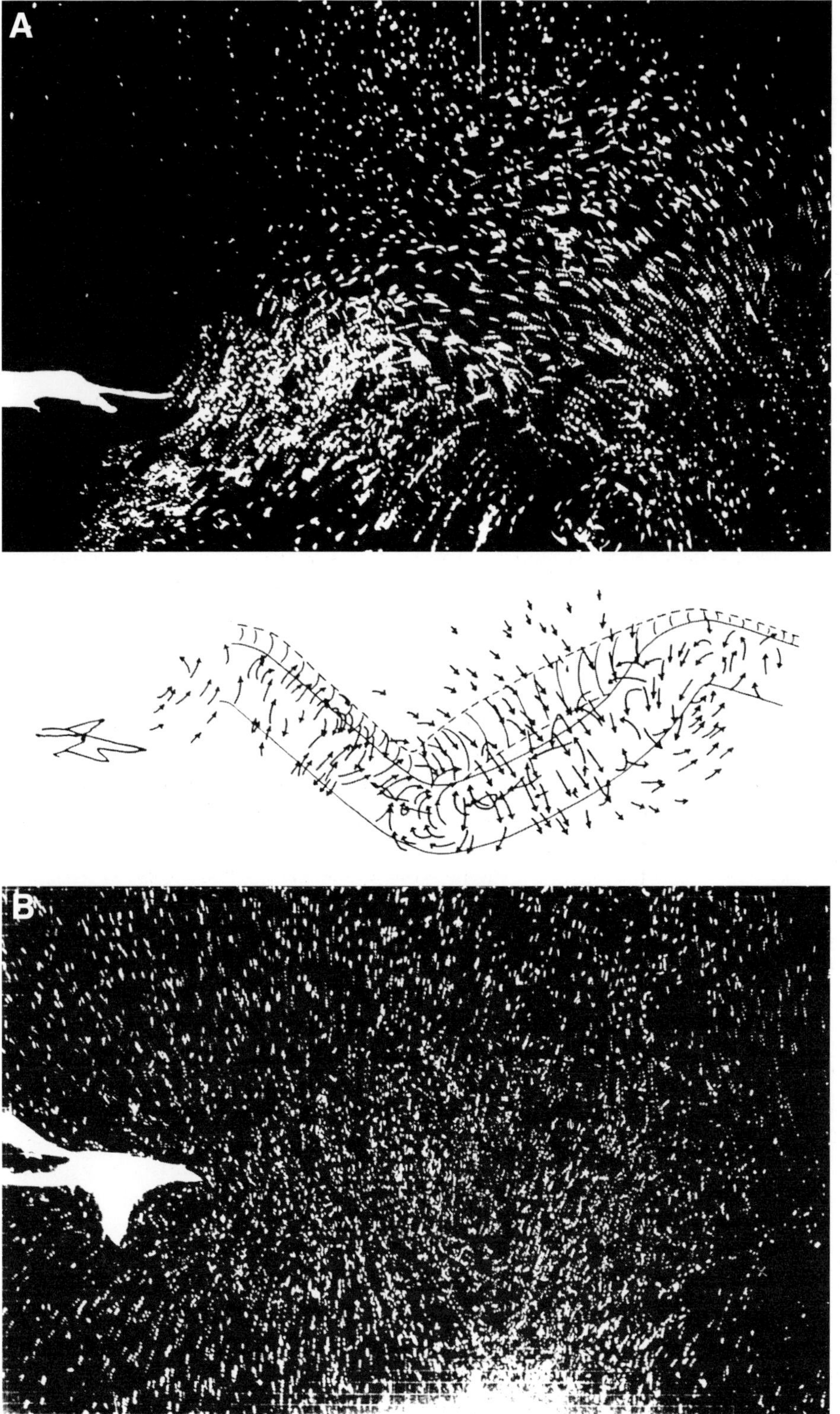

Fig. 2

Fig. 2. Flow visualizations of animals using the continuous vortex gait. (A) European kestrel *Falco tinnunculus* (Falconidae) in cruising flight (from Spedding, 1987*a*). (B) Noctule bat *Nyctalus noctula* (Vespertilionidae) in cruising flight (from Rayner *et al.* 1986); as in the long-eared bat (Fig. 1D), the vortex core diameter is relatively large.

circulation and constant wing span (i.e. with no wing flexure), thrust from the downstroke would be offset by an equal negative thrust from the upstroke and there would be no benefit from flapping the wings. The animal achieves a net forward thrust by reducing wingspan during the upstroke.

Subsequent experiments have revealed that this wake pattern is common, occurring widely in birds with relatively long or high-aspect-ratio wings at cruising speeds. The flow may be thought of as being similar to the planar gliding wake, with the vortices following the path of the wingtips as the wings are flapped. The constant circulation criterion has made this mode tractable to aerodynamic theory (Rayner, 1986, 1993), largely because the unsteady aerodynamic complications expected for large-amplitude flapping with sustained lift can be circumvented (see below); theoretical models predict wake geometry and wingbeat kinematics accurately, and there is no evidence of a momentum anomaly. Comparison with the wing skeleton of the first flying dinosaur *Archaeopteryx* suggests that this mode is primitive in birds, and is consistent with a gliding origin of flapping avian flight (Rayner, 1991).

Wingbeat kinematics and gait in birds and bats

The vortex ring and continuous vortex wake structures are the only patterns we have found in an extensive study of birds and bats of a range of sizes and taxa. Because the patterns are predictable and depend on both morphology and speed, they are referred to as gaits, by analogy with the leg movement patterns of running mammals (Rayner, 1988, 1993; Alexander, 1989).

The continuous vortex gait is used in cruising or steady fast flight by animals with relatively long or high-aspect-ratio wings; it does not occur in species with shorter or more rounded wings and is not used in slow flight. All animals appear to use the vortex ring gait at relatively slow speeds (if they can fly slowly at all), and those with smaller wings use this gait at all speeds. The gaits are distinguished functionally by the lifting action of the upstroke; in the continuous vortex gait, upstroke circulation is equal to downstroke circulation, while in the vortex ring gait upstroke circulation is zero. Gait selection is a trade-off between the weight-supporting benefit and the negative-thrust disbenefit of an active upstroke, compared with the need for enhanced downstroke lift to support weight with an inactive or weaker upstroke. By modelling upstroke lift as a function of speed, I have shown that a lifting upstroke becomes inefficient, because the direction of the lift force is unfavourable and the induced drag is too large, when the parameter:

$$\lambda \propto \boldsymbol{Mg}/[\rho\phi J_0(\phi)b^3fV]$$

exceeds a critical value (Rayner, 1993). ($\boldsymbol{Mg}$ is weight, $2b$ is wingspan, r is air density, ϕ is wingbeat frequency, ϕ is wingbeat amplitude and V is flight speed; J_0 is a Bessel function.) For short-winged animals (low M/b^3) or in slow flight (low $fV/\boldsymbol{g}$), λ is always small, the upstroke should not be used to generate aerodynamic force, and all lift is generated in the downstroke. In birds with relatively large wings, there will be a critical speed above which a lifting upstroke becomes effective: this speed should determine the gait transition.

The gait being used by any animal may readily be determined by high-speed cinematography (Scholey, 1983; Rayner, 1986, 1988, 1993). In the vortex ring gait in birds and bats, the wing flexes substantially during the upstroke, the wrist moves anterior to the shoulder, and the wingtip is brought close to the body to minimize drag and inertia. In the continuous vortex gait, the wing remains much flatter during the upstroke, but the effective span shortens by flexure at the wrist so that the tip is swept back (in birds) or by flexure of the elbow and wrist so that the wingtip is brought towards the body and the wing is shortened (in bats). Recently, Tobalske and Dial (1994) have reported studies of the kinematics of the black-billed magpie *Pica pica* and the pigeon *Columba livia*. The magpie has very short, rounded wings and does not change gait: it generates vortex rings at all speeds, and there is a smooth variation in wingbeat kinematics (e.g. frequency and amplitude) with speed. The pigeon, with longer wings, makes a discrete change in kinematics at between 8 and $10\,\mathrm{m\,s^{-1}}$, corresponding to the gait transition.

The transition between the gaits is rapid, occurring within one or two wingbeats as the animal accelerates (Rayner *et al.* 1986; Fig. 3). There appears to be some hysteresis: an

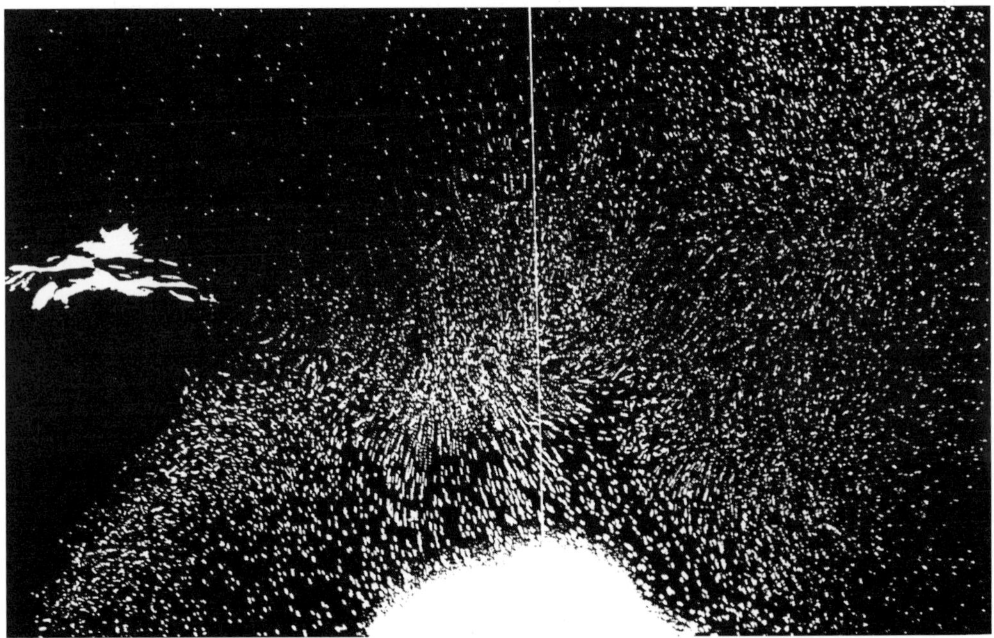

Fig. 3. The transitional wake in accelerated flight of Meyer's conure *Policephalus meyeri* (Psitaccidae). To the right of the image, the wake is a vortex ring; this is followed by a weak transverse vortex and a lifting upstroke, and then by another transverse vortex before the continuous wake begins with a downstroke. The bird is in the middle of the following upstroke. (Photograph by A. L. R. Thomas.)

upward transition (during acceleration) occurs at a higher speed than a downward transition. The speed at which the transition occurs is determined primarily by wing geometry. The gaits are distinguished not only by external (i.e. aerodynamic) force generation and by wing movements, but also by the sequence of force generation in the muscles (Rayner, 1988). Since the wing generates no lift during the upstroke in the vortex ring gait, the animal must raise the wing by active muscle force, primarily using the supracoracoideus. In the continuous vortex gait, the aerodynamic lift during the upstroke will first raise the wing relative to the body; there is a range of speeds in which the supracoracoideus is not needed to raise the wing and in which the speed of the upstroke is controlled by force from a lengthening pectoralis.

Other flapping gaits

Our flow visualization experiments have identified only two gaits in steady flapping flight. There remains the possibility that other gaits may exist in certain animals or under special conditions. Pennycuick (1988) described a possible third gait (his 'ladder' wake) in which upstroke circulation is reduced compared with downstroke circulation, but it is not clear which birds might profit from this configuration, and it is likely to be aerodynamically unfavourable since the concentrated transverse vortices at the extremes of the wingbeat will result in intense induced drag during the upstroke. Analysis of high-speed film suggests that some large birds with relatively short, square wings [e.g. vultures (Accipitridae, Cathartidae)] may develop reduced lift during the upstroke (Rayner, 1988). These birds may be too heavy to support their weight by the downstroke alone, and their kinematics may correspond to a wake similar to Pennycuick's prediction. The wakes of birds of this size have not been visualized. Moreover, because of wake deformation, and because they will interact with the bound wing vortex, the transverse vortices may not persist and may not be obvious in photographs taken some while after they were generated.

An apparently related structure occurs in Lepidoptera and some other insects (Fig. 4; Brodsky and Ivanov, 1984; Brodsky, 1988; Ellington, 1995); here, however, the circulation is completely reversed in the upstroke: air strikes the morphologically dorsal surface of the aerofoil, and the wing generates thrust but negative lift. This gait is dominated by thrust and is likely to be confined to animals with very low wing loading or requiring high thrust (e.g. high acceleration), or to tethered insects, and is unlikely to occur in flying birds or bats in cruising flight.

Two other situations may correspond to additional gaits. As speed increases, friction drag forces become large, and a large thrust is required for steady flight; as a result, induced drag begins to increase at higher flight speeds (Rayner, 1993). In these circumstances, thrust can be large compared with weight, and the animal may need to avoid retardation from a lifting upstroke. But if the downstroke alone is used for thrust and weight support, the vortex rings would be extended along the direction of the flight path and would have a low lift:weight ratio. There is a limit to how far wingbeat frequency and amplitude can be increased to ensure that the rings are configured to contribute usefully to both thrust and weight support. These constraints may impose an upper limit to flight speed (Rayner, 1979*c*), may trigger the use of bounding or undulating

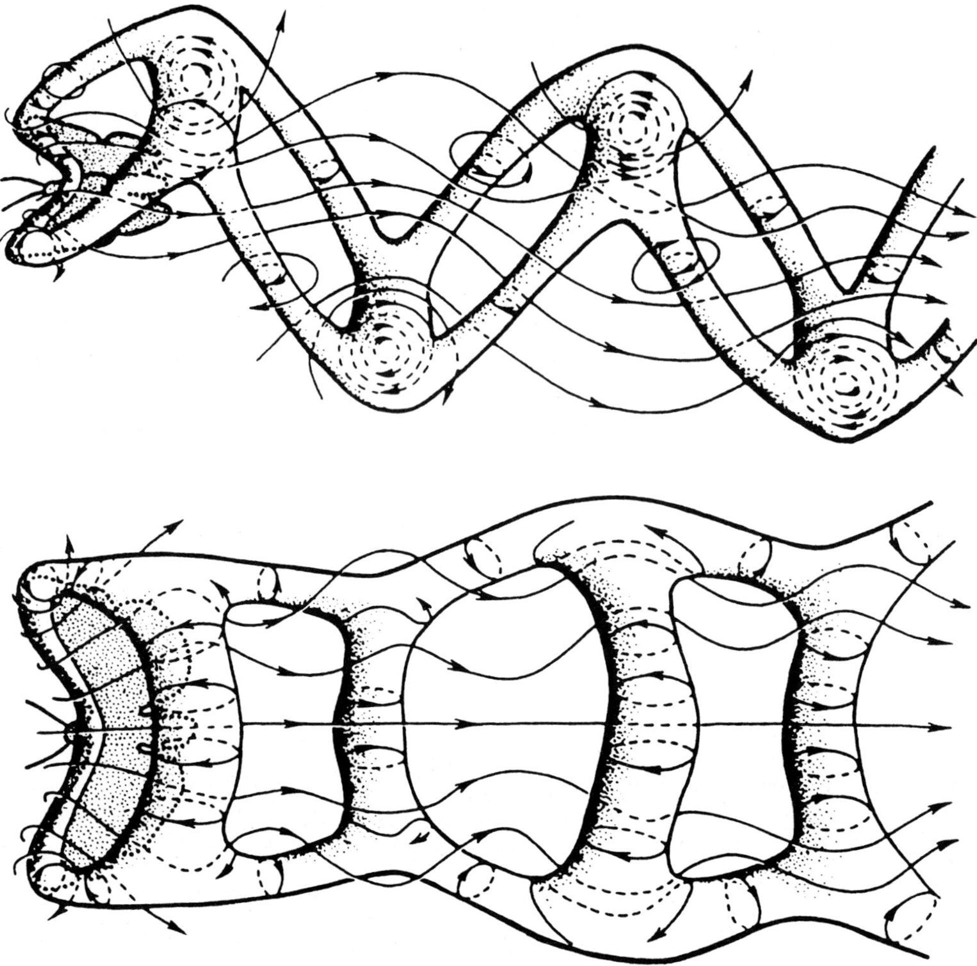

Fig. 4. The vortex wake of the Essex skipper *Thymelicus lineola* (Lepidoptera) in steady forward, but tethered, flight, as reconstructed by Brodsky and Ivanov (1984), seen from above and to the side. According to this model, the sense of the bound vortex reverses between each half-stroke; the resulting interconnecting vortex loops bound a jet which convects momentum backwards, but primarily downwards. The upstroke is used primarily for thrust.

flight (Rayner, 1985*b*) or may require the use of a so-far unknown gait, possibly with unsteady aerodynamic mechanisms to create a thrusting upstroke. This is hypothetical and, even if possible, I do not know whether the transition to this gait would occur within a realistic or achievable range of speeds. This situation has not been visualized; available limited kinematic information from wind-tunnel experiments suggests that intermittent gliding predominates in very fast flight (B. W. Tobalske and K. P. Dial, personal communication).

Some birds have relatively stiff wings which are not readily flexed at the wrist. Swifts (Apodidae, Apodiformes) sweep the entire wing from the wing root and use a variant of the continuous vortex gait (J. M. V. Rayner and A. L. R. Thomas, personal observation). With much higher wingbeat frequencies and relatively shorter wings, the related hummingbirds (Trochilidae, Apodiformes) may use a thrusting (but swept) upstroke in slow flight, varying speed by controlling the inclination of the stroke plane (Greenewalt, 1960) and circulation by controlling wing pitch. At some speeds, upstroke circulation may be negative, as it is in hovering. This situation has also not yet been visualized.

The drag wake

All forces which the animal imposes on its environment must be matched by momentum flows in the surrounding fluid. The greatest external force on the animal is gravity, and the dominant wake flow is the downward vortex-induced flow which matches the vertical component of lift. The drag on the body and wings must also have a reacting airflow but, since flying animals are usually well streamlined, the parasite and profile drag wakes are not intense and are confined to air that has passed relatively close to the body or wing surface and therefore occupies relatively small regions of the wake. By wake sampling, Pennycuick *et al.* (1992) measured the profile drag wake of a Harris' hawk *Parabuteo unicinctus*.

Spedding (1986) and J. M. V. Rayner and A. L. R. Thomas (unpublished) have identified longitudinal flows at the centre of the wake vortices behind animals in both gaits.

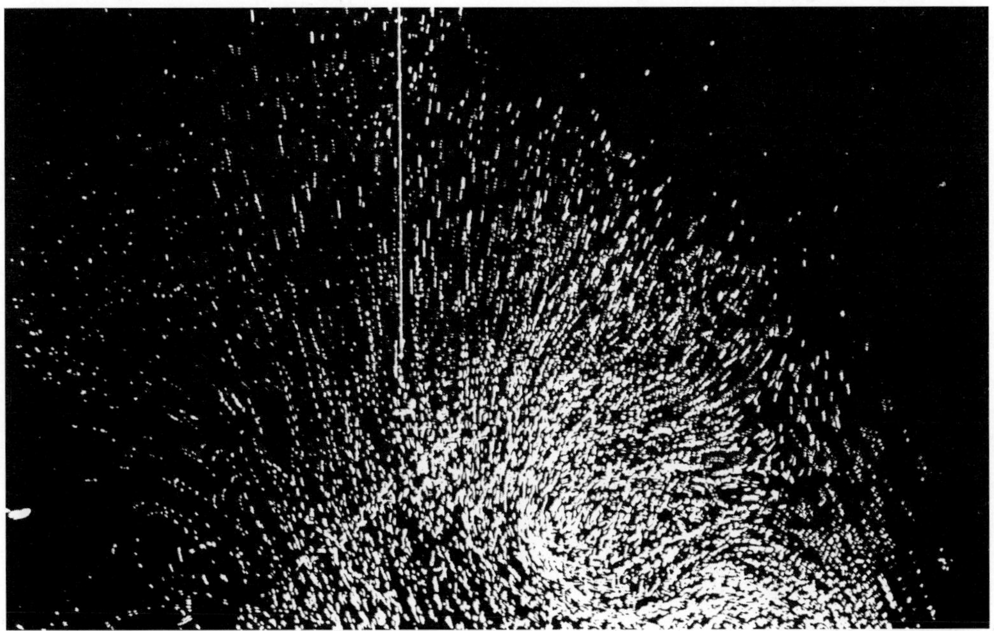

Fig. 5. The vortex ring wake of the fruit bat *Rousettus aegyptiacus* (Megachiroptera) in slow flight, from right to left (J. M. V. Rayner and A. L. R. Thomas, unpublished). A longitudinal flow is clearly visible in the core of the downstroke vortices, and also during the upstroke, following the path of the wingtips, which have moved upwards and slightly backwards relative to the air. This is the viscous drag wake.

These flows are symmetrical and run towards the animal on both sides of the wake. They are part or all of the profile drag wake of the wings which has become trapped within the core of the trailing vortices (Fig. 5).

Hovering and take-off flight

The wake structures in take-off and hovering are less well understood and are the subject of current investigations at Bristol. In these flight modes, it is likely that unsteady aerodynamic force generation is important, and the diversity of wingbeat kinematic patterns suggests that the wake structures are also diverse. Animals often operate close to maximum exertion and to maximum aerodynamic forces, and it is not clear which of these forms the more important constraint. A pigeon in slow flight at 2–3 $m\,s^{-1}$ does not support all of its weight (see above), because it cannot generate sufficient lift – or sufficiently large vortex rings – at this low flight speed; it appears that in this case aerodynamic, rather than energetic, factors limit what the bird can achieve (Rayner, 1993).

Rayner (1979*a*,*c*) predicted that the wake of a hovering bird would be a stack of circular vortex rings each generated by a single downstroke; the complex vortex structures shed during the downstroke would roll up rapidly into circular rings which would be convected below the animal, forming the boundary of an unsteady momentum jet. In most birds, the duration of the wingbeat would ensure that the individual rings would remain largely separate, although their aerodynamic interference would be important in predicting momentum transport and the energy required to sustain the wake. If the upstroke contributed to lift in approximately equal measure to the downstroke, as is the case in many insects and in hummingbirds (Trochilidae), the wake would be similar, but two rings would be generated per wingbeat. The situation would become more complicated if circulation were less in the upstroke than in the downstroke, or according to whether upstroke circulation reversed (as in hovering hummingbirds) or remained of the same sense: alternate rings could be smaller or weaker, and could interact and merge with adjacent rings. In the absence of comprehensive experimental evidence, it is unwise to speculate on the evolution of the wake!

Ellington (1978, 1980) also argued that the hovering wake would consist of stacked rings, but thought that these could not be circular since, in the absence of forward translation, there can be no bound circulation, and hence no lift, near the root of the wings; instead, the rings might take the form of a pair of circular sectors. I suspect that, while the vortex may be shed in this form, this vortex structure is likely to be unstable and would deform rapidly into a more stable, probably circular, configuration.

There is limited experimental evidence. Dathe *et al.* (1984) visualized the wake of a model wing in hovering and found a wake similar to that predicted by Ellington, with vortices shed at wingtip and wing root. However, they used only a single wing with no image plane and, on the grounds of vortex conservation, a trailing vortex must be shed at both ends of the wing; these results are not representative of true hovering birds where the flows on and around the two wings interact. Preliminary flow visualization experiments with birds reveal considerable diversity in wakes in hovering and vertical take-off (J. M. V. Rayner and A. L. R. Thomas, unpublished): in the cockatiel (*Nymphicus hollandicus*), vortices are shed on both the up- and downstroke, and the wake is a vertically oriented sequence of linked rings of alternating sense; the stopping vortex of one half-stroke forms the starting vortex of the next; the wake is similar to that of a flying butterfly (Fig. 4), but oriented vertically. In long-eared bats *Plecotus auritus*, tawny owl *Strix aluco* and pigeon *Columba livia* only the downstroke is aerodynamically active, and each downstroke produces an isolated small-cored vortex ring, as predicted by Rayner (1979*a*,*c*). In small finches and in quail, individual downstroke wake elements are close to one another; the wake appears to approach a turbulent jet, but it has not yet been possible to distinguish individual vortex rings. Since the wingbeat frequencies of these animals are relatively high, this flow may still correspond to Rayner's (1979*a*) prediction. In none of these observations have we found evidence that a trailing vortex is shed from the inner part of the wing.

Unsteady aerodynamics

The question of 'unsteady' aerodynamics is always raised in discussions of flapping animal flight. Intuitively, a flow would be considered unsteady if the periodic variation due to wing flapping is significant compared with the velocities present due to translation, but more normally the term is used in the context of animal locomotion to refer to cases where the prime mechanism of force generation is not steady-state aerofoil action, and the force produced by the aerofoil is not simply the product of bound vortex strength and speed. Unsteady aerodynamic mechanisms, such as delayed stall, wing rotation, the clap-and-fling and the peel (Ellington, 1984, 1995), do not depend on quasi-steady aerofoil action, but may involve intense local vortices shed from the wing leading edge or the wingtips, or vortices trapped on or close to the wings. It can also be important to take account of hysteresis in the development of the circulation about a wing.

However, when applied to birds and bats, I feel the concept of unsteady flow is overworked, and there two particular reasons why it is unhelpful (see also Spedding, 1993). The problem is not directly addressed by visualization of the far wake, since these experiments can say little about conditions on or near to the wings, and transient vortices close to the animal may not persist in the wake, which represents an average of time-varying forces acting on the wings. However, from momentum considerations, all aerodynamic forces experienced by the animal must have reactive flows in the wake.

First, all flows associated with animal movement are 'unsteady' in that they vary with time. There is a continuum from steady flows (i.e. gliding) to flows with intense short-term time variation, such as those that occur in insect hovering (Ellington, 1995). Flows may be called 'quasi-steady' when it is not necessary to invoke unsteady mechanisms to explain the forces they produce; in these cases, conventional slow-speed aerodynamic models are sufficient to explain the flows generated.

Second, unsteady mechanisms are normally understood to apply to wings starting from rest, or with periodic but significant time variation in position, posture or aerodynamic forces. A parameter known as the *reduced frequency* or *advance ratio* (variously defined as the ratio of mean downstroke wingtip speed to forward speed, or as the amplitude of flapping to wing chord) is used to measure the importance of unsteady components; it is implicitly assumed that periodic variation in lift is achieved by periodic variation in the local angle of incidence and circulation. In these conditions, the flow around and behind the wing is essentially two-dimensional (e.g. von Kármán and Sears, 1938; Theodorsen, 1935; von Holst and Küchemann, 1941; Golubyev, 1957) and is dominated by transverse wake vortices shed on each half-stroke.

In birds and bats in cruising flight with the continuous vortex gait, the reduced frequency ($4b\phi f/V$) may be large enough (0.75–1.5; after Rayner, 1993) to imply that unsteady flows (or transverse vortices) should be dominant. However, the flow is probably *not* unsteady in the strict sense since circulation does not vary, and the flow is dominated by longitudinal vortices. The main source of unsteady lift forces (and fortuitously of complication in theoretical modelling) is absent. In this case, a parameter based on the rate of wing deformation (or span reduction) may give a better indication of 'unsteadiness'. Generation and maintenance of the circulation involves an interaction of the local wing posture and the adjacent (locally curved) wake vortices, and as yet this process is not well understood. Since in cruising flight the sectional lift coefficients are normally modest, and at no phase of the wingbeat are large enough to question the quasi-steady hypothesis, it is unlikely that unsteady mechanisms play a major role in this gait.

This certainly does not mean that unsteady flows are absent in flying vertebrates. Mean lift coefficients in hovering or slow flight may greatly exceed the values obtainable by quasi-steady mechanisms (Norberg, 1975, 1976; Rayner, 1979*a*). Many birds use clap-and-fling wingbeats in take-off, or more often in landing (e.g. Muybridge, 1899; Nachtigall and Rothe, 1982; Scholey, 1983; J. M. V. Rayner, personal observation). Lift forces may vary significantly with time in the vortex ring gait (Rayner, 1979*b*; Spedding, 1982, 1986; Spedding *et al.* 1984), and transient or unsteady lift may be important. The 'flick' phase, during which the wing is rapidly adducted during the final part of the upstroke of a slow-flying pigeon (Brown, 1963), probably allows the wing to develop the large circulation that the bird will require for the subsequent downstroke; owing to the Wagner effect, relatively little circulation needs to be shed into the wake at this phase, and none is evident in flow visualizations (Fig. 1B). None the less, estimates of flight energy based on wake structures are unlikely to be significantly affected by unsteadiness, because work done to accelerate the air must persist as wake vortex momentum.

Swimming

Propulsion in most fish is obtained by vortex-induced momentum, and essentially the same physical principles apply to swimming as to flying; however, the mechanisms of vortex generation are more diverse than in birds and are less well understood. Flow visualization experiments have often been confusing. Bird and bat wakes are dominated by the effects of gravity, the predominant flow in the wake is downwards, and the most obvious vortices are longitudinal to the line of flight. Because of the magnitude of gravity, the wake can readily be visualized. By contrast, gravity is absent or negligible in water, and the main wake flow must be backwards and much weaker relative to body mass. The lifting surfaces may be much smaller than those needed for flying; however, since the lifting surface (e.g. a carangiform fish tail) may be of the same scale as the body, there is an opportunity for the drag wake from the body and the lifting wake from the tail to interact. It is this factor that has complicated interpretation of flow patterns in swimming.

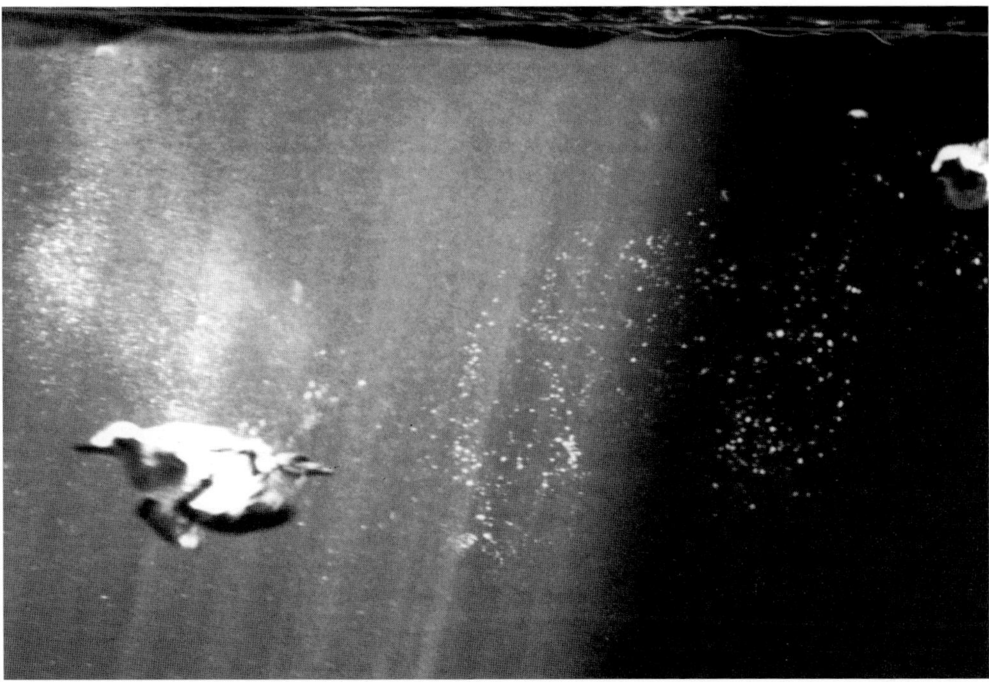

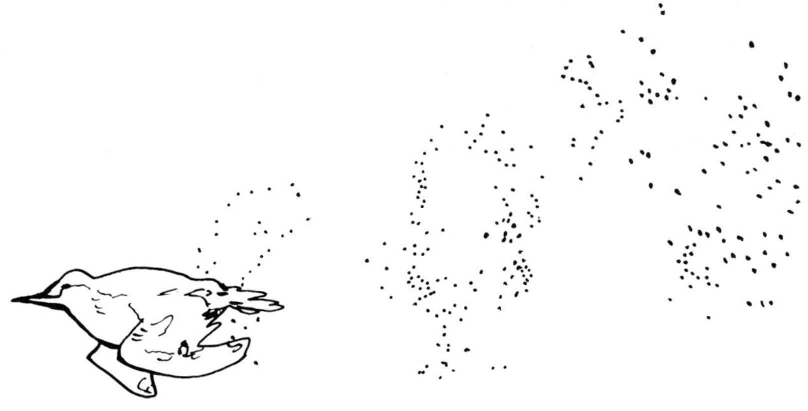

Fig. 6. Air bubbles in the wake of a pigeon guillemot *Cepphus columba* (Alcidae) in underwater 'flight'. The bubbles are forced from the wing covert feathers by water pressure and remain trapped in the vortex. The wake consists of a series of vertically oriented near-circular vortex rings, each formed on a single downstroke. This is similar to the vortex ring gait in flapping flight, but the rings are aligned to produce a thrust alone since the bird is approximately neutrally buoyant. Note the flexed wings with a sharply curved leading edge, which reduce the wing and wake span in swimming.

Swimming birds

It is useful first to consider underwater birds. The wingspan is considerably bigger than the body, so the lift and body drag wakes are separated spatially. Alcids (Fig. 6) swim in water and fly in air, and their wing design and flight morphology reflect this compromise.

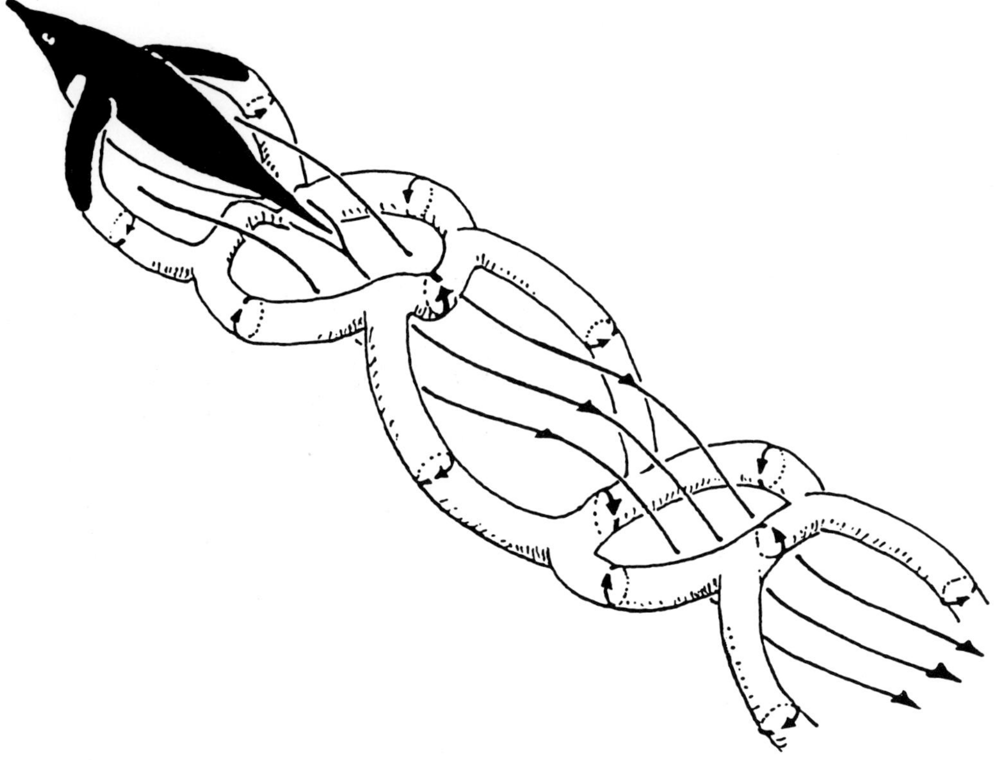

Fig. 7. Wake of a swimming penguin, as predicted by Bannasch (1995). Both up- and downstrokes produce thrust. The flow is similar to that predicted in carangiform fish (see Fig. 8; but orientated dorsoventrally rather than laterally.

It appears that in swimming the upstroke is inactive, as it probably is in flying in these birds. The wake consists of vortex rings, each associated with a single downstroke, but the rings are arranged vertically so that they generate a net thrust with no appreciable vertical component of lift. Bannasch (1995) has predicted that penguins will generate force on the upstroke as well as on the downstroke (Fig. 7); compare this wake with that for Lepidoptera (Fig. 4), where thrust also dominates.

Swimming fish

Most studies on fish hydromechanics have concentrated on flows on or close to the body and/or tail; there have been fewer studies of fish wakes, and there is very little consensus in the literature about the structure of the wake and the mechanisms of its generation. In part this is the result of the technical difficulties in visualizing fish wakes, but there are few predictions with which observations may be compared, and there is little information on which to base a comparative study of the relationships between wake patterns, body movements (or swimming mode) and morphology. Various authors (e.g. Siekmann, 1962; Liebe, 1963; Breder, 1965; Hertel, 1966, 1967; Triantafyllou *et al.* 1991, 1993) have demonstrated how a lateral flexing movement of a fish tail combined with forward

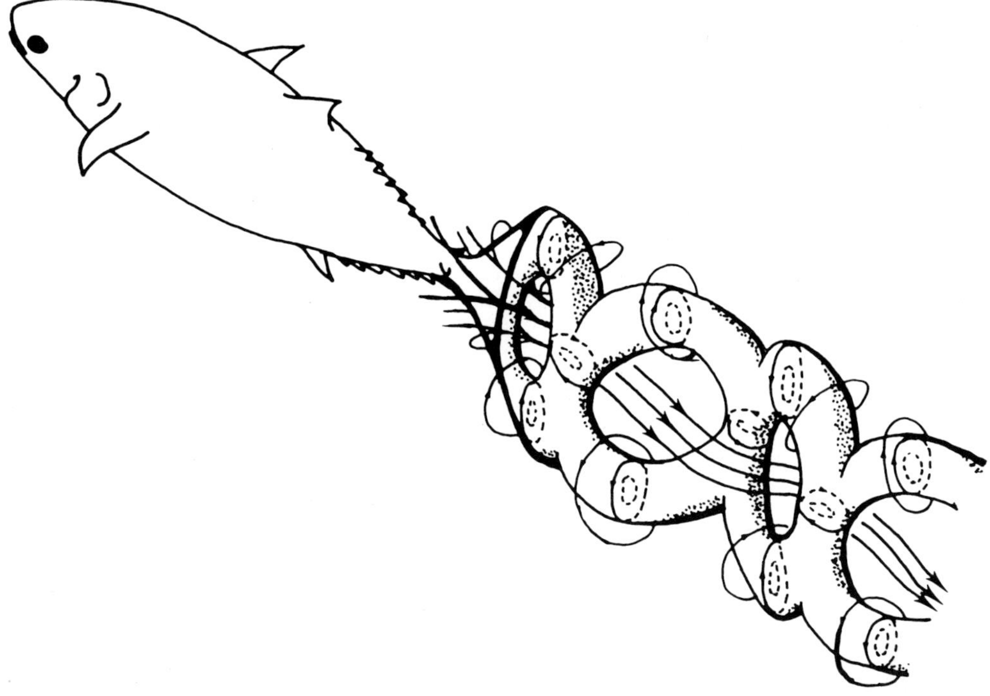

Fig. 8. The probable vortex wake from the tail of a carangiform fish, after Lighthill (1975) and Magnuson (1978), but neglecting possible interactions with the drag wake of the body and with vortex wakes from the other fins. Each beat of the tail sheds a vortex of alternate sense, resulting in a backwardly directed jet with weak lateral flow. Similar wakes probably occur in subcarangiform and anguilliform swimming, but the flow over the body and the mechanisms of vortex generation are more complex. (From Rayner, 1985*a*.)

translation will generate an isolated vortex, and there is extensive experimental evidence from models and from flapping/pitching aerofoils (i) that this is indeed the case, and (ii) that successive oscillations create a wake consisting of alternating vortices (e.g. Bratt, 1950; Hertel, 1966; Golubyev, 1957; Katz and Weihs, 1978; Freymuth, 1990; Ahlborn *et al.* 1991; Panda and Zaman, 1994). Von Kármán and Burgers (1935), Golubyev (1957), Lighthill (1975) and Magnuson (1978) used these arguments to predict the two-dimensional structure of the wake in sustained swimming as a reversed von Kármán vortex street, with alternate vortices generated by each tail stroke (see also Gadd, 1963; Swanson, 1965). Rayner (1985*a*) and Videler (1993) have reconstructed the likely three-dimensional structure of this wake (Fig. 8), emphasizing that the flow is composed of longitudinal as well as transverse vortices. These concepts have been developed primarily for carangiform and subcarangiform swimmers, in which the bulk of force is transmitted to the water at the tail. It is reasonable to expect that the tails of these fish operate as hydrofoils, but three-dimensional and unsteady effects dominate the flow, and neither conventional two-dimensional unsteady nor three-dimensional quasi-steady theoretical models are at all realistic (see Karpouzian *et al.* 1990).

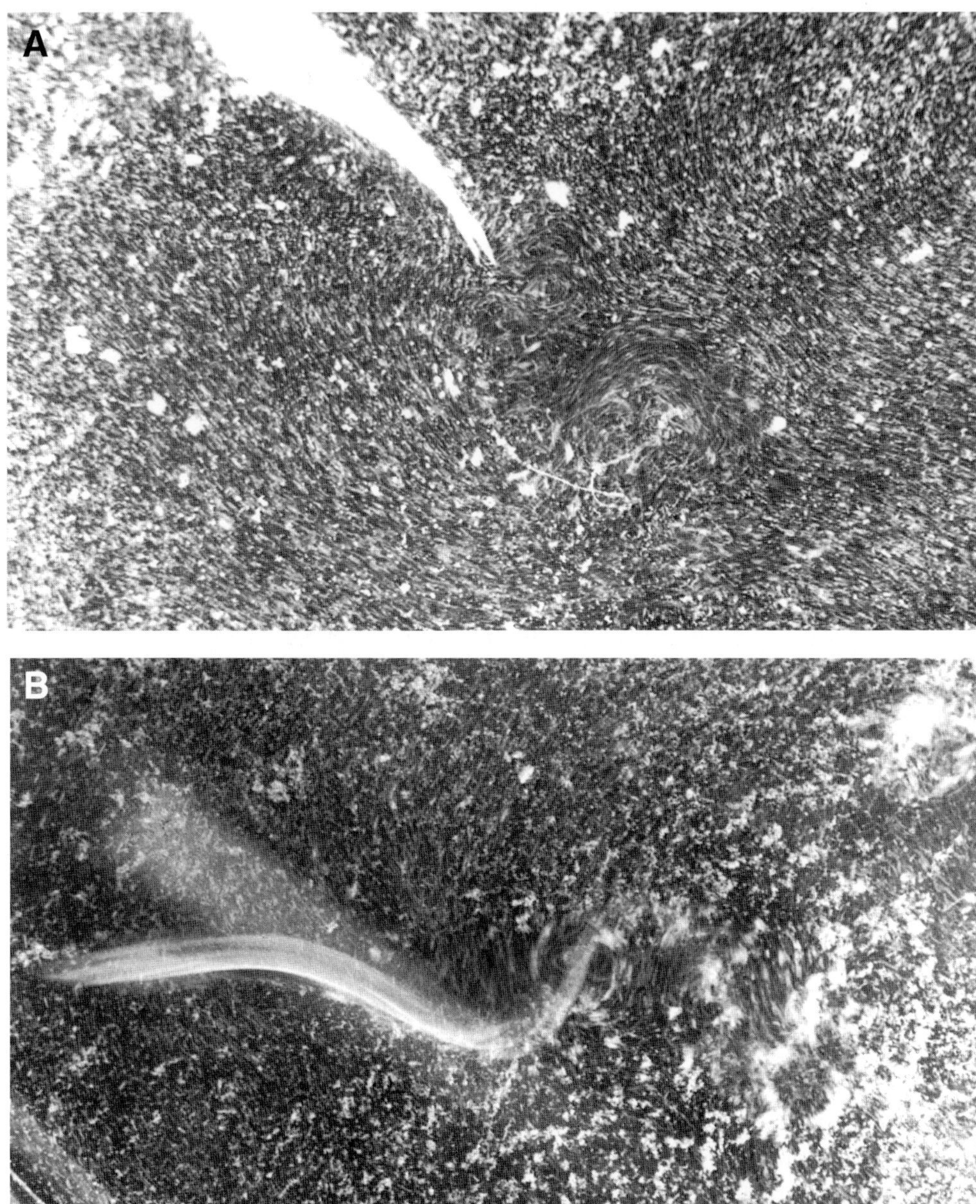

Fig. 9. Flow visualizations of swimming fish, using a suspension of small polyethylene spheres. (A) Blind cave fish *Astyanax mexicanus* swimming in a subcarangiform mode. The fish has generated a thrust wake consisting in cross section of alternately rotating vortices, and there is a trapped vortex adjacent to the body just before the tail. (B) Kuhli loach *Acanthophthalmus kuhli*, an anguilliform swimmer. Trapped vortices are present close to the fish, and the wake consists of a vortex street with intense transverse flows between the wake vortex elements. In neither image was the fish's acceleration controlled.

The limited flow visualization experiments available for fish and other swimmers appear to confirm these models of the wake, although the bulk of this work does little more than confirm that vortices are present as predicted both in carangiform and subcarangiform swimming (including Cetacea) [Hill, 1950; Rosen, 1959, 1962; Allan, 1961; Kent *et al.* 1961; Hertel, 1967; Aleyev and Ovcharov, 1969, 1973; Ovcharov, 1971, 1976, 1978; Wood, 1973; McCutchen, 1976, 1977; Aleyev, 1977; Nakayama and Narasako, 1978; Partridge and Pilcher, 1979; Abe *et al.* 1981 (also in Nakayama, 1993); Rayner, 1985*a*; Yang, 1989; Blickhan *et al.* 1992] and also in anguilliform swimming (fish and snakes) (Hertel, 1966, 1967, 1969; Gray, 1968; Rayner, 1985*a*; Fig. 9).

In carangiform and subcarangiform swimming, vortices are generated at the tail and vortex structures are not normally visible anterior to the tail (e.g. Aleyev, 1977). Anguilliform swimmers generate force along the entire body; the mechanism of vortex generation – and the geometry of the vortices adjacent to the body – is less clear; it seems that potential flow at the body surface generates trapped vortices within the body undulations, and that these travel back towards the tail whence they form the wake. The three-dimensional structure of the vortices and their relationship to the body is not yet apparent: do they, for instance, wrap around the fish? Experimental evidence suggests that, by comparison with carangiform swimmers, anguilliform wakes include more lateral flow between an almost linear row of vortices (Hertel, 1967; Rayner, 1985*a*); Hertel (1967, 1969) has shown that in a swimming eel the vortices become more widely spaced laterally in accelerated swimming, thereby increasing the longitudinal momentum flux. The apparent differences from carangiform wakes may simply reflect experimental conditions or they may be a fundamental difference between the two swimming modes.

The majority of the published illustrations of fish wakes give the impression of an intense backward flow in the wake, and therefore of a strong forward thrust. As for flying birds and bats, the key to understanding the wake is the horizontal force balance between thrust and drag; longitudinal momentum represents useful thrust, while lateral flows do not contribute to propulsion. The drag of a well-streamlined fish (such as a scombrid or the faster sharks) in steady swim–gliding is relatively modest and is due to friction and pressure on the body; in the absence of gravity or acceleration, the reaction of this force alone should appear in the far wake. For a swimming fish, drag is enhanced substantially because of body flapping (estimates range to up to five times the gliding drag; Webb, 1975). The fish must generate thrust to balance this enhanced flapping drag, but this force will not be reflected in the total momentum flow far from the fish if – as seems intuitively reasonable – much of the enhancement is due to induced drag. If the fish is well-streamlined, there may be only a weak thrust wake in steady swimming. Momentum representing the flapping-enhanced profile drag wake will be transported in vortices generated on or close to the body; one explanation for the paradox is that these vortices approach and interact with the lifting vortices at the tail and annihilate one another before reaching the wake (Lighthill, 1975).

The intense wake vortices, and in particular strong lateral flows in the wake, observed in flow visualization experiments probably represent fishes accelerating or in fast starts and turns (e.g. Hertel, 1967; McCutchen, 1977); these factors have rarely been controlled. The wake in steady swimming – for those fish that swim in this way – will normally be much less intense: it may be technically difficult to visualize and measure the vortex strengths present.

Much of the work described in this paper was carried out while I held a Royal Society 1983 University Research Fellowship and has been funded by the SERC and BBSRC. I am grateful to Geoff Spedding, Sue Dow, Gareth Jones, Adrian Thomas and Richard Bonser, without whom the flow visualization experiments could not have been undertaken.

References

ABE, J., YOSHINAGA, A. AND HATANAKA, H. (1981). [Visualization of eddies formed by movement of a fish.] *J. Flow Vis. Soc. Jap* **1**(2), 89–92.

AHLBORN, B., HARPER, D. G., BLAKE, R. W., AHLBORN, D. AND CAM, M. (1991). Fish without footprints. *J. theor. Biol.* **148**, 521–533.

ALEXANDER, R. MCN (1989). Optimization and gaits in the locomotion of vertebrates. *Physiol. Rev.* **69**, 1199–1227.

ALEYEV, YU. G. (1977). *Nekton*. The Hague: W. Junk.

ALEYEV, YU. G. AND OVCHAROV, O. P. (1969). O razvitii protsyessov vikhryeobrazovaniya i kharakhtyerye pogrnichnovo sloya pri dvizhyenii ryib. [On the processes of vortex formation and the character of the boundary layer in moving fishes.] *Zool. Zh.* **48**, 781–790.

ALEYEV, YU. G. AND OVCHAROV, O. P. (1973). [A three-dimensional picture of flow over fish.] *Vopr. Ikhtiol.* **13**(6), 1112–1115.

ALLAN, W. H. (1961). Underwater flow visualization techniques. *U.S. Naval Ord. Test Station tech. Publ.* 2759.

AZUMA, A. (1993). *The Biokinetics of Flying and Swimming*. Tokyo: Springer Verlag.

BANNASCH, R. (1995). *Hydrodynamics of Penguins – An Experimental Approach* (in press).

BLICKHAN, R., KRICK, C., ZEHREN, D., NACHTIGALL, W. AND BREITHAUPT, T. (1992). Generation of a vortex chain in the wake of a subundulatory swimmer. *Naturwissenschaften* **79**, 220–221.

BRATT, J. B. (1950). Flow patterns in the wake of an oscillating aerofoil. *A.R.C. Rep. Mem.* 2773.

BREDER, C. M. (1965). Vortices and fish schools. *Zoologica, N.Y.* **50**, 97–114.

BRODSKY, A. K. (1988). *Mekhanika Polyeta Nasyekomyikh i Evolutsiya Ikh Kryilovovo Apparata*. [*Mechanics of Insect Flight and the Evolution of Their Wings*.] Leningrad: Izdatyel'stvo Leningradskovo Univyersityeta. (Translated 1994, Oxford University Press.)

BRODSKY, A. K. AND IVANOV, V. D. (1984). Rol' vikhryei v polyetye nasyekomyikh. [The role of vortices in insect flight.] *Zool. Zh.* **63**, 197–208.

BROWN, R. H. J. (1963). The flight of birds. *Biol. Rev.* **38**, 460–489.

DATHE, H. H., OEHME, H. AND KITZING, H. (1984). Zur Konfiguration des Hubstrahles rüttelnder Vögel. *Zool. Jb. Abt. Physiol.* **88**, 387–403.

DEMOLL, R. (1918). *Der Flug der Insekten und der Vögel*. Jena: Gustav Fischer.

ELLINGTON, C. P. (1978). The aerodynamics of normal hovering flight: three approaches. In *Comparative Physiology – Water, Ions and Fluid Mechanics* (ed. K. Schmidt-Nielsen, L. Bolis and S. H. P. Maddrell), pp. 327–345. Cambridge: Cambridge University Press.

ELLINGTON, C. P. (1980). Vortices and hovering flight. In *Instationäre Effekte an schwingenden Tierflügeln* (ed. W. Nachtigall), pp. 64–101. Mainz: Franz Steiner.

ELLINGTON, C. P. (1984). The aerodynamics of hovering insect flight. I–VI. *Phil. Trans. R. Soc. Lond. B* **305**, 1–181.

ELLINGTON, C. P. (1995). Unsteady aerodynamics of insect flight. *Symp. Soc. exp. Biol.* **49**, 109–129.

FISH, F. E. (1987). Kinematics and power output of jet propulsion by the frogfish genus *Antennarius* (Lophiiformes: Antennariidae). *Copeia* **1987**, 1046–1048.

FREYMUTH, P. (1990). Thrust generation by an airfoil in hover modes. *Exp. Fluids* **9**, 17–24.

GADD, G. E. (1963). Some hydrodynamical aspects of swimming. *Natl. Phys. Lab. Ship Rep.* 45.

GOLUBYEV, V. V. (1957). *Trudyi po Aerodinamikye* [*Contributions to Aerodynamics*]. Moscow: Gos. Izd. Tekhniko-Tyeoryeticheskoi Lityeraturyi.

GRAY, J. (1968). *Animal Locomotion*. London: Weidenfeld & Nicholson.

GREENEWALT, C. H. (1960). *Hummingbirds*. New York: Doubleday. [Reprinted New York: Dover, 1991]

GRODNITSKY, D. L. AND MOROZOV, P. P. (1993). Vortex formation during tethered flight of functionally and morphologically two-winged insects, including evolutionary considerations on insect flight. *J. exp. Biol.* **182**, 11–40.

HERTEL, H. (1966). *Structure – Form – Movement*. New York: Rheinhold.

HERTEL, H. (1967). Gekoppelte Biege- und Drehschwingungen als Antrieb. *VDI-Z.* **109**, 1215–1221.

HERTEL, H. (1969). Hydrodynamics of swimming and wave-riding dolphins. In *The Biology of Marine Mammals* (ed. H. T. Andersen), pp. 31–63. New York: Academic Press.

HILL, A. V. (1950). The dimensions of animals and their muscular dynamics. *Sci. Prog.* **34**, 450–471.

JONES, R. T. (1980). *Wing Theory*. Princeton: Princeton University Press.

KARPOUZIAN, G., SPEDDING, G. R. AND CHENG, H. K. (1990). Lunate-tail swimming propulsion. Part 2. Performance analysis. *J. Fluid Mech.* **210**, 329–351.

KATZ, J. AND PLOTKIN, A. (1991). *Low-speed Aerodynamics: From Wing Theory to Panel Methods*. New York: McGraw-Hill.

KATZ, J. AND WEIHS, D. (1978). Behaviour of vortex wakes from oscillating airfoils. *AIAA J.* **15**, 861–863.

KENT, J. C., DELACY, A., HIROTA, T. AND BATES, B. (1961). Flow visualization and drag about a swimming fish. *Fish. Res. Inst. Coll. Fish. Univ. Wash. Tech. Rep.* 23pp.

KOKSHAYSKY, N. V. (1979). Tracing the wake of a flying bird. *Nature* **279**, 146–148.

KOKSHAYSKY, N. V. (1980). On the structure of the wake of a flying bird. *Proc. 17th Int. Orn. Congr.* vol. 1, pp. 397–399.

KOKSHAYSKY, N. V. AND PYETROVSKY, V. I. (1979). Pryedvarityel'nyiye dannyiye o kharaktyerye slyeda za lyetashchyei ptitsyei. [Character of the wake of flying birds.] *Dokl. Akad. Nauk SSSR* **244**, 1248–1251. [Translated *Dokl. Biophys.* **244**, 41–43.]

LIEBE, W. (1963). Der Schwanzschlag der Fische. *VDI-Z.* **105**, 1298–1302.

LIGHTHILL, M. J. (1975). *Mathematical Biofluiddynamics*. Philadelphia: SIAM.

LUGT, H. J. (1983). *Vortex Flows in Nature and Technology*. New York: John Wiley.

LUTTGES, M. W. (1989). Accomplished insect fliers. In *Frontiers in Experimental Fluid Mechanics* (ed. M. Gad-el-Hak), pp. 429–456. *Lecture Notes in Engineering* **46**. Heidelberg: Springer Verlag.

MAGNAN, A., PERRILLIAT-BOTONET, C. AND GIRERD, H. (1938). Essais d'enregistrements cinématographiques simultanées dans trois directions perpendiculaires deux à deux à l'écoulement de l'air autour d'un oiseau en vol. *C. r. hebd. Séanc. Acad. Sci., Paris* **206**, 462–464.

MAGNUSON, J. J. (1978). Locomotion by scombrid fishes: hydromechanics, morphology and behavior. In *Fish Physiology*, vol. VII, *Locomotion* (ed. W. S. Hoar and D. J. Randall), pp. 239–313. New York: Academic Press.

MCCUTCHEN, C. W. (1976). Flow visualization with stereo shadowgraphs of stratified fluid. *J. exp. Biol.* **65**, 11–20.

MCCUTCHEN, C. W. (1977). Froude propulsive efficiency of a small fish, measured by wake visualization. In *Scale Effects in Animal Locomotion* (ed. T. J. Pedley), pp. 339–363. New York: Academic Press.

MUYBRIDGE, E. (1899). *Animals in Motion*. New York: Lippincott; London: Chapman & Hall, 1902. [Reprinted New York: Dover, 1957.]

NACHTIGALL, W. AND ROTHE, H. J. (1982). Nachweis eines 'clap-and-fling-Mechanismus' bei der im Windkanal fliegenden Haustaube. *J. Orn., Lpz.* **123**, 439–443.

NAKAYAMA, H. AND NARASAKO, Y. (1978). [On the possibility of thrust by the movement of scale plates.] *Mem. Fac. Fish Kagashima Univ.* **27**, 173–182.

NAKAYAMA, Y. (1993). *Fantasy of Flow* (Flow Visualization Society of Japan). Tokyo: Ohmsha, Amsterdam: IOS Press.

NORBERG, U. M. (1975). Hovering flight in the pied flycatcher *Ficedula hypoleuca*. In *Swimming and Flying in Nature* (ed. T. Y.-T. Wu, C. J. Brokaw and C. Brennen), pp. 869–880. New York: Plenum Press.

NORBERG, U. M. (1976). Aerodynamics of hovering flight in the long-eared bat *Plecotus auritus*. *J. exp. Biol.* **65**, 459–470.

NORBERG, U. M. AND RAYNER, J. M. V. (1987). Ecological morphology and flight in bats (Mammalia,

Chiroptera): wing adaptations, flight performance, foraging strategies and echolocation. *Phil. Trans. R. Soc. Lond. B* **316**, 335–427.

OVCHAROV, O. P. (1971). Vikhryeobrazovaniye v gidrodinamichyeskom slyedye ryibyi pri dvizhyenii. [On vortex formation in the hydrodynamic wake of moving fishes. *Zool. Zh.* **50**, 1755–1758.

OVCHAROV, O. P. (1976). The pattern of flow around the body of the stellate sturgeon *Acipenser stellatus* Pallas. *J. Ichthyol.* **16**, 682–685.

OVCHAROV, O. P. (1978). Some hydrodynamic features of the Black Sea scorpionfish, *Scarpaena porcus*. *J. Ichthyol.* **18**, 153–156.

PANDA, J. AND ZAMAN, K. B. M. Q. (1994). Experimental investigation of the flow field of an oscillating airfoil and estimation of lift from wake surveys. *J. Fluid Mech.* **265**, 65–95.

PARTRIDGE, B. L. AND PILCHER, J. (1979). Evidence against a hydrodynamic function for fish schools. *Nature* **279**, 418–419.

PENNYCUICK, C. J. (1988). On the reconstruction of pterosaurs and their manner of flight, with notes on vortex wakes. *Biol. Rev.* **63**, 209–231.

PENNYCUICK, C. J., HEINE, C. E., KIRKPATRICK, S. J. AND FULLER, M. R. (1992). The profile drag of a hawk's wing, measured by wake sampling in a wind tunnel. *J. exp. Biol.* **165**, 1–19.

RAYNER, J. M. V. (1979*a*). A vortex theory of animal flight. Part 1. The vortex wake of a hovering animal. *J. Fluid Mech.* **91**, 697–730.

RAYNER, J. M. V. (1979*b*). A vortex theory of animal flight. Part 2. The forward flight of birds. *J. Fluid Mech.* **91**, 731–763.

RAYNER, J. M. V. (1979*c*). A new approach to animal flight mechanics. *J. exp. Biol.* **80**, 17–54.

RAYNER, J. M. V. (1980). Vorticity and animal flight. In *Aspects of Animal Movement* (ed. H. Y. Elder and E. R. Trueman), pp. 177–199. *Sem. Ser. Soc. exp. Biol.* **5**. Cambridge: Cambridge University Press.

RAYNER, J. M. V. (1985*a*). Vorticity and propulsion mechanics in swimming and flying animals. In *Konstruktionsprinzipien Lebender und Ausgestorbener Reptilien* (ed. J. Riess and E. Frey), pp. 89–118. Konzepte SFB 230, 4. Universities of Stuttgart and Tübingen.

RAYNER, J. M. V. (1985*b*). Bounding and undulating flight in birds. *J. theor. Biol.* **117**, 47–77.

RAYNER, J. M. V. (1986). Vertebrate flapping flight mechanics and aerodynamics and the evolution of flight in bats. In *Biona Report 5, Bat Flight – Fledermausflug* (ed. W. Nachtigall), pp. 27–74. Stuttgart: Gustav Fischer Verlag.

RAYNER, J. M. V. (1987). The mechanics of flapping flight in bats. In *Recent Advances in the Study of Bats* (ed. M. B. Fenton, P. A. Racey and J. M. V. Rayner), pp. 23–42. Cambridge: Cambridge University Press.

RAYNER, J. M. V. (1988). Form and function in avian flight. *Curr. Orn.* **5**, 1–77.

RAYNER, J. M. V. (1990). The mechanics of flight and bird migration performance. In *Bird Migration* (ed. E. Gwinner), pp. 283–299. Heidelberg: Springer Verlag.

RAYNER, J. M. V. (1991). Avian flight evolution and the problem of *Archaeopteryx*. In *Biomechanics in Evolution* (ed. J. M. V. Rayner and R. J. Wootton), pp. 183–212. *Sem. Ser. Soc. exp. Biol.* **36**. Cambridge: Cambridge University Press.

RAYNER, J. M. V. (1993). On aerodynamics and the energetics of vertebrate flapping flight. In *Fluid Dynamics in Biology* (ed. A. Y. Cheer and C. P. van Dam), pp. 351–400. *Contemporary Mathematics* **141**. Providence: American Mathematical Society.

RAYNER, J. M. V. (1995). Flight mechanics and constraints on flight performance. *Israel J. Zool.* (in press).

RAYNER, J. M. V., JONES, G. AND THOMAS, A. (1986). Vortex flow visualizations reveal change of upstroke function with flight speed in microchiropteran bats. *Nature* **321**, 162–164.

RAYNER, J. M. V. AND THOMAS, A. L. R. (1991). On the vortex wake of an animal flying within a confined volume. *Phil. Trans. R. Soc. Lond. B* **334**, 107–117.

ROSEN, M. W. (1959). Water flow about a swimming fish. *U.S. Naval Ord. Test Station tech. Publ.* 2298.

ROSEN, M. W. (1962). Experiments with swimming fish and dolphins. *Paper Am. Soc. mech. Engrs* 61-WA-203.

SCHOLEY, K. D. (1983). Developments in vertebrate flight. PhD thesis, University of Bristol.

SIEKMANN, J. (1962). Untersuchungen über die Bewegung schwimmender Tiere. *VDI-Z.* **104**, 433–439.

SPEDDING, G. R. (1982). The vortex wake of birds: an experimental investigation. PhD thesis, University of Bristol.

SPEDDING, G. R. (1986). The wake of a jackdaw (*Corvus monedula*) in slow flight. *J. exp. Biol.* **125**, 287–307.

SPEDDING, G. R. (1987*a*). The wake of a kestrel (*Falco tinnunculus*) in gliding flight. *J. exp. Biol.* **127**, 45–57.

SPEDDING, G. R. (1987*b*). The wake of a kestrel (*Falco tinnunculus*) in flapping flight. *J. exp. Biol.* **127**, 59–78.

SPEDDING, G. R. (1992). The aerodynamics of flight. In *Mechanics of Animal Locomotion* (ed. R. McN. Alexander), pp. 52–111. *Adv. comp. env. Physiol.* **11**. Berlin: Springer Verlag.

SPEDDING, G. R. (1993). On the significance of unsteady effects in the aerodynamic performance of flying animals. In *Fluid Dynamics in Biology* (ed. A. Y. Cheer and C. P. van Dam), pp. 401–419. *Contemporary Mathematics* **141**. Providence: American Mathematical Society.

SPEDDING, G. R. AND DELAURIER, J. D. (1995). Animal and ornithopter flight. In *Handbook of Fluid Dynamics and Fluid Machinery* (ed J. A. Schetz and A. E. Fuhs). New York: John Wiley (in press).

SPEDDING, G. R., RAYNER, J. M. V. AND PENNYCUICK, C. J. (1984). Momentum and energy in the wake of a pigeon (*Columba livia*) in slow flight. *J. exp. Biol.* **111**, 81–102.

SWANSON, W. M. (1965). Some observations on fish propulsion: quantitative boundary layer considerations. In *Developments in Mechanics* **2**, 550–564. New York: Plenum Press.

THEORDORSEN, T. (1935). General theory of aerodynamic instability and the mechanism of flutter. *NACA Rep*. 496.

TOBALSKE, B. W. AND DIAL, K. P. (1994). Flight kinematics of black-billed magpies and pigeons over a wide range of speeds. *Am. Zool.* **33**, 134A.

TRIANTAFYLLOU, G. S., TRIANTAFYLLOU, M. S. AND GROSENBAUGH, M. A. (1993). Optimal thrust development in oscillating foils with application to fish propulsion. *J. Fluids Structures* **7**, 205–224.

TRIANTAFYLLOU, M. S., TRIANTAFYLLOU, G. S. AND GOPALKRISHNAN, R. (1991). Wake mechanics for thrust generation in oscillating foils. *Phys. Fluids* A **3**, 2835–2837.

TUCKER, V. A. (1993). Gliding birds: reduction of induced drag by wingtip slots between the primary feathers. *J. exp. Biol.* **180**, 285–310.

VIDELER, J. J. (1993). *Fish Swimming*. London: Chapman & Hall.

VOGEL, S. (1981). *Life in Moving Fluids.* Boston: Willard Grant.

VON KÁRMÁN, T. AND BURGERS, J. M. (1935). General areodynamic theory. In *Aerodynamic Theory*, vol. IIE (ed. W. F. Durand). Berlin: Springer Verlag.

VON KÁRMÁN, T. AND SEARS, W. R. (1938). Airfoil theory for non-uniform motion. *J. aero. Sci.* **5**, 379–390.

VON HOLST, E. AND KÜCHEMANN, D. (1941). Biologische und aerodynamische Probleme des Tierfluges. *Naturwissenschaften* **29**, 348–362. [Translated: Biological and aerodynamical problems of animal flight. *J. R. aeronaut. Soc.* **46**, 39–56, 1942 (abridged) and *NASA tech. Mem.* 75337, 1980.]

WEBB, P. W. (1975). Hydrodynamics and energetics of fish propulsion. *Bull. Fish. Res. Bd Can.* **190**, 1–158.

WOOD, F. G. (1973). *Marine Mammals and Man: the Navy's Porpoises and Sea Lions.* Washington, DC: Luce.

YANG, W.-J. (1989). *Handbook of Flow Visualization*. New York: Hemisphere. (pp. 629–631).

FLUID FLOW THROUGH HAIR-BEARING APPENDAGES: FEEDING, SMELLING AND SWIMMING AT LOW AND INTERMEDIATE REYNOLDS NUMBERS

M. A. R. KOEHL

Department of Integrative Biology, University of California, Berkeley, CA 94720-3140, USA

Summary

Many different types of animals use appendages bearing rows of hairs to capture food or molecules from the surrounding fluid, to locomote or to move fluids past themselves. The performance of these appendages, whose hairs operate at Reynolds numbers (*Re*) of 10^{-5} to 10, depends on how much of the fluid that they encounter flows through the gaps between the hairs rather than around the perimeter of the whole array. We have employed mathematical modeling, microcinematography of hairy appendages on small aquatic animals and flow visualizations around dynamically scaled physical models to elucidate the factors that determine the leakiness of arrays of hairs. We found that rows of hairs operating at very low *Re* function as paddles, whereas those at *Re* near 1 operate like leaky sieves. The *Re* range through which the transition in leakiness occurs depends on the geometry of the appendage. We have discovered that different aspects of morphology and behavior are important in determining the leakiness of a hair-bearing appendage at different *Re*. Our study has revealed conditions under which morphological diversity of hairy appendages has little consequence for performance and other conditions under which simple changes in speed, size or mesh coarseness can lead to novel physical mechanisms of operation.

Introduction

Many animals from different phyla use appendages bearing arrays of hairs to perform important biological functions such as feeding, gas exchange, olfaction and locomotion. For example, a wide variety of suspension-feeding animals employ devices composed of rows of hairs (Fig. 1A, see Fig. 6) to separate food particles from the water around them. Other hair-bearing structures, such as olfactory antennae (Fig. 1B) and filamentous gills (Fig. 1C), capture molecules from the surrounding air or water. Many small animals also use hairy appendages to swim or fly through fluids (Fig. 1D,E) or to produce respiratory or feeding currents (see Fig. 5A). As these examples illustrate, arrays of hairs are important not only because they serve a variety of essential biological functions, but also because they are found in so many different taxa. (Unfortunately, the nomenclature for such hairs and for the appendages that bear them is taxon-specific. For ease of discussion, I will simply refer to them all as 'hairs' or 'bristles' on 'appendages' or 'legs', and I will only indulge in jargon when referring to particular species.)

Key words: suspension feeding, filter, olfaction, copepod, seta, asthetasc, microtrichia, antenna, second maxilla, dynamic scaling.

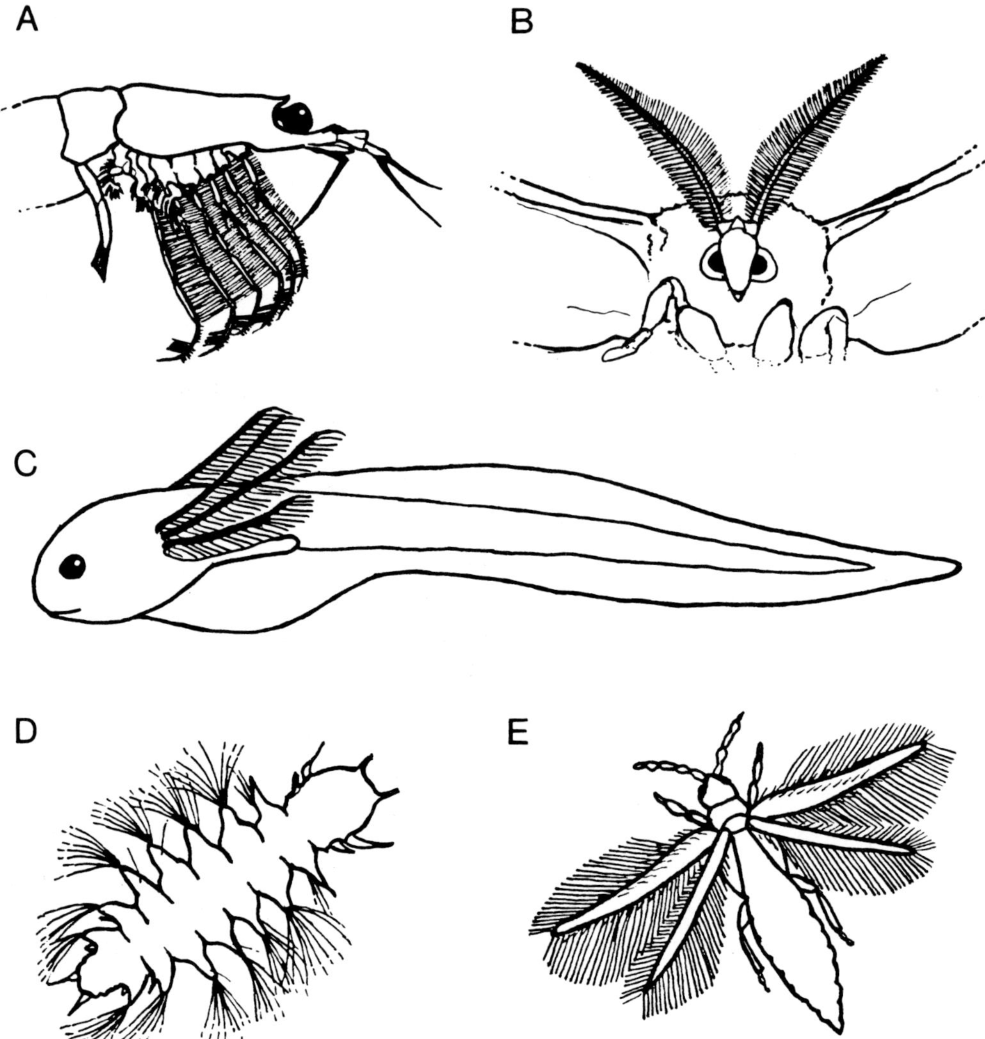

Fig. 1. Examples of hair-bearing appendages that serve different functions: (A) Suspension-feeding legs of a euphausid ('krill'), Phylum Arthropoda; (B) olfactory antennae of a male moth, Phylum Arthropoda; (C) external gills of a larval African lungfish, Phylum Chordata; (D) swimming parapodia of a nereid larva, Phylum Annelida; (E) wings of a thrips, Phylum Arthropoda.

To perform any of the functions listed above, an array of hairs must interact with the water or air around it. Therefore, the first step in figuring out how such an array works is to determine how fluid moves with respect to the hairs when an animal uses the appendage. If we want to move beyond analyses of the mechanisms by which specific appendages of particular organisms work, however, to address broader ecological or evolutionary questions, then we must also ask in more general terms how the performance of an array of hairs depends on defined aspects of its morphology and kinematics. The purpose of this paper is to summarize what we have learned thus far about how the structure and motion of a hair-bearing appendage can affect fluid flow.

Importance of fluid flow near hairs in an array

Most of the types of hairs listed above operate at Reynolds numbers of the order of 10^{-5} to 10 (e.g. reviewed by Rubenstein and Koehl, 1977; LaBarbera, 1984; Cheer and Koehl, 1987*a*; Shimeta and Jumars, 1991; Loudon *et al.* 1994). Reynolds number ($Re=UL/\nu$, where U is velocity, L is a linear dimension, in this case hair diameter, and ν is the kinematic viscosity of the fluid) represents the ratio of inertial to viscous forces for a particular flow situation. At the low and intermediate *Re* at which these hairs operate, viscosity is very important in determining flow patterns, although inertia cannot be ignored for hairs operating at the upper end of this *Re* range. When a viscous fluid flows over a solid surface (such as the surface of a hair), the layer of fluid in contact with the surface does not slip relative to the surface and a velocity gradient develops in the fluid between the object and the freestream flow. The same is true for a body moving through a stationary fluid: some fluid sticks to and moves along with the body, and a velocity gradient develops in the fluid around the object. The lower the *Re*, the thicker this layer of sheared fluid is relative to the dimensions of the body. If the layers of fluid moving along with the hairs in an array are thick relative to the gaps between the hairs, then little fluid may leak through the array.

How much fluid flows through the gaps between hairs on a hair-bearing appendage? We have defined the 'leakiness' of such a gap as the ratio of the volume of fluid that flows through the gap in a unit of time to the volume of fluid that would have flowed (at freestream velocity) through a space of that width if there were no hairs present (Fig. 2) (Cheer and Koehl, 1987*a*). Fluid moves around rather than through a hair-bearing appendage with low leakiness; hence, the appendage is functionally a paddle. In contrast, a hair-bearing appendage with a high leakiness functions like a sieve. Futhermore, at a given speed of appendage motion (i.e. at a given freestream velocity relative to the appendage), the velocity gradient next to the surface of a hair in a leaky appendage is steeper than that next to a hair in a non-leaky array (Cheer and Koehl, 1987*a*; Loudon *et al.* 1994).

The performance of various functions by hair-bearing appendages depends on their leakiness. For example, the amount of water that sticks to and moves with a raptorial appendage determines whether an organism can use that appendage to reach out and grab a food item without pushing it away (Koehl and Strickler, 1981). The effectiveness of a suspension-feeding appendage that filters particulate matter (such as single-celled algae, bacteria or organic particles) from the water also depends on flow through the appendage in several ways: the volume of fluid that can be filtered per unit of time depends on the leakiness of the array of hairs, and the percentage of particles of various physical characteristics that is captured from that volume of fluid depends on the velocity gradients near individual hairs (as described in, for example, Rubenstein and Koehl, 1977; Shimeta and Jumars, 1991). In a similar way, leakiness affects the flux of molecules to the surfaces of hairs in gills and olfactory antennae (e.g. Berg and Purcell, 1977; Murray, 1977;

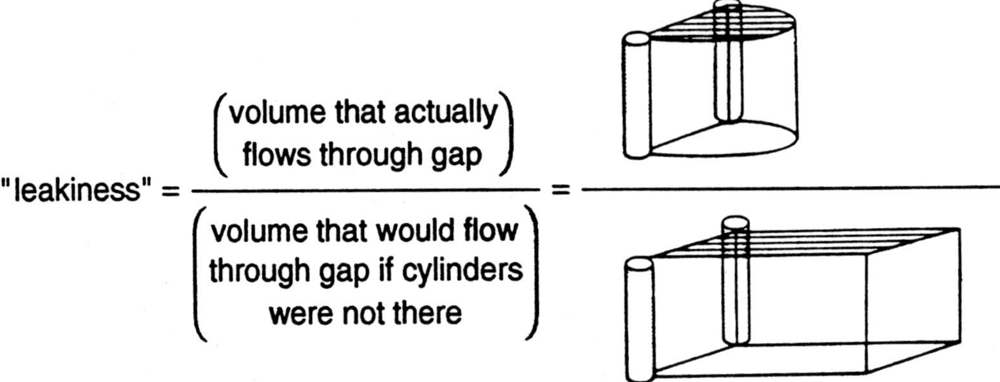

Fig. 2. Leakiness is the ratio of the volume of fluid that actually flows through the gap between a pair of cylinders of unit length in a unit of time (upper diagram) to the volume of fluid that would have flowed through the same area in that unit of time if the cylinders had not been there (i.e. the volume of space between the cylinders across which they sweep in that unit of time; lower diagram) (Cheer and Koehl, 1987*a*).

Schmidt and Ache, 1979; Futrelle, 1984; Atema, 1985; Moore *et al.* 1991). Moreover, the leakiness of hairy locomotory appendages has been assumed to determine their effective area for generating lift and thrust (e.g. Ellington, 1975; Morris *et al.* 1990). Indeed, Leonard (1992) has measured lower drag on arrays of cylinders (at *Re*, based on cylinder diameter, of about 2–200) than on solid plates.

I will use leakiness as a general measure of appendage performance in this paper in order to explore the consequences of morphology and kinematics. Obviously, analyses of particular functions (such as feeding or swimming) should use more relevant measures of performance (e.g. capture rate or cost of transport).

Approaches to studying the fluid flow through arrays of hairs

The flow between hairs can be studied using various empirical and theoretical tools, each with particular advantages and limitations.

First, we can use mathematical models to express quantitatively our theories about the mechanisms underlying a process or to describe quantitatively the behavior of a system. Such models enable us to predict the effects on performance of varying defined parameters, and they also permit us to study combinations of morphology and behavior not found in nature. However, with mathematical models, we are limited to relatively simple geometries and kinematics. Although numerical models run on today's high-speed computers permit us to describe ever more complex systems, they can become very cumbersome and time-consuming.

Second, we can measure the kinematics of, and forces on, real organisms as well as the fluid velocities around them, although many of the technical challenges of doing so for rapidly moving microscopic organisms have not yet been solved. Unfortunately, the diversity available in nature limits our ability to investigate the consequences of particular aspects of morphology or behavior: we cannot systematically vary one parameter while holding all others constant to quantify the effects of each.

Third, we can measure fluid motion around and forces on dynamically scaled physical models. Flow situations characterized by the same geometry and *Re* are dynamically similar; hence, the ratios of velocities and forces at analogous points in the fluid around a model and a prototype, both operating at a given *Re*, are the same. Therefore, a large model moved at a conveniently slow speed in viscous syrup can be used to study the fluid dynamics of a microscopic appendage operating at the same *Re* in water or air. Repeatable velocity and force measurements that cannot be made on uncooperative, delicate microscopic organisms are technically possible with large models. Furthermore, greater spatial and temporal resolution of such measurements can be achieved with large, slow models than is possible with small organisms. Like mathematical models, dynamically scaled physical models have the advantage that parameters can be varied one at a time as the investigator chooses, and combinations that do not exist in nature can be tried. Such physical models, however, can be more complicated in geometry and behavior than is practical for mathematical models. Of course, as with mathematical models, physical models are only as good as their underlying assumptions.

Mathematical models of flow between hairs

Models of flow through filters

Reviews of methods that have been used to calculate fluid motion through mesh-like structures can be found in the literature on filters (e.g. Fuchs, 1964; Davies, 1973; Laws and Livesey, 1978). For example, the two-dimensional flow at low *Re* through an infinite row of cylinders has been modeled (Tamada and Fujikawa, 1957). Since all the fluid must flow through the gaps between hairs in an infinite array, a decrease in gap width leads to an increase in velocity between the hairs. Obviously, such models are not appropriate for hair-bearing legs of finite width since fluid can flow around as well as through such appendages.

One approach to estimating the flow through mesh-like structures of finite width is to treat them like porous plates. Various methods of calculating flow through and around porous screens submerged in a fluid are given by Taylor and Batchelor (1949), Spielman and Goren (1968) and Koo and James (1973). The resistance to flow through biological filters has been estimated using Darcy's law (Cheer and Koehl, 1987*a*) or using a modification of Tamada and Fujikawa's model (Silvester, 1983). Unfortunately, Darcy's law yields leakiness values for various insect filters that are orders of magnitude too low when compared with empirical data (Cheer and Koehl, 1987*b*). The predictions of Silvester's model agree reasonably well with water flow measured through the silk feeding nets spun by aquatic caddisfly larvae (Loudon, 1990), but underestimate flow through feathery moth antennae (by about 50 %) and through feeding fans of aquatic black fly larvae (by several orders of magnitude) (Cheer and Koehl, 1987*b*). Thus, it appears that modeling biological structures composed of rows of hairs as porous screens is only valid when the morphology of the array approximates that of a screen (i.e. when the hairs in a row bear bristles that completely span the gaps between adjacent hairs). A much better match with empirical measurements of flow through hairy appendages has been achieved by the modeling approach of Cheer and Koehl (1987*a*,*b*).

Model of flow between a pair of cylinders

Cheer and Koehl (1987*a*) used a two-dimensional analytical model to calculate fluid movement between and around a pair of circular cylinders at low *Re*. Flow velocities near the hairs were calculated in bipolar coordinates using Stoke's low-*Re* approximation of the Navier–Stokes equations, and flow velocities far from the hairs were calculated in polar coordinates using Oseen's low-*Re* approximation (which takes inertial effects into consideration). A matched asymptotic expansion technique was used to put these two flow fields together.

We used the velocity profiles predicted by this model to determine the leakiness of pairs of hairs operating at a variety of biologically relevant *Re* and spacings. (Throughout this paper, *Re* is based on hair diameter and spacing is represented as the ratio of gap width to hair diameter, *G*/*D*.) Our results (Fig. 3) provide several insights about the functional morphology of hair-bearing appendages.

The leakiness of a pair of hairs depends on *Re*. At *Re* near 1, little fluid is dragged along with the hairs as they move, and a hairy appendage should be sieve-like. In contrast, at very low *Re*, little fluid moves through the gap between adjacent hairs, and a hair-bearing leg should behave more like a paddle. What happens if an organism changes its *Re* (i.e. it grows or changes its speed of appendage motion)? Such a change has little effect on leakiness at very low *Re* ($\leqslant 10^{-3}$); hence, there is great scope in this low-*Re* range for variation in size or behavior without consequences to leakiness. (Of course, increasing speed increases the volume flow rate through an appendage and the steepness of the velocity gradients next to hairs, even if the leakiness of the appendage is unchanged by such a behavioral modification.) In contrast, a change in *Re* in the range between 10^{-2} and 1 produces a substantial change in leakiness and hence in the operation of the appendage as a sieve *versus* as a paddle.

What happens to leakiness if the spacing between adjacent hairs is changed? At a *Re* of 10^{-1} and 10^{-2}, there is a pronounced reduction in leakiness as hairs are moved closer together. At a *Re* of 0.5, however, such a reduction in leakiness only occurs when the hairs are already very close together; there is no effect on leakiness of changing the spacing at a gap:diameter ratio of approximately 15 or greater. At very low *Re* ($\leqslant 10^{-3}$), gap width also has little effect on leakiness. Thus, we see again that there is scope for morphological variation at these very low Reynolds numbers with little consequence to leakiness.

Numerical model of flow through arrays of hairs

The model described in Cheer and Koehl (1987*a*) only deals with two cylinders at *Re*<1, whereas most hairy appendages bear more than two hairs and some animals operate their hairs at *Re*>1. Therefore, Abdullah and Cheer (unpublished results; described in Koehl, 1993) used a numerical model to compute the steady, two-dimensional flow near cylinders at *Re* between 0.5 and 4 to investigate the consequences

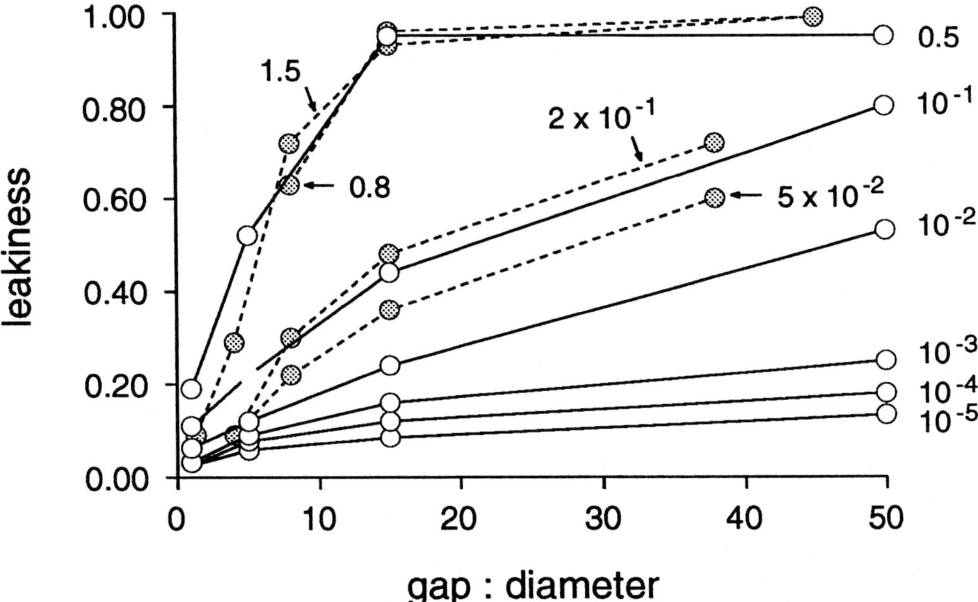

Fig. 3. Plot of leakiness (defined in Fig. 2) as a function of gap:diameter ratio of neighboring hairs. Open circles and solid lines represent the leakiness calculated using the model of Cheer and Koehl (1987*a*). Grey circles and dashed lines represent leakiness measured during towing experiments with the comb-like physical models of Hansen and Tiselius (1992) (see Fig. 8D). Each line represents a different *Re*, as indicated by the numbers near the lines.

of adding more cylinders to a row. Their results have several intriguing biological implications (Koehl, 1993).

As *Re* increases above 1, Abdullah and Cheer's model predicts that the shapes of the velocity profiles between hairs become irregular, with velocity peaks near the cylinders exceeding the freestream velocity (e.g. Fig. 8 in Koehl, 1993). Since the flux of particles or molecules to the capturing surfaces of the hairs on filter-feeding appendages, gills and olfactory antennae is a function of the steepness of the velocity gradients adjacent to the hairs (e.g. Rubenstein and Koehl, 1977; Shimeta and Jumars, 1991; Murray, 1977; Futrelle, 1984), a small change in the speed of a row of hairs operating at *Re* around 1 might make a big difference to its performance.

Abdullah and Cheer's model predicts that the addition of more hairs to a row reduces leakiness if *Re*<1, but increases leakiness if *Re*>1, and measurements of flow through physical models have shown the same phenomenon (Fig. 4). These results suggest that a simple morphological change (a change in the number of hairs on an appendage) can have *opposite* consequences at slightly different *Re*. Although this observation is intriguing,

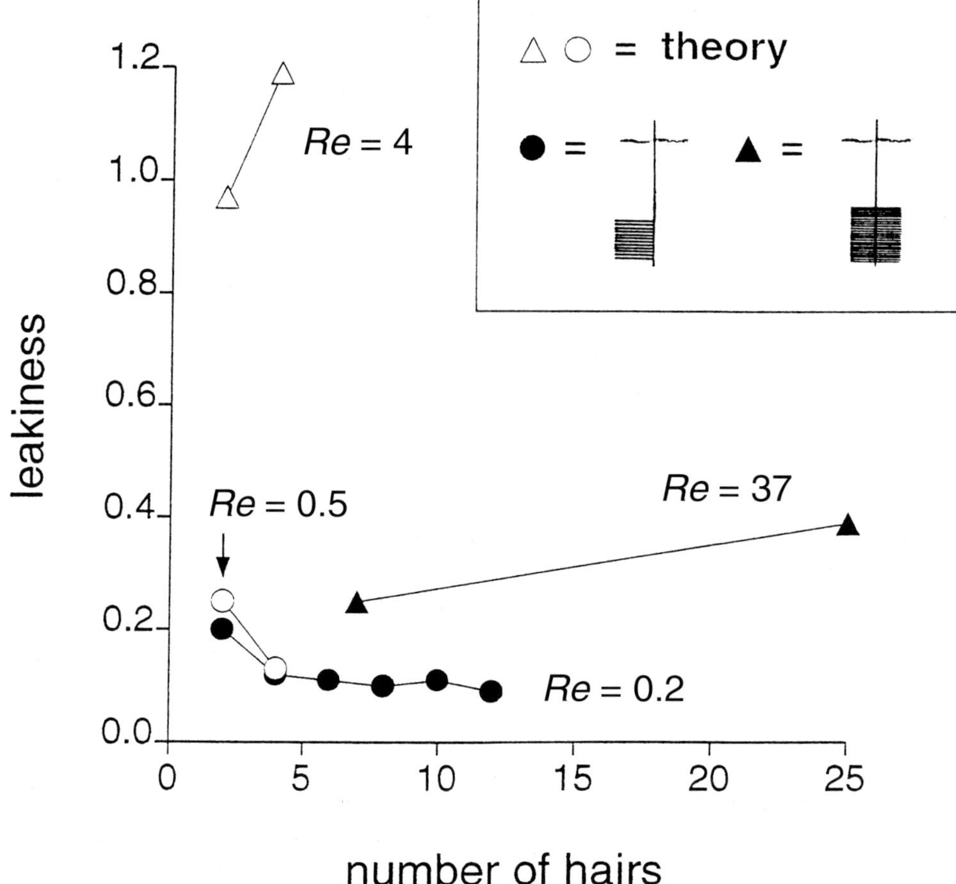

Fig. 4. Leakiness plotted as a function of hair number. Triangles represent $Re>1$ and circles represent $Re<1$. Open symbols are based on calculations of Abdullah and Cheer (cited in Koehl, 1993) and filled symbols are based on measurements for comb-like models (filled triangles, Leonard, 1992; Fig. 8C; filled circles, Hansen and Tiselius, 1992; Fig. 8D).

we must investigate the consequences of hair number over a wider range of *Re* and for arrays bearing more hairs than have thus far been studied before we can speculate about the biological importance of hair number to appendage performance.

While general models such as those described above can point out basic rules about how morphology and behavior ought to affect the performance of hair-bearing appendages, we must turn to real animals to test these ideas.

Measurements of flow through hair-bearing appendages of organisms: second maxillae of calanoid copepods

As described in the Introduction, nature offers a vast array of hairy legs from which to choose study systems to test predictions of the models described above. We have focused on the food-capturing appendages of calanoid copepods, not only because these structures perform a function of tremendous ecological importance, but also because they provide a diversity of morphologies and Reynolds numbers to compare.

Calanoid copepods (Fig. 5A) are small planktonic crustaceans (body lengths of millimeters) than can be extremely abundant in oceans and lakes. Most of these planktonic copepods, which are among the most numerous multicellular animals on earth, feed on unicellular algae and other suspended particulate matter, forming a major link in many aquatic food webs (e.g. Russell-Hunter, 1979; Ruppert and Barnes, 1994). Because of the ecological importance of copepod feeding, many investigators have studied it, often focusing on the rates at which copepods remove various kinds of particles from the water (reviewed in Koehl, 1984). In spite of all this attention, the mechanisms by which copepods capture particulate food were not understood. Textbooks described a specific pair of appendages, the second maxillae (M2s), as filters that strain particles from a current of water forced through them by the beating of four other pairs of feeding legs (reviewed by Koehl, 1984) (Fig. 5A). The M2s, which are composed of hairs ('setae') bearing smaller hairs ('setules'), do indeed look like filters (Fig. 6).

The first step in analyzing copepod feeding was to work out the kinematics of their appendages during feeding and to try to determine the velocity of water flow through the filters (the M2s) when the animals capture different types of particles. Making such measurements posed a number of technical challenges: (1) a copepod is so small that it must be viewed with a microscope, but the flow it creates cannot be studied if the animal is confined to a drop of water on a microscope slide, and (2) a copepod flaps its feeding appendages at such high frequencies that high-speed cinematography is necessary to resolve their motions. Fortunately, Strickler developed an optical system that permitted high-speed microcinematography of zooplankton in large containers of water (e.g. Alcaraz *et al.* 1980). By marking water near feeding copepods with dye released from a micropipette, we were able to use such a system to record water and appendage motions during feeding by several species of copepods (Koehl and Strickler, 1981; Koehl, 1981, 1983, 1993; Koehl *et al.* 1984, and unpublished data).

We discovered that the water current produced by the four pairs of feeding appendages bypasses the M2s; rather than being passive filters, the M2s actively capture food particles from this scanning current (Koehl and Strickler, 1981). During a capture, the M2s fling away from each other (Fig. 5B,C) and then squeeze back together (Fig. 5D,E), as described by Koehl and Strickler (1981). Other microcinematographic studies of the feeding behaviors of copepods have revealed variations in the M2 motions used by different species to capture, manipulate or reject particles (e.g. Alcaraz *et al.* 1980; Paffenhöfer *et al.* 1982; Cowles and Strickler, 1983; Price *et al.* 1983; Price and Paffenhöfer, 1984, 1986; Strickler, 1984; Vanderploeg and Paffenhöfer, 1985). For example, some species use a single fling-and-squeeze to capture large particles, but a series of low-amplitude fling-and-squeeze motions to pump small particles towards the mouth (Price and Paffenhöfer, 1986).

To explore the fluid-mechanical consequences of such differences in M2 motion, we have filmed dye streams around five species of copepods whose M2s differ in speed and in mesh coarseness (examples of three species are shown in Fig. 6) (Koehl *et al.* 1984, and unpublished data; Koehl, 1993). Frame-by-frame analysis of these movies of feeding copepods permitted us to measure the velocities and spacings of the setae on the M2s when the animals captured different sorts of food. We also conducted a morphometric analysis of the second maxillae of these species. Such measurements revealed that the setae on the second maxillae of copeods operate at *Re* ranging from 10^{-2} to 1. Recall that this is the *Re* range in which theory predicts a transition between being a paddle and being a sieve. How leaky are these second maxillae?

We used the model of Cheer and Koehl (1987*a*) to calculate the leakiness of the M2s of various species of copepods (Koehl, 1993; M. A. R. Koehl and A. Y. L. Cheer, unpublished data). The velocity profiles around a seta with a neighbor were calculated for various positions along the length of an M2. Using these velocities as the freestream

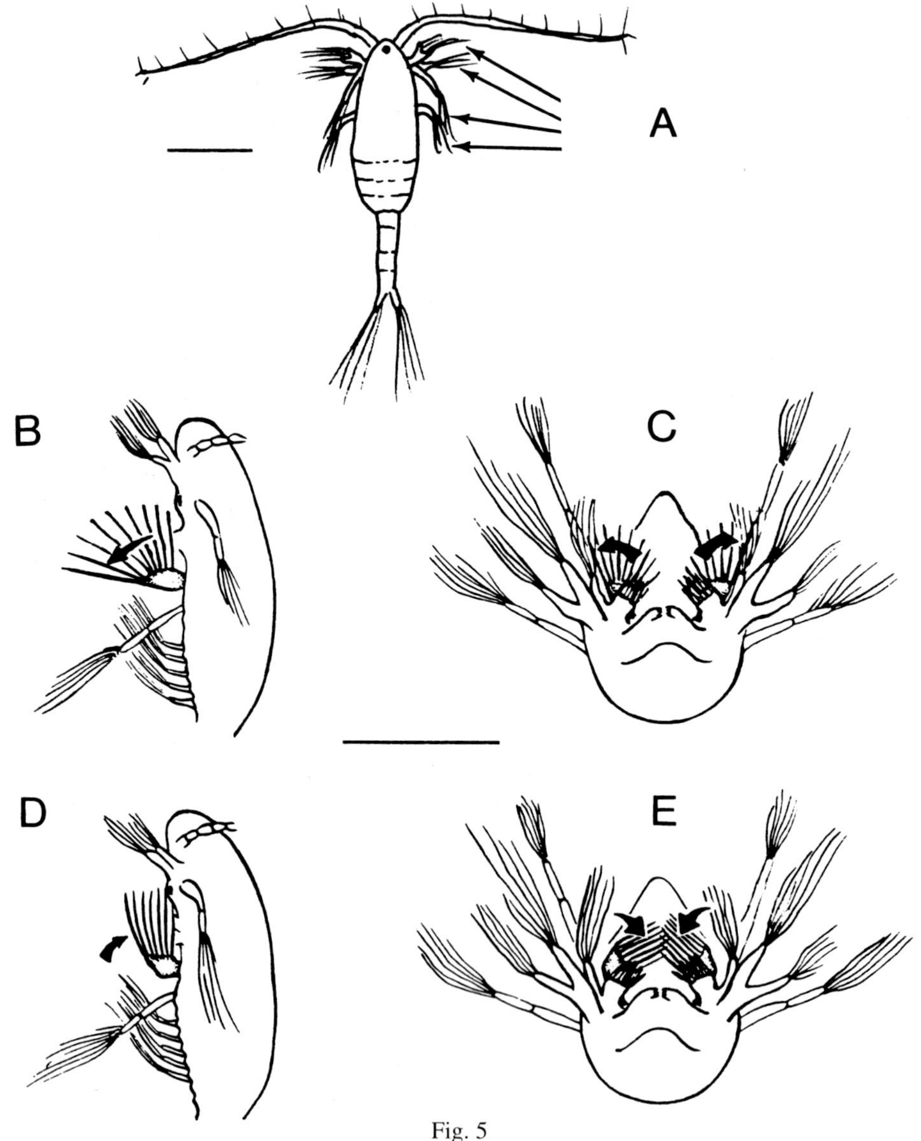

Fig. 5

velocities encountered by the setules, the velocity profiles between pairs of setules were then calculated and used to determine leakiness. These calculations predicted that some species of copepods, such as *Centropages furcatus* (Fig. 6A), whose setae operate at an *Re* of the order of 1, should function like leaky sieves. In contrast, they predicted that other species, such as *Eucalanus pileatus* (Fig. 6B) and *Temora stylifera* (Fig. 6C), whose setae operate at an *Re* of the order of 10^{-2}, should function like non-leaky paddles.

Are these predictions consistent with observations of water flow near second maxillae? If we look at what happens to fine dye streaks in the water when copepods move their second maxillae through them, we do indeed see that the dye flows readily between the setae of *C. typicus* M2s, but moves only slightly between the setae of *E. pileatus* or *T. stylifera* M2s (Koehl, 1993). What mechanisms can appendages characterized by such different leakinesses use to capture particles?

Microcinematography of the motion of particles and dye near the M2s of feeding copepods has revealed two basic types of food capture mechanisms. (1) M2s whose setae operate at an *Re* of the order of 1 during a fling and squeeze filter particles from the water during the squeeze (Koehl, 1993; M. A. R. Koehl and G.-A. Paffenhöfer, unpublished data). (2) M2s whose setae operate at an *Re* of the order of 10^{-2} capture particles by moving the water surrounding the particles. When capturing a particle using a single low-*Re* fling and squeeze, a parcel of water containing the particle is drawn between the M2s during the fling, as described by Koehl and Strickler (1981). When feeding on very small particles by repeatedly flapping the M2s apart and together at low *Re* (Price and Paffenhöfer, 1986), a slowly moving stream of fluid carries the particles towards the mouth. [Childress *et al.* (1987) have modeled various mechanisms by which such appendage motions near a body surface can produce net flow at low *Re*]. These M2s from different species of copepods provide an example of hairy appendages that qualitatively execute similar motions (they fling apart and squeeze together to catch particles), but that capture particles by different physical mechanisms simply because the *Re* at which they move falls on either side of the transition between paddle-like and sieve-like behavior.

Quantitative comparison of model predictions with measured leakinesses of M2s

Although our model's predictions of which M2s operate as filters and which as paddles

---

Fig. 5. Diagrams of a calanoid copepod. (A) Dorsal view of a copepod with its anterior end towards the top of the page. Arrows indicate the four pairs of hairy appendages that produce the feeding current past the animal (second antennae, mandibular palps, first maxillae and maxillipeds), as described in Koehl and Strickler (1981). The food-capturing second maxillae (M2s) (see Fig. 6) and the swimming legs are on the ventral side of the animal and are not visible in this view. Scale bar, 0.25 mm. (B) Lateral view of a copepod flinging its M2s apart from each other and away from the body surface. The black arrow indicates the direction of motion of the left M2. The first maxillae have been omitted from the diagram so that the motion of the M2 could be shown. Scale bar, 0.25 mm for B–E. (C) Head-on view of a copepod flinging its M2s. The ventral surface of the animal is facing the top of the page. Black arrows indicate the directions of motion of the two M2s. The large first antennae have been omitted from the diagram. (D) Lateral view of a copepod squeezing its M2s back together and towards the body. (E) Head-on view of a copepod during an M2 squeezing motion (B–D are based on descriptions in Koehl and Strickler, 1981).

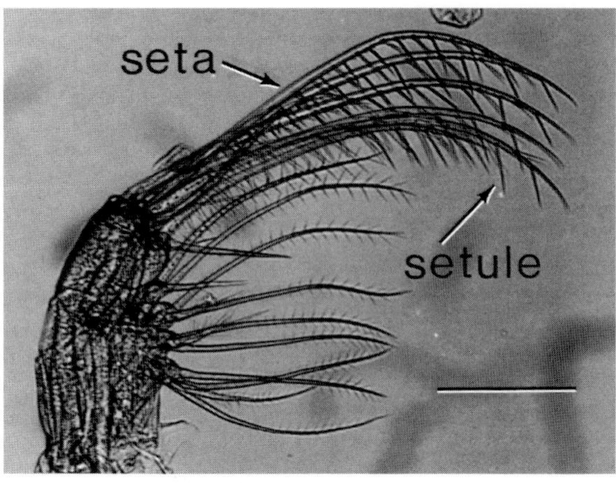

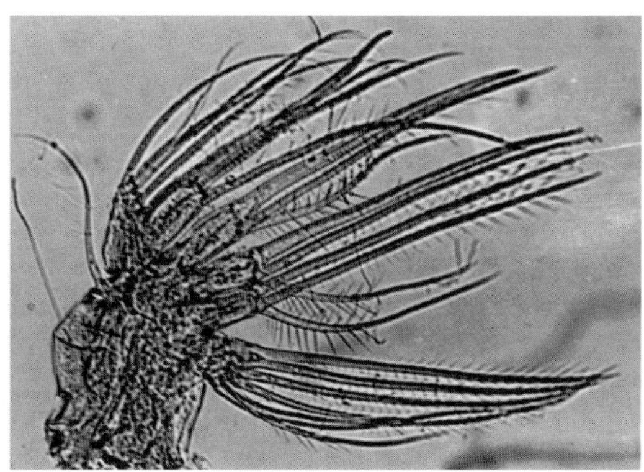

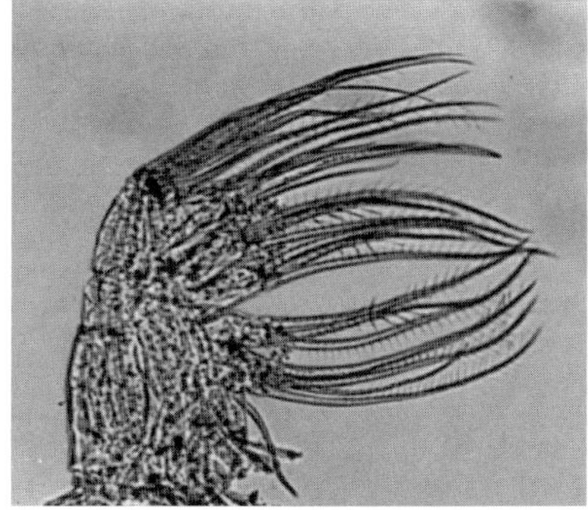

Fig. 6. Light micrographs of the particle-capturing second maxillae (M2s) of several of the species of calanoid copepods we have studied. M2s are composed of large hairs (setae) bearing smaller bristles (setules). The Reynolds numbers (*Re*) reported under each figure indicate the order of magnitude of the *Re* at which the setae operate (based on the diameters and velocities of the distal quarter of the setae). Scale bar, 0.1 mm.

are consistent with observations of dye movements on films of real copepods, our quantitative predictions of leakiness should be compared with those measured through real hair-bearing appendages. Few measurements have been made of the leakiness of

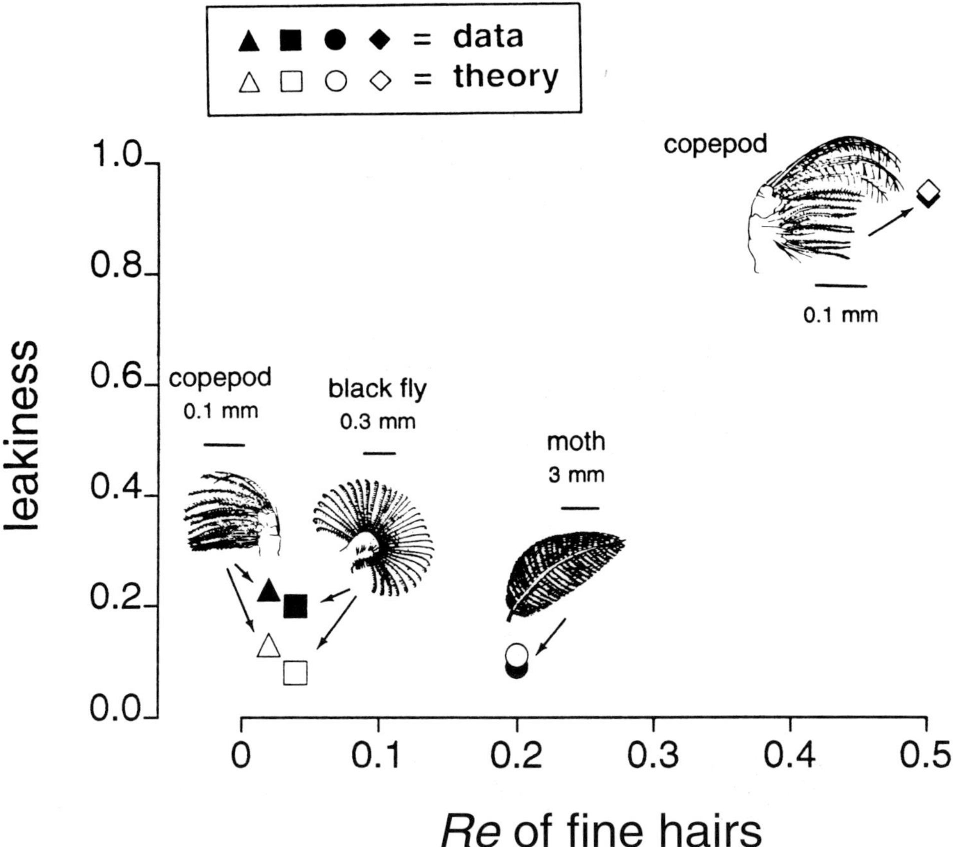

Fig. 7. Leakiness of various hairy appendages plotted as a function of the *Re* of the finest hairs in the mesh of each. Filled symbols represent leakiness measured through real appendages and open symbols represent leakiness calculated using the model of Cheer and Koehl (1987*a*). Triangles, suspension-feeding M2s of the copepod *Eucalanus pileatus* (data and theoretical results from Koehl, 1993); squares, suspension-feeding fans of the aquatic larva of a black fly *Similium vittatum* (data from Craig and Chance, 1982; theoretical results from Cheer and Koehl, 1987*b*); circles, antenna of a male moth *Acitas luna* (data from Vogel, 1983; theoretical results from Cheer and Koehl, 1987*b*); diamonds, suspension-feeding M2s of the copepod *Centropages furcatus* (data and theoretical results from Koehl, 1993).

hair-bearing animal appendages, but the data available are shown in Fig. 7, where they are compared with predictions made using our model. Our predictions for hairs operating at *Re* of 10^{-1} to 1 are in very close agreement with empirical measurements. In contrast, at lower *Re*, the real appendages are leakier than our model predicts. This tells us that there are features of these hairy appendages that affect their leakiness at low *Re* but that we have not incorporated into our model. For example, our model considers hairs in an unbounded fluid, whereas real appendages beat in proximity to the body of the animal to which they are attached. Furthermore, our model is two-dimensional, whereas hairs on real appendages are of finite length and experience three-dimensional flow. As we move to more complicated motions and geometries, it becomes more practical to investigate flow using dynamically scaled physical models rather than very cumbersome numerical models.

Dynamically scaled physical models

A variety of physical models have been used to investigate the fluid motion near hair-bearing appendages (Fig. 8). These models range from simple pairs of cylinders (that can be directly compared with our mathematical model) and comb-like models towed at steady speeds, to more realistic replicas of appendages flapped near walls representing body surfaces. Leakiness was measured in some of these model studies, whereas qualitative observations of flow around or through the models were reported in other studies. I have digitized (using a Jandel digitizing tablet no. 2210 and SigmaScan 3.9 software) the data for comb-like models given in Fig. 6 of Hansen and Tiselius (1992) and in Figs 15 and 16 of chapter 5 in Leonard (1992) so that I could replot their leakiness values along with ours to address various questions posed below.

What are the consequences of moving relative to nearby walls?

We explored the consequences of moving hairs relative to nearby walls (such as the body surface of an animal, the wall of a burrow or the substratum in an animal's habitat) by measuring the leakiness of pairs of cylinders moved along or towards the walls of an aquarium (Fig. 8A) (Loudon *et al.* 1994) and comparing these values with those calculated for pairs of cylinders in an unbounded fluid (Cheer and Koehl, 1987*a*).

We found (Loudon *et al.* 1994) that at a *Re* of 10^{-2} and lower, the leakiness of a pair of cylinders moving through fluid in a tank with walls was higher than that predicted by Cheer and Koehl (1987*a*) for cylinders in an unbounded fluid, even when the cylinders were far away (70 diameters) from the nearest wall. We also found that a change in gap:diameter ratio (*G/D*) could affect the leakiness of a pair of cylinders moving relative to a wall (Loudon *et al.* 1994), whereas Cheer and Koehl (1987*a*) predicted no effect of *G/D* for cylinders operating at such low *Re* in an unbounded fluid. Therefore, a morphological character (i.e. *G/D*) that is of little consequence at low *Re* in an unbounded fluid becomes important when the appendage operates near a wall. We also found that when cylinders operated at $Re \leq 10^{-2}$, leakiness could be increased by moving very close (less than 15 diameters) to a wall (Loudon *et al.* 1994). Although motion at low *Re* relative to a wall also increased the leakiness of cylinders at great distances from the wall, *changes* in distance from the wall did not alter leakiness significantly once the cylinders were farther than about 15 diameters from the wall.

Although we measured pronounced wall effects at very low *Re*, we found that the leakiness of the physical models moving near walls at *Re* of 10^{-1} and 1 matched the theoretical values for cylinders in an unbounded fluid. This suggests that a behavior that is effective at altering leakiness at very low *Re* (i.e. moving close to the body surface or another wall), does not change leakiness at intermediate *Re*.

Our observations about wall effects on leakiness point out some practical considerations for those of us studying flow through hairy appendages. At $Re \leq 10^{-2}$,

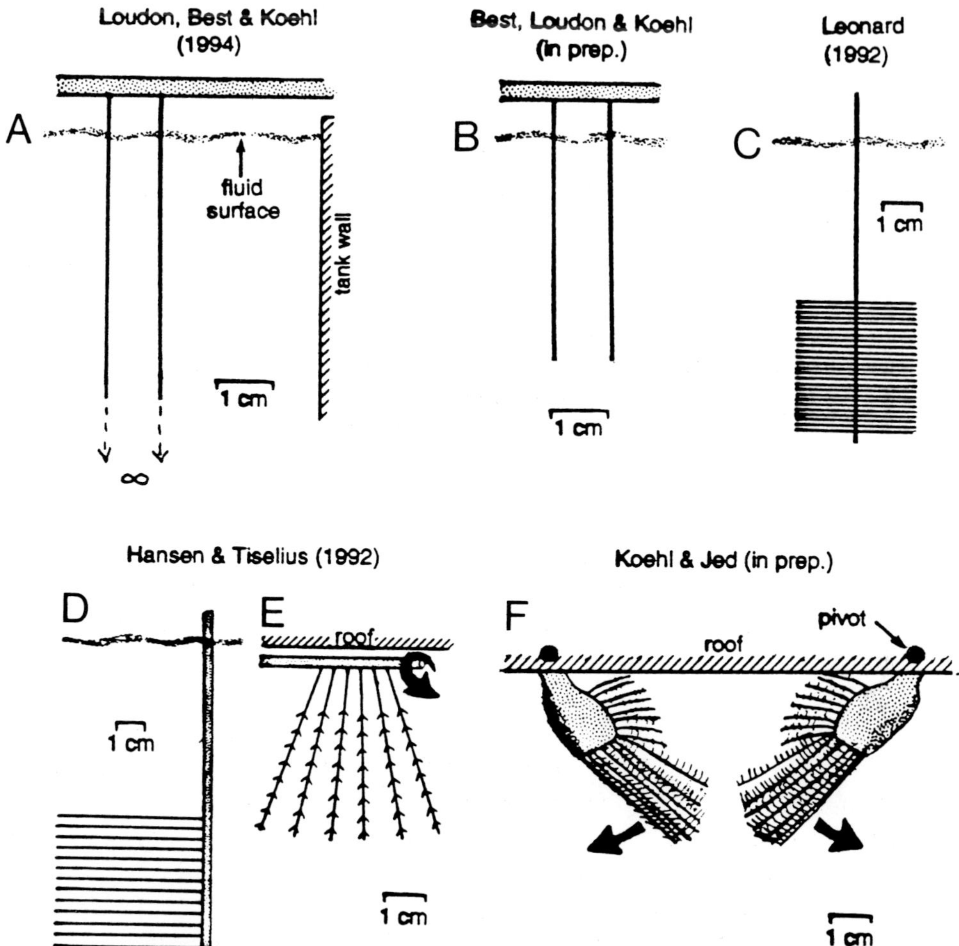

Fig. 8. Diagrams of some of the physical models that have been used to study flow through hair-bearing appendages. (A) Loudon *et al.* (1994) towed pairs of cylinders (which could be compared with the model of Cheer and Koehl, 1987*a*) at steady velocities through a tank of corn syrup solutions. We used 'infinitely long' cylinders (that extended from the floor of the tank to the top of the fluid) to explore the consequences of moving near walls. (B) B. A. Best, C. Loudon and M. A. R. Koehl (in preparation) also towed pairs of cylinders at steady velocities through the same tank to explore the consequences of cylinder length and gap width. (C) Leonard (1992) towed comb-like models at steady velocities through a tank of water or magnesuim sulphate solutions. (D) Hansen and Tiselius (1992) towed comb-like models at steady velocities through a tank of glycerol solutions. (E) Hansen and Tiselius (1992) also rotated in their tank various models of an appendage with six hairs. (F) M. A. R. Koehl and J. Jed (in preparation) used scale models of pairs of M2s from particular species of copepods (Fig. 6). These models executed fling-and-squeeze motions in mineral oil near a roof simulating a copepod body surface.

assuming an unbounded fluid when modeling an appendage that moves relative to an animal's body will result in underestimation of flow velocities through the appendage. Furthermore, at these low values of *Re*, the walls of the tank in which physical models are moved will increase the fluid motion relative to the models. (Note that we have focused on the case of a hair-bearing appendage moving *relative to* a wall. Of course, if a hair is attached to a wall and both move together – or both are stationary in an ambient current – then the wall effect is the opposite of what we have reported: the wall reduces the velocity relative to the hair, which stands partially or fully within the boundary layer of slowed fluid along the surface of the wall.)

What are the consequences of hair length?

The mathematical model of Cheer and Koehl (1987*a*,*b*) is two-dimensional, and the physical models of Loudon *et al.* (1994) are of infinitely long cylinders (i.e. they extend from the bottom of the tank through the surface of the fluid; Fig. 8A); hence, neither study addresses the consequences of fluid flowing around the tips of hairs of finite length. B. A. Best, C. Loudon and M. A. R. Koehl (in preparation) used physical models of pairs of hairs to study the consequences of hair length to leakiness (Fig. 8B). Our results indicate that the leakiness of the gap between cylinders operating at $Re \leqslant 10^{-2}$ is lower if the cylinders are of finite length (Fig. 9) because fluid is free to flow around the tips of the appendage as

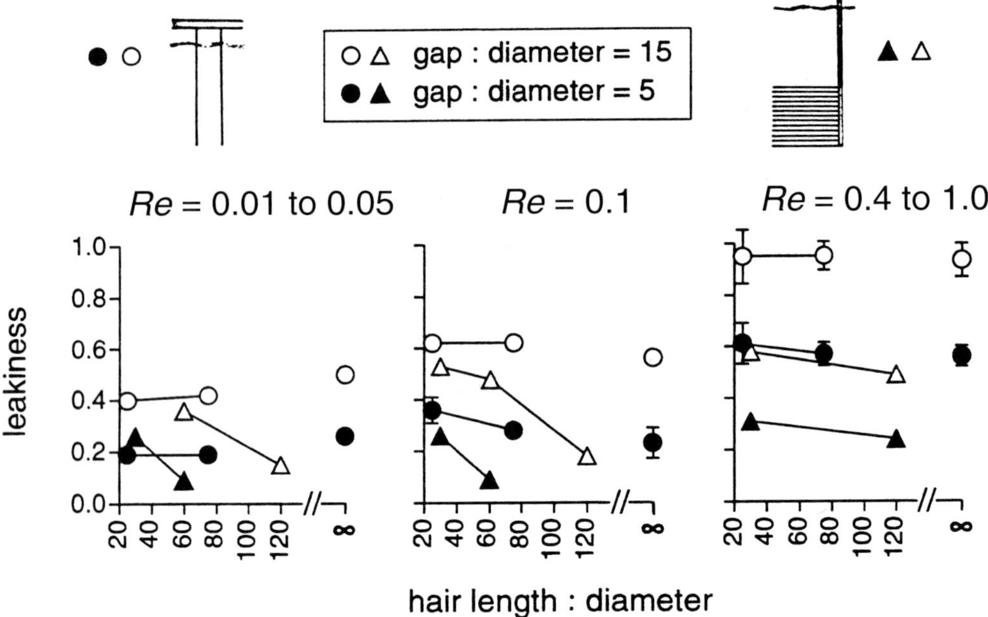

Fig. 9. Leakiness of various models as a function of hair length:diameter ratio. Open symbols represent models with a *G*/*D* of 15; filled symbols represent models with a *G*/*D* of 5; circles represent a pair of cylinders (Fig. 8A,B) at *Re* of 0.01, 0.1 and 1 (∞ indicates cylinders that were 'infinitely' long, extending from the floor of the tank to the top of the fluid). (B. A. Best, C. Loudon and M. A. R. Koehl, in preparation); triangles represent the comb-like models (Fig. 8D) of Hansen and Tiselius (1992) at *Re* of 0.05, 0.1 and 0.4. Error bars, which indicate one standard deviation (S.D., *N*=3–5), are shown for the data of B. A. Best, C. Loudon and M. A. R. Koehl (in preparation) (although in some cases the standard deviations are smaller than the circles used to indicate the mean values); no standard deviations were reported by Hansen and Tiselius.

well as around the sides. In contrast, when models are quite leaky (Re=1), we found no difference in the flow between hairs of finite or infinite length. Our data for pairs of cylinders of finite length show no significant effect on leakiness of changing cylinder length. In contrast, the data of Hansen and Tiselius (1992) for comb-like models (Fig. 8D) indicate that increasing hair length:diameter ratio can decrease comb leakiness (Fig. 9).

What are the consequences of hair Reynolds number?

The results of a variety of physical model studies are consistent with our prediction that a row of hairs operating at $Re \leqslant 10^{-2}$ is paddle-like whereas one moving at a Re of the order of 1 is sieve-like. For example, Gerritsen and Porter (1982) found that no dye passed through their models (plankton netting oscillating in glycerine) of cladoceran feeding appendages whose setules operate at an Re of 10^{-3} to 10^{-4}. Braimah (1987) towed through canola oil scale models of three of the microtrichia-bearing rays (i.e. bristle-bearing cylinders) from the filter-feeding forelegs of larval mayflies and labral fans of larval black flies. He found virtually no flow between the bristles at a bristle Re of 0.02 to 0.07, but increasingly thinner boundary layers and greater flow through the models as bristle Re was raised to 0.8. Similarly, Hansen and Tiselius (1992) used six bristle-bearing cylinders rotated in mixtures of glycerol and water to model a copepod M2 (Fig. 8E). At a Re of the order of 10^{-2}, they observed dye to flow through the models only at the very tips of the cylinders, whereas at $Re \geqslant 1$, they saw dye move through the models all along the length of the cylinders.

What are the consequences of mesh gap:diameter ratio?

Hansen and Tiselius (1992) used comb-like models (Fig. 8D) towed at steady velocities to explore the the leakiness consequences of cylinder spacing. At an Re where the wall effects of the towing tank are not expected to affect leakiness, these comb-like models showed leakinesses very similar to those predicted by Cheer and Koehl (1987*a*) (Fig. 3), the main difference being lower-than-predicted leakinesses at very low values of G/D. (The latter may be due to fluid motion around the tips of the hairs in the three-dimensional models, as well as to the additional resistance of the support rod to fluid motion between the hairs.)

Leonard (1992) and Hansen and Tiselius (1992) tested comb-like models (Fig. 8C,D) at Re higher than those at which the model of Cheer and Koehl (1987*a*) is applicable. As illustrated in Fig. 10A, the critical G/D (the G/D below which gap width affects leakiness) becomes lower as Re is increased. Similarly, for a given gap width, finer hairs yield greater leakiness at a Re of approximately 0.5, whereas this difference is only apparent at narrow gap widths at higher Re (Fig. 10B).

Therefore, both physical and mathematical models show that reducing G/D can lower leakiness at $Re \geqslant 10^{-2}$, although the G/D below which this effect occurs can be quite small at $Re \geqslant 0.5$. As mentioned above, G/D can also affect the leakiness of arrays of hairs operating at $Re \leqslant 10^{-2}$ if they move relative to a wall.

What are the consequences of larger-scale flow around a whole appendage?

Leonard (1992) observed that the leakiness of his comb-like models (Fig. 8C) varied with time even though they were towed at steady velocities. He reported that the fluctuations in flow between hairs occurred as vortices were shed by the whole comb, and that the temporal and spatial pattern of this fluctuating leakiness depended not only on *G*/*D* but also on the *Re* of the whole array. Whether such fluctuating leakiness affects the performance of filters, gills or wings remains to be determined. Nonetheless, Leonard's work illustrates the importance of considering the higher-*Re* flow around whole appendages even if our focus is on the details of the low-*Re* flow around individual hairs.

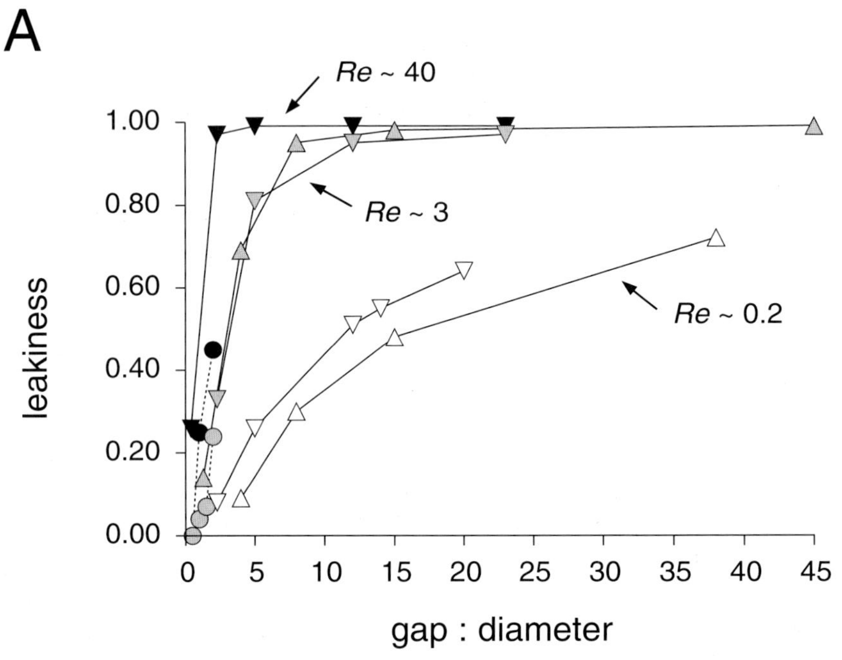

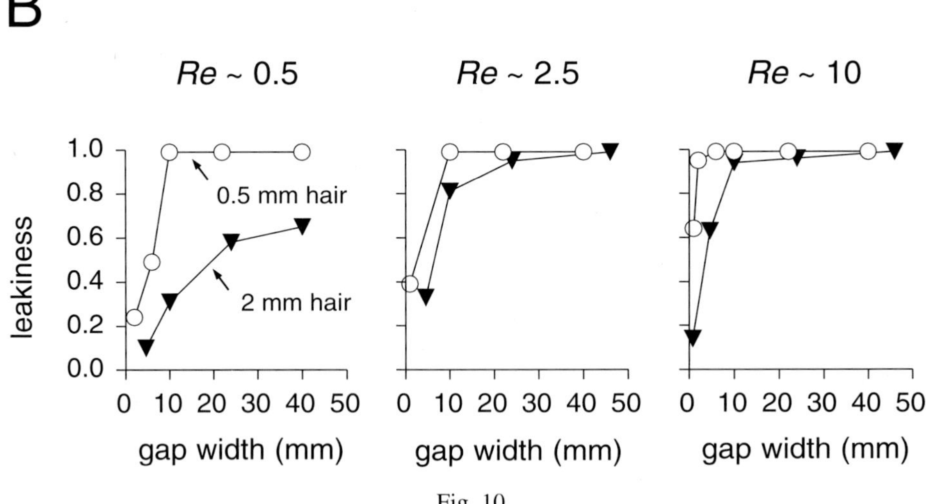

Fig. 10

Physical models of copepod second maxillae

In order to explore how the morphology and motion of copepod M2s affect the water flow through the appendages, we built geometrically similar physical models (Fig. 8F) of the M2s of three species: *C. furcatus, E. pileatus* and *T. stylifera* (Fig. 6). The dimensions of the models (which were 48–57 mm long) were based on morphometric analyses of light micrographs and scanning electron micrographs of the M2s of the animals (M. A. R. Koehl, unpublished data). Each pair of model M2s was mounted on a wall (to simulate the body surface) in a tank of mineral oil (1 m×1 m×0.55 m) and was flapped to mimic the fling-and-squeeze of a copepod (Fig. 5) at *Re* of 1, 10^{-1} and 10^{-2} (all Reynolds numbers in this discussion of M2s are based on the diameter of the setae). A plane (parallel to the length and normal to the width of the M2s) was illuminated through a slit with fiber-optic lamps (Cole Parmer no. 9741) and the fluid was marked with neutrally buoyant particles (*Artemia* cysts). Video records were made of the motion of the models and the marker particles and were digitized using a Peak Performance Video Motion Analysis System (version 5.1.0). These data were used to calculate the velocity of the fluid relative to the appendage (details described in M. A. R. Koehl and J. Jed, in preparation).

Examples of fluid velocities relative to the model M2s of *C. furcatus* (*Re*=1) and *T. stylifera* ($Re=10^{-2}$) are shown in Fig. 11. The differences between the flow patterns relative to the leaky appendage whose setae operate at a *Re* of 1 and the paddle-like appendage whose hairs move at a *Re* of 10^{-2} is striking. As illustrated by the vectors relative to the M2 of *T. stylifera* (Fig. 11), particles move slowly towards the tips of the setae of our model M2s at a *Re* of 10^{-2}; Price and Paffenhöfer (1986) have described similar particle motions near the M2s of copepods feeding at that *Re*.

Fluid velocity (U_{rel}) through the model appendage at some position along its length was divided by the speed (U_{M2}) at which the appendage was traveling at that position to yield a measure of the relative flow through the appendage. Since fluid velocity through the middle of a gap between hairs is a good predictor of leakiness (B A. Best, C. Loudon and M. A. R. Koehl, in preparation), high values of U_{rel}/U_{M2} indicate sieve-like behavior and low values indicate paddle-like function. I will present below a few examples of the questions that can be answered by measuring the effects on U_{rel}/U_{M2} of manipulations of the morphology or kinematics of physical models such as these.

What are the consequences of changing the *Re* (i.e. the size or speed) at which the setae of the M2s of a copepod operate? As illustrated in Fig. 12, the coarse-meshed M2s of *C.*

Fig. 10. Leakiness of comb-like physical models (Fig. 8C,D). (A) Leakiness plotted as a function of *G*/*D* for the models of Hansen and Tiselius (1992) (indicated by triangles) and of Leonard (1992) (indicated by circles). Black symbols represent *Re* of about 40 (*Re*: triangles, 40; circles, 37); grey symbols represent *Re* of about 3 (*Re*: triangles, 2.9 and 3.8; circles, 4), and open symbols represent *Re* of 0.2. (B) Leakiness plotted as a function of gap width (in mm) for the models of Hansen and Tiselius (1992) composed of cylinders that were slim (0.5 mm diameter; represented by open circles) or thick (2.0 mm diameter; represented by black triangles). The *Re* given above each graph is a rough approximation (in the left-hand graph, *Re*: open circles, 0.7, filled triangles, 0.4; in the middle graph, *Re*: circles, 2.2, triangles, 2.9; in the right-hand graph, *Re*: circles, 10.1, triangles, 7.5).

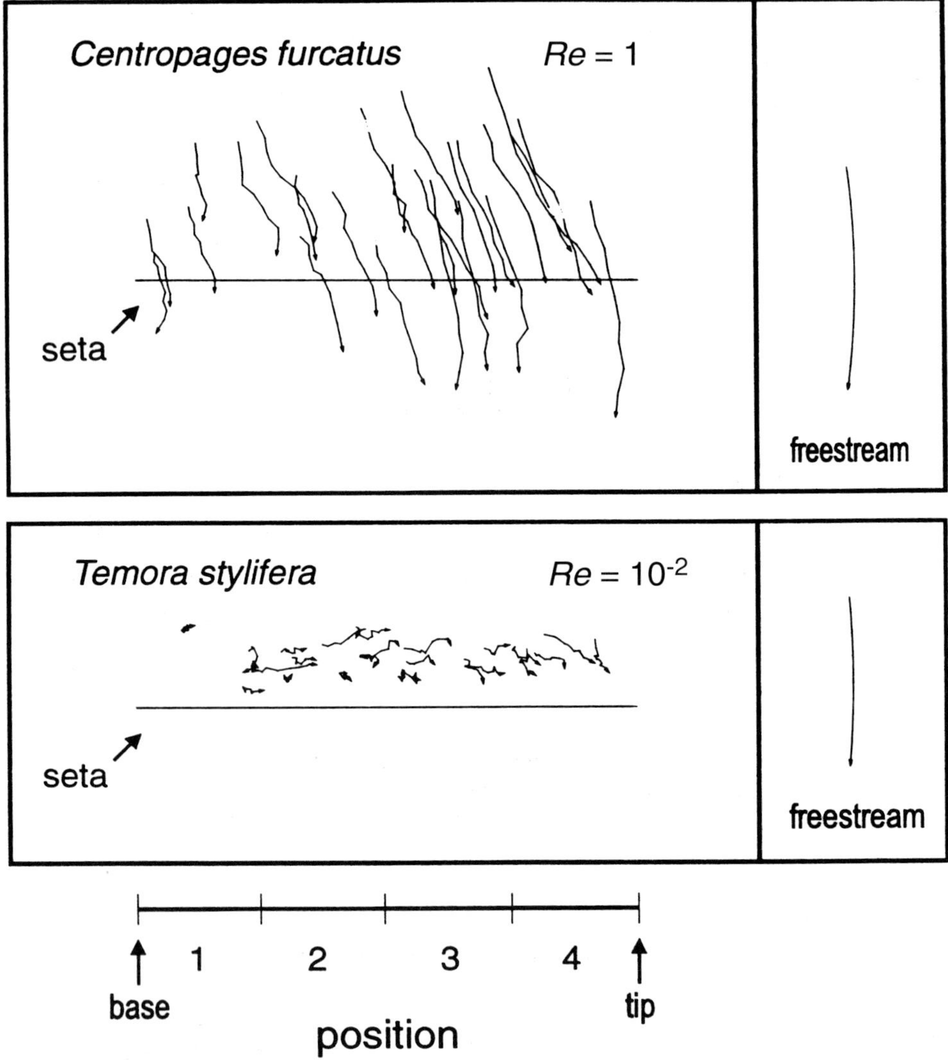

Fig. 11. Velocities of marker particles relative to a marked seta on a dynamically scaled physical model (described in the text and Fig. 8F) of a *C. furcatus* M2 (A) and of a *T. stylifera* M2 (B) during fling motions (Fig. 5B,C). 'Freestream' indicates the velocity relative to the tip of the moving seta of the stationary fluid in the tank. The seta was divided into four regions (indicated by the scale at the bottom of the figure) and the velocity data for each section were pooled to generate graphs such as those in Figs 12 and 14.

furcatus (which normally operate at a *Re* of approximately 1 and are sieve-like) can function as paddles if made to move at a *Re* of 10^{-2}, while the fine-meshed M2s of *T. stylifera* (which normally operate at a *Re* of approximately 10^{-2} and are paddle-like) can leak like sieves if moved at a *Re* of 1. However, the comparison of the three species shown in Fig. 12 reveals that the *Re* range across which the transition from paddle-like to

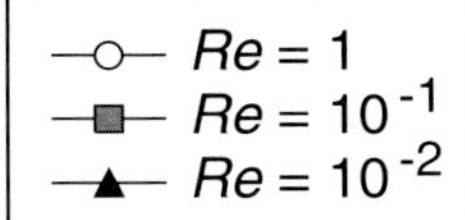

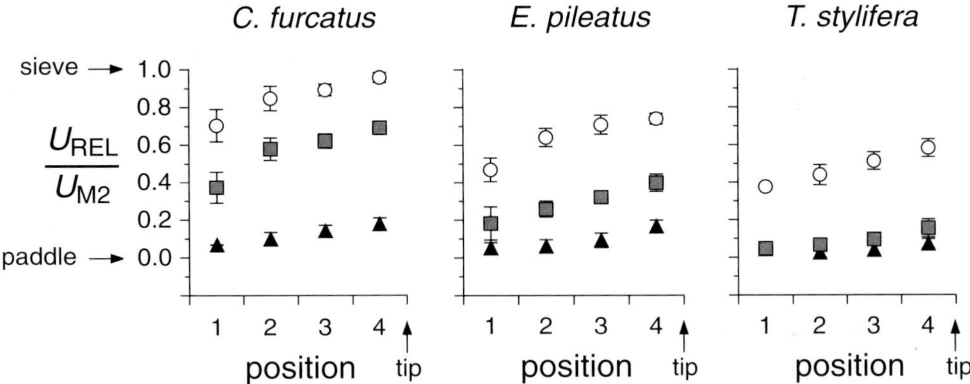

Fig. 12. Fluid movement through models of the M2s of *C. furcatus* (left-hand graph), *E. pileatus* (middle graph) and *T. stylifera* (right-hand graph). Fluid velocity (U_{rel}) through a model appendage at some point along its length was divided by the speed (U_{M2}) at which the appendage was traveling at that point to yield a measure of the relative flow through the appendage ($U_{\mathrm{rel}}/U_{\mathrm{M2}}$). The mean values of $U_{\mathrm{rel}}/U_{\mathrm{M2}}$ for each section of a model (see Fig. 11 for an explanation of positions 1, 2, 3 and 4) are plotted for models run at *Re* of 10^{-2} (black triangles), 10^{-1} (grey squares) and 1 (open circles). Error bars indicate one standard deviation (N=3–12). Kruskal–Wallis tests were used to determine whether the values of $U_{\mathrm{rel}}/U_{\mathrm{M2}}$ at each position for each species were significantly different between *Re* (P<0.05).

sieve-like behavior occurs is higher for the fine-meshed species than for the more coarsely meshed species.

E. pileatus are plastic in their feeding behavior and can change the *Re* at which their M2s operate. For example, they catch particles with single or multiple fling-and-squeeze motions at *Re* of the order of 10^{-2}, but reject unwanted material at *Re* of 10^{-1} (Koehl and Strickler, 1981; Price and Paffenhöfer, 1986; M. A. R. Koehl and G.-A. Paffenhöfer, unpublished data). Our model experiments indicate that a change in *Re* between 10^{-2} and 10^{-1} can produce a large change in leakiness for *E. pileatus* M2s (Fig. 12) (Koehl and Strickler, 1981). Indeed, microcinematographic observations of dye motions near the M2s of *E. pileatus* show that little water moves through the M2s during the various feeding motions (Koehl and Strickler, 1981; Koehl, 1993; M. A. R. Koehl and G.-A. Paffenhöfer, unpublished data), whereas water flows readily through the M2s during the faster rejection, thereby pushing the unwanted material away from the animal as explained in Fig. 13 (Koehl and Strickler, 1981). *E. pileatus* illustrates that an animal's hairy appendage is not constrained by its morphology to be just a paddle or just a sieve *if* it can change its speed across the *Re* range where the transition in leakiness occurs. In contrast, if a *T. stylifera* were to speed up its M2s to an *Re* of 10^{-1}, they would still operate as paddles (Fig. 12) because the leakiness transition occurs at higher *Re* for this fine-meshed species.

What are the consequences to leakiness of differences in the morphology of the M2s?

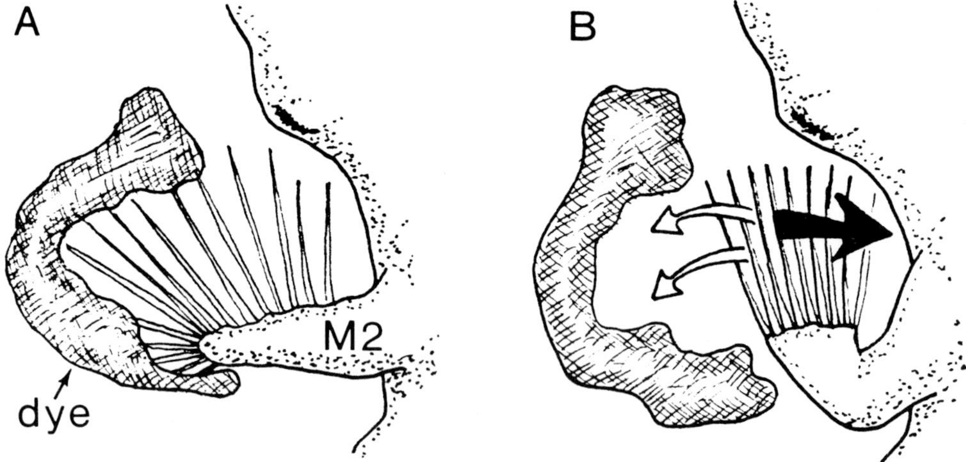

Fig. 13. Diagram of the rejection motion of the M2s of *E. pileatus* (diagrams based on tracings from a film of a feeding *E. pileatus* in Koehl and Strickler, 1981). (A) The copepod scrapes its M2s along the body surface and collects the unwanted material on the backs of the M2s. (B) After pushing the material away from the body, the M2s rapidly squeeze (black arrow) towards the body at an *Re* of 2×10^{-2} (Koehl and Strickler, 1981). The M2s are leaky enough at $Re=10^{-2}$ for water to move (white arrows) between the setae of the M2s, thereby pushing the unwanted material away. The rejected material is then carried off in the feeding current produced by the appendages indicated in Fig. 5A.

Our model experiments show that the coarser the mesh of the M2, the higher the U_{rel}/U_{M2} of the flow through it at *Re* of 1 or 10^{-1} (Fig. 14). However, at *Re* of 10^{-2}, mesh coarseness has no significant effect on leakiness. Hence, once again we see that whether or not morphology affects flow through an array of hairs depends on *Re*.

Conclusions

Many animals from different phyla use appendages composed of arrays of small hairs (*Re* of 10^{-5} to 10) to catch food or molecules from the surrounding water or air and to locomote through or propel fluid. The performance of these various functions depends on the fluid motion around and through the appendages. Physical and mathematical modeling, performed in conjunction with kinematic and morphometric studies of hairy legs on real animals, have revealed a number of patterns in how the flow through arrays of hairs depends on their structure and behavior.

Rows of hairs operating at very low *Re* function as paddles (i.e. little fluid moves between adjacent hairs), whereas those at *Re* near 1 function like leaky sieves. The *Re* range through which the transition in leakiness occurs depends on the geometry of the appendage.

How does the morphology of a row of hairs affect its leakiness? Increasing the gap:diameter ratio (*G*/*D*) of the array has little effect on leakiness at $Re<10^{-2}$, unless the array is moved relative to a nearby wall. In contrast, at *Re* of 10^{-2} and 10^{-1}, leakiness can be greatly increased if gaps are widened relative to hair diameters. However, if *Re* is 1 or

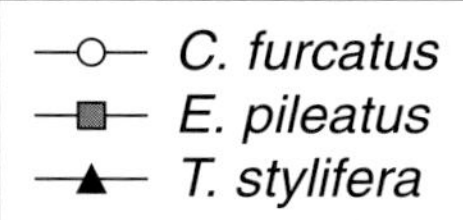

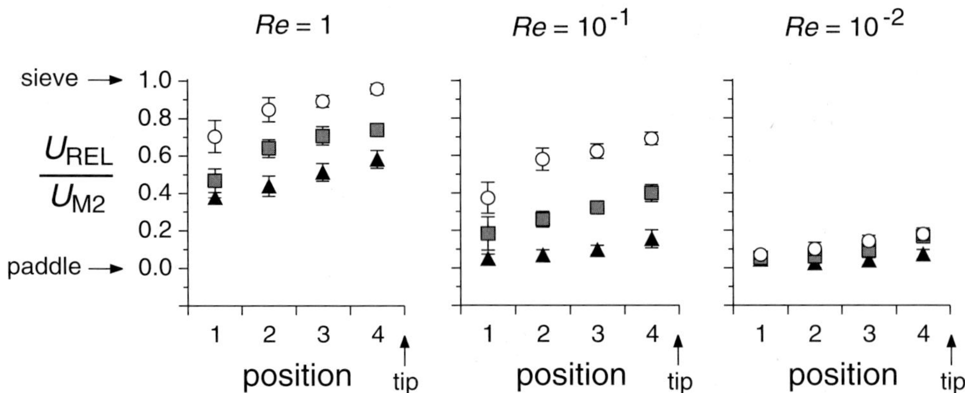

Fig. 14. Fluid movement through models of the M2s of *C. furcatus* (open circles), *E. pileatus* (grey squares) and *T. stylifera* (black triangles). The mean values of U_{rel}/U_{M2} for each section of a model (see Fig. 11 for an explanation of positions 1, 2, 3 and 4) are plotted for models run at *Re* of 1 (left-hand graph), 10^{-1} (middle graph) and 10^{-2} (right-hand graph). Error bars indicate one standard deviation (*N*=3–12). Kruskal–Wallis tests were used to determine whether the values of U_{rel}/U_{M2} at each position for each *Re* were significantly different between species ($P<0.05$).

10, gap width has little effect on leakiness unless *G*/*D* is already very small. This example illustrates that there can be scope for morphological change without performance consequences in one range of *Re*, while in another *Re* range there can be pronounced functional shifts as a consequence of the same structural alteration. Furthermore, a particular morphological change can have the *opposite* consequences at different *Re*. For example, increasing the number of hairs in a row decreases leakiness if *Re* is less than 1, but increases leakiness if *Re* is greater than 1.

How do the kinematics of appendage motion affect leakiness? If an animal whose hairs operate at very low *Re* ($Re\leq10^{-2}$) changes the speed of hair motion, there is no effect on leakiness (although, of course, the absolute speed at which fluid moves through the gap is changed). In contrast, changes in the speed of motion of hairs operating at $Re>10^{-2}$ can produce large changes in leakiness. The coarser the mesh of the appendage, the lower the *Re* at which this transition between paddle-like and sieve-like function occurs. In contrast, the behavior of moving the appendage closer to a wall increases the leakiness of hairs operating at $Re\leq10^{-2}$, whereas at higher *Re* this behavior has no effect. These examples illustrate that different behaviors (i.e. modifying speed *versus* altering distance from a wall) must be used at different *Re* to change leakiness.

These results have interesting implications if we consider the consequences of changing the size (and therefore changing the *Re*) of hair-bearing appendages, either during the growth of an individual or during the evolution of a lineage. Different types of behaviors and morphological features can affect performance at different sizes; therefore, *which* structural and behavioral characters are subject to natural selection might be size-dependent. Furthermore, a simple change in size can lead to a novel function without requiring the development of a novel structure (in this example, we see that it is physically possible for an appendage that was a paddle at smaller size to acquire the ability to filter). Kingsolver and Koehl (1985) have discussed the the evolutionary implications of novel functions resulting from simple size changes.

Our experiments have also revealed some practical issues that should be kept in mind by anyone studying the fluid mechanics of hairs operating at $Re \leq 10^{-2}$. For mathematical models of appendages (which are of finite length and which flap near the surface of an animal's body), the assumption of an unbounded fluid will lead to an underestimation of leakiness, and the use of two-dimensional analyses will lead to an overestimation. For physical models moved through a tank of practical dimensions, the walls of the tank will increase the flow relative to the model. Although this effect is desirable when modeling appendages that move near body surfaces, it may pose problems when modeling organisms swimming in an unbounded fluid. Furthermore, even though suspension-feeding appendages may look like fibrous filters, the mechanism of particle capture by those of very low leakiness may not be filtration, but rather may depend on the movement of the water surrounding the particle.

This research was supported by grants from the National Science Foundation, USA (OCE-820134 and OCE-8917404 to M.A.R.K.; OCE-8117761 to G. Paffenhöfer; OCE-9010115 to A. Cheer), the Office of Naval Research, USA (00014-90-J-1357 to M.A.R.K.), the Hasselblad Foundation (to M.A.R.K. and C. Loudon) and the NASA Ames Research Center (NCC 2-626 to A. Cheer), and by fellowships from the John Simon Guggenheim Memorial Foundation and the John D. and Catherine T. MacArthur Foundation (to M.A.R.K.). I am grateful to D. Abdullah, B. Best, A. Cheer, J. Jed, C. Loudon, G. Paffenhöfer and R. Strickler for collaborating on various aspects of the work cited here; to J. Kingsolver, E. Kwan and W. Ramsey for their work on the devices to tow or flap models; to J. Ahouse, D. Chiu, L. Castillo, F. Dardis, P. Huie, S. Kahane, B. Okamura, M. Piccolo and L. Sutanto for technical help; to K. Johnson and J. Jed for preparing figures and to B. Best and J. Shimeta for comments on this manuscript.

References

ALCARAZ, M., PAFFENHÖFER, G.-A. AND STRICKLER, J. R. (1980). Catching the algae: A first account of observations on filter-feeding calanoids. *Am. Soc. Limnol. Oceanogr. spec. Symp.* **3**, 241–248.

ATEMA, J. (1985). Chemoreception in the sea: Adaptations of chemoreceptors and behavior to aquatic stimulus conditions. *Soc. exp. Biol. Symp*. **39**, 387–423.

BERG, H. C. AND PURCELL, E. M. (1977). Physics of chemoreception. *Biophys. J.* **20**, 193–217.

BRAIMAH, S. A. (1987). Pattern of flow around filter-feeding structures of immature *Simulium bivittatum* Malloch (Diptera: Simuliidae) and *Isonychia campestris* McDunnough (Ephemeroptera: Oligoneuriidae). *Can. J. Zool.* **65**, 514–521.

CHEER, A. Y. L. AND KOEHL, M. A. R. (1987*a*). Paddles and rakes: Fluid flow through bristled appendages of small organisms. *J. theor. Biol.* **129**, 17–39.

CHEER, A. Y. L. AND KOEHL, M. A. R. (1987*b*). Fluid flow through filtering appendages of insects. *IMA J. Math. appl. Med. Biol.* **4**, 185–199.

CHILDRESS, S., KOEHL, M. A. R. AND MIKSIS, M. (1987). Scanning currents in Stokes flow and the efficient feeding of small organisms. *J. Fluid Mech.* **177**, 407–436.

COWLES, T. J. AND STRICKLER, J. R. (1983). Characterization of feeding activity patterns in the planktonic copepod *Centropages typicus* Kroyer under various food conditions. *Limnol. Oceanogr.* **28**, 106–115.

CRAIG, D. A. AND CHANCE, M. M. (1982). Filter feeding in larvae of Simuliidae (Diptera: Culicomorpha): Aspects of functional morphology and hydrodynamics. *Can. J. Zool.* **60**, 712–724.

DAVIES, C. N. (1973). *Air Filtration.* New York: Academic Press.

ELLINGTON, C. P. (1975). Non-steady-state aerodynamics of the flight of *Encarsia formosa*. In *Swimming and Flying in Nature*, vol. 2 (ed. T. Y.-T. Wu, C. J. Brokaw and C. Brennan), pp. 783–796. New York: Plenum.

FUCHS, N. A. (1964). *The Mechanics of Aerosols.* Oxford: Oxford University Press.

FUTRELLE, R. P. (1984). How molecules get to their detectors: The physics of diffusion of of insect pheromones. *Trends Neurosci.* **7**, 116–120.

GERRITSEN, J. AND PORTER, K. G. (1982). The role of surface chemistry in filter feeding by zooplankton. *Science* **216**, 1225–1227.

HANSEN, B. AND TISELIUS, P. (1992). Flow through the feeding structures of suspension feeding zooplankton: A physical model approach. *J. Plankton Res.* **14**, 821–834.

KINGSOLVER, J. G. AND KOEHL, M. A. R. (1985). Aerodynamics, thermoregulation and the evolution of insect wings: Differential scaling and evolutionary change. *Evolution* **39**, 488–504.

KOEHL, M. A. R. (1981). Feeding at low Re by copepods. *Lect. Math. Life Sci.* **14**, 89–117.

KOEHL, M. A. R. (1983). The morphology and performance of suspension-feeding appendages. *J. theor. Biol.* **105**, 1–11.

KOEHL, M. A. R. (1984). Mechanisms of particle capture at low Reynolds numbers: Possible modes of selective feeding. In *Trophic Interactions in Aquatic Ecosystems* (ed. D. L. Meyers and J. R. Strickler), pp. 135–166. Boulder, CO: Westview Press.

KOEHL, M. A. R. (1993). Hairy little legs: Feeding, smelling and swimming at low Reynolds numbers. *Contemp. Math.* **141**, 33–64.

KOEHL, M. A. R., CHEER, A. Y. L. AND PAFFENHÖFER, G.-A. (1984). Water flow around and particle capture by bristled appendages of zooplankton. *EOS Trans. Am. Geophys. Un.* **60**, 925.

KOEHL, M. A. R. AND STRICKLER, J. R. (1981). Copepod feeding currents: Food capture at low Reynolds number. *Limnol. Oceanogr.* **26**, 1062–1073.

KOO, J.-K. AND JAMES, D. F. (1973). Fluid flow around and through a screen. *J. Fluid Mech.* **60**, 513–538.

LABARBERA, M. (1984). Feeding currents and particle capture mechanisms in suspension feeding animals. *Am. Zool.* **24**, 71–84.

LAWS, E. M. AND LIVESEY, J. L. (1978). Flow through screens. *A. Rev. Fluid Mech.* **10**, 247–266.

LEONARD, A. B. P. (1992). The biomechanics, autecology and behavior of suspension-feeding in crinoid echinoderms. PhD dissertation, University of California, San Diego.

LOUDON, C. (1990). Empirical test of filtering theory: Particle capture by rectangular-mesh nets. *Limnol. Oceanogr.* **35**, 143–148.

LOUDON, C., BEST, B. A. AND KOEHL, M. A. R. (1994). When does motion relative to neighboring surfaces alter the flow through arrays of hairs? *J. exp. Biol.* **193**, 133–254.

MOORE, P. A., ATEMA, J. AND GERHARDT, G. A. (1991). Fluid dynamics and microscale chemical movement in the chemosensory appendages of the lobster, *Homarus americanus. Chem. Senses* **16**, 663–674.

MORRIS, M. J., KOHLHAGE, K. AND GUST, G. (1990). Mechanics and energetics of swimming in the small copepod *Acanthocyclops robustus* (Cyclopoida). *Mar. Biol.* **107**, 83–91.

MURRAY, J. D. (1977). Reduction of dimensionality in diffusion processes: Antenna receptors of moths. *In Lectures on Nonlinear-Differential-Equation Models in Biology*, pp. 83–127. Oxford: Oxford University Press.

PAFFENHÖFER, G.-A., STRICKLER, J. R. AND ALCARAZ, M. (1982). Suspension-feeding by herbivorous calanoid copepods: A cinematographic study. *Mar. Biol.* **67**, 193–199.

PRICE, H. J. AND PAFFENHÖFER, G.-A. (1984). Effects of feeding experience in the copepod *Eucalanus pileatus*: A cinematographic study. *Mar. Biol.* **84**, 35–40.

PRICE, H. J. AND PAFFENHÖFER, G.-A. (1986). Capture of small cells by the copepod *Eucalanus elongatus*. *Limnol. Oceanogr.* **31**, 189–194.

PRICE, H. J., PAFFENHÖFER, G.-A. AND STRICKLER, J. R. (1983). Modes of cell capture in calanoid copepods. *Limnol. Oceanogr.* **28**, 116–123.

RUBENSTEIN, D. I. AND KOEHL, M. A. R. (1977). The mechanisms of filter feeding: Some theoretical considerations. *Am. Nat.* **111**, 981–994.

RUPPERT, E. E. AND BARNES, R. D. (1994). *Invertebrate Zoology*. Sixth edition. Fort Worth, TX: Saunders College Publishing.

RUSSELL-HUNTER, W. D. (1979). *A Life of Invertebrates*. New York: Macmillan Publishing Co., Inc.

SCHMIDT, B. C. AND ACHE, B. W. (1979). Olfaction: Responses of a decapod crustacean are enhanced by flicking. *Science* **205**, 204–206.

SHIMETA, J. AND JUMARS, P. (1991). Physical mechanisms and rates of particle capture by suspension feeders. *Oceanogr. mar. Biol. A. Rev.* **29**, 191–257.

SILVESTER, N. R. (1983). Some hydrodynamic aspects of filter feeding with rectangular-mesh nets. *J. theor. Biol.* **103**, 265–286.

SPIELMAN, L. A. AND GOREN, S. L. (1968). Model for predicting pressure drop and filtration efficiency in fibrous media. *Env. Sci. Technol.* **2**, 279–287.

STRICKLER, J. R. (1984). Sticky water: A selective force in copepod evolution. In *Trophic Interactions in Aquatic Ecosystems* (ed. D. L. Meyers and J. R. Strickler), pp. 187–239. Boulder, CO: Westview Press.

TAMADA, K. AND FUJIKAWA, H. (1957). The steady two-dimensional flow of viscous fluid at low Reynolds numbers passing through an infinite row of equal parallel circular cylinders. *Q. J. Mech. appl. Math.* **10**, 425–432.

TAYLOR, G. I. AND BATCHELOR, G. K. (1949). The effects of wire gauze on small disturbances in uniform stream. *Q. J. Mech. appl. Math.* **2**, 1–29.

VANDERPLOEG, H. A. AND PAFFENHÖFER, G.-A. (1985). Modes of algal capture by the freshwater copepod *Diaptomus sicilis* and their relation to food-size selection. *Limnol. Oceanogr.* **30**, 871–885.

VOGEL, S. (1983). How much air passes through a silkmoth's antenna? *J. Insect Physiol.* **29**, 597–602.

HYDRODYNAMICS OF FILTER FEEDING

J. R. BLAKE[1] *and G. R. FULFORD*[2]

[1]School of Mathematics and Statistics, University of Birmingham, Birmingham B15 2TT, United Kingdom *and* [2]Department of Mathematics, Australian Defence Force Academy, Canberra, ACT 2601, Australia

Summary

A fluid mechanical model is developed for the filtering mechanism in mussels that enables estimates to be made of the pressure drop through the gill filaments due to (i) the latero-frontal filtering cilia, (ii) the lateral (pumping) cilia and through the non-ciliated zone at the ventral end of the filament. Calculations indicate that the lateral cilia can generate a sufficient pressure change to 'pump' water through the gill filaments. The velocity profile across the filaments indicates that a backflow can occur in the centre of the channel. Normally the latero-frontal cilia would damp out this backflow but in the case when all the cilia are upright, two 'standing' eddies may form at the mouth of the channel, forcing the incoming water to the side.

Introduction

The filtering mechanism in bivalve molluscs, such as the mussel *Mytilus edulis*, is a complex fluid mechanical problem that is based on three different sets of cilia which have differing functions. The most commonly observed cilia are the latero-frontal cilia (or cirri), which have a feather-like appearance. These are thought to be primarily responsible for filtering out the particles in the incoming stream. There are two sets of these identical cilia: one set covers the opening to the gill filament, the other set is upright for part of the cycle, apparently out of the way and causing no interference to the general flow field. These two sets of latero-frontal cilia interchange positions in a regular cycle. The second set of cilia are the lateral cilia; the 'pump' cilia that provide the motive power to develop the necessary filtering currents. These cilia have dexioplectic metachronal coordination – i.e. the coordinating wave amongst the cilia progresses along the band of cilia to the right (Aiello and Sleigh, 1972; Silvester, 1988). The third set of cilia are the short mucus-carrying cilia that transport the captured particles along the muco-ciliary escalator to the mouth.

However, the capture mechanism for the particles in the incoming stream has continued to fascinate marine biological scientists. It has usually been assumed that the particles are mechanically filtered out by the side branches on the compound latero-frontal cilia and then transferred to the frontal cilia when they open up. Circumstantial evidence, without the assistance of any fluid mechanical theory, would support such a theory. However, such an obvious theory bothered Jørgensen (1982), who proposed the idea of hydrodynamic shear forces that would push the particles sideways in the direction of the mucus-carrying

Key words: filter feeding, low Reynolds number flow, *Mytilus*, cilia.

frontal cilia. The role of the mucus is also extremely fascinating but will not form the basis of this paper, although the interested reader is referred to a recent review paper by Sleigh *et al.* (1988) for further information. While we cannot provide definitive answers to the above speculations, the present paper will develop a qualitative theory that will assist in our understanding of some of the observed phenomena.

Biological background and data

In Fig. 1A a schematic diagram of the water flow pattern in *Mytilus* illustrates the principal features that may be observed (adapted from Silvester and Sleigh, 1984). Inflow into *Mytilus* occurs through the relatively wide inhalant aperture into the mantle cavity. From here, the incoming sea water is 'pumped' through the filtering filaments to the suprabranchial cavity, from which the water is ejected to the outside in a relatively narrow high-speed jet ($2\,\mathrm{cm\,s^{-1}}$). The size of the external openings is under muscular control, which is reflected in the spacing of the filtering filaments inside (Jørgensen, 1983).

Fig. 1B is a schematic illustration of the flow pattern across two gill filaments where the three sets of cilia are clearly identified. The distance between the filaments is usually around 30–40 μm, the length of the latero-frontal cilia 20–30 μm, while the lateral cilia are about 15 μm and the frontal cilia near 6 μm in length. The frontal cilia transport the captured food particles and mucus towards the ventral marginal grooves of the gills. The latero-frontal cilia consist of two alternating sets that cover the opening to the inter-filament canal.

The organisation and coordination of the lateral cilia (the 'pump' cilia) are of particular interest. Silvester (1988) has outlined the principal features of the cilia organisation into a metachronal wave. A schematic illustration of the metachronal wave is shown in Fig. 2A. The length of the cilia is 15 μm while the metachronal wavelength is 12 μm. The metachronal wave is dexioplectic and, since the cilia are facing each other, the metachronal waves move in opposite directions. In Fig. 2B further details are provided on the metachronal wave. The band of lateral cilia has only a total width of 10 μm, while the cilia are 'fanned-out' over a 2.4 μm section in the effective stroke. Further data on the dimensions and frequencies can be found in Table 1.

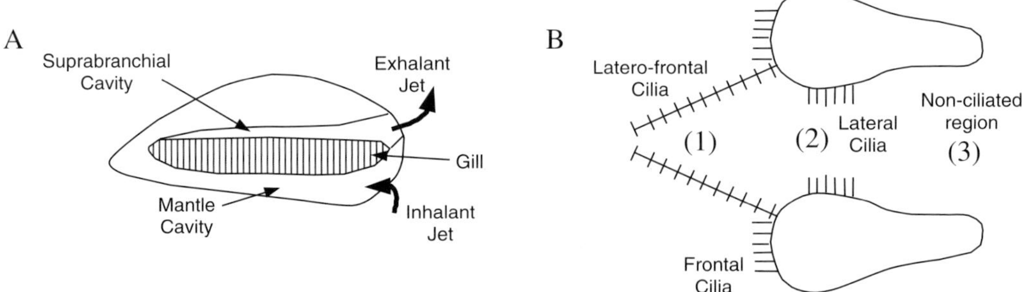

Fig. 1. Schematic diagram of flow through *Mytilus* gills. (A) Overall picture. (B) Gill filament. Adapted from Silvester and Sleigh (1984). Pressure changes across regions 1–3 are described in the text.

Table 1 represents a collection of data on the dimensions, velocities and pressures that have been reported in the literature by Silvester and Sleigh (1984). Jørgensen (1989, 1991) also reports a number of additional interesting features of the flow patterns. If the latero-frontal cilia are inactive, currents produced by the recovery stroke can extend 50 μm or more above the gill surface, whereas when they are functioning normally, these currents barely extend beyond the gill surface. Later we will see that these currents or eddies need not be associated with the recovery stroke but may be due to the pressure generation by the lateral cilia. Another interesting feature is the high observed flow velocities in the inter-filamentary canal, often 2–3 times the ciliary tip speeds. A range of values for the inter-filament canal width have been reported in the literature, from 40 μm (Silvester and Sleigh, 1984; Jørgensen, 1990) to more recent measurements of Jones *et al.* (1992), who reported values ranging from 16 to 35 μm, depending on overall mussel size. Assuming a lateral cilia length of 15 μm, then it is clearly possible for some overlap of the tips of the lateral cilia.

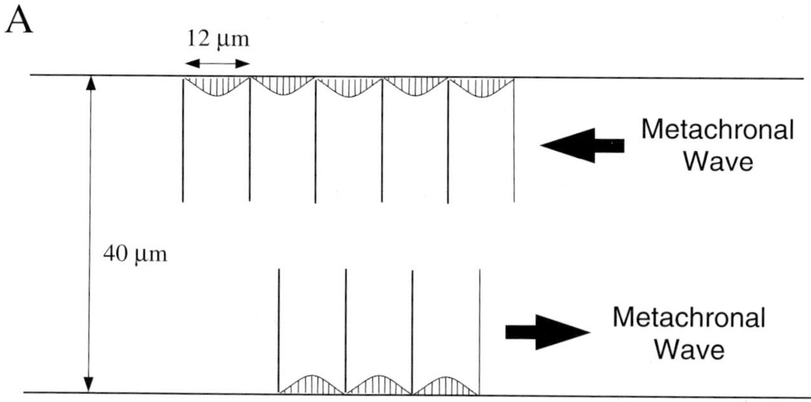

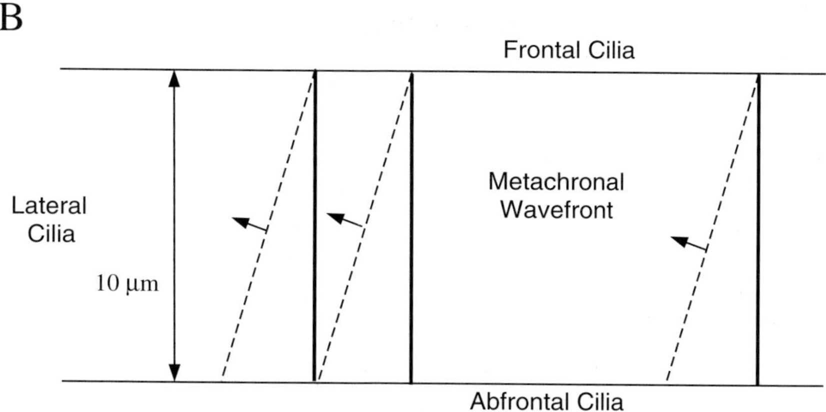

Fig. 2. Metachronal wave on lateral cilia (A) looking through the mouth of the gill filament and (B) looking down on the cilia.

Table 1. *Data on* Mytilus *from Silvester and Sleigh (1984) except for those marked by an asterisk which are from Jones* et al. *(1992)*

Quantity	Symbol	Values
Spacing of cirri branches	d	1.3 μm
Radius of cirri branches	r_0	0.1 μm
Radius of pump cilia	r_p	0.1 μm
Spacing of pump cilia	d_p	0.2 μm
Pump cilium length	l	15 μm
Pump cilium beat frequency	f	15 Hz
Length of ciliated section	L_1	10 μm
Length of non-ciliated section	L_2	190 μm
Half width of 'inner core'	a_0	0.5, 0* μm
Interfilament half-width	b_0	20, 15* μm
Half-distance between filament midpoints	$2h$	40 μm
Viscosity of water	μ	10^{-2} g cm^{-1} s^{-1}
Flow rate through channel	Q_0	0.032 mm^2 s^{-1}

Pressure estimates

The objective of the theoretical model is to obtain estimates of the pressure changes through the gills due to (1) the latero-frontal cilia (the 'filter' cilia), (2) the lateral cilia (the 'pump' cilia) and (3) the non-ciliated region. These regions are clearly indicated in Fig. 1B. The total pressure change across the gill is:

$$\Delta P = \Delta P_1 + \Delta P_2 + \Delta P_3 \tag{1}$$

where ΔP_1 is the pressure change across the latero-frontal cilia, ΔP_2 is the pressure change across the lateral cilia, and ΔP_3 is the pressure change along the non-ciliated region. Note that a negative pressure change corresponds to a positive pressure drop. We now proceed to obtain estimates for these three quantities.

Pressure change across the latero-frontal cilia

The latero-frontal cilia have a well-developed beat pattern that appears to have a rest period when covering the lumen to the gill entrance. These cilia have a feather-like appearance with side branches about 1.3 μm apart. In our analysis, we estimate the pressure drop as that over a single row of stationary parallel cylinders as has been done by previous authors (see, for example, Silvester and Sleigh, 1984; Jørgensen, 1981*a*,*b*). The contribution due to the beat pattern of the latero-frontal cilia is ignored. Thus, a common formula for estimates of this type is:

$$\Delta P_1 = \frac{-8\pi\mu U}{d[1 - 2\ln\tau + 1.6\tau^2 - 144\tau^4 + O(\tau^6)]}, \tag{2}$$

where U is the incident velocity, μ the viscosity, d the cilia branch spacing, r_0 the branch radius and $\tau = 2\pi r_0/d$. In this paper, we will not dwell on this estimate any further but highlight the need for a more detailed fluid mechanical study of the actions of the latero-frontal cilia, perhaps along the line of Cheer and Koehl (1987).

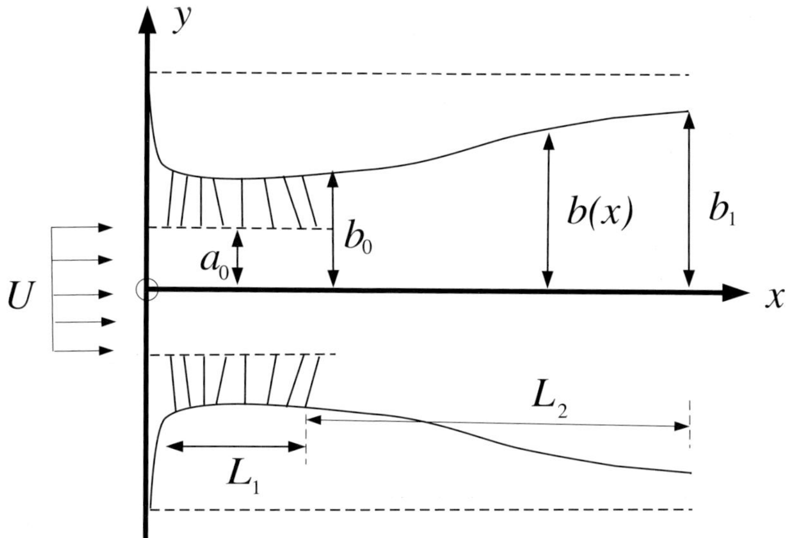

Fig. 3. Model used for lateral cilia pumping characteristics. Here l is the length of the cilia, a_0 is the half-width of the central core between the cilia and water of speed U enters the channel at x=0. Also, L_1 is the length of the ciliated section and L_2 is the length of the non-ciliated section with $b(x)$ as a function describing the half-width of the non-ciliated channel.

Pressure change across the lateral cilia

For the purposes of the mathematical model, we suppose that the edge of the channel is given by $y=\pm b_0$ for $0 \leqslant x \leqslant L_1$ (see Fig. 3). The few lateral cilia of length l are spread out over the section $0 \leqslant x \leqslant L_1$. Thus, the half-width of the 'central core' is $a_0=b_0-l$, the appropriate half-width dimension that is needed in calculating the pressure gradient. We consider separately the flow due to the cilia and the flow due to a pressure gradient. Clearly, even at very low Reynolds number, there will be some channel entry effects, but they will not make any significant change to the overall conclusions of this study.

The velocity field due to the cilia in the absence of a pressure gradient u_c will be approximated by:

$$u_c(y) = \begin{cases} U_c; & 0 \leqslant |y| \leqslant a_0 \\ \dfrac{(b_0 - |y|)U_c}{l}; & a_0 \leqslant |y| \leqslant b_0 \end{cases}, \tag{3}$$

where U_c is the average velocity of the liquid at the tips of the cilia. In many organisms, this is found to be usefully approximated by:

$$U_c \approx 2\pi f l, \tag{4}$$

where f is the beat frequency and l is the length of the cilium (see, for example, Blake, 1972; Blake and Sleigh, 1974; Fulford and Blake, 1986). However, recently authors have claimed that fluid velocities can exceed the tip speed (Sleigh, 1988), so possibly a larger value should be used. The volume flow rate due to the cilia Q_c is:

$$Q_c = U_c(a_0 + b_0) = U_c(2a_0 + l)\,. \tag{5}$$

Now consider the problem of unidirectional flow in a channel of width $2b_0$ under the action of a uniform pressure gradient $\mathrm{d}p/\mathrm{d}x$. To model the resistive effects of the cilia in their recovery strokes, we suppose that attached to the inner surfaces of the channel there is a doubly infinite parallel array of cylindrical rods, height $l = b_0 - a_0$, radius r_0 and spacing of the rods d_p. In the 'inner channel', the flow of the viscous fluid obeys the Stokes flow equations, i.e.:

$$\frac{\mathrm{d}p}{\mathrm{d}x} = \mu \frac{\partial^2 u_p}{\partial y^2}\,, \tag{6}$$

where p is the pressure, μ the viscosity and u_p the velocity in the x-direction, while Darcy's law for flow in a porous medium is applicable for flow through the rods, i.e.:

$$u_p = \frac{-k}{\mu}\frac{\mathrm{d}p}{\mathrm{d}x}\,, \tag{7}$$

where k is the permeability. From Happel and Brenner (1986), page 395, it is possible to obtain an estimate for k for normally oriented rods:

$$k = \frac{d_p^2}{4}\left[\ln\left(\frac{d_p}{r_p}\right) - \frac{1}{2} + \frac{r_p^4}{(d_p^4 + r_p^4)}\right], \tag{8}$$

where d_p is the distance between the 'spacing' cilia and r_p is the radius of these cilia.

The boundary condition on the plane surface between the two regions is a matter of some controversy, but two are commonly used: (i) continuity of velocity between the two regions or (ii) a mixed relationship connecting the shear stress and velocities (Blake *et al.* 1983). Because of the cilia density, the first boundary condition is more appropriate, leading to the following velocity field:

$$u_p(y) = \begin{cases} \dfrac{1}{2\mu}\dfrac{\mathrm{d}p}{\mathrm{d}x}(y^2 - a_0^2) - \dfrac{k}{\mu}\dfrac{\mathrm{d}p}{\mathrm{d}x}\,; & 0 < |y| \leqslant a_0\,, \\[2ex] -\dfrac{k}{\mu}\dfrac{\mathrm{d}p}{\mathrm{d}x}\,; & a_0 < |y| < b_0\,. \end{cases} \tag{9}$$

The volume flow rate per unit length Q_p in the channel is defined as:

$$Q_p = \int_{-b_0}^{b_0} u_p(y)\,\mathrm{d}y\,, \tag{10}$$

yielding:

$$Q_p = -\frac{2}{\mu}\frac{\mathrm{d}p}{\mathrm{d}x}\left(\tfrac{1}{3}a_0^3 + kb_0\right). \tag{11}$$

Thus, the total flow rate Q_0, which is equal to the flow through the lateral frontal cilia, is given by:

$$Q_0 = Q_c + Q_p = U_c(a_0 + b_0) - \frac{2}{\mu}\frac{\mathrm{d}p}{\mathrm{d}x}\left(\tfrac{1}{3}a_0^3 + kb_0\right). \tag{12}$$

Now the pressure change across the lateral cilia may be obtained by exploiting the above formula. Since the gradient is constant, the pressure change is simply obtained by multiplying it by the length of the band of lateral cilia.

$$\Delta P_2 = L_1 \frac{\mathrm{d}p}{\mathrm{d}x} = \frac{\frac{1}{2}\mu L_1}{\frac{1}{3}a_0^3 + kb_0}\,[(2a_0 + l)U_c - Q_0]\,. \tag{13}$$

This equation for the pump characteristics may be expressed as:

$$\Delta P_2 = K(Q_c - Q_0)\,, \tag{14}$$

where Q_c is previously defined in equation 5 and:

$$K = \frac{\frac{1}{2}\mu L_1}{\frac{1}{3}a_0^3 + kb_0}\,. \tag{15}$$

This expression shows the linear characteristic pump behaviour as observed by Jørgensen *et al.* (1988). The zero back pressure condition (ΔP_2=0) yields:

$$Q_0 = Q_c\,, \tag{16}$$

the flow being due entirely to the cilia while setting Q_0=0 yields the back pressure ΔP_{2B} required to stop flow through the gill:

$$\Delta P_{2B} = KQ_c\,. \tag{17}$$

Generally, the value of the porosity is small; thus, high pressures can be generated whenever a_0 becomes small. Jones *et al.* (1992) have suggested that the gap between the tips of the lateral cilia may indeed tend to zero. Fig. 4 shows a dramatic increase in the value of K of several orders of magnitude as the ratio a_0/b_0 decreases from 0.25 to zero.

Pressure change along the non-ciliated region

The theory for calculating the pressure gradient in the non-ciliated region has

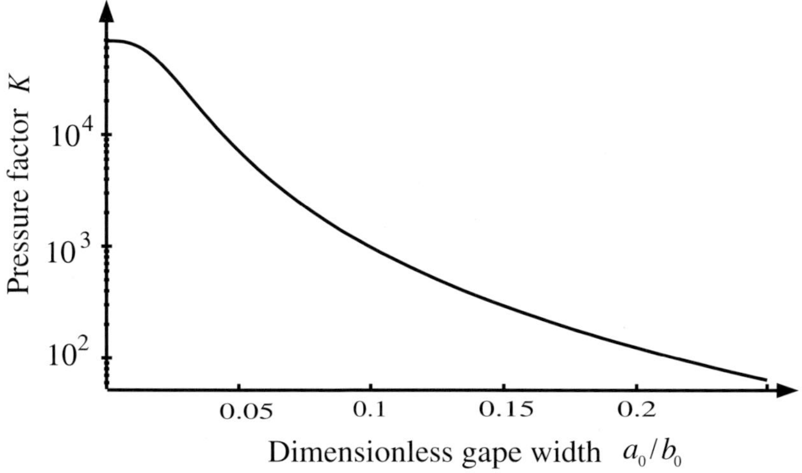

Fig. 4. Plot of pressure factor K (see equation 15) against dimensionless gape width for permeability k=0.5×10^{-5} with other data given in Table 1.

effectively been developed in the previous section where we can set U_c=0, but with the additional complication that the width of the channel is now varying with distance. To simplify the calculations we will suppose that:

$$b(x) = b_0 + (b_1 - b_0)\left(\frac{x - L_1}{L_2}\right)^\gamma, \qquad L_1 \leqslant x \leqslant L_1 + L_2, \tag{18}$$

where γ is the parameter to be specified. Thus, the pressure gradient is given by:

$$\frac{dp}{dx} = \frac{-3\mu Q_0}{2b^3(x)} . \tag{19}$$

Integrating over $L_1<x<L_1+L_2$, and introducing a change of variable $z=(x-L_1)/L_2$, the pressure drop is given by:

$$\Delta P_3 = \frac{-3Q_0\mu L_2}{2b_0^3}\int_0^1 \left[1 + \left(\frac{b_1}{b_0} - 1\right) z^\gamma\right]^{-3} dz, \tag{20}$$

where the term $-3Q_0\mu L_2/(2b_0^3)$ is the pressure change in a channel whose width does not change. In the cases γ=0.5, 1 or 2, simple formulae for the pressure drop may be found – for other values of γ we use numerical quadrature. Typically, $0<\gamma<1$ for a channel where the width increases, along the channel, faster than linearly, as in Fig. 1B.

The results are plotted in Fig. 5. The effect of widening the channel from b_0 to b_1 is to reduce the hydrodynamic resistance. Thus, the pressure difference required to drive the fluid at a given flow rate Q_0 is smaller as the gap width gets bigger. Also, it is advantageous for the gap width to increase more rapidly at the entrance of the channel than at the end, as shown in Fig. 5, where the pressure reduction is greater for larger values of γ. Typically, $b_1/b_2 \approx 2$, giving a relative decrease in pressure ranging from approximately 0.3 for γ=0.5 to 0.2 for γ=0.2.

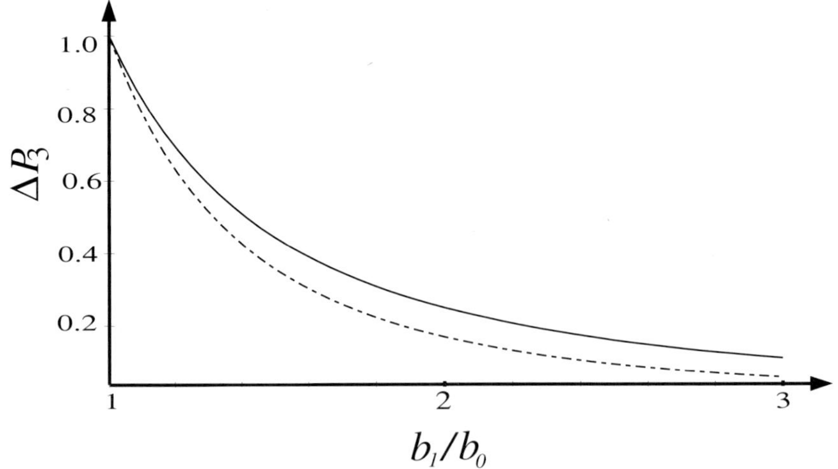

Fig. 5. Plot of pressure in non-ciliated region ΔP_3 against ratio of exit to entrance channel widths b_1/b_0. The pressure has been scaled with respect to the pressure in a channel of constant width b_0. The solid line corresponds to γ=0.5 and the dashed line corresponds to γ=0.2.

Pressure estimates: calculations

Experimentally the pressure in the mantle cavity (p_m) and suprabranchial cavity (p_s) can be measured using a catheter (Jones and Allen, 1986). Typically, p_m is about –5 Pa and p_s is around 12 Pa, giving a pressure change of about 17 Pa across the gill filament. There is a large variation in data for *Mytilus* in the literature (see Jørgensen, 1981*a,b*; Silvester and Sleigh, 1984; Jones and Allen, 1986). Our calculations would suggest that ΔP_1 is in the range –10 to 0 Pa, ΔP_2 can vary from 2 to 500 Pa and ΔP_3 from 3 to 7 Pa. However, the principal objective of this study is to provide a better qualitative understanding of the induced pressures in the inter-filament canal. It should be emphasised that the measured pressures are outside the canal in the mantle cavity and suprabranchial cavity and that both lower and higher pressures could be expected within the canal itself.

The main interest centres around the characteristics of the 'pump cilia'; the lateral cilia. Experimental work of Jørgensen (1981*a,b*) records the pressure/volume flow rate relationship. It is clear that one of the key features is the variability of the gape between the lateral cilia. In our theory, this is associated with the value of a_0.

Flow at the channel mouth

In this section we develop a simple model for the flow of the filtrate near the mouth of a gill filament channel. Here we assume that the latero-frontal cilia are open and inactive, and do not interfere with the flow.

The filtrate passes through one of about 20 parallel gill filaments. We may therefore employ symmetry arguments and consider the incident flow as occurring through the periodic structure as indicated on the left-hand side of Fig. 6.

Thus, we wish to consider flow in a semi-infinite ($x \leqslant 0$) channel of width $2h$ ($|y| \leqslant h$). Far upstream ($x \to -\infty$) the velocity is uniform across the width of the channel. Because the gill filament system is periodic, we require symmetry conditions on the 'boundaries'. In terms of the velocities we have:

$$\frac{\partial u}{\partial y} = 0 \quad \text{and} \quad v = 0 \quad \text{at} \quad y = \pm h, \tag{21}$$

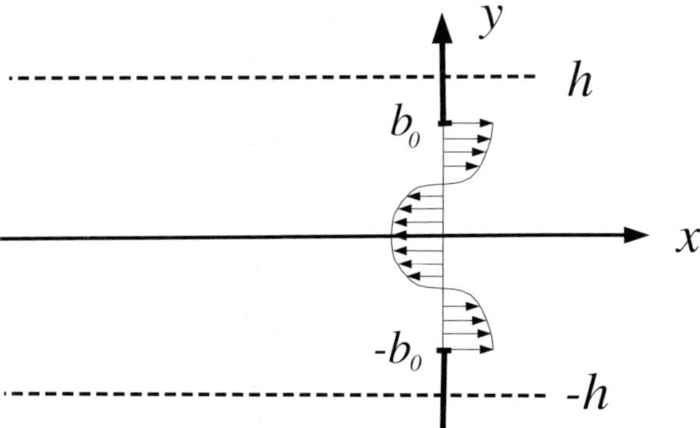

Fig. 6. Model used for investigation of capture eddies when latero-frontal cilia are inactive.

where u is the velocity in the x-direction and v the velocity in the y-direction. On the end boundary $x=0$, at the upstream end of the lateral cilia, we have mixed conditions: the no-slip condition on the solid boundary and a prescribed velocity profile produced by the lateral cilia over the remainder.

It is convenient at this stage to write the velocity field in the lateral cilia section as consisting of three components as follows:

$$u(y)=u_{\mathrm{c}}(y)+u_{\mathrm{p}}^{(1)}(y)+u_{\mathrm{p}}^{(2)}(y)\,, \tag{22}$$

where the velocity field $u_{\mathrm{c}}(y)$ due to the cilia alone is defined in (3) while the next two expressions on the right-hand side of equation 22 are obtained by splitting the pressure gradient flow field into the 'open channel' $u_{\mathrm{p}}^{(1)}(y)$ and 'porous medium' $u_{\mathrm{p}}^{(2)}(y)$ components as follows:

$$u_{\mathrm{p}}^{(1)}(y)=\begin{cases}\dfrac{1}{2\mu}\dfrac{\mathrm{d}p}{\mathrm{d}x}(y^2-a_0^2) & \text{for } 0\leqslant|y|\leqslant a_0\,,\\[2ex] 0 & \text{for } a_0\leqslant|y|\leqslant b_0\,,\end{cases} \tag{23}$$

and

$$u_{\mathrm{p}}^{(2)}(y)=-\frac{k}{\mu}\frac{\mathrm{d}p}{\mathrm{d}x}\qquad\text{for } 0\leqslant|y|\leqslant b_0\,. \tag{24}$$

We also require that $v(0,y)=0$ on the plane boundary and $u(y)=0$ for $b_0\leqslant|y|\leqslant h$, the no-slip condition.

It is, however, convenient to express the Stokes flow equations in terms of the stream function Ψ, which is related to the velocities as follows:

$$u=\frac{\partial\Psi}{\partial y}\quad\text{and}\quad v=-\frac{\partial\Psi}{\partial x}\,, \tag{25}$$

which, when substituted into the vorticity equation, yields the biharmonic equation:

$$\nabla^4\Psi=0 \tag{26}$$

for the stream function. In terms of Ψ, the boundary conditions become:

$$\Psi(x,y)\rightarrow\frac{Q_0}{2h}y\quad\text{as}\quad x\rightarrow-\infty\,, \tag{27}$$

while on $y=h$:

$$\Psi(x,h)=\frac{Q_0}{2}\quad\text{and}\quad\frac{\partial^2\Psi}{\partial y^2}(x,h)=0\,, \tag{28}$$

and on $y=-h$

$$\Psi(x,-h)=\frac{-Q_0}{2}\quad\text{and}\quad\frac{\partial^2\Psi}{\partial y^2}(x,-h)=0\,. \tag{29}$$

This second condition can be omitted on symmetry arguments. Thus, the flux through the system is Q_0. On $x=0$ we have:

$$\frac{\partial \Psi}{\partial x}(0,y)=0.$$

It is also possible to exploit symmetry in this problem and if we let Ψ=0 and y=0, we need only solve for the region $0 \leqslant y \leqslant h$ and $x \leqslant 0$. Thus, we may integrate equation 22 to yield the value for the stream function on x=0 as:

$$\Psi(0,y)=\begin{cases} U_c y+\dfrac{1}{2\mu}\dfrac{\mathrm{d}p}{\mathrm{d}x}\left(\tfrac{1}{3}y^3-a_0^2 y\right)-\dfrac{k}{\mu}\dfrac{\mathrm{d}p}{\mathrm{d}x}y, & 0\leqslant y\leqslant a_0 \\ \left[b_0 y-\tfrac{1}{2}(y^2+a_0^2)\right]\dfrac{U_c}{l}-\dfrac{k}{\mu}\dfrac{\mathrm{d}p}{\mathrm{d}x}y-\dfrac{1}{3\mu}\dfrac{\mathrm{d}p}{\mathrm{d}x}a_0^3, & a_0\leqslant y\leqslant b_0 \\ \dfrac{Q_0}{2}, & b_0\leqslant y\leqslant h \end{cases} \qquad (30)$$

with $\Psi(0,-y)=-\Psi(0,-y)$.

A solution is given by the series:

$$\Psi(x,y)=\frac{Q_0}{2h}y+\sum_{n=1}^{\infty}A_n\sin\frac{n\pi y}{h}\left(1-\frac{n\pi x}{h}\right)e^{n\pi x/h}, \qquad (31)$$

where

$$A_n=A_n^{(c)}+A_n^{(1)}+A_n^{(2)}, \qquad (32)$$

where each component on the right-hand side of equation 32 matches the respective contributions to the lateral cilia velocity profile in equation 22. Here:

$$\begin{aligned} A_n^{(c)}&=\frac{2h^2U_c}{l}\left[\frac{\cos(n\pi a_0/h)-\cos(n\pi b_0/h)}{(n\pi)^3}\right] \\ A_n^{(1)}&=\frac{2h^2}{\mu}\frac{\mathrm{d}p}{\mathrm{d}x}\left[\frac{n\pi a_0\cos(n\pi a_0/h)-h\sin(n\pi a_0/h)}{(n\pi)^4}\right] \\ A_n^{(2)}&=\frac{-2kh}{\mu}\frac{\mathrm{d}p}{\mathrm{d}x}\left[\frac{\sin(n\pi b_0/h)}{(n\pi)^2}\right]. \end{aligned} \qquad (33)$$

This solution is not uniformly valid as $x\to 0$, leading to divergent series for the velocities. However, as we know the values of Ψ in x=0, this does not create a problem. These potential difficulties can be overcome by developing biorthogonal series expansions along the line discussed by Joseph and Sturges (1978).

The calculations are more meaningful if we express all variables in domensionless form. Thus, we use:

$$\Psi'=\frac{\Psi}{Q_c}, \qquad Q'=\frac{Q_0}{Q_c},$$

and

$$x'=\frac{x}{h}, \quad y'=\frac{y}{h}, \quad \alpha_0=\frac{a_0}{h}, \quad \beta_0=\frac{b_0}{h}, \quad k_0=\frac{k}{h^2}, \quad l_0=\frac{l}{h},$$

where lengths are scaled with respect to h and the stream function with regard to Q_c, the mean flow rate due to the cilia alone. The problem is therefore fully specified by the four dimensionless parameters Q', α_0, β_0 and k_0 where:

$$\Psi'(x',y') = \frac{Q'y'}{2} + \sum_{n=1}^{\infty} A_n \sin n\pi y'(1-n\pi x')\mathrm{e}^{n\pi x'}, \tag{34}$$

where $A_n = A_n^{(c)} + A_n^{(1)} + A_n^{(2)}$. It also proves convenient to express $\mathrm{d}p/\mathrm{d}x$ in terms of Q' using equation 12, thus yielding:

$$\begin{aligned} A_n^{(c)} &= \frac{2}{(\beta_0^2-\alpha_0^2)}\left[\frac{\cos(n\pi\alpha_0)-\cos(n\pi\beta_0)}{(n\pi)^3}\right], \\ A_n^{(1)} &= \frac{1-Q'}{\frac{1}{3}\alpha_0^3+k_0\beta_0}\left[\frac{n\pi\alpha_0\cos(n\pi\alpha_0)-\sin(n\pi\alpha_0)}{(n\pi)^4}\right], \\ A_n^{(2)} &= \frac{-k_0(1-Q')}{\frac{1}{3}\alpha_0^3+k_0\beta_0}\left[\frac{\sin(n\pi\beta_0)}{(n\pi)^2}\right]. \end{aligned} \tag{35}$$

The significant dimensionless parameter is Q', which is the ratio of the 'through flow' to that which may be generated entirely by cilia in the absence of a pressure gradient.

Fig. 7A–C shows some typical stream function plots. We have taken $\alpha_0=0.125$, $\beta_0=0.5$ and the porosity parameter $k_0=0.5\times10^{-5}$. As the dimensionless flow rate parameter Q' decreases, we see that two eddies appear at the mouth of the channel. The eddies grow in magnitude as $Q'\to0$.

Backflow or eddies can occur in front of the filaments provided that:

$$Q' < 1 - \frac{\frac{4}{3}\alpha_0^3+4k_0\beta_0}{(\alpha_0+\beta_0)(\alpha_0^2+2k_0)}, \tag{36}$$

which was obtained from equations 30 and 12 by seeking criteria for the velocity u_1 at $y=0$ and $x=0$ to change sign. In the examples illustrated in Fig. 7, a range of values of Q' is included to illustrate the possible flow pattern that can develop in particular circumstances. In these examples, the critical value of Q' for eddies to appear is $Q'\approx0.733$. Above this value the throughflow is sufficiently strong that no eddies occur, but below this value the flow produced by the lateral cilia induces a sufficiently strong backflow in the channel that opposes the incoming stream to form a pair of eddies at the mouth of the channel.

Constant values of the stream function provide the trajectories of fluid motion which will coincide with the trajectories for 'small' food particles. These calculations highlight the range of phenomena that may occur and give an improved interpretation of the observations of Jørgensen (1982) with regard to the reported eddy behaviour.

In Jørgensen's (1982) paper, eddy patterns were also reported for isolated patches of cilia from *Mytilus* in the presence of a slide and coverslip. The patterns observed closely resemble those predicted theoretically for this experimental arrangement by Blake *et al.* (1982) and Liron and Blake (1981). It needs to be emphasized that these eddies are the

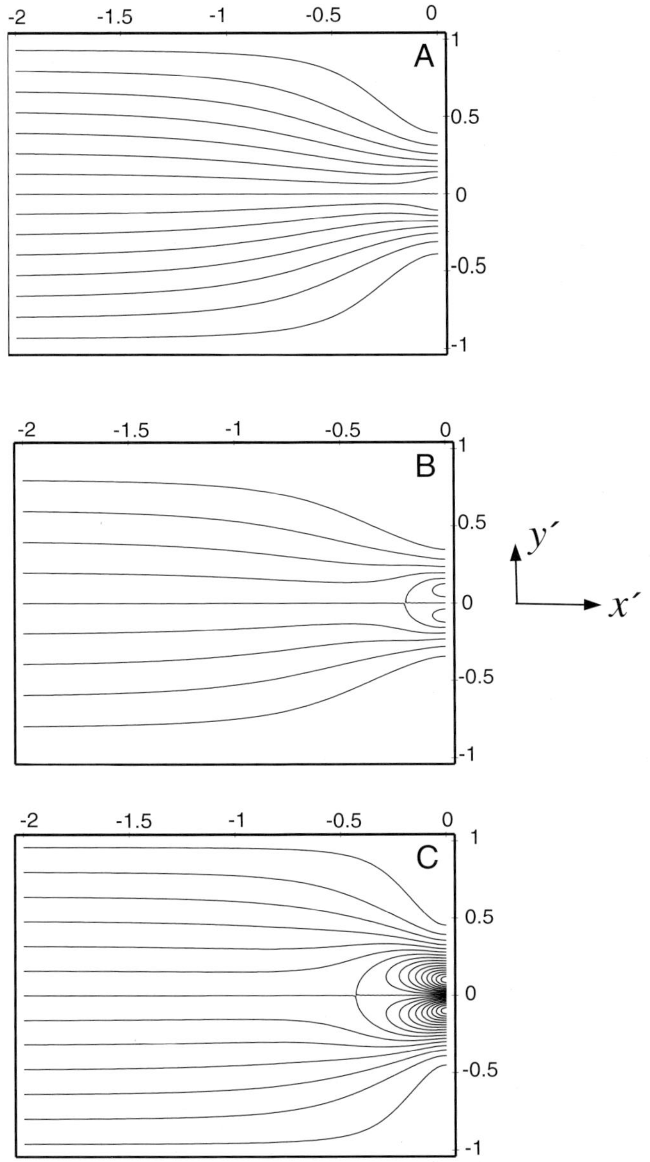

Fig. 7. Stream function plots for the stream function in equation 33. (A) Q'=0.75, (B) Q'=0.5 and (C) Q'=0.25.

result of the presence of the slide and coverslip and not any special features that may be attributed to the cilia.

Discussion

This paper has developed a qualitative understanding of features related to filter feeding in *Mytilus*. One of the principal controversies over the last decade has been the magnitude of the pressure changes in the gills. This paper develops a quantitative model that enables marine biologists and modellers better to understand the observed variations in measured pressures in the system. This variability is primarily associated with the gape between the tips of the lateral cilia, the principal pump in the system (abfrontal cilia would appear to provide some limited pumping as well, Jones *et al.* 1990).

Jørgensen (1982) has reported eddies in front of the latero-frontal cilia when they are open and inactive. This paper would suggest that this is entirely consistent with fluid dynamical theory in this special chemically induced example. However, when the latero-frontal cilia are active, this phenomenon is likely to be eliminated, since the moving latero-frontal cilia will interfere with the flow and reduce the effect of the backflow from the channel which produces the eddies.

The theory presented in this paper is an introductory model for the pressure changes in the inter-filament canal. Improved models will clearly need to be developed for specific features of the system, most notably the filter mechanism associated with the latero-frontal cilia, perhaps by extending the theory of Cheer and Koehl (1987) and the metachronally coordinated oblique beating pattern of the lateral cilia. A more detailed model of the hydrodynamics of the flow near the lateral cilia tips is needed in view of our result concerning greatly increased pressures when the cilia tips are close together. There is some evidence that fluid velocities may be higher than maximum ciliary tip speed, which suggests a new mechanism for ciliary propulsion (Sleigh, 1988) other than the envelope and cilia sublayer models previously reported in the literature (Blake and Sleigh, 1974).

The authors wish to acknowledge the valuable insight into filter feeding in *Mytilus* that has been gained from discussions with Professor M. A. Sleigh and Dr H. Jones.

References

AIELLO, E. AND SLEIGH, M. A. (1972). The metachronal wave of *Mytilus edulis. J. Cell Biol.* **54**, 493–506.

BLAKE, J. R. (1972). A model for the micro-structure in ciliated micro-organisms. *J. Fluid Mech.* **55**, 1–23.

BLAKE, J. R., LIRON, N. AND ALDIS, G. K. (1982). Flow patterns around micro-organisms and in ciliated ducts. *J. theor. Biol.* **98**, 127–141.

BLAKE, J. R. AND SLEIGH, M. A. (1974). Mechanics of ciliary locomotion. *Biol. Rev.* **49**, 85–125.

BLAKE, J. R., VANN, P. AND WINET, H. (1983). A model of ovum transport. *J. theor. Biol.* **102**, 145–166.

CHEER, A. Y. L. AND KOEHL, M. A. R. (1987). Paddles and rakes: Fluid flow through bristled appendages of small organisms. *J. theor. Biol.* **129**, 17–39.

FULFORD, G. R. AND BLAKE, J. R. (1986). Muco-ciliary transport in the lung. *J. theor. Biol.* **121**, 381–402.

HAPPEL, J. AND BRENNER, H. (1986). *Low Reynolds Number Hydrodynamics.* Martinus Nijhoff.

JONES, H. D. AND ALLEN, J. R. (1986). Inhalant and exhalant pressures in *Mytilus edulis* L. and *Cerastoderma edule* (L). *J. exp. mar. Biol. Ecol.* **98**, 231–240.

JONES, H. D., RICHARDS, O. G. AND HUTCHINSON, S. (1990). The role of ctenidial abfrontal cilia in water pumping in *Mytilus edulis* L. *J. exp. mar. Biol. Ecol.* **143**, 15–26.

JONES, H. D., RICHARDS, O. G. AND SOUTHERN, T. A. (1992). Gill dimensions, water pumping rate and body size in the mussel *Mytilus edulis* L. *J. exp. mar. Biol. Ecol.* **155**, 213–237.

JØRGENSEN, C. B. (1981*a*). A hydromechanical principle for particle retention in *Mytilus edulis* and other ciliary suspension feeders. *Mar. Biol.* **61**, 277–282.

JØRGENSEN, C. B. (1981*b*). Feeding and cleaning mechanisms in the suspension feeding bivalve *Mytilus edulis*. *Mar. Biol.* **65**, 159–163.

JØRGENSEN, C. B. (1982). Fluid mechanics of the mussel gill: The lateral cilia. *Mar. Biol.* **70**, 275–281.

JØRGENSEN, C. B. (1983). Fluid mechanical aspects of suspension feeding. *Mar. Ecol. Prog. Ser.* **11**, 89–103.

JØRGENSEN, C. B. (1989). Water processing in ciliary feeders with special reference to the bivalve filter pump. *Comp. Biochem. Physiol.* **94**A, 383–394.

JØRGENSEN, C. B. (1991). *Bivalve Filter Feeding: Hydrodynamics, Bioenergetics, Physiology and Ecology*. Denmark: Olsen and Olsen.

JØRGENSEN, C. B., LARSEN, P. S., MØHLENBERG, F. AND RIISGÅRD, H. U. (1988). The mussel pump: properties and modelling. *Mar. Ecol. Prog. Ser.* **35**, 205–216.

JOSEPH, D. D. AND STURGES, L. (1978). The convergence of biorthogonal series for biharmonic and Stokes' flow edge problems. Part II. *SIAM J. appl. Math.* **34**, 7–26.

LIRON, N. AND BLAKE, J. R. (1981). Existence of viscous eddies near boundaries. *J. Fluid Mech.* **107**, 109–129.

SILVESTER, N. R. (1988). Hydrodynamics of flow in *Mytilus* gills. *J. exp. mar. Ecol.* **120**, 171–182.

SILVESTER, N. R. AND SLEIGH, M. A. (1984). Hydrodynamic aspects of particle capture by *Mytilus*. *J. mar. Biol. Ass. U.K.* **64**, 859–879.

SLEIGH, M. A. (1988). Filter feeding by bivalve molluscs. In *Yearbook of Science and Technology*. McGraw Hill.

SLEIGH, M. A., BLAKE, J. R. AND LIRON, N. (1988). The propulsion of mucus by cilia. *Am. Rev. respir. Dis.* **137**, 726–741.

INSECT SOUND PRODUCTION: TRANSDUCTION MECHANISMS AND IMPEDANCE MATCHING

H. C. BENNET-CLARK
Department of Zoology, South Parks Road, Oxford OX1 3PS, UK

Summary

The chain of sound production in insects can be summarised as: (1) muscle power → (2) mechanical vibration of the sound-producing structure → (3) acoustic loading of this source → (4) sound radiation. At each link (→) optimal impedance matching is desirable but, to meet other acoustic requirements, each stage has special properties.

The properties of sound waves are discussed in the context of impedance matching between sources of different sizes or configurations and the surrounding fluid medium.

Muscles produce high pressures over small areas, but sound sources produce low pressures over large areas. Link 1→2 requires a change in the force:area ratio between the muscle and the sound source. Because the source size is necessarily small, sounds tend to be produced at a higher frequency than that of the driving muscle contraction, so link 1→2 may involve a frequency multiplication mechanism. This can also be regarded as a mechanism of impedance matching between the aqueous muscle and the structure from which the insect produces sound.

Stage 2 typically involves a resonant structure that determines the song frequency and is excited by link 1→2. If link 2→3 provides good impedance matching, the mechanical resonance is likely to be damped, with loss of song purity. So it is desirable for the stage 2 resonance to be sustained by coherent excitation and for the acoustic loading (link 2→3) to maintain the dominant frequency between stages 2 and 4. Examples where this occurs are cricket wings and cicadas.

At stage 3, the source size or configuration should allow impedance matching between the sound source (3) and its load (4). A variety of acoustic devices are exploited, leading to loud, efficient sound production. Examples that use resonant loads, tuned to the insects' song frequency, are the burrows of mole crickets and the abdomens of cicadas.

Overall, the mechanisms of sound production of many insects are capable of producing songs of high species-specificity that act as long-range signals.

Introduction

Many singing insects produce loud, long-range, pure-tone signals. The prime roles of such songs are to attract conspecific mates or in aggressive encounters, where loudness and the ability to sing persistently may be paramount. Insects are small animals, on the whole, so there is only a limited amount of muscle available to power the sound

Key words: insect song, bioacoustics, transduction, impedance matching, frequency control.

production. It is usually the males that sing, so sound production may lead to major anatomical and behavioural specialisations in this final adult stage.

In acoustic communication, as with the use of wireless or other long-range signals, specificity and range may be enhanced if the signal is sharply tuned. The receptor can then be tuned to the same frequency, to the exclusion of extraneous noise and the enhancement of the important signal. For such a communication, it is important that the signal causes a receptor response; here there are two main requirements. First, the signal should last long enough to allow the receptor's response to build up to above its threshold. If the receptor is sharply tuned, the signal must persist for longer and *vice versa*. But if the receptor is sharply tuned, its steady-state sympathetic response may be many times that of the driving signal, so it will be more sensitive. Second, in order for the receptor response to build up steadily during the signal, the signal waveform should be coherent; in other words, there should be no rapid changes in phase or amplitude during the signal.

The range of song frequencies that can be produced by insects is limited by such constraints as their body size and transmission losses in the fluid medium; since many species of insects sing, there is, in effect, acoustic congestion of the frequency bands. This leads to a further level of coding for species-specificity: the structure of the song. Insects' songs usually consist of a train of pulses, where the period of the pulses and the structure of the sequence of pulses are specific; this song structure is important for song recognition (see, for example, Huber *et al.* 1989).

Thus, the song of such insects as crickets or cicadas may be a long complex train of sound pulses. This pulse train can be reduced to its fundamental elements of pulses or tone bursts which are more-or-less sharply tuned to a single frequency in which the pulse can be regarded as a low-frequency modulation or tone burst of a higher-frequency carrier wave.

This review is concerned with the problems of converting muscle power into sound power. Problems of this type can be reduced to a series of functional steps. At each step, transduction occurs; and at each step, optimal impedance matching is desirable.

A general model of insect sound production

It may be useful to think of sound production as the following chain of events. (1) Muscle power is a series of contractions, initiated by a neural pattern that programs the song pulse. This causes (2) mechanical vibration of some structure, usually exoskeletal, which may or may not be the major sound source. This vibration is arranged to allow (3) acoustic loading of the vibrating structure, which involves transduction between the solid structure and the surrounding fluid medium. This stage of impedance matching leads to (4) sound radiation. At each link, optimal impedance matching is desirable but, to meet other acoustical and biological requirements, each stage has special properties.

Because each link in the chain is dependent on both its predecessor and its successor, the reductionist approach can only be carried so far. The justification for the approach is that parts of insects can often be made to function in isolation, so the role of a link can be examined both independently and as a component of the system.

Problems of acoustic impedance matching

A sound wave propagates as cycles of compression and rarefaction that proceed from the source at the velocity of sound, which varies from medium to medium. As the wave propagates, it also causes local cycles of fluid movement, termed the 'particle velocity'. The loudness of the sound can be expressed as its power or intensity, in $\mathrm{W\,m^{-2}}$; conventionally, $10^{-12}\,\mathrm{W\,m^{-2}}$ is taken as a threshold or reference level of 0 dB (see Olson, 1957).

Sound intensity can be expressed as the products of its components, the sound pressure p, measured in Pa (or $\mathrm{N\,m^{-2}}$), and the particle velocity u, measured in $\mathrm{m\,s^{-1}}$. A comparison can be drawn with electrical power, which is the product of volts (which can be regarded as an analogue of pressure) and current (which can be regarded as an analogue of velocity); the power in a known resistive load can also be expressed in terms of either the voltage across the load or the current flowing through it. In the same way, sound intensity can also be expressed in terms of the specific acoustical resistance of the medium, which is the product of the density of the medium ρ and the velocity of sound in it, c:

$$\text{Sound intensity} = pu = p^2/\rho c = u^2 \rho c\,. \qquad (1)$$

According to the maximum power transfer theorem, for optimal source-to-load coupling the source and load resistances should be equal (Langford-Smith, 1957). If the source and load have reactive components, these should be equal in magnitude but opposite in sign; in electrical terms, if the source impedance has an inductive component, this should be balanced by a capacitative load reactance; by acoustical or mechanical analogy, if the source has an inertial reactive component, the load should have a matching compliant component. The theorem has important implications for efficient sound radiation from a solid surface, such as an insect wing, into a surrounding fluid medium.

The specific acoustic impedance of a source depends on its shape and configuration but, for the present purpose, most insect sound radiators can be reduced to two cases. First is a vibrating disc or piston set in a baffle or wall, of which sound radiation from within the body of a cicada is an example. Second is a free-edged vibrating piston, on which the wings of a cricket or a fruit fly might be modelled. The acoustic impedance of either source can be reduced to its resistive and reactive components.

Owing to the rapid spherical spreading of the sound wave near to the source, acoustic 'near-field' effects occur out to a distance of about one-third of the sound wavelength λ. In the near field, the magnitude of the particle velocity relative to the sound pressure greatly exceeds that in the 'far-field' plane wave conditions farther away from the source. In a plane wave, the particle velocity is in phase with the sound pressure. Close to a very small sound source, however, the phase of the particle velocity leads the sound pressure by an angle that asymptotes to 90° as the source is approached (Beranek, 1949; Olson, 1957).

Similarly, the specific acoustic impedance of a source depends on its size relative to the sound wavelength (Figs 1, 2) (Olson, 1957). The specific acoustic resistance of a small vibrating piston in a baffle (which can be regarded as a monopole source), doubles as the source size doubles (or the sound frequency doubles), reaching that of the surrounding

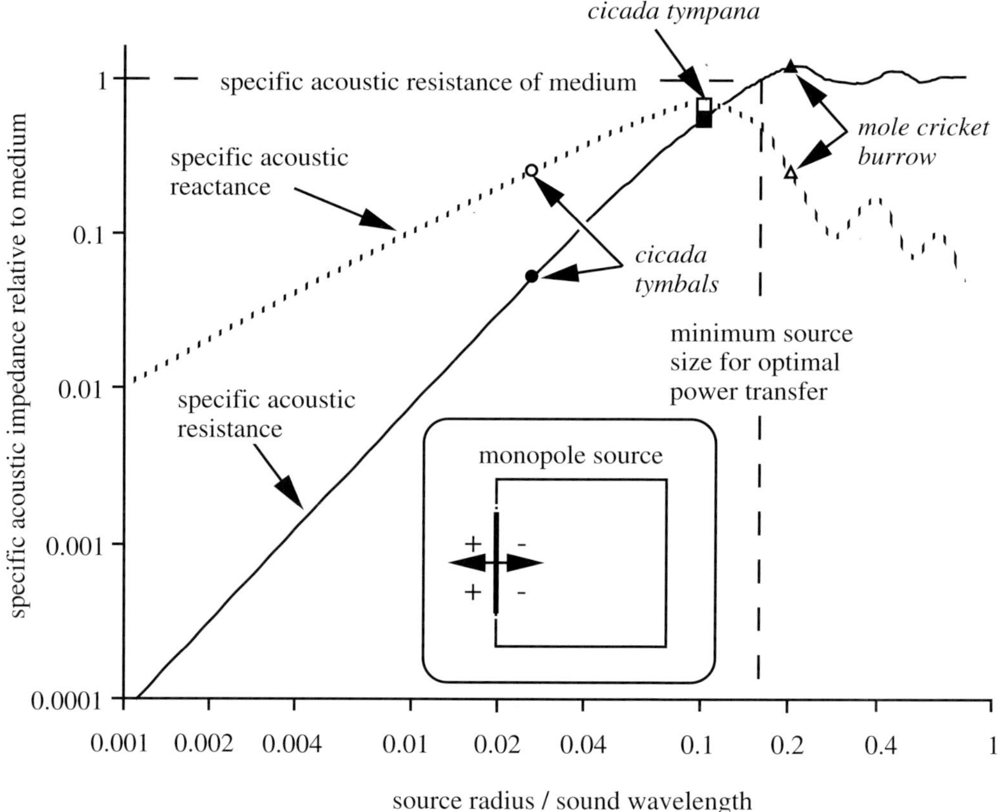

Fig. 1. Graph of the specific acoustic impedance (shown as the resistive and reactive components) of a monopole sound source or a vibrating piston set in an infinite baffle (for the configuration, see the inset), relative to that of the fluid medium, against the source radius/sound wavelength (λ). The symbols show the dimensions and specific acoustic impedance of examples discussed in the text (redrawn, with additions, from data in Olson, 1957).

medium in the far field at a source radius of about 0.16λ (Fig. 1). With a small piston vibrating freely in the medium (which can be regarded as a dipole source or two antiphase sources close together), there is substantial size-dependent acoustic current leakage from front to back. The specific acoustic resistance quadruples as the source size doubles, reaching that of the surrounding medium at a source radius of about 0.23λ (Fig. 2).

The reactive component of the source impedance also depends on the source size. With a monopole source smaller than about 0.1λ radius, the reactance is effectively inductive and exceeds the source resistance (Fig. 1), but with increasing source size the reactance becomes capacitative and is less than the source resistance. Thus, the loading is predominantly reactive for small sources but becomes predominantly resistive above the critical source radius of 0.16λ. If the source radius exceeds this critical value, its acoustic loading will be close to optimal. Similar considerations apply to dipole sources, but here

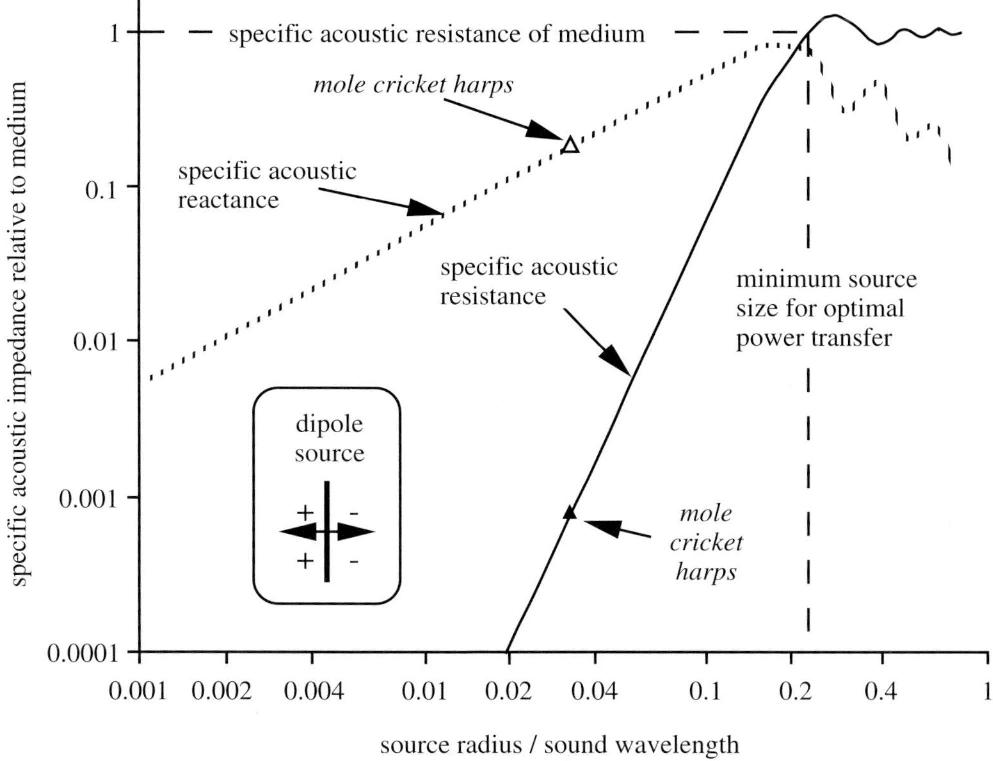

Fig. 2. Graph of the specific acoustic impedance (showing the resistive and reactive components) of a dipole sound source or a free-edged vibrating piston (for the configuration, see the inset), relative to that of the fluid medium, against the source radius/sound wavelength (λ). The symbols show the dimensions and specific acoustic impedance of an example discussed in the text (redrawn, with additions, from data in Olson, 1957).

the reactive component of a small source vastly exceeds its resistance (Fig. 2). As many insects, such as crickets, sing from free-edged vibrating structures that can be modelled as small dipole sources, it is important to consider their acoustic loading. One immediate consequence is that, for a good match to occur between the small wing and the surrounding air, the song wavelength should be short or, in other words, the song frequency should be high and should be even higher in smaller insects.

A singing insect can increase the specific acoustic resistance of a small sound-producing structure and thus improve the coupling between it and the medium in a variety of ways. The commonest is to place a free-edged piston source in some form of baffle: only a small part of a cricket's wing (*Gryllus* spp.) vibrates, and the rest of the wing acts as a baffle; tree crickets (*Oecanthus* spp.) sing far more loudly when they place their wings across a hole in a large leaf (Prozesky-Schulze *et al.* 1975). Another trick is to increase the effective source area: mole crickets place their wings across the throat of a horn-shaped acoustic burrow that has large openings at the surface of the ground (Bennet-Clark, 1970); in cicadas, the small tymbals cause pressure changes within the abdomen of the insect which are radiated as sound through the far larger abdominal tympana or eardrums (Young, 1990). The special cases of mole crickets and cicadas are explored in more detail later.

The problem of acoustic impedance matching also has relevance for the transmission of a sound wave from water to air (or *vice versa*), in which the specific acoustic resistances differ markedly; this is discussed below.

Transduction of muscle power into mechanical vibration

Muscle produces relatively low-frequency pulses of mechanical power. The highest frequency for direct muscle action in a singing insect is about 500 Hz, but such muscles are highly specialised (Josephson and Young, 1985). More typical song-producing muscles contract more slowly: those of the cricket *Gryllus campestris*, also used in flight, contract at about 30 Hz, and those of many cicadas contract at 100–200 Hz. The carrier frequencies of cicada songs, however, range typically from about 4 to 15 kHz (for reviews, see Dumortier, 1963*b*; Bennet-Clark, 1989; Bennet-Clark and Young, 1994).

Frequency multipliers

In many insects, such as crickets or cicadas, a single muscle contraction produces a song pulse which is a toneburst of many cycles of the song frequency. Other insects, such as the bush cricket *Ephippiger*, can produce many discrete song pulses from a single muscle contraction. Notable exceptions to this pattern are the short-range low-frequency wing-flapping communication of such small insects as fruit flies (see Bennet-Clark, 1971, 1975, for discussions of their acoustics).

In most crickets (Orthoptera – Ensifera: Gryllidae, Tettigoniidae etc.), contraction of the sound-producing muscles causes a closing movement of the partially opened forewings. The wings of the male are highly specialised, with a file on one wing and a plectrum or scraper on the other. The cycle of catch and release of a file tooth by the plectrum causes buckling of the 'harp' or 'mirror' of the wing, which in turn leads to a sequence of buckling movements. The file varies from species to species in length and number of teeth from about 35 to over 300 teeth (for reviews, see Dumortier 1963*a*; Bennet-Clark, 1989). In practice, one wing-closing stroke covers up to three-quarters of the length of the file, so the mechanism provides a frequency multiplication from 20-fold to over 200-fold (Table 1).

In crickets, the plectrum and file mechanism excites and sustains resonance of part of the wing. There are two principal mechanisms.

In gryllids and their relatives, in which the left and right forewings are similar, the harp areas (Fig. 3A) of both wings are set into vibration by the mechanical escapement of the file and plectrum (Elliott and Koch, 1985). The harp region can, independently, be excited into resonance by sound (Fig. 3B). The harp's resonant frequency varies from species to species: a range from 4.2 to 4.85 kHz has been found in *Gryllus campestris* (Nocke, 1971) and about 2.8 kHz was reported in *Scapteriscus acletus* (Bennet-Clark, 1987); these frequencies correspond closely with those of the insects' songs, 4.7 kHz and 2.7 kHz

Table 1. *Song frequency multiplier mechanisms in insects*

	Gryllotalpa vineae (Orthoptera: mole cricket)	*Cyclochila australasiae* (Hemiptera: cicada)
Mechanism	File teeth on wing trip in sequence	Tymbal ribs buckle in sequence
Song pulse rate	approx. 65 Hz	240 Hz
Song frequency	3.5 kHz	4.3 kHz
Song pulse duration	8 ms	3 ms
1/pulse duration	125 Hz	330 Hz
Multiplication factor	28×	14×

The multiplication factor is taken as the song frequency × pulse duration.

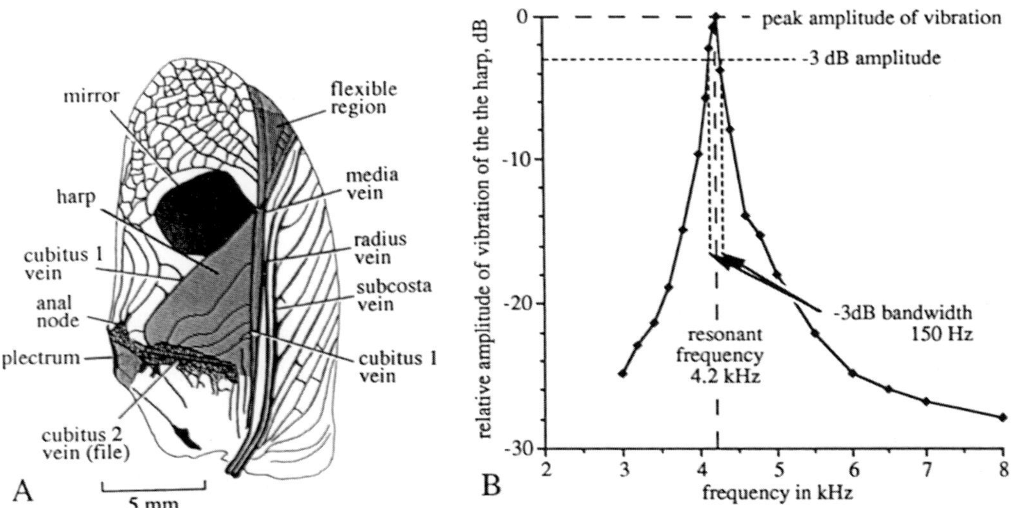

Fig. 3. (A) Drawing of the underside of the right forewing of the cricket *Gryllus campestris* to show the plectrum that engages in the file teeth of the contralateral wing. Successive tripping of the file teeth excites resonant vibration of the harp area of both wings. The vein nomenclature follows the Comstock–Needham convention (Ragge, 1955) (relabelled from Bennet-Clark, 1989). (B) Frequency–energy spectrum of the vibration of the harp of *Gryllus campestris* when excited by sound. The harp resonance shows a peak at 4.2 kHz. The quality factor Q, calculated from equation 2 in the text, is 28 (redrawn from data in Nocke, 1971).

respectively. The harp area of the wing can be modelled accurately as an elastic plate clamped at the edges (Pierce, 1948; Nocke, 1971).

In tettigoniids, the two forewings differ markedly; the wing bearing the file is robust while that with the plectrum has a thin membrane surrounded by a discrete U-shaped sclerotised frame. The plectrum appears to excite a resonance in the U-shaped frame, causing sound radiation from the thin membrane (Bailey, 1970). The frame has been modelled as a vibrating bar (Bailey, 1970); with such vibrating bars, which include tuning forks, the resonant frequency is proportional to $1/l^2$, where l is a characteristic length.

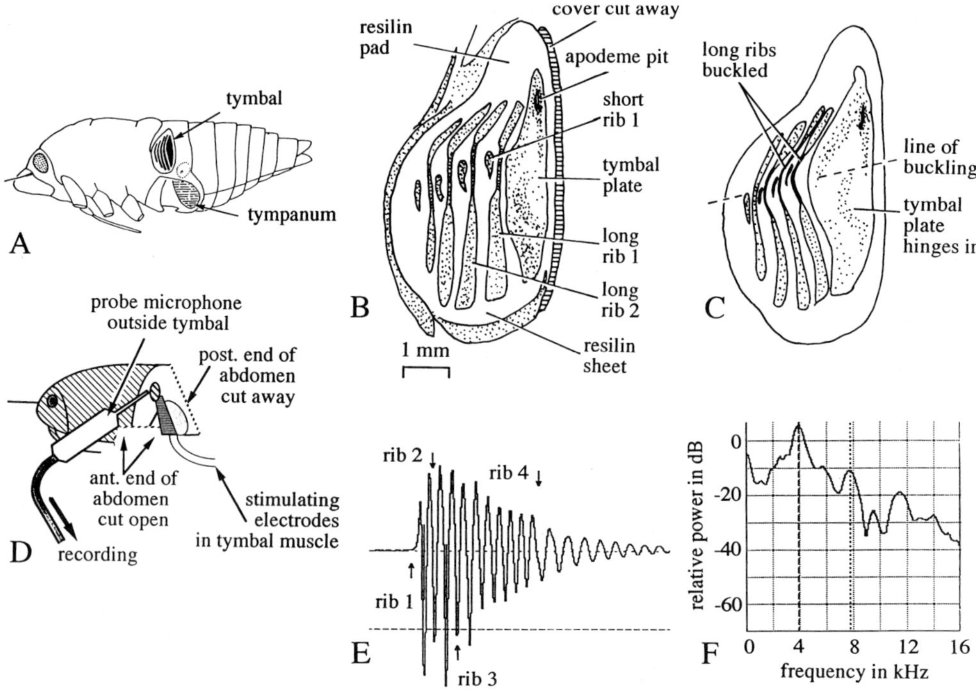

Fig. 4 (A) View of the left side of the cicada *Cyclochila australasiae* to show the tymbal which excites the abdominal resonator and the thin tympanal membrane through which sound is radiated from the abdomen (by kind permission of Dr David Young). (B) The left tymbal of the cicada *Cyclochila australasiae.* The tymbal plate is pulled inwards by the tymbal muscle, which inserts at the apodeme pit and causes sequential buckling of the long ribs from back to front. The resilin pad restores the shape of the tymbal after relaxation of the tymbal muscle. (C) The tymbal, showing buckling of three tymbal long ribs. As each rib buckles inwards, it produces a resonant click (B and C are tracings from a video record). (D) Diagram of an experimental cicada preparation, with parts of the thorax and abdomen cut away, used to stimulate and record the sound of tymbal clicks with minimal influence from the cicada body. (E) Oscillogram of a sound pulse produced by stimulation of the tymbal muscle causing sequential buckling of the tymbal ribs in a cut-away cicada preparation (D). The sequence of buckling of the tymbal ribs (C) is deduced from the shape of the pulse envelope and the frequency–energy spectrum of the pulse. (F) Frequency–energy spectrum of the sound pulse shown in E, showing the 4 kHz dominant frequency of a train of tymbal clicks of the cicada *Cyclochila australasiae.* The 8 kHz sideband is produced by the modulation of the pulse envelope every second cycle (see E) (E and F are modified from data used in Young and Bennet-Clark, 1995).

Taking a standard linear dimension of the harp frame, this model gives a good prediction of song frequency for a wide range of tettigonioid species (Sales and Pye, 1974).

A very different mechanism is found in cicadas, which have paired tymbals in the anterior abdominal tergites (Fig. 4A,B). The domed tymbal is driven by a large muscle which brings about sequential inward buckling of a series of convex sclerotised ribs (Fig. 4B,C) (Pringle, 1954; Simmons and Young, 1978). Recent work with *Cyclochila* has shown that, as each tymbal rib buckles inwards, a pulse of sound or click is produced and that the tymbal resonates at the 4 kHz (Fig. 4F) of the insect's song (Fig. 4E,F) (Young and Bennet-Clark, 1995). During a single contraction of the tymbal muscle, successive ribs of the tymbal buckle at the same phase but at every second (Fig. 4E) or third cycle, so that the sequential rib clicks contribute to the production of a long coherent song pulse (Fig. 4E).

Although the mechanisms differ between the different groups, they share various common features (Table 1). A single slow muscle contraction brings about many cycles of mechanical vibration of part of the insect exoskeleton; there is frequency multiplication between the driving muscle contraction and the resulting vibration. The driven region is also typically the resonator that determines the song carrier frequency.

Force:area and liquid-phase:gas-phase relationships

Compared with sounds, muscle contraction produces relatively high pressures. Values of 300 kPa in tetanus and 30–100 kPa in a muscle twitch are typical (Alexander, 1983); 1 atmosphere is 10^5 Pa, so peak muscle pressures are around 2 atmospheres. A sound wave in air with a pressure difference of 2 atmospheres equates to a sound pressure of 194 dB, which is explosively loud! Normal air-borne acoustic communication occurs at far lower levels, between typical thresholds of 30–40 dB and maximum levels of 80–100 dB.

Since muscle is predominantly water, its density, the propagation velocity of a sound wave in it and its specific acoustic resistance (see Olson, 1957) differ markedly from those of the air into which the insect is singing (Table 2). According to the maximum power transfer theorem, the source and load resistances should be the same, for optimal source-to-load coupling, but between muscle and air there is a 3650:1 specific acoustic resistance mismatch. From equation 1, for a sound wave of a given intensity, impedance matching would require sound pressures in water that are 60 times those in air and particle velocities in air that are 60 times those in water.

This can be regarded as a problem of impedance conversion or transformation, but one for which it is difficult to make a formal model. In many singing insects, a muscle of small cross-sectional area and high-pressure contraction is used to drive a piston of large area, e.g. the harp of the cricket forewings, with consequent pressure transformation. Although the amplitude of vibration of the harp is probably quite small, the frequency multiplier mechanism of the file and plectrum (Table 1) as well as the resonance of the

Table 2. *Acoustic properties of water and air*

	Water		Air
Density ρ (kg m^{-3})	1000		1.2
Velocity of sound c (m s^{-1})	1500		340
Specific acoustic resistance ρc (kg m^{-2} s^{-1})	1.5×10^6		410
Ratio of specific acoustic resistances	3650	to	1
Sound pressure ratio	60.4	to	1
Particle velocity ratio	1	to	60.4

See equation 1 for the relationship between the terms used in this table.

harp allow a single muscle contraction at low velocity to produce vibration at a far higher frequency, with a consequent increase in vibration velocity.

Impedance conversion of this type but in the opposite direction, from air to water, occurs in vertebrate hearing (for a review, see Fletcher, 1992).

Mechanical drive to the vibrating structure

The design requirements for a domestic loudspeaker differ significantly from those for an insect sound radiator. The loudspeaker should transduce all frequencies and respond rapidly to transient signals, so it should have a non-resonant response but, because electronic amplifier power is readily available, the loudspeaker can be inefficient. By contrast, since insect song pulses do not show rapid changes of amplitude, the sound-producing structure can be sharply tuned and sound radiation can be optimised to the song frequency. Because muscle power may be limited and costly, high transduction efficiency is desirable.

Sharpness of tuning and the quality factor Q

The sharpness of tuning of a resonant system can be expressed using the quality factor Q (sometimes known as Q_{3dB}). The effective gain in the amplitude of the response at resonance is Q times that at a frequency far below the resonant frequency.

Q can be measured in several ways (Morse, 1948; Langford-Smith, 1957); for example, from the change of amplitude (or of phase) with frequency:

$$Q = \frac{\text{resonant frequency}}{\text{bandwidth at } -3\text{ dB}} \qquad (2)$$

(-3 dB is half peak power). The easiest way of determining the Q of insect song pulses or their resonators is to measure the amplitude of successive cycles at the build-up at the start or free decay following a driven oscillation. Q is then given by the slope of a plot of ln(increment) or ln(decrement) per cycle:

$$Q = \frac{\pi}{\ln(\text{increment})} = \frac{\pi}{\ln(\text{decrement})}\ . \qquad (3)$$

The vibration of a high-Q resonator takes a long time to build up and decay, compared with that of a low-Q resonator (Fig. 5), because $1/Q$ of the energy is gained or lost in successive cycles of the vibration. So long as energy is supplied at this rate, the amplitude of vibration will not decay.

The songs of insects are confined to relatively narrow frequency bands, suggesting that they have a sharply tuned resonant system (Table 3). Thus, their sound-producing mechanism must be able to provide mechanical power to replace the power that is radiated as sound.

Maintaining the vibration and its coherence

This is the role of the escapement of a clock – and this analogy has been made for the role of the file and plectrum of the cricket wing resonator (Elliott and Koch, 1985). Such

Table 3. *Dominant frequency and sharpness of tuning (as Q) of the songs of various insects*

Insect	Order	Dominant song frequency (kHz)	Song Q
Gryllotalpa vineae	Orthoptera, Ensifera	3.4	18
G. gryllotalpa	Orthoptera, Ensifera	1.6	16
Gryllus campestris	Orthoptera, Ensifera	4.7	10
Cyclochila australasiae	Hemiptera, Homoptera	4.3	>10

Data are taken from Bennet-Clark (1975) and Bennet-Clark and Young (1992).

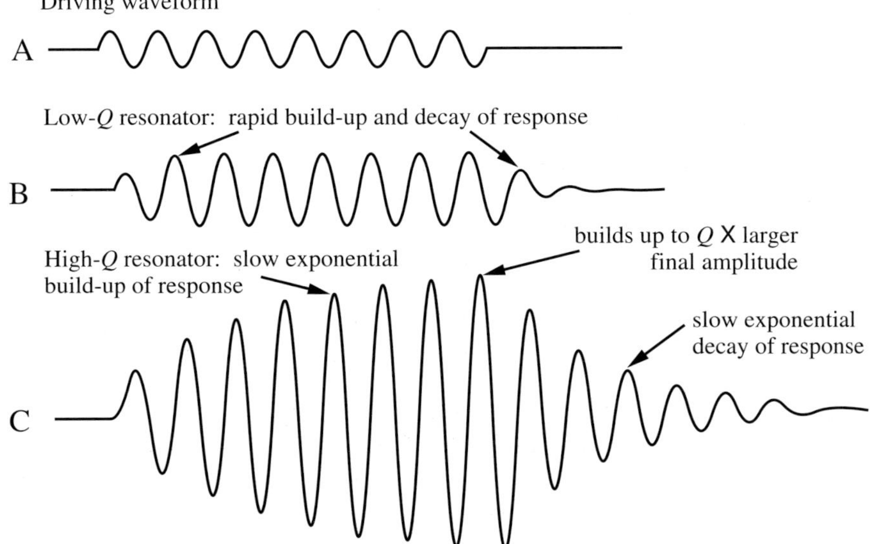

Fig. 5. Diagram of the response of resonators to a sinusoidal drive. (A) The driving tone-burst. (B) The response of a low-Q resonator builds up rapidly to a small peak amplitude and then decays rapidly. (C) The response of a high-Q resonator builds up slowly to a far larger peak amplitude and then decays slowly.

an escapement has two important functions: first, because energy is only supplied to the resonator at a particular phase in the vibration, the coherence of the vibration is maintained; second, the energy can be fed to the resonator as a series of quanta to replace the energy that is dissipated in each cycle.

The first of these functions has been observed in crickets, where the vibration of the harp is sustained at every cycle by the catch–release action of the plectrum on the teeth of the file (Fig. 6A,B) (Elliott and Koch, 1985) and where the harps of the two wings are driven in-phase, one directly by the file and the other *via* the plectrum, which acts as a phase inverter (Fig. 6C,D). In cicadas, coherent excitation of the tymbal resonance occurs

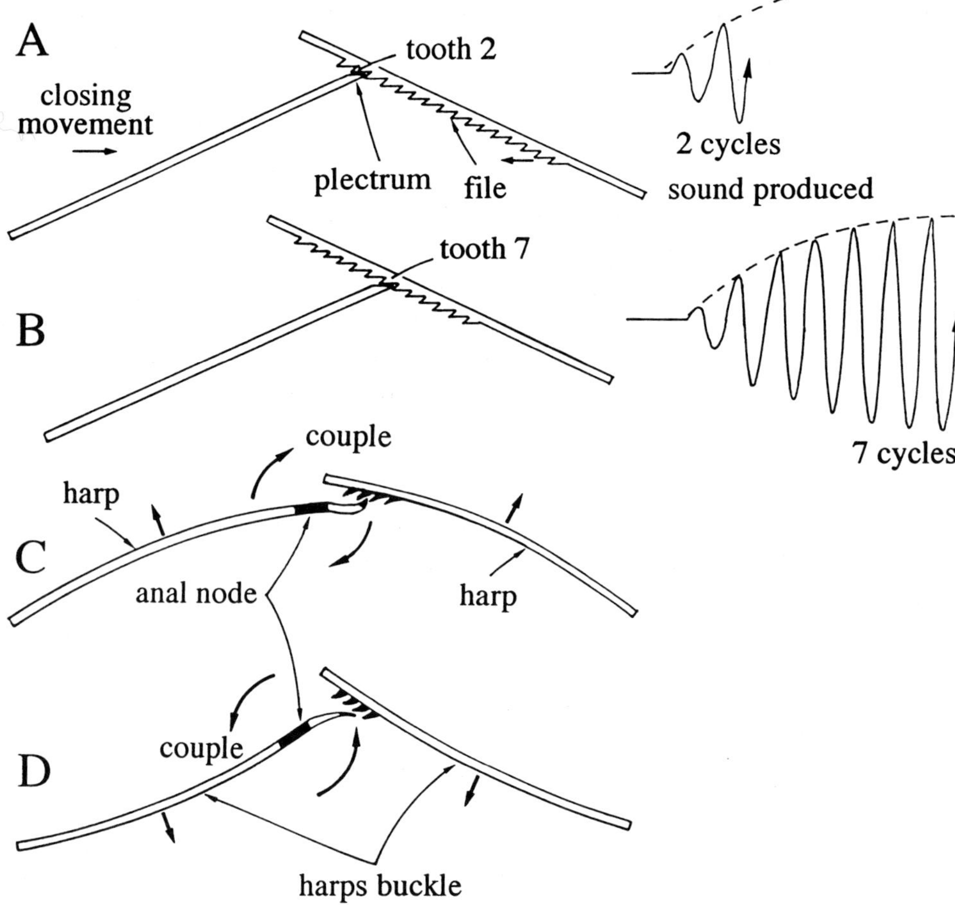

Fig. 6. A model of the excitation of the harp of gryllid crickets by the file-and-plectrum mechanism. A and B show how successive catch and release of the plectrum on the teeth of the file leads to the build-up of a succession of cycles of the song pulse. Note that the catch and release action of one tooth leads to the production of one cycle of the sound. C and D show how the plectrum might act as a phase inverter by producing a couple around the anal node (see Fig. 3A) of the left wing. The catch and release of teeth on the harp of the right-hand wing by the plectrum then causes the harps of both wings to be excited simultaneously and in the same phase. Because both harps are resonant at the same frequency, the mechanism produces a coherent waveform at the resonant frequency (from Bennet-Clark, 1989).

by the buckling of successive tymbal ribs at the same phase of the waveform but at intervals of two or three cycles of the vibration (Fig. 4E) (Bennet-Clark and Young, 1992; Young and Bennet-Clark, 1995).

Evidence that the energy is supplied continuously during the song pulse to replace the energy that is dissipated as sound is given by the close correspondence between the instantaneous amplitude of the song pulse envelope and the spacing of the teeth of the file in two species of mole cricket (Bennet-Clark, 1970, 1987).

Since many of the insects that use mechanisms of this type are also noisy for their size, their sound-producing mechanisms must be capable of efficient transduction of mechanical vibration into sound power.

Acoustic loading of the vibrating structure

The paradox of loud pure-tone sounds

If a sound source radiates large amounts of power, it suggests that there is a large resistive or damping load; since many insects are noisy, this rule must apply. However, a damping load lowers the Q of the resonator, so its sharpness of tuning will fall. Many noisy insects produce pure-tone sounds, which implies that the resonant structure is lightly damped; at face value, this rule is incompatible with the first rule.

This paradox appears to be resolved, but in slightly different ways, in two groups of insects: mole crickets and cicadas.

Horns as acoustic impedance-matching devices

Mole crickets have a resonant region of the forewings, the harp, that is small relative to the sound wavelength. They sing from specialised horn-shaped burrows (Bennet-Clark, 1970, 1987) (Fig. 7). Early studies of this burrow showed that the outer horn-shaped region flared exponentially in cross-sectional area (Bennet-Clark, 1970), suggesting that this region acted as an acoustic impedance converter – a megaphone. This presents the acoustic resistance of the large mouth of the horn at the ground surface to the small insect wings, which are placed at the narrow throat of the burrow. The design seems to be common to the burrows of other mole cricket species (Bennet-Clark, 1987; A. G. Daws, personal communication).

Since the horn region is quite short, its throat impedance has a significant inertial reactive component. However, Klipsch (1941) has shown that this reactance can be matched by a compliant reactive component placed on the other side of the sound source. In his study, Klipsch calculated the volume required for a compliant component on the source side of the radiating horn to match the inertance of a horn of a given throat area and rate of flare, so as to present a purely resistive impedance at the horn throat. The volume of the bulb region (Fig. 7) of the burrow of three species of mole crickets is compatible with this role (Bennet-Clark, 1970, 1987), but recent work (A. G. Daws, H. C. Bennet-Clark and N. H. Fletcher, in preparation) suggests that the horn may be operating in a higher-order resonant mode than in the Klipsch design.

Tests with burrows of the mole cricket *Scapteriscus acletus*, using a dipole source located in the plane at which the insect places its wings, were used to examine the burrow acoustics (Bennet-Clark, 1987). The burrow is resonant at the insect's song frequency of 2.7 kHz, with a Q of about 3. It also provides an effective gain of about 24 dB, equivalent to a 240-fold increase in the sound power output of the doublet source. This may be explained as follows: the burrow acts as a series resonant circuit, or acceptor circuit, that provides a pure resistive load to the small wings of the insect; it also acts as an acoustic transformer that provides good acoustic matching, at the large mouth of the horn, between the wings and the air into which sound is radiated.

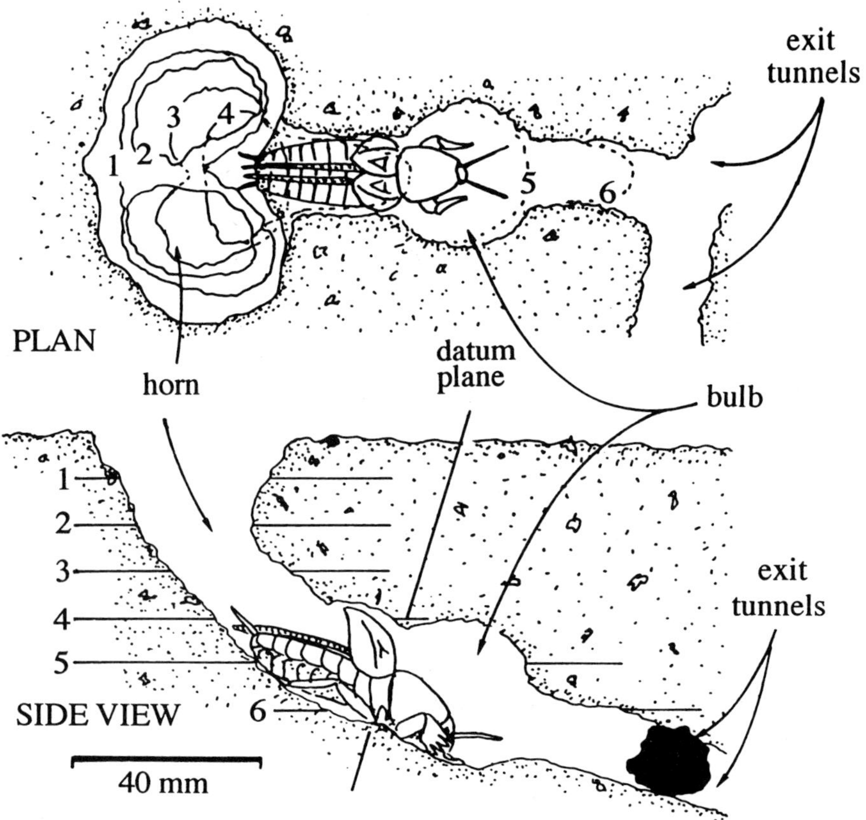

Fig. 7. Scale drawings of the singing burrow of the mole cricket *Gryllotalpa vineae* showing the outer horn, the position of the singing insect and the inner bulb (from Bennet-Clark, 1989). The plan shows the contours of the burrow at the depths shown on the side view.

Recent experiments with model mole cricket burrows (A. G. Daws, H. C. Bennet-Clark and N. H. Fletcher, in preparation) have shown that the sound pressures in the bulb are of similar magnitude but opposite in phase and have also shown that phase inversion of the sound pressure occurs at the plane at which the insect places its wings. As the insect's wings can be regarded as a small dipole source (which has equal but opposite phase on its two sides), they provide an appropriate current drive at the horn throat and, in turn, the horn provides at its throat a resonant acceptor circuit that provides a resistive load to the insect's wings.

Some further evidence that a system of this type is operating here is given by the relationship between the spacing of the file teeth and the shape of the song pulse. At the start of the song pulse, the amplitude builds up rapidly and it decays rapidly at the end of the pulse but, in the middle of the pulse, the pulse amplitude closely follows the tooth spacing. This is consistent with a model in which the muscle power that is transduced into vibration at each file tooth impulse is then dissipated as sound power from the mouth of the burrow.

Thus, overall, the system provides the impedance-matching conditions that allow a small sound source to radiate loud sounds; the mole cricket *Gryllotalpa vineae* produces an average sound level of 88 dB at 1 m range above its burrow and can be heard from a range of about 0.5 km.

Impedance matching via a Helmholtz resonator

Although the paired tymbals have been regarded as the primary sound-producing structures of cicadas, the sound radiated from their outer surfaces is quieter than that radiated through the tympana or ear drums (Young, 1990).

Most of the abdomen of a male cicada is filled with a large air sac. This extends to the inside surfaces of the tymbals and of the large tympana or eardrums on the ventral surface. The tympanal cuticle in most species is very thin, but the tympana are covered ventrally by a pair of opercula which are extensions of the metathoracic sternum. In the singing position, the insect raises and extends its abdomen and at the same time opens the opercula away from the tympana (Young, 1990).

It has been shown experimentally that the integrity of the abdomen and its air sac are important for the purity and loudness of the song; when the posterior part of the abdomen is cut away, leaving the tymbals and their muscles intact, the insect will still sing, but the song is quieter and its loses the tonal purity (Young, 1990).

This and later experimental work (Bennet-Clark and Young, 1992) suggested that the abdominal air sac and the tympana formed the components of a Helmholtz resonator. In such a resonator, the cavity acts as a compliance and the neck acts as an inertance. The resonant frequency, f_0, is determined by:

$$f_0 = \frac{c}{2\pi} \sqrt{\frac{a}{lv}}, \tag{4}$$

where c is the speed of sound air, a is the area of the neck, l is the length of the neck and v is the volume of the cavity. In the present case, where the cavity has two holes, a minor modification to the general equation is required (Seto, 1971). Overall, the volume of the abdominal air sac and the dimensions of the paired tympana give good prediction of the sound frequency for *Cyclochila* (Fig. 8) and for two other species of cicada (Bennet-Clark and Young, 1992). Since the song frequency of a variety of other cicada species scales closely with the reciprocal of body length, the Helmholtz resonator model may apply widely among cicadas (Bennet-Clark and Young, 1994).

Experimental tests with cicada bodies and with models that have the dimensions of cicada abdomens have confirmed that these act as acoustic resonators with a Q of about 6, resonant at or close to the observed dominant frequency of the insect's song.

It thus appears that the resonant clicks produced by the tymbals cause pressure changes in the abdominal air sac that excite a sympathetic acoustic resonance within the abdomen. Sound power is then radiated from the abdominal resonator through the tympana (Young, 1990) (Figs 4A, 8).

The click sounds produced by the the buckling of successive tymbal ribs (Fig. 4E) cohere to form a sound pulse with a somewhat ragged envelope. The song pulses produced *via* the tympana in the intact insect show far smoother envelopes, suggesting

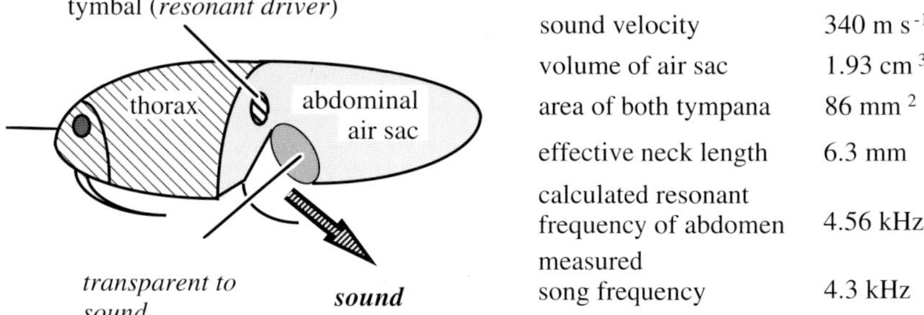

sound velocity	340 m s^{-1}
volume of air sac	1.93 cm^{3}
area of both tympana	86 mm^{2}
effective neck length	6.3 mm
calculated resonant frequency of abdomen	4.56 kHz
measured song frequency	4.3 kHz

Fig. 8. A diagrammatic model of cicada sound production to show the drive from the tymbal and the elements of the abdominal Helmholtz resonator discussed in the text. Dimensions for the cicada *Cyclochila australasiae* are taken from Bennet-Clark and Young (1992). The resonant frequency is calculated from equation 4, with corrections for the presence of two tympana and their short necks.

that one important role of the cicada abdomen is to accept signals at the resonant frequency and to reject (or filter out) the higher and lower frequencies that modulate the dominant frequency. This was tested using an earphone, as a small sound source, which was fitted with a removable model cicada abdomen. When the model was driven with a coherent train of clicks, each separated by one or two cycles at the model's resonant frequency, the model sound output became a long smooth pulse. Thus, the slow build-up or decay of the response of the abdominal resonator (or its action as an acoustic filter) acts as a mechanism to produce the long smooth coherent sound pulses required as recognisable long-range signals (see Introduction).

The acoustic impedance of the sound source

In both insects considered here, the small-area primary resonator, either the harp of the wings of mole crickets or the tymbals of cicadas, is used to provide an internal closely coupled drive to a secondary resonator from which sound power is then radiated. The advantage of this arrangement is that the drive from the internal resonator excites the secondary resonator with little or no power loss; the impedance matching in such a closed system appears to be very good.

Thus, in both cases, the secondary resonator can be regarded as an acoustic transformer that dissipates sound power where it opens to the surrounding fluid medium. However, the vibrating mass of fluid associated with the secondary resonator and the dimensions of its openings can be far larger than their equivalents for the primary resonator, so the system can be regarded as allowing the small vibrating surface of the primary resonator to excite the sympathetic resonance of a large volume of fluid.

Returning to the maximum power transfer theorem (see *Problems of impedance matching*), it is desirable that the sound-radiating surface is large enough to provide a close match with the specific acoustic resistance of the surrounding air (Figs 1, 2). This appears to be met well by the singing burrows of mole crickets (Table 4). The harp areas of the two forewings of *Gryllotalpa vineae* may be regarded as a dipole source of approximately 3 mm radius, which at 3.5 kHz is 1/30 of the sound wavelength (λ); from

Table 4. *Dimensions of insect primary and secondary sound sources*

	Gryllotalpa vineae Orthoptera (mole cricket)	*Cyclochila australasiae* Hemiptera (cicada)
Dominant sound frequency	3.5 kHz	4.3 kHz
Sound wavelength	97 mm	79 mm
Primary source and configuration	Harps on forewings (dipole)	Tymbal in abdomen (monopole)
Primary source size	5×3 mm per harp (paired and synchronous)	5×3 mm per tymbal (act alternately)
Effective primary source radius	2 mm	2 mm
Minimum optimum source radius (Figs 1 and 2) if monopole	15.5 mm	12.5 mm
Secondary source and configuration	Mouth of burrow (monopole)	Tympana (eardrums) (monopole)
Secondary source size	30×50 mm	10×22 mm
Effective secondary source radius	20 mm	7.5 mm

Data are taken from Bennet-Clark (1970), Josephson and Young (1981) and Bennet-Clark and Young (1992).

Fig. 2, it can be seen that the specific acoustic resistance of a source of this size is about 0.001 that of air, so there is a considerable impedance mismatch. However, the mouth of the burrow has an effective radius of about 20 mm and acts as a monopole source radiating from the surface of the ground; this source radius is about 0.2λ, which is large enough to allow a good impedance match between the mouth of the singing burrow and the surrounding air (Fig. 1). An estimate of the efficiency of conversion of muscle power to acoustic power in *Gryllotalpa vineae* singing from its burrow gives values of 17–35 % (Bennet-Clark, 1970), suggesting that the impedance matching along the chain is good.

In the cicada *Cyclochila australasiae*, each tymbal can be regarded as a monopole source of about 2 mm equivalent radius, or 0.025λ (Table 4) so its specific acoustic resistance is about 0.05 that of air (Fig. 1). The paired tympana have an effective source radius of about 7.5 mm, or about 0.1λ, so their specific acoustic resistance is about 0.6 that of air (Fig. 1), which represents an 11-fold increase. Measurements have shown that the sound radiated near to the outer surface of the tymbal is 9 dB quieter than that radiated *via* the tympana, which is consistent with the difference between the relative size and specific radiation resistance of these two sound sources.

Power losses

It is useful at this point to consider other power losses in acoustic systems that may reduce transduction efficiency.

In the absence of information, it is hard to quantify the losses within the muscles due to their inertia and viscosity. At the link between the muscle and the mechanical resonator it excites, there are the costs of moving the non-resonant components, such as the muscle apodemes of cicadas or non-resonant wing areas of crickets. In the cicada tymbal mechanism, the tymbal muscle attaches to the tymbal plate *via* a thin circular cuticular disc and a thin flexible strap-like apodeme. These structures move at the muscle contraction velocity and, because the inward buckling of the tymbal de-tenses the apodeme, they are unlikely to cause appreciable damping of the tymbal vibration. In crickets, the wing-closing movement is transmitted up the anterior veins of the forewing *via* a flexible region to drive the resonant harp; once again, the driving structure moves relatively slowly and is mechanically de-coupled from the vibrating structure, so the energy losses at this stage are likely to be quite small.

Further energy losses are likely from the internal damping of the primary resonator. Again, these are hard to quantify, but a Q of 13 has been measured for the unloaded tymbal of *Cyclochila* compared with a Q of 5 from the same tymbal when acoustically loaded by the insect's abdominal resonator (Young and Bennet-Clark, 1995); this implies that the internal resistive losses in the primary resonator are fairly small. The fact that the Q value of the tymbal resonance falls to rather less than half its unloaded value implies that the total damping in the chain has more than doubled, so the extra damping due to the acoustic resistance during sound radiation is equal to, or somewhat greater than, the internal damping of the tymbal; but this, of course, is expected from a well-matched system.

It can be inferred that there are substantial transduction losses between the harp and burrow resonators of mole crickets. One source of such loss is sound leakage through the pores of the earth in which the burrow is dug; mole crickets sing more loudly on wet days or from burrows dug in damp soil (Bennet-Clark, 1970, 1987).

With the enclosed system of the cicada abdomen, the biggest losses are those through the outside of the tymbal (about 10 % of the total: see above) or through the cuticle of the abdominal tergites and sternites. Here the losses seem to be small; Young (1990) found that the sound pressure levels over the general surface of the abdomen were 12–16 dB lower than those measured at the tympana, and he was unable to detect any significant vibration of the abdominal cuticle during singing in *Cyclochila*.

Sound production as a system

Both cicadas and mole crickets use coupled resonators to produce loud pure-tone songs. They do this by supplying mechanical power from a primary resonator at an appropriate phase, over a number of cycles of the sound pulse, to a well-designed secondary structure that is resonant at the same frequency. By supplying power at a rate comparable to that at which it is dissipated, they are able to produce sound pulses with smooth envelopes.

How general is this system? Parallels can be found throughout the engineering of radio communication (Langford-Smith, 1957) as well as in the design of musical instruments. There are also accounts of similar systems in vertebrates, but these do not appear to have been analysed formally.

One tantalising vertebrate mechanism is the sound production of frogs, where air passing through the small vocal cords produces the fundamental frequency that is modulated by the arytenoids of the larynx. The resulting vibratory air flow causes pulsations of the wall of the subspherical vocal sac, which acts as a large sound-radiating surface (Gans, 1973); it is not known whether the thin-walled vocal sac is resonant at the song frequency. A pulsating sphere has a specific radiation resistance similar to that of a monopole source of the same radius, so the mechanism found in frogs appears to have a similar role of acoustic impedance conversion to that found in cicadas.

Thus, we can re-specify the elements of the sound production chain to take account of the mechanisms that are described here. (1) Muscle contraction provides power at low frequency and high pressure to drive an escapement or other frequency-multiplier mechanism that retains waveform coherence. (2) A high-frequency mechanical oscillator, which can be a large-mass small-area resonator that defines the sound frequency and is coupled to (3) a large resonant sound radiator, which maintains the sound frequency and provides impedance matching between stages 2 and 4. The power fed from stage 1 to stage 2 to stage 3 is dissipated from stage 3 as (4) a loud pure-tone sound wave.

It is tempting to see whether the maximum power transfer theorem can be applied more generally to effector mechanisms. There are few good examples for animals where the question of power transfer from source to load has been treated in this way, but Alexander (1973) has surveyed the muscle loading in a variety of strenuous tasks from blood-sucking to swimming and concludes that, in many cases, muscles are loaded so that they can contract at the velocity and stress that allow them to produce maximum power. This suggests that the problems of transduction and impedance matching in sound production that are discussed here are merely a special case of a general problem of animal design.

Much of the work on cicada sound production described here has been done either by or in collaboration with Dr David Young, of the University of Melbourne. This has been, for me, a very happy and fruitful collaboration; it is with pleasure that I acknowledge my gratitude to him and also to the University of Melbourne for hospitality and financial support during the course of this work.

References

Alexander, R. McN. (1973). Muscle performance in locomotion and other strenuous activities. In *Comparative Physiology. Locomotion, Respiration, Transport and Blood* (ed. L. Bolis, K. Schmidt-Nielsen and S. H. P. Maddrell), pp. 1–21. Amsterdam: North Holland.

Alexander, R. McN. (1983). *Animal Mechanics* (2nd edn). Oxford: Blackwell Scientific Publications.

Bailey, W. J. (1970). The mechanics of stridulation in bush crickets (Tettigonioidea, Orthoptera). I. The tegminal generator. *J. exp. Biol.* **52**, 495–505.

Bennet-Clark, H. C. (1970). The mechanism and efficiency of sound production in mole crickets. *J. exp. Biol.* **52**, 619–652.

Bennet-Clark, H. C. (1971). Acoustics of insect song. *Nature* **234**, 255–259.

Bennet-Clark, H. C. (1975). Sound production in insects. *Science Progr.* **62**, 263–283.

Bennet-Clark, H. C. (1987). The tuned singing burrow of mole crickets. *J. exp. Biol.* **128**, 383–409.

Bennet-Clark, H. C. (1989). Songs and the physics of sound production. In *Cricket Behavior and Neurobiology* (ed. F. Huber, T. E. Moore and W. Loher), pp. 227–261. Ithaca: Cornell University Press.

Bennet-Clark, H. C. and Young, D. (1992). A model of the mechanism of sound production in cicadas. *J. exp. Biol.* **173**, 123–153.

Bennet-Clark, H. C. and Young, D. (1994). The scaling of song frequency in cicadas. *J. exp. Biol.* **191**, 291–294.

Beranek, L. L. (1949). *Acoustic Measurements*. New York: John Wiley and Sons.

DUMORTIER, B. (1963*a*). Morphology of sound emission apparatus in Arthropoda. In *Acoustic Behaviour of Animals* (ed. R. G. Busnell), pp. 277–345. Amsterdam: Elsevier.

DUMORTIER, B. (1963*b*). The physical characteristics of sound emissions in Arthropoda. In *Acoustic Behaviour of Animals* (ed. R. G. Busnel), pp. 346–373. Amsterdam: Elsevier.

ELLIOTT, C. J. H. AND KOCH, U. T. (1985). The clockwork cricket. *Naturwissenschaften* **72**, 225–227.

FLETCHER, N. H. (1992). *Acoustic Systems in Biology.* Oxford: Oxford University Press.

GANS, C. (1973). Sound production in the Salientia: mechanism and evolution of the emitter. *Am. Zool.* **13**, 1179–1194.

HUBER, F., MOORE, T. E. AND LOHER, W. (1989). (eds.) *Cricket Behavior and Neurobiology.* Ithaca: Cornell University Press.

JOSEPHSON, R. K. AND YOUNG, D. (1981). Synchronous and asynchrononous muscles in cicadas. *J. exp. Biol.* **91**, 219–237.

JOSEPHSON, R. K. AND YOUNG, D. (1985). A synchronous insect muscle with an operating frequency greater than 500 Hz. *J. exp. Biol.* **118**, 185–208.

KLIPSCH, P. W. (1941). A low frequency horn of small dimensions. *J. acoust. Soc. Am.* **13**, 137–144.

LANGFORD-SMITH, F. (1957). *Radio Designer's Handbook* (4th edn, 4th impression with addenda). London: Iliffe and Sons, Ltd.

MORSE, P. M. (1948). *Vibration and Sound.* New York: McGraw-Hill.

NOCKE, H. (1971). Biophysik der Schallerzeugung durch die Vorderflügel der Grillen. *Z. vergl. Physiol.* **74**, 272–314.

OLSON, H. F. (1957). *Acoustical Engineering.* Princeton, NJ: Van Nostrand.

PIERCE, G. W. (1948). *The Songs of Insects.* Harvard, MA: Harvard University Press.

PRINGLE, J. W. S. (1954). A physiological analysis of cicada song. *J. exp. Biol.* **32**, 525–560.

PROZESKY-SCHULZE, L., PROZESKY, O. P. M., ANDERSON, F. AND VAN DER MERWE, G. J. J. (1975). Use of a self-made sound baffle by a tree cricket. *Nature* **255**, 142–143.

RAGGE, D. R. (1955). *The Wing Venation of the Orthoptera Saltatoria.* London: British Museum (Nat. Hist.).

SALES, G. D. AND PYE, J. D. (1974). *Ultrasonic Communication in Animals.* London: Chapman and Hall.

SETO, W. W. (1971). *Theory and Problems of Acoustics.* New York: McGraw-Hill.

SIMMONS, P. AND YOUNG, D. (1978). The tymbal mechanism and song patterns of the bladder cicada *Cystosoma saundersii. J. exp. Biol.* **76**, 27–45.

YOUNG, D. (1990). Do cicadas radiate sound through their ear-drums ? *J. exp. Biol.* **151**, 41–56.

YOUNG, D. AND BENNET-CLARK, H. C. (1995). The role of the tymbal in cicada sound production. *J. exp. Biol.* **198**, 1001–1020.

HIGH REYNOLDS NUMBER FLOW IN TUBES OF COMPLEX GEOMETRY WITH APPLICATION TO WALL SHEAR STRESS IN ARTERIES

T. J. PEDLEY

Department of Applied Mathematical Studies, University of Leeds, Leeds LS2 9JT, UK

Summary

The arterial systems of mammals contain many generations of branching, curved, elastic tubes, and the flow in them is unsteady. The flow details are important in determining the distribution of wall shear stress in arteries, a major factor in atherogenesis. The purpose of this paper is to point out that unsteady flow at realistic values of the Reynolds number (several hundred) and frequency parameter is much more complicated than a knowledge of steady flow in simpler geometries would suggest. Three-dimensional effects in curved, branched or indented tubes introduce secondary motions and horseshoe vortices, under which the wall shear can remain high for a considerable distance downstream. Unsteady flow in two-dimensional, non-uniform tubes can lead to regions of flow separation far from the non-uniformity, again associated with high wall shear, not low shear as for two-dimensional, steady, separated flow. Moreover, both two- and three-dimensional flows can be non-unique, so that the same driving pressures in the same geometry can lead to different flow patterns, depending on the initial conditions. There is great sensitivity to small geometric and temporal perturbations, making it very difficult to predict flow in one arterial bifurcation from a knowledge of another, or even at a particular site in one subject from a knowledge of another. Vessel elasticity is an additional complicating factor whose effects remain to be assessed in detail.

Introduction

Material transport from one part of the body to another, in vertebrates or other large animals, involves fluid (liquid or gas) flowing along, and across the walls of, systems of tubes. The most widely studied tube systems are the mammalian cardiovascular and ventilatory systems.

For steady flow in a long, straight, circular tube, every element of a viscous fluid flows in a straight line with a constant speed, and the velocity profile is parabolic. The relationship between the driving pressure drop per unit length and the flow rate through the tube is linear, the ratio of the two (the viscous resistance) being inversely proportional to the fourth power of the tube diameter (Poiseuille's Law). Such a smooth, laminar flow

Key words: blood flow, arterial wall stress, atherosclerosis, high Reynolds number flow, unsteady flow, flow in complex geometry.

will break down into turbulence if the Reynolds number exceeds a critical value of about 2000; the Reynolds number Re is defined by:

$$Re = \rho\bar{u}d/\mu\,, \tag{1}$$

where ρ and μ are the fluid density and viscosity, d is the tube diameter and $\bar{u}$ is the average fluid velocity within it ($\bar{u}$=$4Q/\pi d^2$, where Q is the volume flow rate).

Unfortunately, Poiseuille flow is not to be found anywhere in the human body. Blood vessels and airways are typically short, curved, branched and elastic, and the flow is not steady (and blood is not a Newtonian viscous fluid, though this is probably not important in the large blood vessels with which I shall be concerned). In short tubes, the flow does not become fully developed, and high velocity gradients occur in thin boundary layers near their entrance, which enhances the rate at which energy is dissipated and therefore increases the pressure drop for a given flow rate (Prandtl, 1952). In curved tubes, secondary motions are generated, which distort the primary velocity profile (Dean, 1927, 1928) and also enhance the energy dissipation (White, 1929). Flow in a bifurcation combines the main features of entry flow and curved tube flow (Schroter and Sudlow, 1969).

The details of unsteady viscous flow are significantly different from those of steady flow, whatever the geometry, as long as the dimensionless frequency parameter α is not small, where:

$$\alpha^2 = \rho\omega d^2/4\mu \tag{2}$$

and ω is the dominant radian frequency of the unsteadiness (Womersley, 1955). Moreover, a time-dependent pressure, such as that generated by a pumping heart, causes the dimensions of an elastic tube to vary with time, and this is responsible for the propagation of pressure waves along the tube (Young, 1809). Physiological fluid flows, in fact, are very complicated and a lot of effort is required to measure or calculate all the details. Whether it is worth doing so depends on what we want to know.

In general terms, the reasons for studying physiological fluid dynamics are fourfold: (i) pure physiology, understanding how the fluid flow systems work in normal animals; (ii) patho-physiology, understanding the origin and effects of disease processes such as atherosclerosis or bronchitis; (iii) diagnosis, i.e. designing and interpreting measurements of mechanical quantities, such as blood pressure, heart sounds, breath sounds, etc; (iv) cure, or the bio-engineering of prosthetic devices (heart-valves, dialysis machines) or surgical techniques (e.g. coronary artery bypass surgery).

In the context of large arteries, the principal topics that have been subjected to fluid dynamic study are as follows: (a) pulse wave propagation and reflection, leading to a determination of the load against which the heart must act, the diagnosis of severe constrictions (stenoses), and the design of cardiac assist devices (McDonald, 1974; Pedley, 1980, chapter 2; Elzinga and Westerhof, 1991); (b) the distribution in space and time of the viscous shear stress exerted by the flowing blood on the artery wall, because of its importance in atherogenesis (Fry, 1987; Giddens *et al.* 1993; Friedman, 1993); (c) mass transport across the arterial endothelium and within the vessel wall, the detailed mechanisms for which are also of fundamental importance in atherogenesis (Yuan *et al.*

1991; Weinbaum and Chien, 1993); (d) the functioning of natural and artificial heart valves (Lee and Talbot, 1979); and (e) fluid–structure interaction phenomena associated with flow in a collapsible tube under external compression (Kamm and Pedley, 1989), such as an artery under a sphygmomanometer cuff (some workers believe that Korotkoff sounds are a manifestation of flow-induced flutter). Arteries do not normally collapse, of course, but veins do, above the level of the heart, which means that the heart has to pump blood up to the level of the top of the jugular vein; this explains why the central arterial blood pressure in a giraffe has to be as inconveniently high as 33 kPa (250 mmHg) (Seymour *et al.* 1993).

It is the wall shear stress (topic b) that I shall concentrate on here; space constraints prohibit discussion of the others, or of gas flow in the pulmonary airways, although it is in many respects similar to blood flow in arteries and veins (see Pedley *et al.* 1977).

It has often been adequate to use highly idealised descriptions in analysing physiological flows. For example, in both pulse wave propagation and collapsible tube problems, one-dimensional models have been used in which the internal pressure and velocity along the pipe have been taken not to vary across the tube, just along it. Uniform curved tubes are used as a paradigm for non-uniformly curved arteries. Such models are extremely useful, permitting relatively simple mathematics and computing and leading to useful predictions whose physical basis is clearly understood. In some cases, however, predictions based on simple models do not provide adequate explanations of experimental observations, and intuition based on them can be actually misleading. Then, the models have to be refined to take account of real effects which had previously been explicitly ignored.

Atherosclerosis and arterial wall shear stress

The distribution of wall shear stress in arteries is a topic in which I believe that the fluid mechanical details are important but are not yet fully understood. The evidence linking wall shear to atherogenesis has been reviewed many times, and I shall not rehearse it in detail here; the excellent recent articles by Giddens *et al.* (1993), Friedman (1993) and Fry (1987) are to be especially recommended.

The results of several *in vivo* studies show that, if a normal artery, with an intact endothelium, is altered so that the mean wall shear stress (*WSS*) changes, then over a period of months the artery wall remodels itself to restore the mean *WSS* to its normal value (Zarins *et al.* 1987). The normal shear stress, as estimated from the assumption of Poiseuille flow, is usually in the range 1–2 $\mathrm{N\,m^{-2}}$, the actual value depending on the species and the vessel. Such long-term adaptation is thought to be important during angiogenesis and growth, determining artery diameters in response to flow rate demands. The only signal related to flow rate that the endothelial cells could detect is the *WSS*. If it rises, then the response of the vessel is to increase its luminal diameter while retaining the same wall thickness. However, if the *WSS* falls below about 1 $\mathrm{N\,m^{-2}}$, the diameter is reduced by means of a marked relative thickening of the intimal part of the wall.

It has been established that early atheromatous plaques are associated with intimal thickening and that they tend to develop in regions believed to have low mean wall shear stress (Caro *et al.* 1971; Zarins *et al.* 1983). This raises the interesting possibility that the initial development of an atheromatous plaque may be little more than the normal adaptive response in a region of low mean *WSS*, though it should be noted that short-term time-dependence, and in particular periodic reversal, of the *WSS* has also been observed to affect intimal thickening at certain sites (Zarins *et al.* 1983; Ku *et al.* 1985). Subsequent plaque development will, of course, depend on the mechanism by which endothelial cells and the intima behind them respond to changes in *WSS*, and will be mediated by a range of biochemical, genetic and other factors. However, a necessary precondition to understanding the process is a knowledge of the normal distribution of mean and time-dependent *WSS* in regions known to be susceptible to atherogenesis and some understanding of how that distribution will change as the plaque grows. The main purpose of this paper is to show that the necessary understanding is hard to come by, and that there are several pitfalls into which it is easy for even an expert fluid dynamicist to fall.

Flow separation and wall shear stress

The original 'low wall shear stress' hypothesis, by Caro *et al.* (1971), was based on a visual correlation between sites in large arteries susceptible to atherogenesis and places where the wall shear stress was expected to be low. The sites in question, mostly in the aorta and its major branches, were on the inside of bends, on the outer walls of bifurcations, on the wall opposite a side branch and in regions of cross-sectional area expansion such as the carotid sinus.

Steady flow

Simple steady flow experiments in a cast of the aorta confirmed that the wall shear is low and that flow separation may occur at the susceptible sites (Caro *et al.* 1971).

Intuition about flow separation is often based on steady, two-dimensional flow, at a realistic arterial value of the Reynolds number ($300<Re<2000$, say), in a simple expansion in a two-dimensional channel (Fig. 1): as the flow passes through the expansion, it experiences a deceleration which is associated with a pressure rise (Bernoulli's Theorem). This causes the flow to separate, leaving a closed recirculating eddy beneath. Fluid elements remain in the eddy for a long time (they can escape only by diffusion), the velocity is low and hence so is the wall shear stress.

The geometry of arteries is of course three-dimensional, and the flow resembles its two-dimensional counterpart only on planes of symmetry, if they exist. Off the plane of symmetry, however, the flow is quite different in three dimensions. We have already noted that secondary motions arise in a uniform curved tube, since the faster-moving fluid near the centre is swept towards the outside of the bend, to be replaced at the inside by the slower-moving fluid near the walls. The consequence is that a steep gradient of axial velocity is generated near the outside wall, and for some distance around the circumference, resulting in relatively high wall shear there but a much reduced wall shear on the inside part of the wall. The details depend on the values of the Reynolds number *Re* and the curvature ratio δ, given by:

$$\delta = a/R, \tag{3}$$

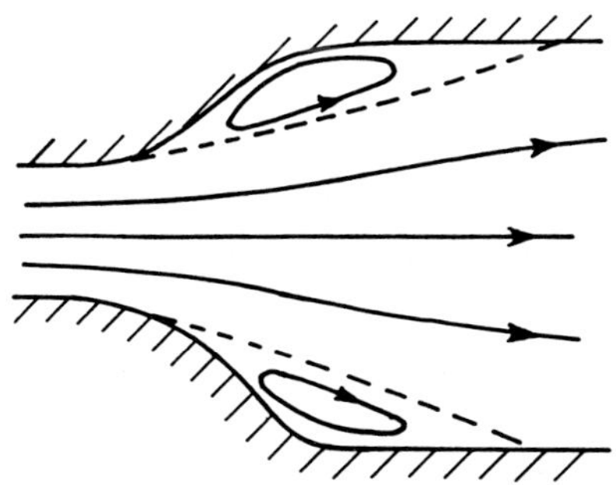

Fig. 1. Steady flow separation at an abrupt expansion in a two-dimensional channel, illustrated by a symmetrical expansion, at which a symmetrical flow may be possible.

a being the tube radius and R the radius of curvature of the centre line. If δ is large enough, the wall shear can become very low on the inside wall, especially if the tube curvature is not uniform or the flow not fully developed (see Talbot and Wong, 1982, for example). (A fully developed flow is one in which the fluid velocities are independent of distance along the tube.)

Steady flow in a symmetrical bifurcation depends on a number of parameters, including the branch angle and the area ratio (of combined daughter tubes to parent tube) in addition to *Re* and curvature ratios. If the flow divider is sharp and the area ratio is 1, the bifurcation can be regarded as two curved tubes stuck together; the wall shear stress at the outside of the bends (the inner wall of the bifurcation) is enhanced further because new boundary layers with steep velocity gradients develop downstream from the flow divider as it splits the oncoming velocity profile (Fig. 2). Separation is not usually seen if the area ratio is 1 or less (as at the aortic bifurcation) unless the curvature of the outer wall (inside of the bend) is relatively sharp (Walburn and Stein, 1980). If the area ratio exceeds 1, so that there is an overall expansion, or if the distribution of flow rate in the daughter tubes is markedly unequal, flow separation can be found at the outer wall in one or both daughters (Zeller *et al.* 1970; Walburn and Stein, 1980).

When the geometry of the bifurcation is not symmetrical, flow separation is more likely. The extreme case is that of a perpendicular side branch of a parent artery (Fig. 3). Regions of separated flow are seen just inside the daughter tube and on the wall of the parent tube opposite the branch. The trajectories of individual fluid elements can be very complex (Karino *et al.* 1979), as can the shear stress distribution (Lutz *et al.* 1977). Another asymmetric geometry that has been widely studied is the carotid bifurcation, where the expansion of the carotid sinus is particularly prone to separation and to atheroma (Ku, 1988).

The separated eddy at a site of steady three-dimensional flow separation is rather different from a two-dimensional one. Fluid elements that are not precisely on a plane of symmetry follow spiral trajectories that carry them out of the eddy a finite time after entering it, so their residence times in the eddy are low and the eddy can be thought of as 'open' rather than 'closed'. In many cases, nevertheless, the fluid velocities and wall shear stress remain low.

Some 'open' separated flow regions, however, have a very different character and are

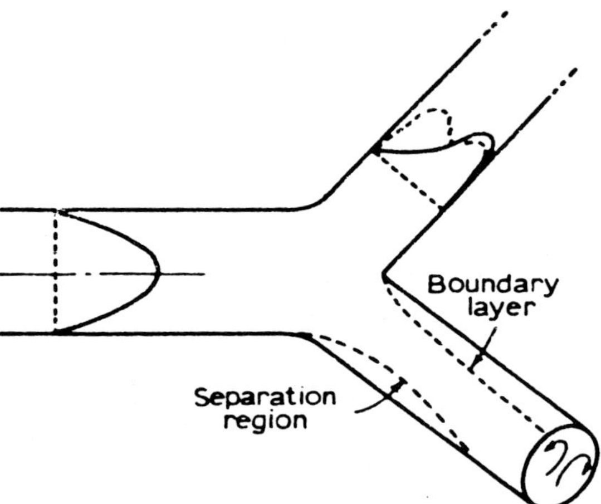

Fig. 2. Sketch of flow downstream of a symmetrical bifurcation with Poiseuille flow in the parent tube. Secondary motion, a new boundary layer and a possible separation region are indicated in the lower branch; distorted velocity profiles in the plane of the junction (solid curve) and in the perpendicular plane (broken curve) are sketched in the upper branch. (From Pedley *et al.* 1977.)

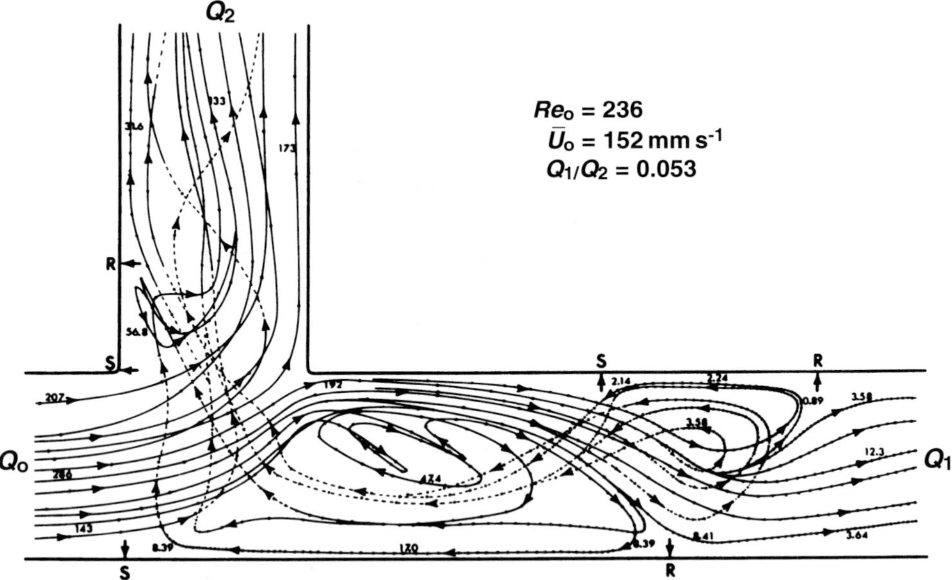

Fig. 3. Flow patterns in an asymmetric, three-dimensional branch. Projections of three-dimensional particle paths in a right-angled branch when most of the flow goes down the side branch. The subscript 'o' denotes parameter values in the parent tube. (From Karino *et al.* 1979.)

known as 'horseshoe' (or 'hairpin') vortices. This name was introduced into the arterial literature by Fukushima and Azuma (1982). Consider flow over a smooth boundary encountering an abrupt protuberance (Fig. 4). If the flow were two-dimensional, a region

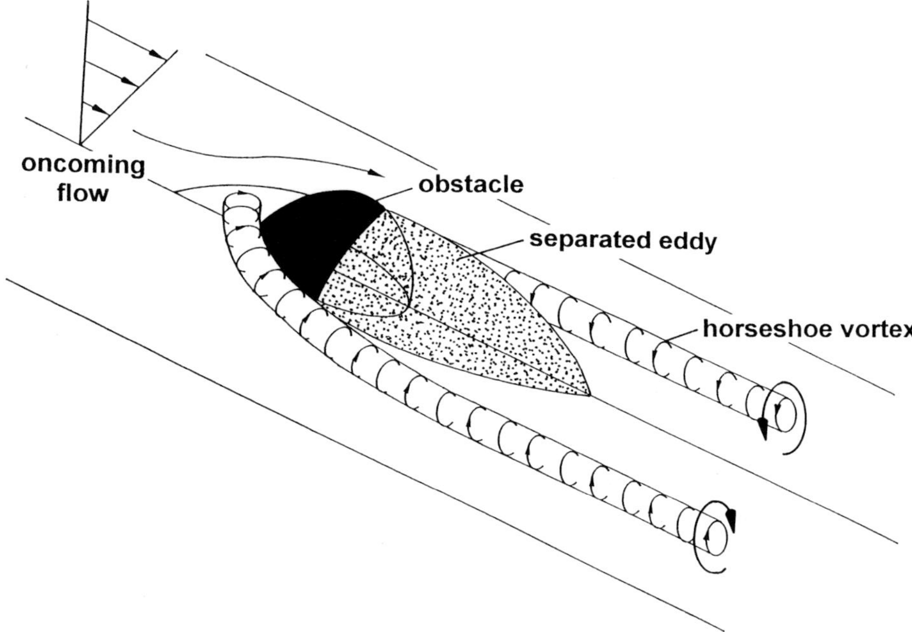

Fig. 4. Sketch of the generation of a horseshoe vortex when the flow over a wall or in a pipe encounters a three-dimensional protuberance. See text for further details. (After Fukushima and Azuma, 1982.)

of flow separation would occur upstream of the protuberance as well as downstream, and in it the recirculating flow would be sluggish and the *WSS* low. In three dimensions, however, fluid not on the plane of symmetry is swept round the sides of the obstacle. Now, it is a property of fluid flow that vorticity is carried along with fluid elements. (Vorticity is the vector quantity that measures the rate of rotation of a fluid element.) If the line of fluid elements parallel to the local vorticity vector is stretched, then the intensity of the vorticity is proportionately increased until limited by viscous effects. Such vortex line stretching is the main mechanism by which intense vortices are formed, over a bath-plug or in a tornado, for example. In the case depicted in Fig. 4, a transverse line of fluid elements near the wall is parallel to the vector of vorticity associated with the velocity gradient in the boundary layer near the wall. As that line approaches the protuberance, the fluid on the plane of symmetry is brought to rest, but the fluid elements to either side are swept downstream, carrying with them and intensifying the associated vorticity. The consequence is that a pair of intense counter-rotating vortices is formed downstream of the protuberance; they are joined together in front of the obstacle and are called the horseshoe vortex. On the wall underneath the vortex is a region of high wall shear, directed approximately transversely to the flow in the wake region downstream of the protuberance. Thus, scanning across the wake, we would find normal, longitudinal wall shear outside it; high, transverse shear under the horseshoe vortices; and (probably) low, three-dimensional shear in the sluggish region between the horseshoe vortices.

It should be noted that the original protuberance needs to be sufficiently abrupt for upstream flow separation to occur in order that intense horseshoe vortices can form. A smooth protuberance will affect the wall shear distribution, but not in so dramatic a way. Thus, one would expect horseshoe vortices to be generated by severe atherosclerotic plaques but not by early intimal thickening.

Intense longitudinal vortices are also formed downstream of a pair of small side branches, such as intercostal arteries coming off the aorta, by a similiar mechanism (see Van Dyke, 1982, Fig. 99) A further example discussed by Fukushima and Azuma (1982) was of flow in a symmetrical bifurcation with a blunt flow divider. If the plane of the bifurcation is taken to be horizontal, fluid above the horizontal plane of symmetry and impinging on the flow divider will be deflected upwards as it is simultaneously swept downstream in one or other of the daughter tubes (see Pedley *et al.* 1977, Fig. 22). Thus, the horseshoe vortex mechanism can set up the observed secondary motions further upstream than could the curved-tube, centrifugal force mechanism acting alone. This more vigorous secondary flow may have the effect of diminishing, or sweeping away altogether, a separated flow region that would otherwise occur on the outside wall of the bifurcation (depending on the area ratio). In this case, the presence or otherwise of a sluggish separated flow eddy depends on the extremely complicated details of the three-dimensional flow.

We conclude that, in three-dimensional steady flow, regions of flow separation may not occur where two-dimensional intuition says they should; they may occur some distance away from the geometrical disturbances that cause them to exist (e.g. horseshoe vortices). The wall shear in these regions may be very high, not very low, and it may not be parallel to the mainstream flow. The wall shear distribution is very sensitive to small variations in the geometry of bifurcations or of (atherosclerotically generated) protuberances.

Unsteady flow: two-dimensional

Although the long time-scale for atherogenesis suggests that it is the distribution of time-mean wall shear stress that is important, there is, as we have seen, some evidence that short time-scale phenomena also have an effect (Ku *et al.* 1985). In any case, the mean wall shear stress in a highly pulsatile flow will not normally be the same as the wall shear stress in a steady flow with the same mean flow rate (this is a mathematical property of nonlinear systems in general). Therefore, a discussion of unsteady flows is required. We start with two-dimensional geometry, following the same approach as Pedley *et al.* (1988).

It should be noted first that even in parallel-sided vessels, the ratio of the amplitude of the wall shear oscillation to the mean is much greater than the same ratio for flow rate (Pedley, 1976). This is because the slow-moving fluid near the wall responds more rapidly to a change in pressure gradient than does the flow in the core. It follows that the adverse pressure gradient required to decelerate the bulk flow can cause reversal of the velocity near the wall even when the overall flow rate remains positive.

We now consider two examples of time-dependent flow in a long two-dimensional channel. In the first example, the channel is rigid and parallel-sided apart from a segment of one wall which moves in and out in a prescribed way; the flow far upstream is steady (Fig. 5). In the second example, the flow is pulsatile and the channel rigid but either

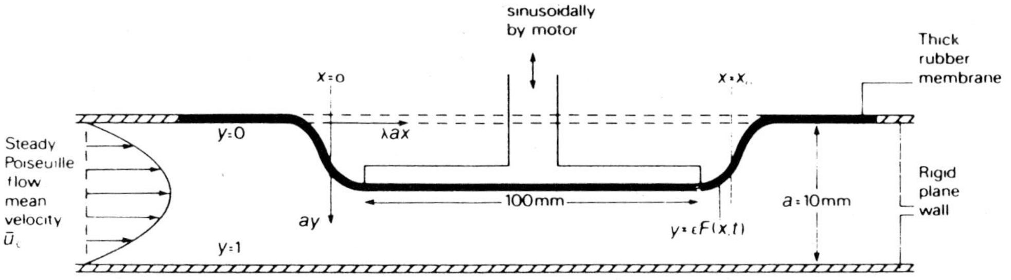

Fig. 5. Experimental apparatus for observing flow in an approximately two-dimensional channel with a section of one wall which can be moved in and out; there is steady, Poiseuille flow upstream.

stepped, so that one half is narrower than the other, or indented by a localised constriction.

First, we consider steady flow past a moving indentation. The flow is determined by the values of three dimensionless parameters: ϵ, the maximum ratio of indentation height to undisturbed channel width d; upstream Reynolds number Re (equation 1); and frequency parameter α (equation 2) or, equivalently, the Strouhal number St, given by:

$$St = d/\bar{u}T = 2\alpha^2/\pi Re\,, \tag{4}$$

where T is the oscillation period. Experimental observations were presented by Pedley and Stephanoff (1985) for values of Re in the range 480–1200, St in the range 0.005–0.077, and ϵ up to 0.57; these values of Re and α^2 are typical of moderately large arteries (Caro *et al.* 1978). The following description of what occurs during one oscillation period is based on the experimental observations in one particular case; the flow is illustrated in Fig. 6 using streamline plots subsequently computed from a direct numerical integration of the Navier–Stokes equations for the same parameter values (Ralph and Pedley, 1988). Agreement between experimental and computational results was excellent.

The cycle begins with the indentation flush with the rigid wall; half-way through (t=0.5) the obstruction to the flow is maximal; at the end of the cycle (t=1), the indentation is once more flush. During the first third of the cycle, a single separated flow eddy develops in the lee of the indentation, as it would if the flow were quasi-steady. However, by t=0.40, the core streamlines have developed a dip downstream of the primary eddy, and a second flow separation region is apparent on the opposite rigid wall. A little later on (t=0.45), another eddy has appeared on the indented wall, and so on: as time progresses, more and more eddies are generated and the core streamlines become more and more wavy. However, towards the end of the cycle, new disturbances cease to be generated and all the old ones are washed away downstream so that the flow is undisturbed at the start of the new cycle. The crests and troughs of the waves, called vorticity waves, and the eddies associated with them propagate gradually downstream, at about one-third of the propagation speed of the wave front (beyond which there is no disturbance) as predicted by a relatively simple mathematical theory (Pedley and Stephanoff, 1985).

From the present point of view, the most interesting feature of the flow is the wall shear

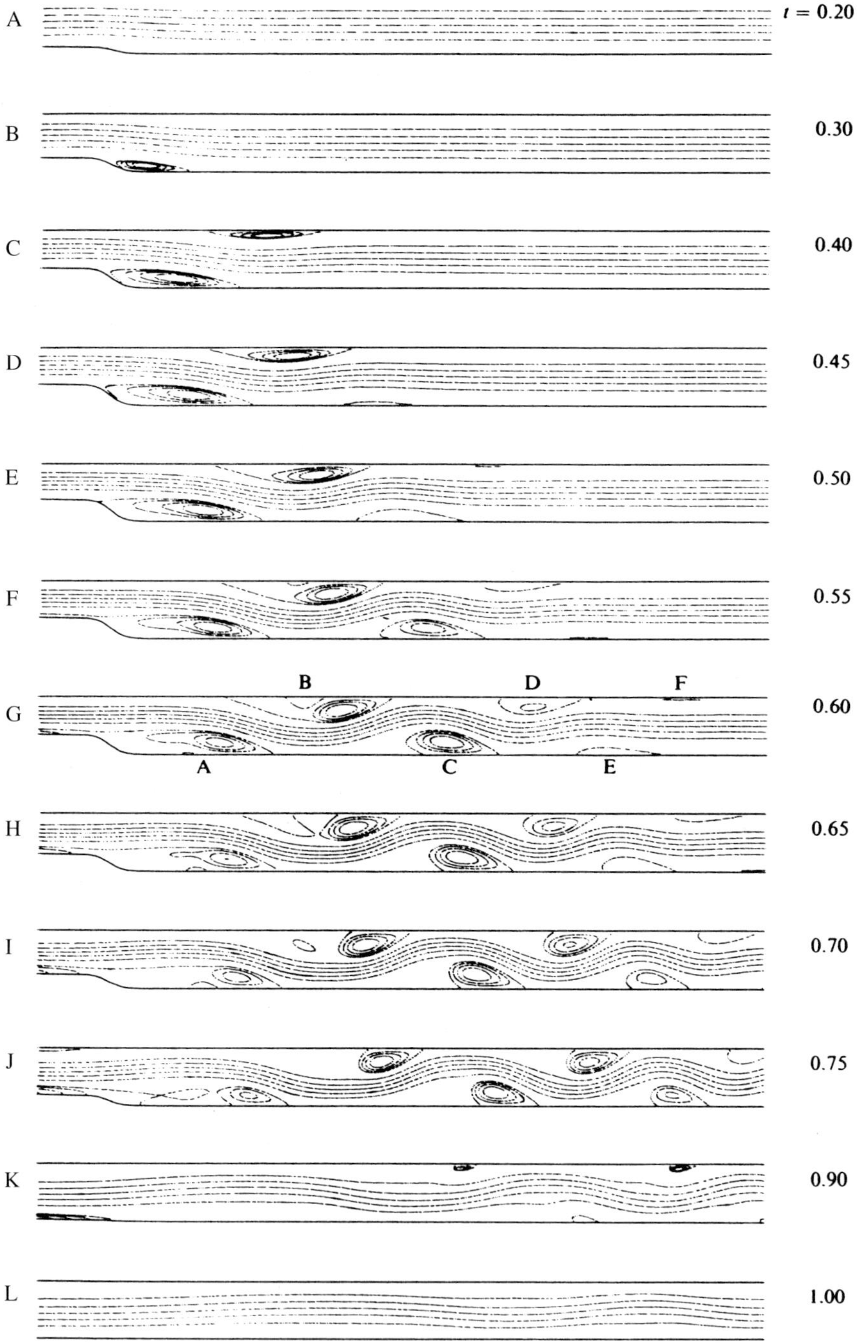

Fig. 6. Computed instantaneous streamlines downstream of the oscillating indentation of Fig. 5 with Re=507, St=0.037 and ϵ=0.4. Time t is scaled with the cycle period. At t=0 the indentation is flush with the rigid part of the wall; it then moves in and back and is flush again at t=1. Note the successive generation and propagation of alternate separated flow regions on the walls. (From Ralph and Pedley, 1988.)

in the separated-flow eddies associated with the waves. Near the downstream end of each eddy, under the region of rapid recirculation, the magnitude of the *WSS* rises to approximately six times the value associated with the mean flow, as shown in Fig. 7. The regions of lowest wall shear also occur under the separated flow eddies, towards the rear. Both the high- and the low-shear zones propagate downstream with the eddies.

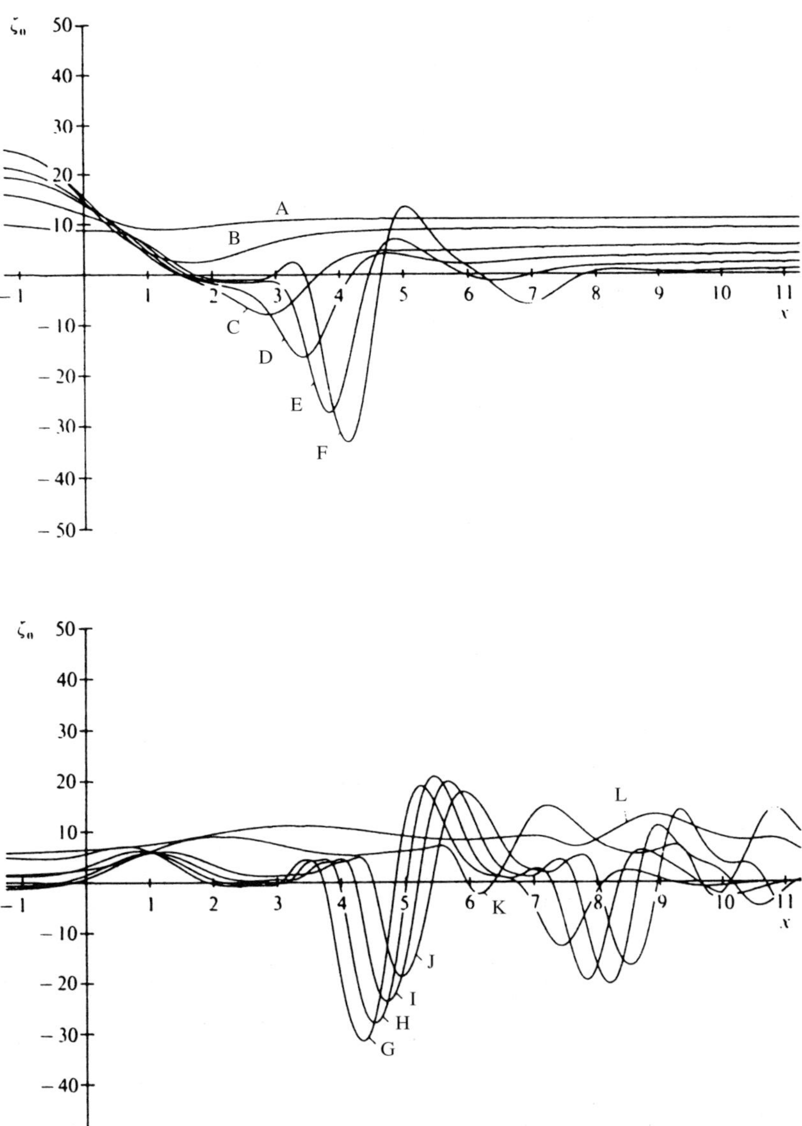

Fig. 7. Computed graphs of dimensionless wall shear rate ζ_0 on the plane wall against downstream distance x (scaled with the undeformed channel width) at different times t. Top graph: t= (A) 0.20, (B) 0.30, (C) 0.40, (D) 0.45, (E) 0.50, (F) 0.55. Bottom graph: t = (G) 0.60, (H) 0.65, (I) 0.70, (J) 0.75, (K) 0.90, (L) 1.00. Other parameters as for Fig. 6. (From Ralph and Pedley, 1988.)

Another experiment performed with the apparatus of Fig. 5 was to set up a steady indentation, and then give it a small-amplitude oscillation, as it might be from a stenosis in an elastic-walled vessel (Ralph and Pedley, 1990). After some initial adjustments, vorticity waves were again set up, with amplitudes corresponding to the mean indentation height not to the amplitude of the forced oscillation. Presumably, therefore, localised areas of high and low wall shear stress would occur in the associated eddies, but computations have not been made for this example.

The second flow to be considered is purely oscillatory flow past a fixed (and still asymmetric) indentation; that is, a step separating two channels of different widths. The experiments have been done by Sobey (1985) and the corresponding computations by Tutty and Pedley (1993). Once again, waves are generated downstream of the indentation during each cycle but, in this case, the crests propagate only a little way downstream before moving upstream again, although the wave front still moves rapidly downstream. Again, however, eddies are formed under the wave crests, and they have a similar structure to those in the previous case. The maximum and minimum wall-shear magnitudes are comparable with those shown in Fig. 7.

A similarly complex flow was found in the more physiological case of pulsatile flow (oscillatory but with non-zero mean equal to the amplitude, so that the flow rate falls to zero each cycle but does not reverse) past a localised asymmetric stenosis (Fig. 8). In this case, the only published study was computational (Tutty, 1992), although there have been some unpublished experiments (Park, 1989). In the computations, both non-sinusoidal and sinusoidal oscillations in flow rate were used. In both cases, vorticity waves of a variety of wavelengths were generated each cycle, with the wave front propagating rapidly downstream. However, the wave crests themselves and the associated separation points remained approximately stationary, as did regions of low wall shear just downstream of the separation points. The high wall shear regions at the downstream ends of the separated eddies fluctuated in position quite significantly, so the wall shear over a given segment of wall oscillated between large positive and negative values.

To summarise the situation for two-dimensional time-dependent flows in non-uniform channels, we can say that several regions of flow separation can develop, at some distance from the geometric non-uniformity that generates them. The highest wall shear stress in the flow, as well as the lowest, tends to occur under the separated flow eddies. In cases of oscillatory flow past fixed non-uniformities, the separation region remains approximately stationary, so that low and fluctuating high wall shear zones occur on the same segments of wall each cycle.

Unsteady flow: three-dimensional

The complexity of steady flow in three dimensions and of time-dependent flow in two dimensions suggests, rightly, that unsteady three-dimensional flow will be extremely complicated. General principles, by which the flow pattern and wall shear stress distribution (in a new geometry or with a new flow rate distribution) can be predicted from previous studies, appear not to be available. As a result, there have been, and continue to be, numerous experimental and computational studies on pulsatile flow in a wide range of different circumstances, all giving information that is interesting and useful

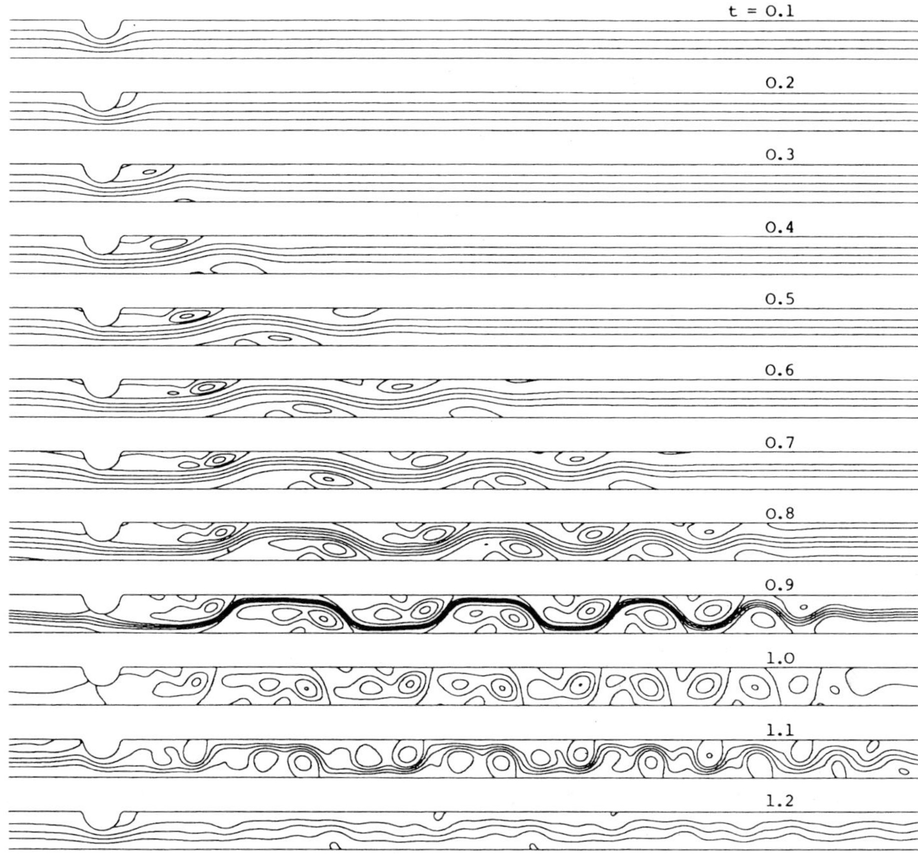

Fig. 8. Computed instantaneous streamlines for pulsatile flow past a localised indentation in one wall of a two-dimensional channel. Maximum $Re = 750$, $St = 0.024$. (From Tutty, 1992.)

but is not susceptible to global interpretation (Ku *et al.* 1985; Ku and Giddens, 1987; Lou and Yang, 1992; Perktold *et al.* 1991; van Steenhoven *et al.* 1992).

Even in the highly idealised geometry of a uniform curved tube of circular cross section, far from the ends so that the flow is fully developed, with a sinusoidally pulsatile flow rate, there are four relevant dimensionless parameters and the flow depends sensitively on them. The four parameters are as follows: curvature ratio δ (equation 3), Reynolds number *Re* (equation 1) associated with the mean or the maximum flow rate, ratio of maximum to mean flow rate (say A), and frequency parameter α (equation 2). At small curvature ($\delta \ll 1$) and in steady flow ($A=1$, $\alpha=0$), we have seen that the secondary flow is directed towards the outside of the curve in the core of the tube, and back towards the inside near the walls (though this is itself an oversimplified picture – see next section). When the flow rate is purely oscillatory at high frequency (i.e. when A is infinite and α is also large), there is again a mean secondary flow, but in the opposite direction, inwards in the core and outwards at the walls (Lyne, 1971). Thus, somewhere in between, for a pulsatile flow with non-zero mean, there will be a conflict between the tendency for outward mean secondary motion in the core, driven by the mean flow rate, and that for inward mean secondary motion in the core, driven by the flow rate oscillation. This case was studied by Smith (1975) and Blennerhassett (1976); the most interesting results were those of Blennerhassett (see Pedley, 1980, section 4.2), who found that more than one flow was obtainable for the same values of the governing parameters. Such non-uniqueness in the flow is discussed more fully in the next section.

Another idealised geometry is that of the symmetrical bifurcation, although here a number of additional parameters have to be considered, as we saw above. Studies have ranged from those in which the flow was not very different from the equivalent steady flow (e.g. Walburn and Stein,1980, 1982; Menon *et al.* 1984) to those in which dramatic differences could be seen. For example, Jan *et al.* (1989) studied purely oscillatory flow in a symmetrical bifurcation typical of the pulmonary airways and showed that, while the flow was relatively streamlined, with little or no flow separation, at the times of maximum flow rate in either direction, dramatic disturbances developed around the times of flow reversal. Such flow patterns, if they are to be found in arteries, would have considerable implications for the wall shear stress distribution, because a separated eddy generated near the junction during one half-cycle would be totally disrupted by the vigorous mixing at flow reversal.

Because of the complexity of unsteady flow, even in idealised three-dimensional geometries, and the significant effect that small geometric perturbations can have, the question arises as to the relevance of studies in idealised geometries. If no generally applicable understanding can be gained, giving a qualitative idea of the flow in a wide range of arterial bifurcations, then surely it is necessary to investigate the precise geometry of interest? Experimental and computational studies on flow in a cast of the carotid bifurcation have revealed a wealth of detail on flow separation and wall shear stress that could not have been obtained from symmetrical bifurcations (Ku *et al.* 1985; Ku and Giddens, 1987; van Steenhoven *et al.* 1992). Again, of course, flow in a cast or model from a different individual is likely to give different results (Friedman, 1993). There is a strong desire to make generalisations from results which are difficult and time-consuming to obtain, but it is necessary to treat any such generalisations with great caution.

Non-uniqueness of flow in channels and tubes

A further difficulty in predicting the flow in airways and arteries is the fact, already alluded to, that it may not be unique. In a given geometry with a given pressure gradient driving the flow (steady or pulsatile), different flow and wall shear patterns can be obtained depending on the initial conditions. This is related to, but not the same as, instability, in which one (typically steady) solution of the governing equations is unstable to small disturbances and gives rise either to an unsteady or turbulent state or to another steady flow, which is stable. The latter is common in closed systems, such as a finite volume of fluid set into convective motion by heating. 'Open' systems, such as pipe flows with fluid entering at one end and leaving at the other, are usually thought to break down rapidly into turbulence once the critical state is reached. However, the situation envisaged here is one in which more than one stable flow exists, possibly as well as an unstable one.

One of the most familiar examples (in an 'open' system) is that of steady, two-dimensional flow in a channel with a symmetrical expansion (Fig. 1). One might at first suppose that a symmetrical flow would develop, with a separated flow zone on each wall, as sketched in Fig. 1. However, except at very low values of the Reynolds number, such a symmetrical flow is not seen; instead, the flow tends to hug one wall or the other, leaving a single, large separated flow region on the opposite side (Reneau *et al.* 1967; Sobey, 1985; Durst *et al.* 1993), as shown in Fig. 9. In each of these cases, the symmetrical flow presumably exists, in the sense that it is a solution of the steady-flow equations, but it is unstable and gives way to one of two coexisting stable states. The choice between those two states depends on how the flow was initially set up, or on barely discernible geometric imperfections.

Moreover, it is not necessary for the geometric configuration to be symmetrical for two stable states to coexist (Borgas and Pedley, 1990; Bujurke *et al.* 1995). Fig. 10 shows two steady flows computed at the same Reynolds number in a channel with one plane wall and one expanding wall (Bujurke *et al.* 1995); the first point of flow separation can occur on either wall. The flow that hugs the curved wall was more difficult to obtain than the other one, as it would be in an experiment, but given suitable initial conditions it could be observed. The difference between the wall shear distributions in the two cases is obvious.

A more interesting example, from the point of view of arteries, is that of fully developed flow in a uniform curved tube, as revealed by computational studies (Dennis and Ng, 1982; Yanase *et al.* 1989; Daskopoulos and Lenhoff, 1989). If the centre line is only gently curved, so that the curvature ratio δ (equation 3) is much less than 1, it can be shown that steady flow depends on the value of a single parameter, the Dean number D:

$$D = 4\sqrt{2} Re \delta^{1/2} . \tag{5}$$

Here Re is given by equation 1, with the velocity $\bar{u}$ being the average velocity for flow in a straight pipe driven by the same pressure gradient (the average velocity is somewhat less in a curved pipe); the numerical factor $4\sqrt{2}$ is put in so that the present notation agrees with that of the papers to be discussed.

When D is sufficiently small, the steady-flow equations have just one solution and there is a single secondary-flow vortex in each half of the tube. Fig. 11A shows contours of axial velocity and secondary flow streamlines in half the tube for D=500; the secondary flow is still approximately symmetrical (left–right), but has carried the faster-moving fluid towards the outside of the bend, and the axial velocity distribution is far from symmetrical.

A similar two-vortex flow has been computed for quite large values of D, up to at least 6000. The axial velocity contours and secondary streamlines for D=5000 are shown in Fig. 11B; these were computed by Daskopoulos and Lenhoff (1989), but agree closely with those of Collins and Dennis (1975) and Dennis and Ng (1982). However, there is a critical value of D, say D_1, above which more than one steady solution to the equations exists; Dennis and Ng (1982) found D_1 to be about 956, a value confirmed by Daskopoulos and Lenhoff (1989) and Yanase *et al.* (1989). Daskopoulous and Lenhoff computed two more solutions for D in excess of D_1, and two more again for D greater than another critical value D_2 (approximately 2500). The contour and streamline plots for

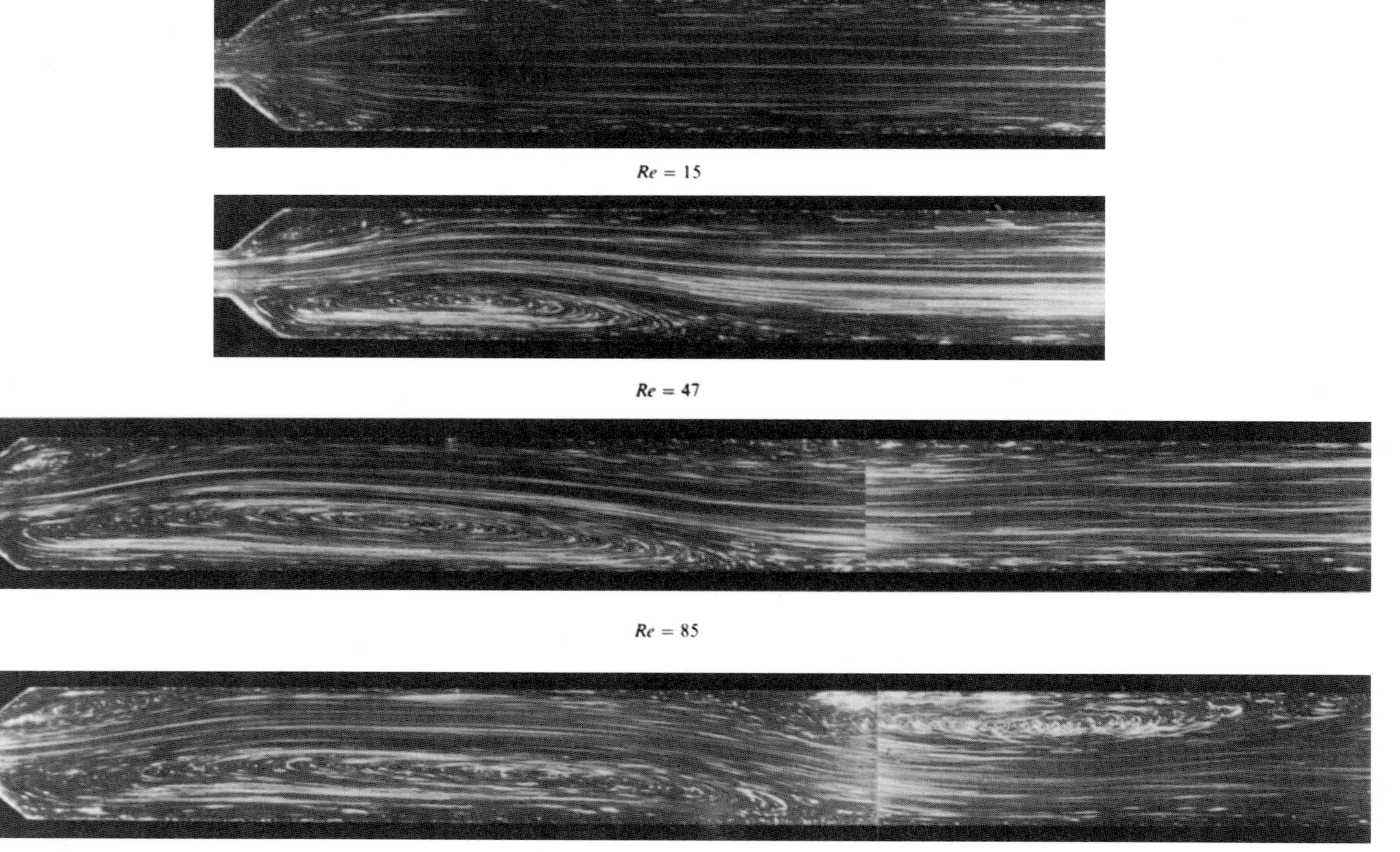

Fig. 9. Visualisation of steady flow through a symmetrical two-dimensional 45° expansion at various values of Reynolds number *Re*, showing that asymmetric flow occurs except at the lowest *Re*. (From Sobey, 1985.)

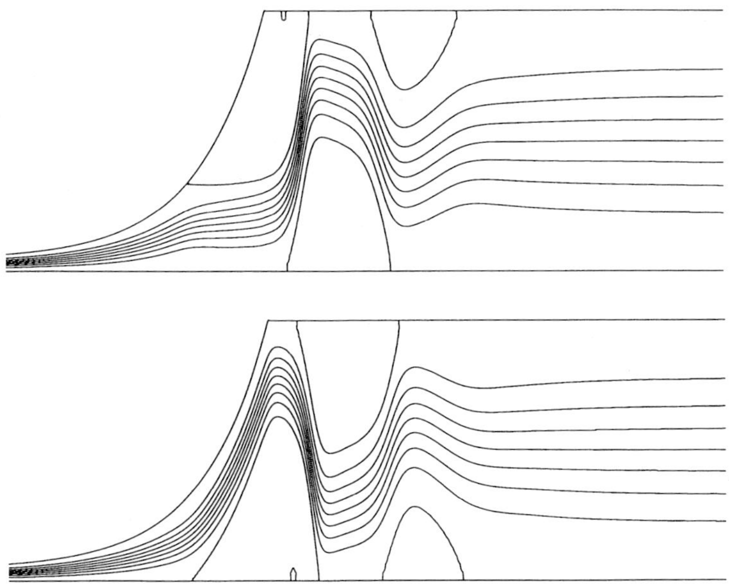

Fig. 10. Computed streamlines for steady flow through an asymmetric expansion, showing that two different steady flows are possible at the same value of the Reynolds number, Re = 500. (From Bujurke *et al.* 1995.)

all four solutions are given in Fig. 12, of which A and B are the two solutions that exist for $D>D_1$ (at D=3000) and C and D are those that exist only for $D>D_2$ (at D=3100). All these solutions are four-vortex in character (two vortices in each half of the tube) and do not look very different from each other. However, Daskopoulos and Lenhoff investigated their stability, and found that the only stable four-vortex flow for $D>D_1$ is that depicted in Fig. 12A; the others are all unstable. This result suggests that, for $D>D_1$, the flow that will actually be observed in an experiment will be either the two-vortex solution (Fig. 11) or the four-vortex solution such as that of Fig. 12A. Presumably, if the Dean number is gradually increased from a low value, the two-vortex flow will persist, but a suitably violent perturbation could result in the four-vortex flow being set up. [We should note that Yanase *et al.* (1989) developed a slightly more general stability analysis and concluded that the four-vortex flow is unstable after all, and therefore not observable. In contrast, in the experiments of Cheng and Mok (1986), the four-vortex flow was observed, and hence presumably stable, for a range of values of Dean number when the curvature ratio δ was not very small.]

It may be thought that whether a unique, stable steady flow exists for a certain geometry and Reynolds (or Dean) number is not particularly important when the real flows of interest are time-dependent anyway. Starting from a given initial state, with a given time-dependent pressure gradient, surely the flow will be well determined as a solution of the Navier–Stokes equations? In principle that is correct, but the existence of more than one steady solution, stable or unstable, means that the outcome can depend very sensitively on the initial or boundary conditions. A small change in geometry, or a small change in the pressure-gradient waveform, may lead to a substantially different

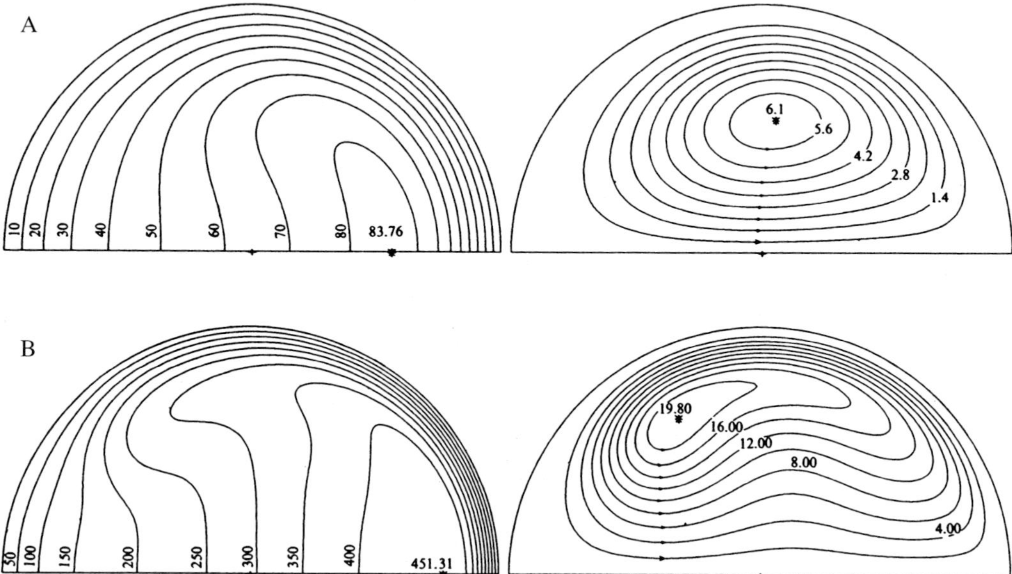

Fig. 11. Computed axial velocity contours (left) and two-vortex secondary flow streamlines (right) for steady flow in a curved tube of small curvature at two values of the Dean number. (A) D=500; (B) D=5000. (From Daskopoulos and Lenhoff, 1989.)

pattern of flow and wall shear. The pattern could vary from one cycle to the next, in a manner described technically as chaotic. As far as I know, there have not yet been any studies that examine flow in branched tubes from this point of view, and perhaps there should be. The concept of chaos has already been proved to be important in the cardiovascular system, in the context of cardiac or vascular smooth muscle (Winfree, 1983; Griffiths and Edwards, 1994*a*,*b*).

The influence of elasticity

The detailed flow studies reviewed in the last two sections have all been performed in rigid tubes, or in channels in which the wall moves in a prescribed way. The fact that wall motion can have interesting and unexpected consequences suggests that the elastic nature of arteries and airways may have a significant effect on the details of the flow and the shear stress distribution. That is known to be strongly true in circumstances when the difference between internal and external pressure becomes negative, so that the vessel tends to collapse (see Kamm and Pedley, 1989). Except under an inflated cuff, however, the pressure within arteries is normally well above the external (atmospheric) pressure and collapse is not a danger. Abnormally, arterial collapse may occur; the decrease in internal pressure at an atherosclerotic stenosis may lead to substantial deformation of the vessel wall just downstream, and the associated stresses could result in plaque rupture and thromboembolism (Ku *et al.* 1990). Nevertheless, it should be recognised that relatively small pulsations of a segment of an artery wall may have a considerable influence on the wall shear distribution, both locally and at a distance.

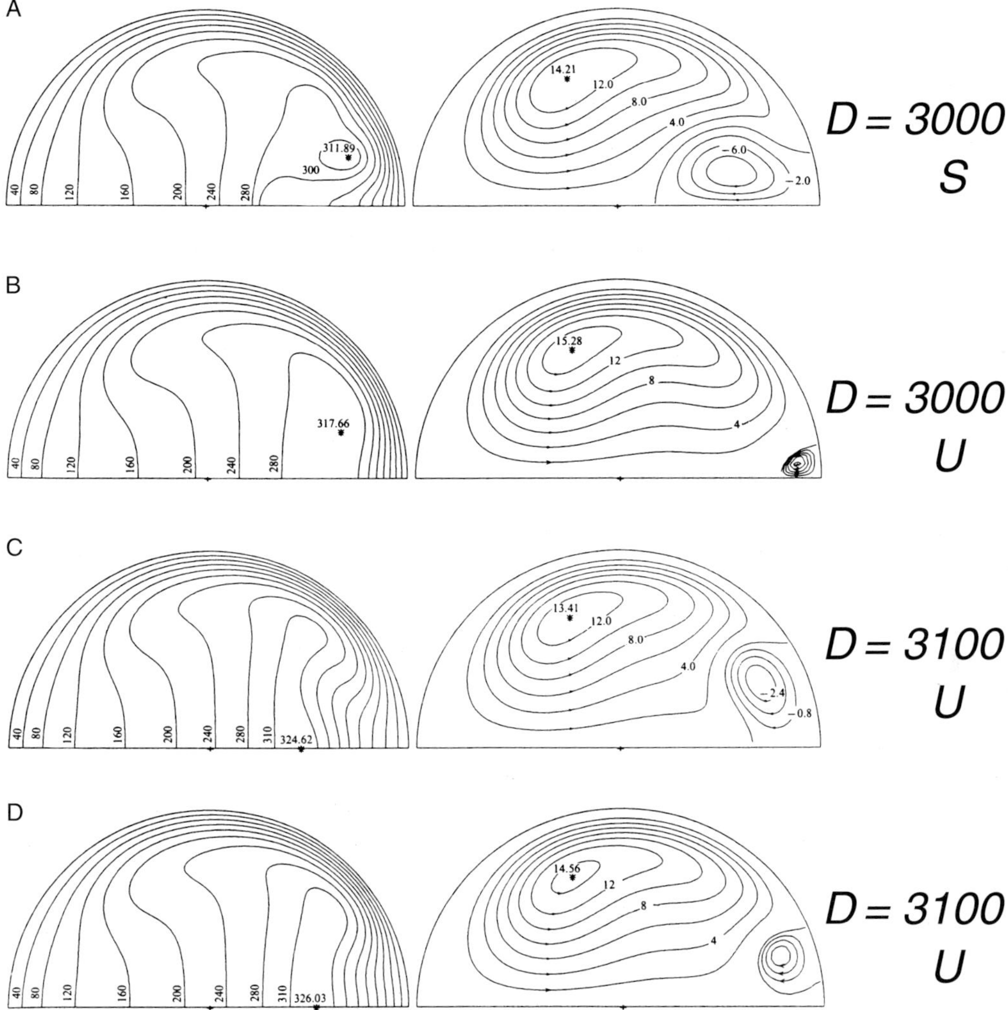

Fig. 12. Computed axial velocity contours (left) and secondary flow streamlines (right) for steady flow in a curved tube of small curvature at comparable values of the Dean number D, showing the non-uniqueness of the flow. The flows marked S are stable, those marked U are unstable. (From Daskopoulos and Lenhoff, 1989.)

Such possibilities have only recently been recognised, and there have been few relevant studies. Some of the first experimental studies were by Liepsch and Moravec (1984) and Ku and Liepsch (1986), who looked at the effect of elasticity on flow at a bifurcation (modelling side branches from the aorta) and found that wall shear was reduced by about 25 % below its value in a rigid bifurcation. More recent studies on the carotid bifurcation have shown a large effect (Anayiotos *et al.* 1994): measurements in a realistically elastic model and an otherwise identical rigid model give estimates of mean wall shear that are uniformly reduced by about 30 %, because the mean vessel diameter was increased, but peak wall shear was reduced by up to 100 %. These conclusions conflict somewhat with those of Friedman *et al.* (1992).

Complete computations to confirm this effect have not yet proved feasible, because of the enormous computer resources required for the solution of the time-dependent Navier–Stokes equations in complex three-dimensional geometry when the boundary positions are not known *a priori*. A two-dimensional elastic bifurcation has been studied by Lou and Yang (1993), and they indeed found a reduction in maximum wall shear, though only by around 10 %. A preliminary three-dimensional computation in an elastic model of the carotid bifurcation has been made by Reuderink (1991) on the assumption that only the propagating pressure pulse, and not the local hydrodynamic stresses, was of importance in determining vessel dimensions. He concluded that wall shear would be reduced by up to 30 %.

A conceptually important additional point has been made by Dutta *et al.* (1992), who pointed out that, for pressure pulse propagation in a straight elastic tube, the mean wall shear stress is very sensitive to the phase difference between the wave forms of pressure and of flow rate. It follows that, *in vivo*, there will be great sensitivity to the magnitude and phase of any reflected waves present and, hence, to peripheral haemodynamic conditions.

Concluding remarks

I hope I have made it clear that the fluid dynamical study of flow in vessels of complex geometry, at Reynolds numbers characteristic of large airways and arteries, is far from complete. The three-dimensionality of the geometry, the time-dependence of the driving pressure gradient, the transverse motions of the vessel walls and the potential non-uniqueness of the flow all imply that there is great sensitivity to small perturbations in either geometry or wave form. The more it is necessary to know the wall shear distribution in detail, in order to examine the response (say) of individual endothelial cells to their dynamic environment, the less will it be adequate to use idealised conditions, or conditions in one particular individual, as suitable models for conditions in another individual subject. Idealised models still have their place, as the source of general insights such as those discussed here, but detailed individual simulations will increasingly be required.

There is another trend in biological fluid dynamics, well exemplified by many of the contributions to this Symposium, to which I would like to allude in conclusion. Increasingly, the hydrodynamic study of the fluid flow in a vessel of a certain geometry is coupled to a parallel study of how that geometry is itself governed by the flow. Solid mechanical studies of passively elastic (or viscoelastic) vessels are at one end of the spectrum envisaged here, in which the wall shape responds more or less instantaneously to the hydrodynamic stresses. At the other end are the very-long-time-scale studies of vessel remodelling in response to enhanced or diminished mean wall shear stress. In between, however, are a range of other time scales which are important for a range of reasons: hormonal (time scales of a day, or a month), pharmacological (time scale dictated by human intervention) and physiological. Prominent in the last category are studies involving vascular smooth muscle whose contraction (time scale of seconds or minutes) can be stimulated by, and in turn can influence, fluid mechanical events.

Examples arise in reactive hyperaemia (Smye and Bloor, 1994) and in the chaotic pressure oscillations that can occur in small arteries as a response to variations in the calcium ion fluxes into (or out of) the smooth muscle cells (Griffiths and Edwards, 1994*a*,*b*). Somewhat analogous are investigations of peristaltic pumping in the ureter or gut. Observing the hydrodynamic consequences (of the muscle contraction, say), using well-established measurement techniques, leads in many cases to enhanced understanding of the intrinsic biological processes at work in the vessel wall.

References

ANAYIOTOS, A. S., JONES, S. A., GIDDENS, D. P., GLAGOV, S. AND ZARINS, C. K. (1994). Shear stress at a compliant model of the human carotid bifurcation. *J. Biomech. Eng.* **116**, 98–106.

BLENNERHASSETT, P. (1976). Secondary motion and diffusion in unsteady flow in a curved pipe. PhD thesis, Imperial College, London.

BORGAS, M. S. AND PEDLEY, T. J. (1990). Non-uniqueness and bifurcation in annular and planar channel flow. *J. Fluid Mech.* **214**, 229–250.

BUJURKE, N. M., PEDLEY, T. J. AND TUTTY, O. R. (1995). Comparison of series expansion and finite-difference computations of internal flow separation. *Phil. Trans R. Soc. Lond. A* (submitted).

CARO, C. G., FITZ-GERALD, J. M. AND SCHROTER, R. C. (1971). Atheroma and arterial wall shear: observation, correlation and proposal of a shear dependent mass transfer mechanism for atherogenesis. *Proc. R. Soc. Lond. B***177**, 109–159.

CARO, C. G., PEDLEY, T. J., SCHROTER, R. C. AND SEED, W. A. (1978). *The Mechanics of the Circulation.* Oxford: Oxford University Press.

CHENG, K. C. AND MOK, S. Y. (1986). In *Fluid Control and Measurement*, vol. 2 (ed. M. Harada), pp. 765–773. New York: Pergamon.

COLLINS, W. M. AND DENNIS, S. C. R. (1975). The steady motion of a viscous fluid in a curved tube. *Q. Jl Mech. appl. Math.* **28**, 133–156.

DASKOPOULOS, P. AND LENHOFF, A. M. (1989). Flow in curved ducts: bifurcation structure for stationary ducts. *J. Fluid Mech.* **203**, 125–148.

DEAN, W. R. (1927). Note on the motion of fluid in a curved pipe. *Phil. Mag. Ser. 7,* **4**, 208–223.

DEAN, W. R. (1928). The streamline motion of fluid in a curved pipe. *Phil. Mag., Ser. 7,* **5**, 673–695.

DENNIS, S. C. R. AND NG, M. (1982). Dual solutions for steady laminar flow through a curved tube. *Q. Jl Mech. appl. Math.* **35**, 305–324.

DURST, F., PEREIRA, J. C. F. AND TROPEA, C. (1993). The plane symmetric sudden-expansion flow at low Reynolds numbers. *J. Fluid Mech.* **248**, 567–581.

DUTTA, A., WANG, D. M. AND TARBELL, J. M. (1992). Numerical analysis of flow in an elastic artery model. *J. Biomech. Eng.* **114**, 26–33.

ELZINGA, G. AND WESTERHOF, N. (1991). Matching between ventricle and arterial load: an evolutionary process. *Circulation Res.* **68**, 1495–1500.

FRIEDMAN, M. H. (1993). Atherosclerosis research using vascular flow models: from 2-D branches to compliant replicas. *J. Biomech. Eng.* **115**, 595–601.

FRIEDMAN, M. H., BARGERON, C. B., DUNCAN, D. D., HUTCHINS, G. M. AND MARK, F. F. (1992). Effects of arterial compliance and non-Newtonian rheology on correlations between intimal thickness and wall shear. *J. Biomech. Eng.* **114**, 317–320.

FRY, D. L. (1987). Mass transport, atherogenesis and risk. *Arteriosclerosis* **7**, 88–100.

FUKUSHIMA, T. AND AZUMA, T. (1982). The horseshoe vortex: a secondary flow generated in arteries with stenosis, bifurcations and branchings. *Biorheology* **19**, 143–154.

GIDDENS, D. P., ZARINS, C. K. AND GLAGOV, S. (1993). The role of fluid mechanics in the localization and detection of atherosclerosis. *J. Biomech. Eng.* **115**, 588–594.

GRIFFITHS, T. M. AND EDWARDS, D. H. (1994*a*). EDRF suppresses chaotic pressure oscillations in isolated resistance artery without influencing intrinsic complexity. *Am. J. Physiol.* **266**, H1786–H1800.

GRIFFITHS, T. M. AND EDWARDS, D. H. (1994*b*). Fractal analysis of the role of smooth muscle Ca fluxes in genesis of chaotic arterial pressure oscillations. *Am. J. Physiol.* **266**, H1801–H1811.

JAN, D. L., SHAPIRO, A. H. AND KAMM, R. D. (1989). Some features of oscillatory flow in the lung. *J. appl. Physiol.* **67**, 147–159.

KAMM, R. D. AND PEDLEY, T. J. (1989). Flow in collapsible tubes: a brief review. *J. Biomech. Eng.* **111**, 177–179.

KARINO, T., KWONG, H. H. M. AND GOLDSMITH, H. L. (1979). Particle flow behaviour in models of branching vessels. I. Vortices in 90° T-junctions. *Biorheology* **16**, 231–248.

KU, D. N. (1988). A review of carotid duplex scanning. *Echocardiography* **5**, 53–69.

KU, D. N. AND GIDDENS, D. P. (1987). Laser Doppler anemometer measurements of pulsatile flow in a model carotid bifurcation. *J. Biomech.* **20**, 407–421.

KU, D. N., GIDDENS, D. P., ZARINS, C. K. AND GLAGOV, S. (1985). Pulsatile flow and atherosclerosis in the human carotid bifurcation: positive correlation between plaque location and low and oscillating shear stress. *Arteriosclerosis* **5**, 293–302.

KU, D. N. AND LIEPSCH, D. (1986). The effects of non-Newtonian viscoelasticity and wall elasticity on flow at a 90° bifurcation. *Biorheology* **23**, 359–370.

KU, D. N., ZEIGLER, M. N. AND DOWNING, J. M. (1990). One-dimensional steady inviscid flow through a stenotic collapsible tube. *J. Biomech. Eng.* **112**, 444–450.

LEE, C. S. F. AND TALBOT, L. (1979). A fluid-mechanical study of the closure of heart valves. *J. Fluid Mech.* **91**, 41–63.

LIEPSCH, D. AND MORAVEC, ST. (1984). Pulsatile flow of non-Newtonian fluid in distensible models of human arteries. *Biorheology* **21**, 571–586.

LOU, Z. AND YANG, W.-J. (1992). Biofluid dynamics at arterial bifurcations. *Crit. Rev. biomed. Eng.* **19**, 455–493.

LOU, Z. AND YANG, W.-J. (1993). A computer simulation of the blood flow at the aortic bifurcation with flexible walls. *J. Biomech. Eng.* **115**, 306–315.

LUTZ, R. J., CANNON, J. N., BISCHOFF, K. B. AND DEDRICK, R. L. (1977). Wall shear stress distribution in a model canine artery during steady flow. *Circulation Res.* **41**, 391–399.

LYNE, W. H. (1971). Unsteady viscous flow in a curved pipe. *J. Fluid Mech.* **45**, 13–31.

MCDONALD, D. A. (1974). *Blood Flow in Arteries* (2nd edn). London: Edward Arnold.

MENON, A. S., WEBER, M. E. AND CHANG, H. K. (1984). Model study of flow dynamics in human central airways. III. Oscillatory velocity profiles. *Respir. Physiol.* **55**, 255–275.

PARK, D. K. (1989). A biofluid mechanics study of arterial stenoses. MSc thesis, Lehigh University, Bethlehem, Pennsylvania.

PEDLEY, T. J. (1976). Viscous boundary layers in reversing flow. *J. Fluid Mech.* **74**, 59–79.

PEDLEY, T. J. (1980). *The Fluid Mechanics of Large Blood Vessels.* Cambridge: Cambridge University Press.

PEDLEY, T. J., RALPH, M. E. AND TUTTY, O. R. (1988). Unsteady, separated laminar flow in non-uniform vessels. In *Role of Blood Flow in Atherogenesis* (ed. Y. Yoshida, T. Yamaguchi, C. G. Caro, S. Glagov and R. M. Nerem), pp. 97–102. Tokyo: Springer.

PEDLEY, T. J., SCHROTER, R. C. AND SUDLOW, M. F. (1977). Gas flow and mixing in the airways. In *Bioengineering Aspects of the Lung* (ed. J. B. West), pp. 163–265. New York: Dekker.

PEDLEY, T. J. AND STEPHANOFF, K. D. (1985). Flow along a channel with a time-dependent indentation in one wall: the generation of vorticity waves. *J. Fluid Mech.* **160**, 337–367.

PERKTOLD, K., NEREM, R. M. AND PETER, R. O. (1991). A numerical calculation of flow in a curved tube model of the left main coronary artery. *J. Biomech.* **24**, 175–189.

PRANDTL, L. (1952). *The Essentials of Fluid Dynamics* (3rd edn, translated). Glasgow: Blackie & Son.

RALPH, M. E. AND PEDLEY, T. J. (1988). Flow in a channel with a moving indentation. *J. Fluid Mech.* **190**, 87–112.

RALPH, M. E. AND PEDLEY, T. J. (1990). Flow in a channel with a time-dependent indentation in one wall. *J. Fluids Eng.* **112**, 468–475.

RENEAU, L. R., JOHNSTON, J. P. AND KLINE, S. J. (1967). Performance and design of straight, two-dimensional diffusers. *J. basic Eng.* **89**, 141–150.

REUDERINK, P. (1991). Analysis of the flow in a 3D distensible model of the carotid artery bifurcation. Doctoral dissertation, Eindhoven Technical University.

SCHROTER, R. C. AND SUDLOW, M. F. (1969). Flow patterns in models of the human bronchial airways. *Respir. Physiol.* **7**, 341–355.

SEYMOUR, R. S., HARGENS, A. R. AND PEDLEY, T. J. (1993). The heart works against gravity. *Am. J. Physiol.* **265**, R715–R720.

SMITH, F. T. (1975). Pulsatile flow in curved pipes. *J. Fluid Mech.* **71**, 15–42.

SMYE, S. W. AND BLOOR, M. I. G. (1994). An elastic porous tube model of reactive hyperaemia. *Med. biol. Eng. Comput.* **32**, (in press).

SOBEY, I. J. (1985). Observation of waves during oscillatory channel flow. *J. Fluid Mech.* **151**, 395–426.

TALBOT, L. AND WONG, S. J. (1982). A note on boundary-layer collision in a curved pipe. *J. Fluid Mech.* **122**, 505–510.

TUTTY, O. R. (1992). Pulsatile flow in a constricted channel. *J. Biomech. Eng.* **114**, 50–54.

TUTTY, O. R. AND PEDLEY, T. J. (1993). Oscillatory flow in a stepped channel. *J. Fluid Mech.* **247**, 179–204.

VAN DYKE, M. (1982). *An Album of Fluid Motion*. Stanford: Parabolic Press.

VAN STEENHOVEN, A. A., JANSSEN, J. D. AND VAN CAMPEN, D. H. (1992). Cardiovascular fluid mechanics. In *Theoretical and Applied Mechanics* (ed. S. R. Bodner, J. Singer, A. Solan and Z. Hashin), pp. 407–422. Amsterdam: North-Holland.

WALBURN, F. J. AND STEIN, P. D. (1980). Flow in a symmetrically branched tube simulating the aortic bifurcation: the effects of unevenly distributed flow. *Ann. Biomed. Eng.* **8**, 159–173.

WALBURN, F. J. AND STEIN, P. D. (1982). The shear rate at the wall in a symmetrically branched tube simulating the aortic bifurcation. *Biorheology* **19**, 307–316.

WEINBAUM, S. AND CHIEN, S. (1993). Lipid transport aspects of atherogenesis. *J. Biomech. Eng.* **115**, 602–610.

WHITE, C. M. (1929). Streamline flow through curved pipes. *Proc. R. Soc. Lond. A* **123**, 645–663.

WINFREE, A. T. (1983). Sudden cardiac death: a problem in topology. *Scient. Am.* **248**, 144–161.

WOMERSLEY, J. R. (1955). Method for the calculation of velocity, rate of flow and viscous drag in arteries when the pressure gradient is known. *J. Physiol., Lond.* **127**, 553–563.

YANASE, S., GOTO, N. AND YAMAMOTO, K. (1989). Dual solutions of the flow through a curved tube. *Fluid Dyn. Res.* **5**, 191–201.

YOUNG, T. (1809). On the functions of the heart and arteries. *Phil. Trans. R. Soc. Lond.* **99**, 1–31.

YUAN, F., CHIEN, S. AND WEINBAUM, S. (1991). A new view of convective–diffusive transport processes in the arterial intima. *J. Biomech. Eng.* **113**, 314–329.

ZARINS, C. K., GIDDENS, D. P., BHARADVAJ, B. K., SOTTIURAI, V. S., MABON, R. F. AND GLAGOV, S. (1983). Carotid bifurcation atherosclerosis: quantitative correlation of plaque localization with flow velocity profiles and wall shear stress. *Circulation Res.* **53**, 502–514.

ZARINS, C. K., ZATINA, M. A., GIDDENS, D. P., KU, D. N. AND GLAGOV, S. (1987). Shear stress regulation of artery lumen diameter in experimental atherogenesis. *J. vasc. Surg.* **5**, 413–420.

ZELLER, H., TALUKDER, N. AND LORENZ, J. (1970). Model studies of pulsating flow in arterial branches and wave propagation in blood vessels. In *Fluid Dynamics of Blood Circulation and Respiratory Flow*, AGARD Conference Proceedings no. **65**.

ARTERIAL WINDKESSELS IN MARINE MAMMALS

ROBERT E. SHADWICK[1] *and JOHN M. GOSLINE*[2]

[1]Marine Biology Research Division, Scripps Institution of Oceanography, La Jolla CA 92093-0204, USA *and* [2]Department of Zoology, University of British Columbia, Vancouver, BC, Canada V6T 1Z4

Summary

In marine mammals, the aortic arch is enlarged relative to the descending aorta to varying degrees in different species. The ratio of maximal diameter of the arch to that of the thoracic aorta is about 2.3 in the harbour seal (*Phoca vitulina*), 3.6 in the Weddell seal (*Leptonychotes weddelli*) and 3.2 in the fin whale (*Balaenoptera physalus*), compared with only 1.4 in the dog. This anatomical specialisation probably provides increased volume capacitance in the arterial circulation as an adaptation to diving bradycardia. Data on the morphometric and mechanical properties of aortic tissues from seals and fin whale are compared. In the harbour seal, more than 80 % of the volume change in the entire thoracic aorta that results from a pressure pulse occurs in the bulbous arch, and this is more than 90 % in the Weddell seal and fin whale. The enhanced capacitance of the arch in the harbour seal is primarily due to its larger diameter, as the relative wall thickness and elasticity of the arch and thoracic aorta are the same. A similar situation appears to exist in the larger Weddell seal, although extrapolation of the pressure–volume curves suggests that the arch might be somewhat less stiff than the thoracic aorta. In addition to being greatly expanded, the aortic arch of the fin whale is also much more distensible than the relatively thin-walled and much stiffer descending aorta. At the estimated mean blood pressure, the elastic modulus of this vessel is 12 MPa, or 30 times that of the aortic arch. The major haemodynamic consequence of this type of arterial modification is that the aortic arch acts as a Windkessel, i.e. the capacitance of the aorta is increased significantly close to the heart, leading to a reduced characteristic impedance and probably reduced pulsatility in the descending aorta. In the extreme case of the whale, the arterial capacitance is shifted entirely to the arch, and the impedance change at the entrance to the thoracic aorta is so high that this probably represents the major reflection site in the arterial tree.

Introduction

The mechanical properties of arteries and their influence on arterial haemodynamics are well understood. In general, the aorta has a non-uniformly distributed compliance and it expands and recoils elastically with each pulse of blood ejected by the heart. This smoothes the pulse and helps to maintain flow to the peripheral vessels during diastole. The aorta is an elastic structure that becomes progressively stiffer and smaller in diameter

Key words: artery wall, aortic arch, elasticity, haemodynamics, Windkessel, impedance, circulatory mechanics, diving mammal, seal, whale.

with increasing distance from the heart. These properties contribute to an increase in the characteristic pressure wave velocity (c_0) and hydraulic impedance (Z_0), both being important determinants of pressure and flow dynamics. In the dog, for example, the distal portion of the abdominal aorta is two times stiffer and 2.4 times smaller than the aortic arch, while c_0 and Z_0 increase by twofold and ninefold, respectively (Caro *et al.* 1978). These features are known as the elastic and geometric tapers of the arterial tree. Along with blood pressure, these aortic mechanical properties are relatively constant among terrestrial species.

An interesting morphological feature of the aorta of diving mammals is an enlargement of the arch to form a structure called the aortic bulb. Drabek (1975) provided quantitative comparisons of aortic arch dimensions in several Antarctic seal species and he, as well as others (Elsner, 1969; Strauss, 1969, cited in Drabek, 1975), suggested that this was an adaptation to diving bradycardia. They proposed that the enlarged aortic arch was an elastic reservoir, or Windkessel, that acted as a passive pump to maintain blood flow to the brain and coronary arteries during long diastolic periods of bradycardia. Using a mathematical model of a mammalian arterial system with an enlarged aortic arch that matched the dimensions in harbour seals, Campbell *et al.* (1981) concluded that the function of the aortic bulb was primarily to reduce input impedance and peak systolic pressure, thereby reducing cardiac work and oxygen consumption.

In two instances, the morphometric and mechanical properties of aortas from marine mammals have been investigated (Rhode *et al.* 1986; Shadwick and Gosline, 1994), and these data provide the basis for a discussion of arterial design and haemodynamics presented here. Comparison of small harbour seals (*Phoca vitulina*, approximately 70 kg) and large Weddell seals (*Leptonychotes weddelli*, approximately 400 kg) with very large fin whales (*Balaenoptera physalus*, approximately 40 000 kg) indicates that there are substantial differences in the relative contribution of the enlarged aortic arch to the total system compliance and that these differences may be related to diving capabilities. In the case of the small harbour seals, the storage capacitance of the aorta is greatly increased by the enlargement of the arch, while in the large whales the descending aorta is so stiff that virtually all the arterial capacitance is concentrated in the expansible aortic arch. The large, deep-diving Weddell seals appear to take a somewhat intermediate position.

Aortic dimensions and distensibility

Table 1 shows how different the arterial dimensions are in marine mammals compared with those of a typical terrestrial species, and also how much more dominant the arch becomes in terms of size and system capacitance with increasing body mass. The ratio of maximal diameter of the arch to that of the thoracic aorta is about 1.4 in the dog, 2.3 in the harbour seal, 3.6 in the Weddell seal and 3.2 in the fin whale (Table 1). The enhanced volume storage capacity provided by the enlarged aortic arch is indicated by the volume capacitance ratio, which reaches a remarkably high value of 0.98 in the fin whale. Two interesting observations made by Rhode *et al.* (1986) are that the aortic volume of a 95 kg harbour seal is greater than that of a 460 kg horse and that the volume of the seal's arch alone is greater than the volume of the entire aorta of a human of similar body mass.

Table 1. *Dimensions of the aorta in terrestrial and diving mammals*

Species (mass)	Arch			Thoracic aorta			Volume capacitance ratio
	D	*h*	*h/r*	*D*	*h*	*h/r*	
Dog[a] (20 kg)	1.9	0.16	0.17	1.33	0.10	0.18	0.48
Harbour seal[b] (70 kg)	3.76	0.27	0.17	1.62	0.13	0.19	0.83[a]
Weddell seal[b] (405 kg)	10.2	0.5	0.11	2.8	0.22	0.19	0.94
Fin whale[c] (approximately 40 000 kg)	28.2	4.5	0.47	8.8	0.3	0.07	0.98

Dimensions for external diameter (D) and wall thickness (h) are in cm. Wall thickness ratio (h/r) is derived using internal radius ($r=D/2-h$). Volume capacitance ratio is the ratio of the capacitance of the aortic arch to the capacitance of the arch and descending thoracic aorta together, where capacitance is defined as volume change per unit pressure change within the physiological pressure range.

[a]Data from Campbell *et al.* (1981); [b]calculated from Rhode *et al.* (1986) for mean of 15 harbour seals and one Weddell seal; [c]data from Shadwick and Gosline (1994) and unpublished.

Among the species compared here and by Drabek (1975), aortic arch enlargement is most extreme in the Weddell seal and fin whale. An interesting difference between these two species is that the Weddell seal has a relatively thin-walled aortic arch, and that the whale has a thick-walled arch and an extremely thin-walled thoracic aorta. In the latter, the transition from arch to thoracic aorta is anatomically abrupt, occurring over a distance about equal to the diameter of the descending vessel. While the data in Table 1 point out the varying degrees of morphological modification found in the diving mammals, the functional consequences are more clearly appreciated by considering the mechanical properties of these vessels. Examples of pressure–volume curves for vessel segments taken from seals and fin whales are compared in Fig. 1. In each species, the unpressurised volume is greater in the aortic arch than in the entire descending thoracic aorta, by about twofold in the whale and harbour seal and by nearly sixfold in the Weddell seal. Assuming that the normal physiological blood pressure is in the range 10–15 kPa, as in other mammals (Rhode *et al.* 1986), it is also apparent that the volume change during a cardiac cycle is much larger in the arch than in the descending thoracic aorta, particularly in the fin whale (approximately 35 litres *versus* 0.6 litres, respectively), where the volume compliance of the thoracic aorta is negligible compared with that of the large distensible arch (Table 1).

The astonishing differences in size and distensibility of the arch and thoracic aorta in the fin whale are highlighted in Fig. 2 by diagrams of calculated cross-sectional dimensions of these vessels at pressures of 0, 10 and 15 kPa. Over the physiological pressure range, the aortic arch expands greatly, both in circumference and in length, resulting in a volume increase of more than 60 % between 10 and 15 kPa (Shadwick and

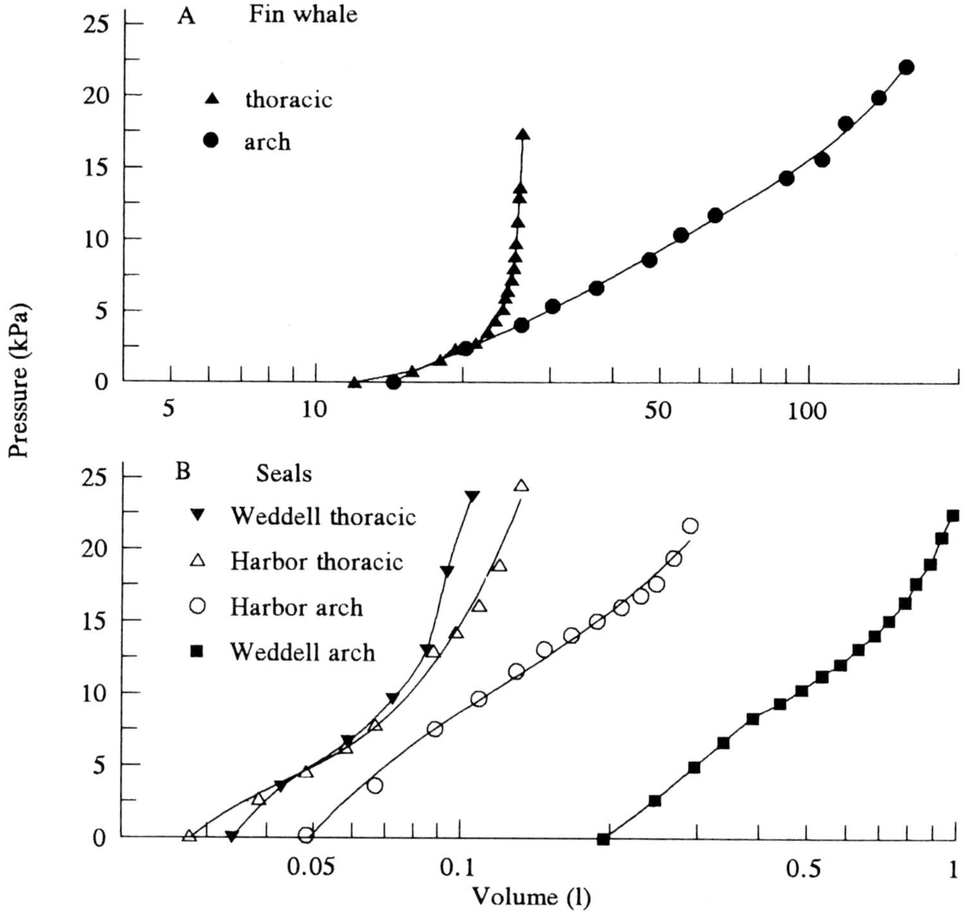

Fig. 1. Pressure–volume curves for *in vitro* inflations of the aorta from marine mammals, comparing the bulbous aortic arch with the descending thoracic aorta. (A) Fin whale aortic arch and thoracic aorta from 18 m and 19.8 m animals, respectively, estimated at 35 000–40 000 kg. (B) Arch and thoracic aorta from a 86 kg harbour seal and a 405 kg Weddell seal (redrawn from Rhode *et al.* 1986). Note that the volume scales are logarithmic.

Gosline, 1994). By contrast, the thoracic aorta changes by less than 1 % in radius and less than 2 % in volume, indicating again that the compliance of this arterial system resides virtually entirely within the arch.

Arterial wall material properties

The material properties of blood vessels can be quantified from inflation data in terms of circumferential stress and strain. From these, the elastic modulus, an index of vessel stiffness, can be derived. The formulation of elastic modulus varies depending on whether the pressurised cylinder is held at a fixed length, such as the thoracic aorta, or untethered, such as the aortic arch (see Shadwick and Gosline, 1985, 1994). In the

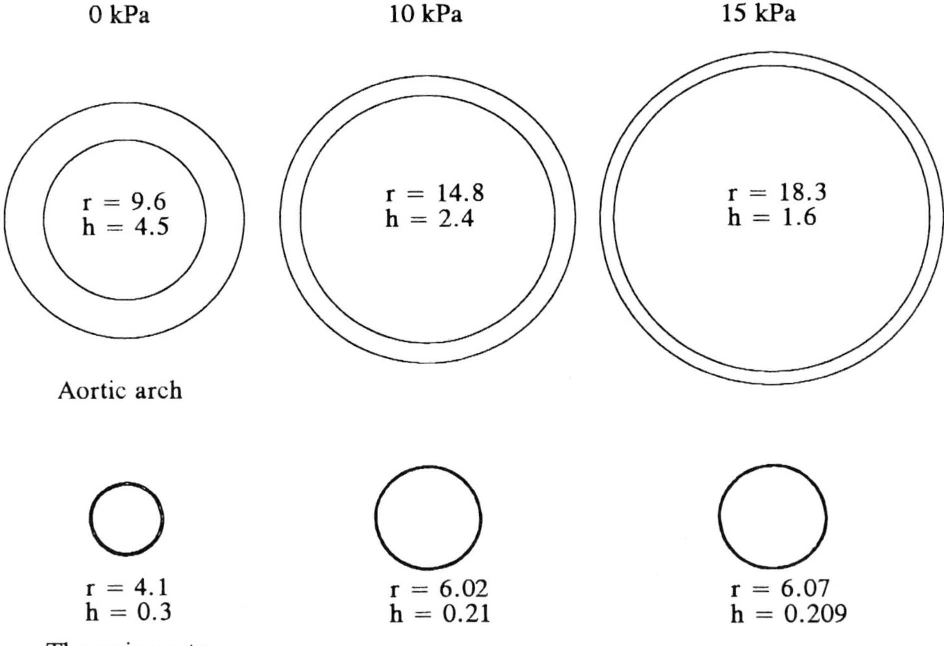

Fig. 2. Illustration of the difference in size and distensibility of the fin whale aortic arch and thoracic aorta. The diagrams show calculated cross-sectional dimensions of these vessels at pressures of 0, 10 and 15 kPa. Dimensions of wall thickness (h) and internal radius (r) are in centimetres. Note that, in the arch, longitudinal strains are approximately equal to circumferential strains, while in the tethered thoracic aorta, length changes are negligible.

absence of details on tethering for the inflation experiments on harbour seal arteries conducted by Rhode *et al.* (1986), we calculated the elastic modulus from their stress–strain data according to Bergel's method (Bergel, 1961). Details of these calculations for the whale vessels are given by Shadwick and Gosline (1994). Fig. 3A shows the circumferential elastic modulus plotted as a function of strain. At their predicted *in vivo* mean strains, the whale thoracic aorta is about 30 times stiffer than the arch, while in the seal these vessels are materially similar. Thus, in the harbour seal, the levels of stress, strain and elastic stiffness are comparable in the arch and thoracic aorta, and the differences in distensibility of these vessels can be attributed solely to their different geometry (Rhode *et al.* 1986). This includes the difference in longitudinal tethering as well as size. The *in vivo* tethering of the thoracic aorta restricts volume changes to radial expansion, while the arch can increase in length as well as in diameter. In the aortic arch of the whale, longitudinal and circumferential strains during inflation are approximately equal, so that the volume increase is much greater than radial expansion alone would provide.

Stress–strain and modulus data have not been reported for the vessels in the Weddell seal. However, if we assume that length changes which occur during inflations of the aortic segments are similar in the Weddell seal and the whale, then the pressure–volume

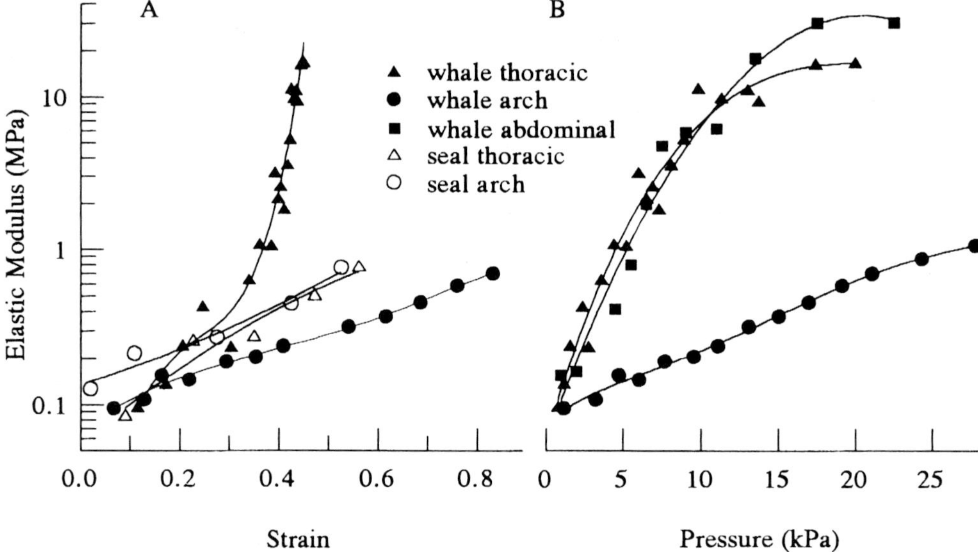

Fig. 3. Elastic modulus as a function of circumferential strain for fin whale and harbour seal aortas (A) and as a function of inflation pressure for aortic arch, thoracic and abdominal aortic segments of the fin whale (B). Based on an estimated mean resting blood pressure of 13 kPa, the corresponding *in vivo* mean strains would be about 0.43 for the whale thoracic aorta and 0.5 for the whale arch and the harbour seal vessels. Seal data in A are based on stress–strain curves given by Rhode *et al.* (1986); curves in B are redrawn from Shadwick and Gosline (1994).

data of Rhode *et al.* (1986) can be used to estimate values of stress, strain and elastic modulus. When this is done, we find that the material properties of the arch and descending thoracic aorta of the Weddell seal appear to be similar to those of the harbour seal, with perhaps slightly higher stiffness in the thoracic tissue. These conclusions must be regarded as only tentative and await further investigation.

The high stiffness of the thoracic aorta in the whale at physiological pressures is mimicked by the abdominal aorta (Fig. 3B) and, presumably, also by the continuation of the aorta in the caudal region. This means that, in contrast to the relatively gradual 'elastic taper' found in terrestrial mammals (Fig. 4), and perhaps the seals, the whale has a very abrupt transition from a highly compliant Windkessel proximal to the heart to a very rigid conduit that delivers blood to the posterior portion of the body. This unique mechanical specialization has not been described in the aorta of any other mammal.

Haemodynamics

Wave propagation

A fundamental property of the circulation is that the pressure pulses generated by the heart travel through the system as waves. The intrinsic pressure wave velocity in an elastic tube (c_o) is dependent on the wall thickness ratio and elastic modulus and can thus

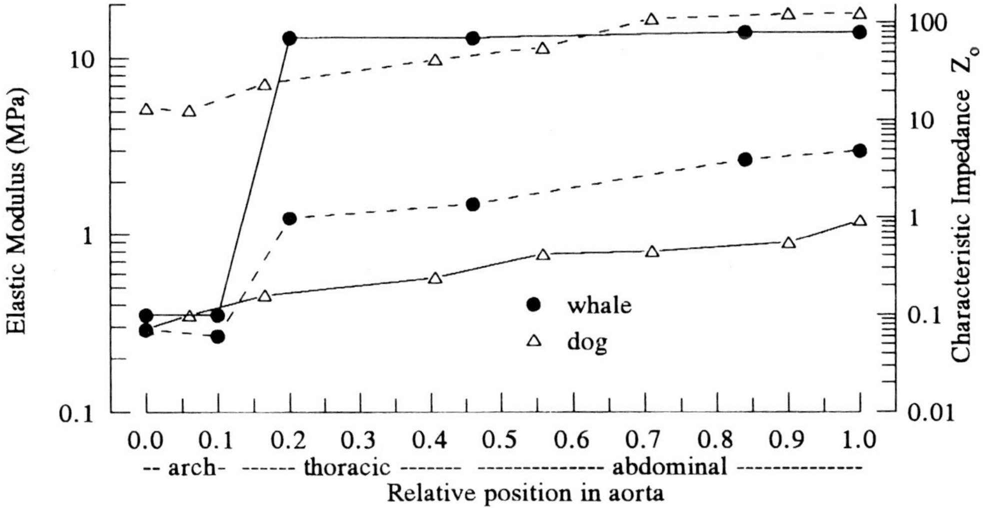

Fig. 4. Circumferential elastic modulus (solid lines) and characteristic impedance (broken lines) at estimated mean blood pressure (13 kPa) as a function of the relative position along the aorta in the dog and the fin whale. The gradual increase in modulus with distance from the heart exhibited by the dog aorta is typical of the elastic taper in mammalian systems. The abrupt change in stiffness by a factor of 30 at the transition from the aortic arch to the descending thoracic aorta in the fin whale is a unique feature that localises the aortic compliance entirely within the arch. Data for the dog are summarised from Caro *et al.* (1978) and Milnor (1982).

Table 2. *Haemodynamic parameters for fin whale and harbour seal*

Artery segment	L (m)	E (MPa)	c_o ($m\,s^{-1}$)	Z_o ($MPa\,s\,m^{-3}$)	Γ
Whale arch	1.3	0.4	4.7	0.057	
					0.92
Whale thoracic	2.5	12	14.8	1.3	
Whale abdominal	4.5	12	15.9	4.1	
Seal arch	0.08	0.6	4.5	2.4	
					0.67
Seal thoracic	0.22	0.6	5.1	13.3	

Length (L), circumferential elastic modulus (E), pressure wave velocity (c_o) and characteristic impedance (Z_o) for aortic segments were determined for a mean blood pressure of 13 kPa.

Reflection ratio (Γ) is for junction between arch and thoracic aorta.

Parameters for the seal were derived from data given in Rhode *et al.* (1986). Equations used from Caro *et al.* (1978) and Milnor (1982) are: $c_o^2=Eh/2\delta r$, where δ is blood density, $Z_o=\delta c_o/A$, where A is the cross-sectional area of the lumen, and $\Gamma=(1-x)/(1+x)$, where $x=Z_{o(arch)}/Z_{o(thoracic)}$.

be calculated (Table 2). In the fin whale, c_o increases abruptly from about $5\,m\,s^{-1}$ in the arch to about $15\,m\,s^{-1}$ in the thoracic and abdominal aortas, as a direct consequence of the increase in circumferential stiffness. In other mammals, including the harbour seal, c_o rises only slightly from about $4\,m\,s^{-1}$ in the aortic arch to about $5\,m\,s^{-1}$ in the thoracic aorta (Milnor, 1982).

The characteristic impedance Z_o is related to c_o divided by the lumen cross-sectional area. This parameter defines the ratio of pressure to flow in the absence of reflected waves and thus it links the flow dynamics in a blood vessel to its physical properties. Impedance is important haemodynamically because, as it changes along the arterial tree, partial wave reflections result. Z_o is predicted to increase dramatically (23-fold) at the entrance to the thoracic aorta in the whale, but much less so (fivefold) in the harbour seal (Table 2). In the dog, only a twofold increase in Z_o from the arch to thoracic aorta occurs (Fig. 4). As a comparison with Z_o calculated from the arterial properties, we also predicted the aortic Z_o from allometry (Westerhof and Elzinga, 1991). Doing so yields values of $0.02\,MPa\,s\,m^{-3}$ for the whale and $7\,MPa\,s\,m^{-3}$ for the harbour seal. In the case of the seal, the allometric prediction falls between the calculated values for arch and thoracic segments, whereas in the whale the predicted Z_o is close to that calculated for the arch. In most mammals, the peripheral resistance R_p is about 20 times Z_o for the input to the aorta (Milnor, 1982). In the whale, the calculated value of R_p (see below) is also about 20 times Z_o for the arch (Table 2; Fig. 4), making it equivalent to Z_o for the thoracic aorta. This suggests that in the whale the capacitive portion of the aorta is limited to the arch and that the remainder of the aorta can be considered as being functionally part of the peripheral resistance. It seems likely, therefore, that the pulsatility of flow into the thoracic aorta would be much reduced by the damping effect of the bulbous arch. In the harbour seal, this effect would probably be much less pronounced because of the relatively small rise in impedance at the descending thoracic aorta.

Wave propagation in the arterial tree is dominated by the presence of reflected waves. Partial reflections occur at points of impedance mismatch, such as the bifurcation of the abdominal aorta to the femoral arteries in terrestrial mammals. The net result of the interaction of incident and reflected waves in the central circulation is an increase in amplitude and a change in shape of the pressure waves as they travel distally from the heart. A widely held view is that the mammalian heart rate and aortic length are matched so that the major components of the pulse wave reflect at nearly one-quarter of a wavelength from the heart. This produces a minimum value of impedance at the input and lowers the load on the heart (Noordergraaf *et al.* 1979). In the simple Windkessel model, wave propagation effects are neglected because it is assumed that the pressure pulse is similar in amplitude and shape and is synchronous in time at all locations, i.e. it is propagated instantaneously (Caro *et al.* 1978). While this condition is not met in terrestrial mammals, it is closely approximated in many ectotherms, where heart rates are relatively low and the aortic length is much shorter relative to the length of the fundamental pressure wave. In these animals, wave propagation effects do not dominate, and the elastic vessels in the central circulation function as a single-capacitance structure or Windkessel (Shelton and Burggren, 1976; Langille and Jones, 1977; Shadwick *et al.* 1987; Gibbons and Shadwick, 1991), which functions to smooth the pulsatile pressure and flow from the heart much as a capacitor can be used in an electrical circuit to filter alternating current components from an electrical signal.

In the absence of an abdominal bifurcation in the fin whale, and given the large increase in impedance that occurs abruptly between the aortic arch and the descending aorta, the major arterial reflection site must occur at this point. In fact, based on the values of Z_o in Table 2, we calculate a reflection ratio (Γ) of 0.92 at this junction, which should serve to isolate the downstream vessel from most of the pulsatility produced by the heart (Shadwick and Gosline, 1994). The reflection ratio at the same junction in the harbour seal is only 0.67. By comparison, Γ for the abdominal bifurcation in a dog, regarded as the major aortic reflection site in terrestrial mammals, is about 0.44 (Caro *et al.* 1978). Data for the Weddell seal indicate an approximately threefold decrease in diameter between the arch and the descending thoracic aorta (Rhode *et al.* 1986). Even if these two segments have similar elastic moduli, the impedance will increase by a factor of 9 as a result of the reduction in diameter (i.e. Z_o varies as $1/r^2$; see Table 2). Such a pronounced impedance mismatch should give a reflection ratio of 0.8, suggesting that the aortic arch in the Weddell seal may function more like that in the whale than that in the smaller harbour seal. To assess whether the aortic arch in the whale functions as a Windkessel *in vivo* requires an estimate of the pressure wavelengths, which can be calculated from c_o and heart rate.

Scaling of the arterial time constant and heart rate

In the arterial system of mammals, the peripheral resistance (R_p) and the system capacitance (C) determine the time constant of exponential pressure decay in diastole (τ), i.e. $\tau = R_pC$. Mean blood pressure and mean pulse pressure are relatively constant among species. Since end-diastolic aortic pressure depends on the end-systolic pressure and on the rate of pressure decay and duration of diastole (T_d), it was proposed by Westerhof and Elzinga (1991) that the ratio of diastolic to systolic pressure is the same in mammals of different sizes because the ratio T_d/τ is held relatively constant at about 0.25 (i.e. diastolic pressure decays as an exponential function of T_d/τ). In other words, as heart rate decreases with increasing body mass, T_d increases proportionally and so must τ in order to maintain the same end-diastolic pressure level. This is important because it is the diastolic pressure head that drives myocardial perfusion (Westerhof and Elzinga, 1991). We can use this relationship to predict τ and T_d, and therefore heart rate, in the whale.

Assuming that virtually all the arterial capacitance is in the arch, we calculate C from Fig. 1 as about 8 litres kPa^{-1}. Cardiac output, estimated from scaling relationships (Peters, 1983) for a 40 000 kg animal is about 13 litres s^{-1}. If mean pressure is 13 kPa, then R_p (=pressure/flow)=1 $\mathrm{MPa\,s\,m^{-3}}$. The time constant τ is thus estimated to be 8 s, requiring T_d to be about 2 s. Since the diastolic period is about 60 % of the cardiac cycle (Westerhof and Elzinga, 1991), this suggests a heart rate of 0.3 Hz or 18 min^{-1}. Estimates based directly on the allometry of heart rate in mammals (Peters, 1983) yield values ranging from 12 to 17 min^{-1} for the whale (Shadwick and Gosline, 1994).

The aortic arch as a Windkessel

Based on a predicted heart rate of 0.2–0.3 Hz (12–18 min^{-1}) and wave velocity of 4.7 $\mathrm{m\,s^{-1}}$ in the aortic arch, the wavelength of the fundamental cardiac frequency will be 16–24 m, or up to 20 times longer than the arch itself. This is in contrast to the situation in terrestrial mammals, where the fundamental pressure wavelength is only 4–6 times longer than the distance from the heart to the major arterial reflecting site, and significant propagation effects occur (Noordergraaf *et al.* 1979; Milnor, 1982). Consequently, the time for the pressure wave to travel through the whale's arch is a negligible fraction of the heart period, and thus pressure changes should be uniform and virtually simultaneous throughout. If heart rate falls during extreme dives, the ratio of pressure wavelength to the length of the arch will increase further. A similar situation probably exists in the Weddell seal and to a much lesser extent in the harbour seal. Differences in the extent to which the aortic arch acts as a Windkessel may be correlated with diving ability and the degree of diving bradycardia experienced, although more data are needed to support this hypothesis. Thus, the relatively simple Windkessel model, which is considered to be inadequate to describe haemodynamics in terrestrial mammals, appears to be applicable to the circulation in these marine mammals.

References

Bergel, D. H. (1961) The static elastic properties of the arterial wall. *J. Physiol., Lond.* **156**, 445–457.

Campbell, K. B., Rhode, E. A., Cox, R. H., Hunter, W. C. and Noordergraaf, A. (1981). Functional consequences of expanded aortic bulb: a model study. *Am. J. Physiol.* **240**, R200–R210.

Caro, C. G., Pedley, T. J., Schroter, R. C. and Seed, W. A. (1978). *The Mechanics of the Circulation.* Oxford: Oxford University Press.

Drabek, C. M. (1975). Some anatomical aspects of the cardiovascular system of antarctic seals and their possible functional significance in diving. *J. Morph.* **145**, 85–106.

Elsner, R. W. (1969). Cardiovascular adjustments to diving. In *The Biology of Marine Mammals* (ed. H. T. Anderson), pp. 117–145. New York: Academic Press.

Gibbons, C. A. and Shadwick, R. E. (1991). Circulatory mechanics in the toad *Bufo marinus*. II. Haemodynamics of the arterial Windkessel. *J. exp. Biol.* **158**, 291–306.

Langille, B. L. and Jones, D. R. (1977). Dynamics of blood flow through the hearts and arterial systems of anuran amphibia. *J. exp. Biol.* **68**, 1–17.

Milnor, W. R. (1982). *Hemodynamics*. Baltimore: Williams and Wilkens.

Noordergraaf, A., Li, J. K. and Campbell, K. B. (1979). Mammalian hemodynamics: a new similarity principle. *J. theor. Biol.* **79**, 485–489.

Peters, R. H. (1983). *The Ecological Implications of Body Size*. Cambridge: Cambridge University Press.

Rhode, E. A., Elsner, R., Peterson, T. M., Campbell, K. B. and Spangler, W. (1986). Pressure–volume characteristics of aortas of harbor and Weddell seals. *Am. J. Physiol.* **251**, R174–R180.

Shadwick, R. E. and Gosline, J. M. (1985). Mechanical properties of the octopus aorta. *J. exp. Biol.* **114**, 259–284.

Shadwick, R. E. and Gosline, J. M. (1994). Arterial mechanics in the fin whale suggest a unique hemodynamic design. *Am J. Physiol.* **267**, R805–R818.

Shadwick, R. E., Gosline, J. M. and Milsom, W. K. (1987). Arterial haemodynamics in the cephalopod mollusc *Octopus dofleini*. *J. exp. Biol.* **130**, 87–106.

Shelton, G. and Burggren, W. (1976). Cardiovascular dynamics of the chelonia during apnoea and lung ventilation. *J. exp. Biol.* **64**, 323–343.

Westerhof, N. and Elzinga, G. (1991). Normalized input impedance and arterial decay time over heart period are independent of animal size. *Am. J. Physiol.* **261**, R126–R133.

THE DYNAMICS OF COLLAPSIBLE TUBES

C. D. BERTRAM

Graduate School of Biomedical Engineering, University of New South Wales, Sydney 2052, Australia

Summary

The importance of collapsible-tube phenomena derives primarily from blood, air and urine flows in mammals, although similar principles underlie invertebrate jetting and the avian syrinx. Biological fluid conduits have flexible walls and many experience higher external than internal pressures during physiological manoeuvres. The tube typically becomes noncircular, and large shape and cross-sectional area changes occur for small transmural pressure change. Two consequences ensue: a highly nonlinear constitutive relationship, and strong coupling between the fluid and solid mechanics. Depending on how flow is controlled, the tube can exhibit flow-rate-independent pressure-drop, or pressure-drop-independent flow-rate, or a locally negative slope to the pressure-drop to flow-rate relationship. At sufficiently large Reynolds number, these behaviours are accompanied by self-excited oscillation in a surprising variety of modes, including aperiodic ones. Chaotic behaviour has been predicted numerically, but not unequivocally demonstrated. Intrinsic chaotic oscillation must be distinguished from sensitivity to turbulent through-flow. To this end, the response to periodic upstream forcing is currently being investigated.

Steady flow

Biological conduits for fluid flow are typically tubes of more or less circular cross section. Most have rather flexible walls, being supported by surrounding tissue rather than by their own structure. The structural properties of the wall are mainly devoted to resisting distension by pressure within. When the transmural pressure (p_{tm}) is thus positive, the conduit has circular shape if its wall is uniform. In the course of physiological manoeuvres, such conduits also experience negative transmural pressure; the external pressure exceeds that within, and the wall is subjected to circumferential compressive stress. The result is buckling, and commonly the adoption of a twin-lobed cross-sectional shape, where the opposite sides may touch; this process is called collapse. The twin-lobed shape is the lowest-energy configuration for a uniformly flexible wall except close to end-constraints (see, for example, Fung and Sobin, 1972), but small tissue conduits with relatively thick walls may close completely (Fig. 1). An example of the constitutive relationship between p_{tm} and cross-sectional area (A) for a collapsing tube, the 'tube law', is shown in Fig. 2. When $p_{tm}>0$, i.e. the tube is being distended, the compliance is low: relatively little area change attends a given pressure change. At a critical negative p_{tm}, the tube buckles, and thereafter the compliance is high until the

Key words: blood vessels, chaos, flow limitation, nonlinear dynamics, pulmonary airways, self-excited oscillation, venous return.

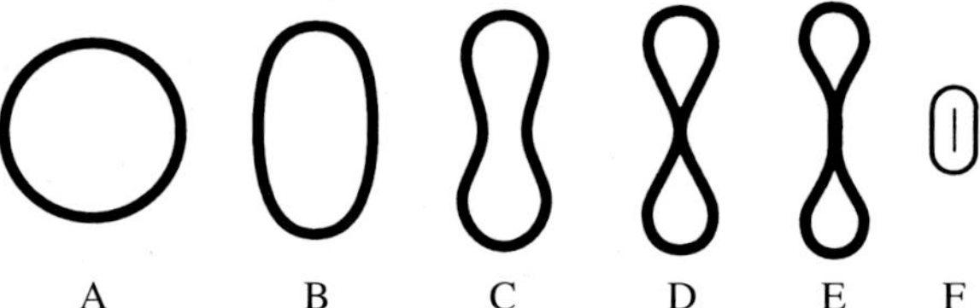

Fig. 1. The five generic stages in collapse of a thin membrane as p_{tm} becomes more negative: (A) distended, (B) oval, (C) indented, (D) opposite-wall point contact, (E) line contact. Complete closure, which involves folding, is achieved by small thick-walled biological vessels (F).

opposite walls make contact. The curve is thus sigmoidal, describing a highly nonlinear relationship.

This nonlinearity, and more especially the high compliance between buckling and opposite-wall contact, is the key to collapsible-tube dynamics. The small pressure differences associated with the fluid flow within the tube suffice to alter the cross-sectional shape considerably. The shape of the conduit and the nature of the flow thus acquire an unusually high degree of coupling; viscous and inertial pressure losses act in concert to cause a uniform tube conveying a flow to become progressively more collapsed towards the downstream end.

Fig. 3 shows qualitatively the behaviour that stems from this coupling. Whereas the flow rate (Q) through a rigid or distended tube depends only on the axial pressure

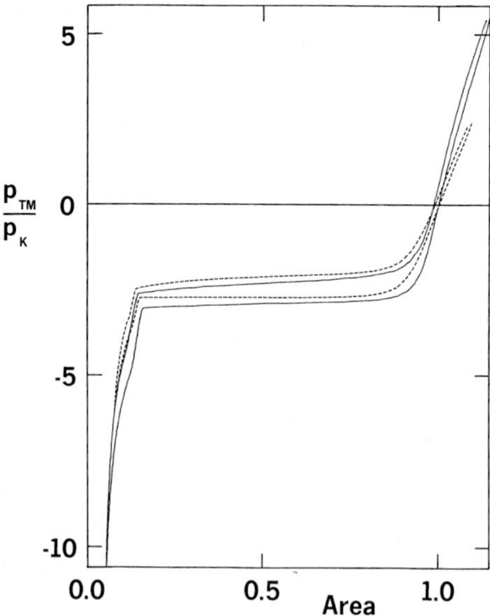

Fig. 2. The relationship beween p_{tm} and A for tubes of two different wall thicknesses (thinner one: solid line), showing that the threshold p_{tm} at which buckling occurs is independent of wall thickness when p_{tm} is normalised by a factor p_k based on the bending stiffness.

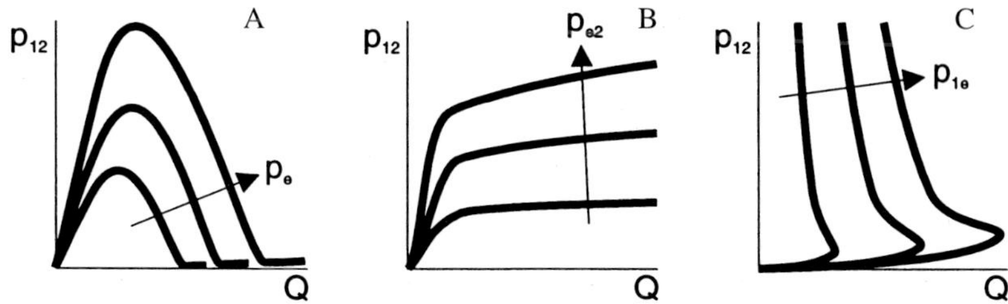

Fig. 3. The relationship between p_{12} and Q. Each curve represents a constant value of p_e (A), of p_{e2} (B) and of p_{1e} ($=-p_{e1}$) (C). The arrows show the direction in which the curves move as the parameter in question is increased.

gradient, as set by the pressures p_1 upstream and p_2 downstream, now the external pressure p_e also matters. Three distinct types of relationship between $p_{12}=p_1-p_2$ and Q are possible. In the most obvious experiment, p_e is held constant, and p_1 and p_2 are allowed to find their own levels as Q is varied. The family of curves shown in Fig. 3A results, each curve corresponding to a different p_e. Starting from low Q, initially the tube is collapsed along its whole length, and p_{12} increases rapidly with Q; the tube resistance p_{12}/Q is high. At the peak of the curve, p_1 begins to exceed p_e, and thereafter the tube progressively becomes less collapsed from the upstream end with increasing Q. The resistance falls, and the incremental resistance dp_{12}/dQ is negative. Eventually p_2 exceeds p_e and the foot of the curve is reached; thereafter, the whole tube is distended and its resistance is low, while $dp_{12}/dQ>0$ again.

The behaviour shown in Fig. 3B results if data are collected at fixed values of $p_{e2}=p_e-p_2$. A protocol for this would be to set a range of Q values, each time then adjusting p_e to yield the desired value of p_{e2}. Each curve in Fig. 3B corresponds to a different value of p_{e2}. The curves exhibit a plateau where p_{12} is constant, the value of p_{12} at which this occurs depending on the value of p_{e2}. This is *pressure-drop limitation*; p_{12} depends only on p_{e2} and is thus independent of p_1, which now influences only the flow rate.

The dual behaviour, *flow-rate limitation*, results if $p_{e1}=p_e-p_1$ is kept constant. Under these conditions, each curve (Fig. 3C) exhibits a region where Q is independent of the value of p_{12} and its value depends on the value of p_{e1}. A suitable protocol for conducting such an experiment would be to set a series of values of upstream head p_u, each time adjusting p_e to yield the desired value of p_{e1}. For those values of p_u leading to the limitation region of the curves, reaching the required p_{e1} will be found to have restored Q to the flow-limited value. Equally validly, one might start with a set of values of far-downstream (exit) pressure. In general, p_1 and p_2 are not identical to p_u and exit pressure if there is intervening hydraulic resistance.

Depending on experimental conditions, such as the length and wall thickness of the tube relative to its diameter, both flow-rate limitation and pressure-drop limitation may be somewhat approximate; the limited Q will tend to decrease with p_{12} (one reason for the negative effort dependency of maximal forced expiration), and the limited p_{12} will tend to increase with Q. Both ways of expressing the tube behaviour are more fundamental than that in Fig. 3A, in that both sets of curves are independent of the settings of parameters external to the tube. In contrast, each curve in Fig. 3A becomes a family of curves if an external parameter, such as resistance downstream of the tube, is varied (Conrad, 1969).

Although pressure-drop limitation is equally important theoretically, flow-rate limitation has proved of greater interest to biologists. This is partly because the use of one pressure drop to influence another is less spectacular than the control of flow rate and partly because positive constant values of p_{e1} tend to occur naturally. The required circumstances are approximated in the lung on expiration: an elevated external pressure compresses both a highly compliant reservoir and the flexible outflow conduit (Fry *et al.* 1954; Shapiro, 1977*a*). Then $p_1 \approx p_e$, and $p_2 < p_1$ as a result of both viscous drag and the conversion of static pressure to kinetic energy (in turn promoting further collapse in a positive feedback).

A simple model of flow-rate limitation can be constructed on the basis of viscous drag alone, using a highly idealised collapsible tube: one in which there is Poiseuille flow ($\Delta p \propto Q/A^2$) at all axial positions (x) and which collapses discontinuously from A=1 to a smaller cross section (A=0.2, say) at the position where $p(x)-p_e$ first falls below a threshold negative value as a result of flow-induced pressure drop. The model needs one extra feature to portray collapsible-tube behaviour accurately, namely that the compliance remain finite after collapse. This yields the sloping line in the tube law shown in Fig. 4A. Fig. 4B shows $p(x)$ for a series of values of p_2 in this tube (relative to p_e).

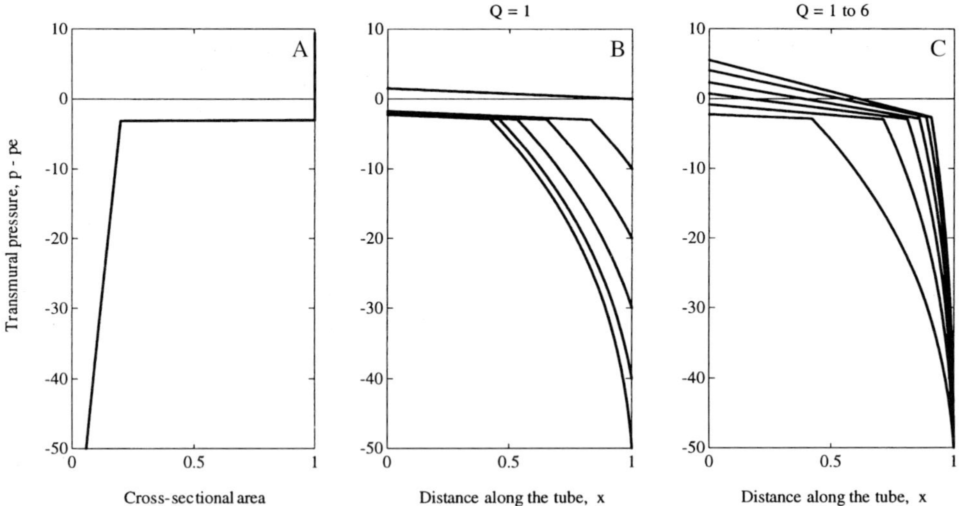

Fig. 4. (A) The relationship between p_{tm} and A, or tube law, applicable to the simplified model of a collapsible tube consisting of two sections in which there is fully developed laminar viscous flow, with finite compliance after collapse. (B) The variation of $p(x)$ with distance x, for various values of p_2, both relative to p_e. The collapsed section of the tube tapers (A decreases as x increases), and the same Q and p_{1e} result for all p_{2e} values corresponding to downstream collapse. (C) The flow-limited Q is independent of p_{2e} but a sensitive function of p_{1e}; at constant p_{2e}, a sixfold range of Q_{max} is the result of a relatively small range of p_{1e} values.

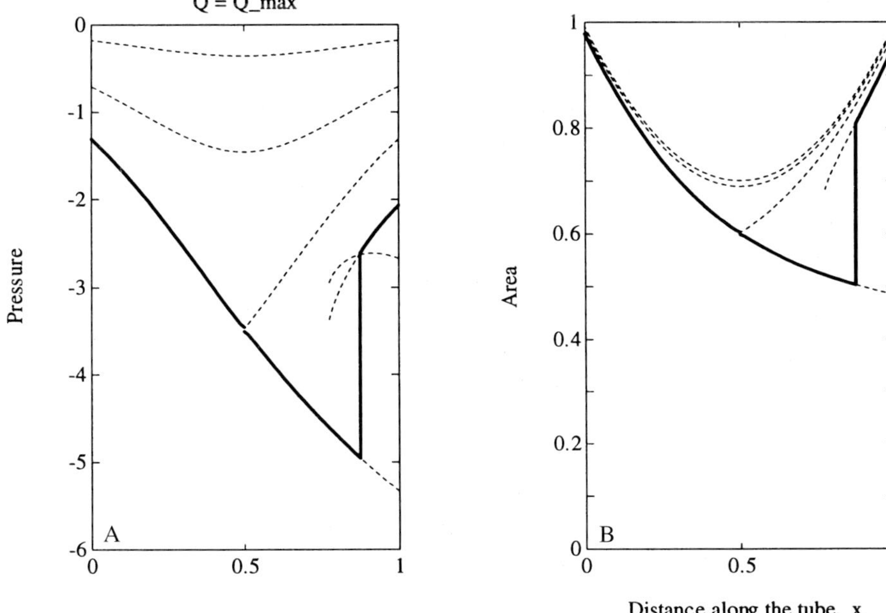

Fig. 5. (A) The bold line shows $p(x)$ in a tube which has minimum undisturbed area at x=0.5, in which there is inviscid flow at the wave-speed-limited Q. Dashed lines extending from x=0 to x=1 show subcritical flows up to Q_{max}. The flow becomes supercritical at x=0.5, the choke point, and returns to subcritical at a point determined by p_2, in this case at x=0.875, where the energy dissipated across the shock is of the right magnitude for subcritical flow downstream to meet the given p_2. (B) The corresponding $A(x)$ curves. The prescribed values of p_2 and Q_{max} determine the area at all points downstream of the shock, which is located where the area discontinuity furnishes the pressure rise needed to intersect the prescribed subcritical $p(x)$. After Wilson *et al.* (1986).

Constant flow rate can be inferred from the similar slope of all $p(x)$ curves in the A=1 region, the length of which decreases as p_2 decreases. Q and p_1 are now completely independent of p_2 for all p_{e2} values above the collapse threshold, and successive equal reductions in p_2 produce progressively smaller increases in the length of the collapsed part of the tube. Fig. 4C shows, for a fixed p_2, how a wide range of limited flow rates is the result of a rather small range of p_{1e} values.

Flow-rate limitation in the absence of significant viscous drag occurs theoretically when the flow velocity at some point x reaches the velocity of propagation of small pressure waves, c. Since c^2 is proportional to $A\mathrm{d}p/\mathrm{d}A$, the wave velocity reaches low values in the high-compliance region of the tube law, although Bertram and Raymond (1991) showed that the required $\mathrm{d}p/\mathrm{d}A$ is not simply the tube law slope. The simple model of Wilson *et al.* (1986), which has pressure varying according to Bernoulli's law, then predicts that $Q_{max}=A_c c_c$, where A_c and c_c both pertain to the site x_c at which the choking condition first occurs. Shapiro (1977*a*) shows that some axial non-uniformity is required, simulated in the model (Fig. 5) by a central $A(x)$ minimum. Downstream of the choking site, flow is supercritical [$Q_{max}/A(x)>c(x)$], returning to subcriticality by way of a shock, a sudden tube expansion analogous to a hydraulic jump downstream of a weir, at which turbulent energy dissipation is allowed. Kamm *et al.* (1991) have postulated a dynamical alternative whereby the flow smoothly regains the subcritical condition it must have at the rigid-pipe exit, but their experimental evidence is equivocal.

Unsteady flow

At Reynolds numbers exceeding a threshold ranging from about 300 in the case of extremely diaphanous tubes (Ohba *et al.* 1989) to about 5000 in the case of the thick-walled tubes investigated by Bertram *et al.* (1990), self-excited oscillation is observed. The oscillation derives its energy from the (steady) upstream head propelling the flow. The site of maximum oscillation amplitude is the tube 'throat' at the downstream end where A is smallest, immediately before the tube re-expands to meet the downstream boundary condition. This is usually a circular rigid pipe of diameter corresponding to that of the collapsible tube at p_{tm}=0, but Bertram *et al.* (1989) have shown that oscillation also occurs when the collapsed segment is defined by a smoothly varying external pressure applied to the central section of a longer tube, as in the case of a sphygmomanometer cuff.

Oscillation is associated with the regions of Fig. 3B,C providing pressure-drop and flow-rate limitation respectively, and with the region of decreasing resistance in Fig. 3A. The oscillation can be thought of as presenting a time-varying resistance to flow. Its vigour is related to the Reynolds number; usually the time-varying $p_2(t)$ is far from sinusoidal, featuring a brief large negative-going spike once per cycle. Oscillation frequency is inversely related to the inertial impedance presented downstream, and to a lesser extent upstream, and increases discontinuously with p_e, so that several distinct modes may be identified. The existence of more than one mode was first noted by Bonis (1979), and this aspect of behaviour has been further investigated since (Bertram *et al.* 1990, 1991; Bertram and Butcher, 1992). Since the stability depends on external factors, Fig. 3B and Fig. 3C now lose their generalising power, and Fig. 6 presents a depiction of modes as closed regions in a space defined by $\bar{p}_{e2}=p_e-\bar{p}_2$ and p_u. Within a given region, oscillation frequency is a weakly increasing function of both these parameters, but across region boundaries it changes abruptly. Jensen (1990) has shown how the existence of such multiple modes may be predicted theoretically, and Kamm *et al.* (1993) have remarked on how the mode influences flow-limited flow rate. Because $p_2(t)$ varies dramatically during a cycle, the instantaneous $p_{e2}(t)$ would span all the regions at that p_u value. Fig. 6 also shows the existence of unattainable zones; the mode change across that zone entails a discontinuity in $\bar{p}_{e2}$. The most prominent of these zones is associated with the abrupt onset of collapse and oscillation as p_e is gradually raised past the threshold in Fig. 4A.

The fact that collapsible-tube oscillations always start and stop abruptly, rather than, for example, growing and dying away gradually as a parameter is varied, leads to the probable topology shown in Fig. 7. The axes of this figure are abstract, but can be approximately identified with p_e and A. The smooth S-bend is then a flow-induced distortion of the tube law of Fig. 2. Starting at the top left and increasing p_e, the stable equilibrium at values of A just less than 1 eventually disappears by folding under, leaving

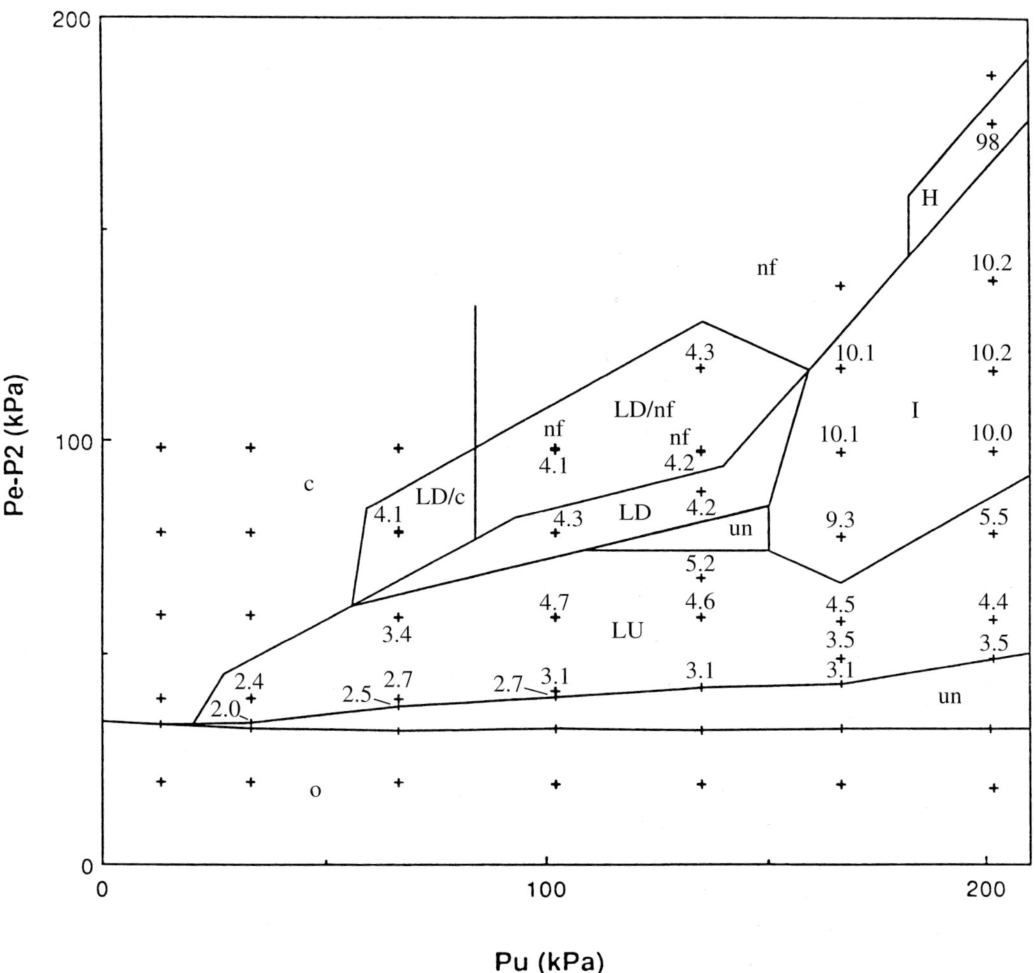

Fig. 6. Control-space diagram showing how the individual operating points investigated can be regarded as examples within closed regions, each of which corresponds to a different mode (o, steady flow, open tube; c, steady flow, collapsed tube; L, low-frequency oscillation, in which modes U and D have different waveshapes; I, intermediate-frequency oscillation; H, high-frequency oscillation; nf, small-amplitude noise-like fluctuation; un, unattainable zone). A number by a point denotes oscillation frequency in Hz.

the oscillatory path as the only stable one. If p_e is subsequently reduced, the oscillatory path is followed until it meets the folded-under (unstable) part of the S, where it disappears in a well-known bifurcation type called a 'blue-sky catastrophe'.

Biological examples

The biological instances of collapsible-tube phenomena have been reviewed by Shapiro (1977*b*) and Kamm (1987). Mammalian circulatory and respiratory examples

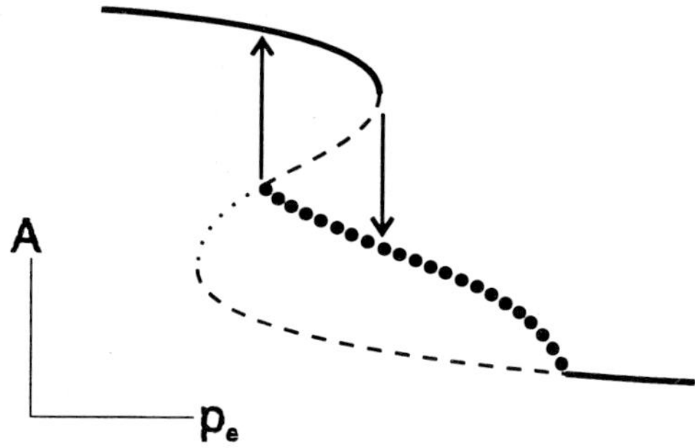

Fig. 7. The topology of the initiation and cessation of oscillation as the control parameter p_e is varied. Solid curves, stable operating points with steady flow. Broken curves, unstable (unattainable) operating points with one (dashed) or two (dotted) degrees of instability. Filled circles describe the locus of stable oscillatory operating points. Arrows depict transitions from one stable state to another as the stability or existence of the first ceases.

dominate, although similar principles underlie all situations where a fluid flows through a passage subjected to external pressure. Zoological examples include the muscular expulsion of water, by squid for propulsion or by ascidians (sea-squirts) as part of filter-feeding. The avian syrinx is a true collapsible tube, in that a membrane forming part of the bronchus is compressed externally by air-sac pressure. In the functionally similar mammalian larynx (Berke *et al.* 1991), the vocal 'cords' (a misnomer that seems to transcend language barriers) more closely resemble the lips of the player of a brass musical instrument.

Collapsible tubes are generically known as 'Starling resistors' to physiologists, after the device used by Knowlton and Starling (1912) to provide a crude, but readily adjustable, simulation of the arterial load in experiments on cardiac function. In the same field, it was gradually realized that the collapse of extrathoracic veins limited the maximum flow rate at which blood returns to the right heart and is thus a powerful determinant of cardiac output. The venous return issue is nowadays normally identified with Guyton, although he acknowledged many earlier workers (see, for example, Guyton and Adkins, 1954) and the explicit link with collapsible tubes was made by Holt (1941).

Venous collapse is of course widespread; it can be observed in the back of the hand held above the head, and sometimes prominently by the pulsation of the skin over the jugular of recumbent dogs. The particular instance of the giraffe jugular has been discussed by Pedley (1987). Ultrasound allows one to observe the collapse of the abdominal and thoracic inferior vena cava in response to Müller and Valsalva manoeuvres. Oscillatory inferior vena cava collapse has occasionally been reported (Brecher, 1952; Matsuzaki, 1986). Intramuscular veins and arteries are routinely subject to high external pressures, both in skeletal (Arnoldi, 1965) and cardiac (Guiot *et al.* 1990) muscle, leading to closure and flow interruption. Collapse of the major pulmonary veins has been shown (Rajagopalan *et al.* 1979) to prevent transmission of right heart pulsatility to the left atrium when thoracic pressure is positive. Within the lung lobes, Fung and Sobin (1972) showed that collapse of the pulmonary capillaries starts when alveolar pressure exceeds that at the venular end of the capillaries, and that collapse all the way along and flow shut-off occur when it exceeds that at the arteriolar end.

Several therapeutic interventions act by promoting the collapse of vessels: of veins during external limb compression for preventing blood stasis, of arteries during external limb compression for cardiac assistance (Lueptow *et al.* 1981), and of all the major intrathoracic vessels during 'cardiac massage' (Beyar *et al.* 1984). Intra-aortic balloon counterpulsation makes effectively an annular collapsible tube (Bonis and Ribreau, 1981; Walsh *et al.* 1991) of part of the aorta. Vascular collapse also largely sets the duration of dialysis and other haemo-exchange procedures, by limiting the maximum flow rate obtainable by arteriovenous anastomosis.

Flow limitation in the maximal forced expiration manoeuvre for assessment of pulmonary airway function was documented by Fry *et al.* (1954), and a theoretical description in terms of choking was given by Lambert and Wilson (1972). However, the wave-speed mechanism had already been introduced to urology by Griffiths (1969, 1971), who remains the authority for urethral flow limitation. Elad *et al.* (1987) have explored expiratory flow limitation for non-uniform airways. The oscillatory consequence of small-airway collapse (wheezing) has been extensively investigated by Grotberg and colleagues (see, for example, Grotberg and Gavriely, 1989). Large-airway oscillation has been the subject of experimental simulation and theoretical modelling by Walsh *et al.* (1991). With geometrical allowances akin to those for the larynx, snoring can also be considered as a collapsed-tube oscillation, and successful sleep apnœa therapy has been based on preventing collapse by positive-pressure ventilation (Wilcox *et al.* 1993).

Complex oscillations

The several modes of periodic oscillation described in the section on unsteady flow do not yet complete the range of observable dynamics. Modes can coexist: a large-amplitude low-frequency oscillation that brings the opposite walls in contact once per cycle may include a high-frequency flutter at that time. Nonlinear systems such as this can, in general, be expected to display certain universal behaviours. One of these is hysteresis, or overlap of mode regions, whereby the mode observed at a given point (in terms of the two controlling parameters, p_u and p_{e2} in this case; see Bertram *et al.* 1991) depends on how the point was approached. This behaviour was observed by Bertram *et al.* (1990).

Another is chaos, typically to be expected at the margins of regions of periodic oscillation. A chaotic oscillation is aperiodic, has a broad frequency spectrum and, when viewed in the appropriate cross section, has fractal dynamics. However, demonstrating all three of these properties for an observed oscillation is not easy, owing to the confounding presence of noise. Aperiodic oscillations are indeed observed at the boundaries between regions (Bertram *et al.* 1991). Since in these experiments the Reynolds number is such that the flow through the tube is turbulent, the possibility arises that aperiodicity is a result of heightened sensitivity to random turbulent forcing at these points rather than to the operation of a chaotic system. Thus, the challenge is to show underlying order in what is sceptically supposed to be stochastic aperiodicity. Direct demonstration of fractal properties has not been achieved so far, and may not be achievable in a system that cannot be perfectly controlled (see below). Tools for detecting or quantifying chaotic properties, such as local dimension calculation (Bertram *et al.* 1991) or searching for unstable periodic points (Smith, 1990), have given equivocal results. Some candidate traces have been shown to have toroidal topology, representing the simultaneous operation of two modes, as in amplitude modulation. Theory indicates that this is one precursor of the chaotic state; a third simultaneous mode would immediately cause chaos. Jensen (1992) has emulated such toroidal modes in a numerical model of a collapsible tube that also displays intermittency, another chaotic behaviour. However, intermittency (mode-changing at irregular intervals) is only weak evidence of chaos in an experiment, because it does not, of itself, represent a demonstration of order. Characteristic patterns of change in the intermittency as a parameter is varied are needed to demonstrate order, and such patterns have yet to be found numerically, let alone experimentally.

Fractal dynamics make stringent demands on any experiment in respect of the degree to which variable parameters must be tightly controlled, and the influence of possibly confounding outside variables must be eradicated. Collapsible tubes are poor candidates for such control. Factors that are difficult to reproduce perfectly or to hold constant include the rheological behaviour of the tube material and the axisymmetric mounting of the tube. In consequence, aperiodic modes are not always reproducible. To extend the range of parameter space in which aperiodic modes can reliably be excited, periodic forcing, giving the fluid supply to the tube a pulsatile component, has been adopted (Bertram and Sheppeard, 1991). This leads to mode-locked interactions in most cases, whereby the collapsed-tube oscillation is constrained to adapt to the forcing, giving rise to long-period oscillation involving integer ratios of tube cycles and forcing cycles. Aperiodic oscillation is observed at certain forcing frequencies. It is believed that this work-in-progress will yield hard evidence for the expected chaotic behaviour.

References

ARNOLDI, C. C. (1965). Venous pressures in the leg of healthy human subjects at rest and during muscular exercise in the nearly erect position. *Acta chir. scand.* **130**, 570–583.

BERKE, G. S., GREEN, D. C., SMITH, M. E., ARNSTEIN, D. P., HONRUBIA, V., NATIVIDAD, M. AND CONRAD, W. A. (1991). Experimental evidence in the *in vivo* canine for the collapsible tube model of phonation. *J. acoust. Soc. Am.* **89**, 1358–1363.

BERTRAM, C. D. AND BUTCHER, K. S. A. (1992). A collapsible-tube oscillator is not readily enslaved to an external resonator. *J. Fluids Structures* **6**, 163–180.

BERTRAM, C. D. AND RAYMOND, C. J. (1991). Measurements of wavespeed and compliance in a collapsible tube during self-excited oscillations: a test of the choking hypothesis. *Med. Biol. Eng. Comput.* **29**, 493–500.

BERTRAM, C. D., RAYMOND, C. J. AND BUTCHER, K. S. A. (1989). Oscillations in a collapsed-tube analog of the brachial artery under a sphygmomanometer cuff. *ASME J. Biomech. Eng.* **111**, 185–191.

BERTRAM, C. D., RAYMOND, C. J. AND PEDLEY, T. J. (1990). Mapping of instabilities for flow through collapsed tubes of differing length. *J. Fluids Structures* **4**, 125–153.

BERTRAM, C. D., RAYMOND, C. J. AND PEDLEY, T. J. (1991). Application of nonlinear dynamics concepts to the analysis of self-excited oscillations of a collapsible tube conveying a fluid. *J. Fluids Structures* **5**, 391–426.

BERTRAM, C. D. AND SHEPPEARD, M. D. (1991). Interaction of self-excited oscillation and pulsatile upstream forcing in a collapsible tube conveying a flow. *Med. Biol. Eng. Comput.* **29** (Suppl.), 259.

BEYAR, R., KISHON, Y., SIDEMAN, S. AND DINNAR, U. (1984). Computer studies of systemic and regional blood flow mechanisms during cardiopulmonary resuscitation. *Med. Biol. Eng. Comput.* **22**, 499–506.

BONIS, M. (1979). Ecoulement visqueux permanent dans un tube collabable elliptique. Thèse de doctorat d'état, Université de Technologie de Compiègne.

BONIS, M. AND RIBREAU, C. (1981). Wave speed in noncircular collapsible ducts. *ASME J. Biomech. Eng.* **103**, 27–31.

BRECHER, G. A. (1952). Mechanism of venous flow under different degrees of aspiration. *Am. J. Physiol.* **169**, 423–433.

CONRAD, W. A. (1969). Pressure–flow relationships in collapsible tubes. *IEEE Trans. Biomed. Eng.* **16**, 284–295.

ELAD, D., KAMM, R. D. AND SHAPIRO, A. H. (1987). Choking phenomena in a lung-like model. *ASME J. Biomech. Eng.* **109**, 1–9.

FRY, D. L., EBERT, R. V., STEAD, W. W. AND BROWN, C. C. (1954). The mechanics of pulmonary ventilation in normal subjects and in patients with emphysema. *Am. J. Med.* **16**, 80–97.

FUNG, Y. C. AND SOBIN, S. S. (1972). Pulmonary alveolar blood flow. *Circulation Res.* **30**, 470–490.

GRIFFITHS, D. J. (1969). Urethral elasticity and micturition hydrodynamics in females. *Med. Biol. Eng.* **7**, 201–215.

GRIFFITHS, D. J. (1971). Hydrodynamics of male micturition. *Med. Biol. Eng.* **9**, 581–596.

GROTBERG, J. B. AND GAVRIELY, N. (1989). Flutter in collapsible tubes: a theoretical model of wheezes. *J. appl. Physiol.* **66**, 2262–2273.

GUIOT, C., PIANTA, P. G., CANCELLI, C. AND PEDLEY, T. J. (1990). Prediction of coronary blood flow with a numerical model based on collapsible tube dynamics. *Am. J. Physiol.* **258**, H1606–H1614.

GUYTON, A. C. AND ADKINS, L. H. (1954). Quantitative aspects of the collapse factor in relation to venous return. *Am. J. Physiol.* **177**, 523–527.

HOLT, J. P. (1941). The collapse factor in the measurement of venous pressure: the flow of fluid through collapsible tubes. *Am. J. Physiol.* **134**, 292–299.

JENSEN, O. E. (1990). Instabilities of flow in a collapsed tube. *J. Fluid Mech.* **220**, 623–659.

JENSEN, O. E. (1992). Chaotic oscillations in a simple collapsible tube model. *ASME J. Biomech. Eng.* **114**, 55–59.

KAMM, R. D. (1987). Flow through collapsible tubes. In *Handbook of Bioengineering* (ed. R. Skalak and S. Chien), pp. 23.1–23.19. New York: McGraw-Hill.

KAMM, R. D., ELAD, D., JAEKLE, D. E. AND SHAPIRO, A. H. (1991). Theory and experiments on smooth transitions through the critical state (S=1) in collapsible tube flow. *Adv. Bioeng. ASME BED* **20**, 329–332.

KAMM, R. D., PATEL, N. AND ELAD, D. (1993). On the effect of flow-induced flutter on flow rate during a forced vital capacity maneuver. *FASEB J.* **7**, A11.

KNOWLTON, F. P. AND STARLING, E. H. (1912). The influence of variations in temperature and blood-pressure on the performance of the isolated mammalian heart. *J. Physiol., Lond.* **44**, 206–219.

LAMBERT, R. K. AND WILSON, T. A. (1972). Flow limitation in a collapsible tube. *J. appl. Physiol.* **33**, 150–153.

LUEPTOW, R. M., KARLEN, J. M., KAMM, R. D. AND SHAPIRO, A. H. (1981). Circulatory model studies of external cardiac assist by counterpulsation. *Cardiovasc. Res.* **15**, 443–455.

MATSUZAKI, Y. (1986). Self-excited oscillation of a collapsible tube conveying fluid. In *Frontiers in Biomechanics* (ed. G. Schmid-Schönbein, S. Woo and B. Zweifach), pp. 342–350. New York: Springer-Verlag.

OHBA, K., SAKURAI, A. AND OKA, J. (1989). Self-excited oscillation of flow in collapsible tube. IV. Laser Doppler measurement of local flow field. *Technol. Rep. Kansai Univ.*, no. **31**.

PEDLEY, T. J. (1987). How giraffes prevent œdema. *Nature* **329**, 13–14.

RAJAGOPALAN, B., FRIEND, J. A., STALLARD, T. AND LEE, G., DE J. (1979). Blood flow in pulmonary veins. II. The influence of events transmitted from the right and left sides of the heart. *Cardiovasc. Res.* **13**, 677–683.

SHAPIRO, A. H. (1977*a*). Steady flow in collapsible tubes. *ASME J. Biomech. Eng.* **99**, 126–147.

SHAPIRO, A. H. (1977*b*). Physiologic and medical aspects of flow in collapsible tubes. *Proc. 6th Canad. Congr. Appl. Mech.*, Vancouver, pp. 883–906.

SMITH, L. A. (1990). Quantifying chaos with predictive flows and maps: locating unstable periodic orbits. In *Measures of Complexity and Chaos* (ed. N. B. Abraham, A. M. Albano, A. Passamante and P. E. Rapp), pp. 359–366. New York: Plenum.

WALSH, C., SULLIVAN, P. A. AND HANSEN, J. S. (1991). Subcritical flutter in collapsible tube flow: a model of expiratory flow in the trachea. *ASME J. Biomech. Eng.* **113**, 21–26.

WILCOX, I., GRUNSTEIN, R. R., HEDNER, J. A., DOYLE, J., COLLINS, F. L., FLETCHER, P. J., KELLY, D. T. AND SULLIVAN, C. E. (1993). Effect of nasal continuous positive airway pressure during sleep on 24-hour blood pressure in obstructive sleep apnea. *Sleep* **16**, 539–544.

WILSON, T. A., RODARTE, J. R. AND BUTLER, J. P. (1986). Wave-speed and viscous flow limitation. *Handbook of Physiology*, section 3, vol. III, (ed. P. T. Macklem and J. Mead), pp. 55–61. Bethesda, MD: American Physiological Society.

A GENERAL METHOD FOR THE COMPUTER SIMULATION OF BIOLOGICAL SYSTEMS INTERACTING WITH FLUIDS

CHARLES S. PESKIN and DAVID M. McQUEEN

Courant Institute of Mathematical Sciences, New York University, 251 Mercer Street, New York, NY 10012, USA

Summary

At this Symposium on Biological Fluid Dynamics, it is appropriate to ask whether there is any common theme that unites the diverse problems that arise in the study of living systems interacting with fluids. The answer that immediately comes to mind is this: biological fluid dynamics invariably involves the interaction of elastic flexible tissue with viscous incompressible fluid. (In many cases the tissue is not only elastic, it is also active, i.e. capable of doing work on the fluid.) This paper describes the immersed boundary method, which is a general framework for the computer simulation of biofluid dynamic systems. This method has already been applied to blood flow in the heart (including the computer-assisted design of prosthetic cardiac valves), platelet aggregation during blood clotting, aquatic animal locomotion, wave propagation along the basilar membrane of the inner ear, and flow in collapsible tubes. In the immersed boundary method, the elastic (and possibly active) biological tissue is treated as a part of the fluid in which additional forces (derived from the tissue stresses) are applied. Because the tissue is represented in terms of its force field, the method remains straightforward, even when the geometry of the biological tissue is complicated, dynamic and not known in advance.

Introduction

This paper is intended as a tutorial on the immersed boundary method, which has been applied to a wide range of problems, mostly in biofluid dynamics, including blood flow in the heart (Peskin, 1972, 1977, 1980, 1992; Peskin and McQueen, 1980, 1989, 1992*a*,*b*; McQueen and Peskin, 1983, 1985, 1989, 1990, 1991; McQueen *et al.* 1982; McCracken and Peskin, 1980; Meisner *et al.* 1985; Peskin and Printz, 1992), platelet aggregation during blood clotting (Fogelson, 1984, 1985; Fauci and Fogelson, 1993), flow of suspensions (Fogelson and Peskin, 1988; Sulsky and Brackbill, 1991), fluid dynamics of the inner ear (Beyer, 1992), aquatic animal locomotion (Fauci and Peskin, 1988; Fauci, 1990; Fauci and Fogelson, 1993), and flow in collapsible tubes (Rosar, 1994). Generally speaking, the method is applicable to any problem in which a fluid interacts with an elastic material. The elastic material may be an active one, as in the case of cardiac muscle or a swimming fish.

The philosophy of the immersed boundary method is to treat the elastic material as a

Key words: computer simulation, immersed boundary method, heart, blood flow, platelet aggregation, aquatic animal locomotion, inner ear, collapsible tube, Navier–Stokes equations, Fast Fourier Transform, Dirac delta function, heart valves, prosthetic cardiac valves.

part of the fluid in which additional forces (arising from the elastic stresses) are applied. The fluid equations are solved on a regular cubic lattice, the structure of which is not modified in any way by the presence of the immersed elastic bodies, the geometry of which may be quite complicated. The elastic material is tracked in Lagrangian fashion, by following a collection of representative material points. The spatial configuration of these points is used to compute elastic forces, which are applied to the nearby lattice points of the fluid. The fluid velocity is updated under the influence of these forces, and the new velocity is then interpolated at the elastic material points, which are moved at the interpolated velocity to complete the time step.

The various applications of the immersed boundary method have been listed above (with references), but the following remarks may give the reader a more detailed picture of what has already been done. The method has been used to design a prosthetic cardiac valve, for which a patent has been issued. It has been used to create a detailed model of the platelet aggregation process during blood clotting, a model that includes the platelets themselves, the blood plasma in which they are immersed, elastic interplatelet links as well as links between a platelet and the injured vessel wall, secretion of adenosine diphosphate (ADP) that occurs upon platelet activation, the convection and diffusion of ADP in the flowing blood, and the activation of platelets that experience an above-threshold level of ADP as well as platelets that encounter the injured region of the vessel wall. Because the immersed boundary method is used, the fluid dynamics automatically adapt to the changing geometry of the flow region as the platelet aggregate grows. The immersed boundary method has also been used to study the swimming of various creatures, from undulating eels to algae that do the breast stroke. Interactions of swimming spermatozoa with each other and with elastic channel walls has also been studied. Because the immersed boundary method is used, these studies automatically include the mechanical feedback influence of the hydrodynamics on the swimming motions of the creature in question. The deformations of the creature are not rigidly prescribed but are influenced by hydrodynamic forces. In sedimentation problems, the immersed boundary method makes it possible to study the effects of particle elasticity, and also to study large numbers of interacting particles, since the computational effort grows only linearly with the number of immersed particles. Wave propagation along the basilar membrane of the inner ear and flow in collapsible tubes are two problems for which a variety of idealized models have been introduced and studied. In such problems, the immersed boundary method opens up the prospect of raw simulation, almost akin to experiment, in which something approaching the full complexity of the system is allowed to operate in the model.

The next section of this paper describes a mathematical formulation of the equations of motion of a viscous incompressible fluid containing an immersed system of elastic fibers. This formulation forms the foundation of the immersed boundary method, which is then described in the subsequent section. At the core of the immersed boundary method is a smoothed approximation to the Dirac delta-function, the construction of which is given next. The paper concludes with an example application which is qualitatively discussed (with computer-generated figures): blood flow in a three-dimensional computer model of the mammalian heart.

Mathematical formulation

Consider a viscous incompressible fluid containing an immersed system (a continuum) of elastic fibers. The fibers are pure force-generators. By themselves, they have neither mass nor volume but, together with the fluid in which they are immersed, they form an incompressible viscoelastic material. This material is highly anisotropic, since the fiber stress points always in the fiber direction.

Let the unknown motion of the fibers be described in Lagrangian form:

$$\mathbf{x}=\mathbf{X}(q,r,s,t), \tag{1}$$

in which (q,r,s) defines a material point and (q,r) defines a fiber. The unit tangent $\boldsymbol{\tau}$ to the fibers is given by:

$$\boldsymbol{\tau}=\frac{\partial\mathbf{X}/\partial s}{|\partial\mathbf{X}/\partial s|} \tag{2}$$

and the fiber tension T is given by a generalized Hooke's law:

$$T=\mathcal{S}\left(\left|\frac{\partial\mathbf{X}}{\partial s}\right|;q,r,s,t\right). \tag{3}$$

Here $T\,\mathrm{d}q\,\mathrm{d}r$ is the force transmitted by the bundle of fibers $\mathrm{d}q\,\mathrm{d}r$, and $|\partial\mathbf{X}/\partial s|$ determines the local fiber strain, from which this force is computed. The explicit dependence of $\mathcal{S}$ on q, r, s, t allows for different stress–strain relationships at different locations and times. In particular, the explicit time dependence makes possible the representation of active materials, such as muscle.

Let B be some arbitrary region of the (q,r) parameter plane. This defines a bundle of fibers. Consider the segments of these fibers defined by $s_1 \leqslant s \leqslant s_2$. Since the fibers are massless, the total force acting on these segments must be zero. This total force includes both the force of the fluid on the fibers and also the force transmitted across the surfaces $s=s_1$ and $s=s_2$ by the fibers themselves. Thus:

$$0=\text{force of fluid on fiber segments}+\int_B (T\boldsymbol{\tau})\Big|_{s_1}^{s_2}\,\mathrm{d}q\,\mathrm{d}r. \tag{4}$$

Using Newton's law of equal and opposite forces, and also the fundamental theorem of calculus, we may rewrite this equation as follows:

$$\begin{aligned}\text{force of fiber segments on fluid} &= \int_B (T\boldsymbol{\tau})\Big|_{s_1}^{s_2}\,\mathrm{d}q\,\mathrm{d}r\\ &= \int_{s_1}^{s_2}\int_B \frac{\partial}{\partial s}(T\boldsymbol{\tau})\,\mathrm{d}q\,\mathrm{d}r\,\mathrm{d}s.\end{aligned} \tag{5}$$

Since B, s_1 and s_2 are arbitrary, this shows that the density of the fiber force $\mathbf{f}$ with respect to the measure dq dr ds is given by:

$$\mathbf{f} = \frac{\partial}{\partial s}(T\boldsymbol{\tau}). \tag{6}$$

Expanding the derivative, we see that the fiber force density has a tangential component and a component in the direction of the principal normal to the fibers:

$$\begin{aligned} \mathbf{f} &= \frac{\partial T}{\partial s}\boldsymbol{\tau} + T\frac{\partial \boldsymbol{\tau}}{\partial s} \\ &= \frac{\partial T}{\partial s}\boldsymbol{\tau} + T\left|\frac{\partial \mathbf{X}}{\partial s}\right| K\mathbf{n}, \end{aligned} \tag{7}$$

where $K = |\partial\boldsymbol{\tau}/\partial s| / |\partial\mathbf{X}/\partial s|$ is the fiber curvature and $\mathbf{n} = (\partial\boldsymbol{\tau}/\partial s)/|\partial\boldsymbol{\tau}/\partial s|$ is the principal normal. There is no component of the fiber force in the binormal direction $\boldsymbol{\tau}\times\mathbf{n}$.

We may now formulate equations of motion for the fiber-fluid system. Let the fluid have density ρ and viscosity μ, and let $\mathbf{u}(\mathbf{x},t)$, $p(\mathbf{x},t)$ be the velocity and pressure of the fluid. Note that these are expressed in Eulerian form; they are functions of the fixed position $\mathbf{x}$ and the time t. The equations of motion are as follows:

$$\rho\left(\frac{\partial \mathbf{u}}{\partial t} + \mathbf{u}\cdot\nabla\mathbf{u}\right) = -\nabla p + \mu\nabla^2\mathbf{u} + \mathbf{F}, \tag{8}$$

$$\nabla\cdot\mathbf{u} = 0, \tag{9}$$

$$\mathbf{F}(\mathbf{x},t) = \int \mathbf{f}(q,r,s,t)\,\delta[\mathbf{x} - \mathbf{X}(q,r,s,t)]\,\mathrm{d}q\,\mathrm{d}r\,\mathrm{d}s, \tag{10}$$

$$\begin{aligned} \frac{\partial \mathbf{X}}{\partial t} &= \mathbf{u}[\mathbf{X}(q,r,s,t),t], \\ &= \int \mathbf{u}(\mathbf{x},t)\,\delta[\mathbf{x} - \mathbf{X}(q,r,s,t)]\,\mathrm{d}\mathbf{x}, \end{aligned} \tag{11}$$

$$T = \mathcal{S}\left(\left|\frac{\partial \mathbf{X}}{\partial s}\right|; q, r, s, t\right), \tag{12}$$

$$\boldsymbol{\tau} = \frac{\partial\mathbf{X}/\partial s}{|\partial\mathbf{X}/\partial s|}, \tag{13}$$

$$\mathbf{f} = \frac{\partial}{\partial s}(T\boldsymbol{\tau}). \tag{14}$$

Equations 8–9 are the familiar Navier–Stokes equations of a viscous incompressible fluid (in Eulerian form). The applied force density **F** is here used to express the effect of the fibers acting in the fluid, see below. Equations 12–14 determine the fiber forces. (These equations have been derived and discussed above and are repeated here in order to display the entire system of fiber-fluid equations in one place.) Note that these fiber equations are in Lagrangian form: **X**, $\boldsymbol{\tau}$ and **f** are functions of the Lagrangian parameters q, r, s (and of the time t).

Equations 10–11 are the interaction equations which couple the fibers and the fluid. In these equations δ denotes the three-dimensional Dirac delta function. Equation 10 expresses the fiber force density as a sum (integral) of point forces applied at the locations of the fiber points. To see more clearly the meaning of this equation, we integrate both sides over an arbitrary region Ω which may or may not contain some of the fibers:

$$\begin{aligned}\int_{\Omega} \mathbf{F}(\mathbf{x},t)\,\mathrm{d}\mathbf{x} &= \int \mathbf{f}(q,r,s,t) \int_{\Omega} \delta[\mathbf{x}-\mathbf{X}(q,r,s,t)]\,\mathrm{d}\mathbf{x}\,\mathrm{d}q\,\mathrm{d}r\,\mathrm{d}s \\ &= \int_{\mathbf{X}(q,r,s,t)\in\Omega} \mathbf{f}(q,r,s,t)\,\mathrm{d}q\,\mathrm{d}r\,\mathrm{d}s\,, \qquad (15)\end{aligned}$$

which simply says that the total force of the fibers on the region Ω at time t can be found by integrating over all of the fiber segments (if any) that happen to lie within the region Ω at time t.

Equation 11 is the no-slip condition of a viscous fluid, which here plays the role of an equation of motion for the fibers. It states that the fibers move at the local fluid velocity. The reason for writing this out in terms of the Dirac delta function (the second form of equation 11) will become clear when we consider the numerical scheme that is used to solve the fiber-fluid equations.

It is important to note that the formulation given above still makes sense when the fibers are confined to a surface (a heart valve leaflet, for example) instead of filling up a region of space. In that case, we merely drop one of the Lagrangian parameters (say q), and equations 10–11 become:

$$\mathbf{F}(\mathbf{x},t) = \int \mathbf{f}(r,s,t)\,\delta[\mathbf{x}-\mathbf{X}(r,s,t)]\,\mathrm{d}r\,\mathrm{d}s\,, \qquad (16)$$

$$\frac{\partial \mathbf{X}}{\partial t} = \int \mathbf{u}(\mathbf{x},t)\,\delta[\mathbf{x}-\mathbf{X}(r,s,t)]\,\mathrm{d}\mathbf{x}\,. \qquad (17)$$

The delta function appearing in these equations is still three-dimensional, but equation 16 now involves only a double integral. It therefore defines **F** as a delta-function layer with support along the immersed elastic boundary only. Although **F** is now infinite on this internal boundary, its integral over any (finite) volume is finite. (Equation 17, by contrast, involves a triple integral which gives directly a finite result without any further integration.)

The immersed boundary method

We now consider the numerical solution of equations 8–14. Let time proceed in steps of duration Δt and let superscripts denote the time step index. Thus, $\mathbf{u}^n(\mathbf{x})=\mathbf{u}(\mathbf{x}, n\Delta t)$. At the beginning of the time step, $\mathbf{u}^n$ and $\mathbf{X}^n$ are known. We shall describe the computation of $\mathbf{u}^{n+1}$ and $\mathbf{X}^{n+1}$.

The fluid equations are discretized on a cubic lattice of mesh width h. The following difference operators are applied to functions defined on this lattice:

$$(D_\alpha^+\phi)(\mathbf{x}) = \frac{\phi(\mathbf{x}+h\mathbf{e}_\alpha)-\phi(\mathbf{x})}{h}, \tag{18}$$

$$(D_\alpha^-\phi)(\mathbf{x}) = \frac{\phi(\mathbf{x})-\phi(\mathbf{x}-h\mathbf{e}_\alpha)}{h}, \tag{19}$$

$$(D_\alpha^0\phi)(\mathbf{x}) = \frac{\phi(\mathbf{x}+h\mathbf{e}_\alpha)-\phi(\mathbf{x}-h\mathbf{e}_\alpha)}{2h}, \tag{20}$$

$$\mathbf{D}^0 = (D_1^0, D_2^0, D_3^0), \tag{21}$$

where α=1, 2, 3 and where $\mathbf{e}_1$, $\mathbf{e}_2$ and $\mathbf{e}_3$ are unit vectors in the coordinate directions.

Similarly, the fiber equations are discretized on a rectangular lattice in the (q, r, s) space of the Lagrangian parameters (but note that this is some curvilinear lattice in physical space, and that the physical locations of the fiber lattice points are not, typically, those of the fluid lattice). Let Δq, Δr and Δs be the three fiber-lattice spacings. For any function $\psi(q, r, s)$, let the central difference operator D_s be defined by:

$$(D_s\psi)(q,r,s) = \frac{\psi\left(q,r,s+\frac{\Delta s}{2}\right)-\psi\left(q,r,s-\frac{\Delta s}{2}\right)}{\Delta s}. \tag{22}$$

Each time step proceeds as follows. First, compute the fiber force $\mathbf{f}^n$ from the fiber configuration $\mathbf{X}^n$. This is done using the following equations:

$$T^n = S^n(|D_s\mathbf{X}^n|; q, r, s), \tag{23}$$

$$\boldsymbol{\tau}^n = \frac{D_s\mathbf{X}^n}{|D_s\mathbf{X}^n|}, \tag{24}$$

$$\mathbf{f}^n = D_s(T^n\boldsymbol{\tau}^n). \tag{25}$$

Suppose $\mathbf{X}^n$ is defined at integer points $s=k\Delta s$. Then T^n and $\boldsymbol{\tau}^n$ are defined at half-integer points $s=(k+\frac{1}{2})\Delta s$. Finally $\mathbf{f}^n$ is defined once again at the integer locations.

The next step is to evaluate the fiber force density $\mathbf{F}^n$ as follows:

$$\mathbf{F}^n(\mathbf{x}) = \sum_{q,r,s} \mathbf{f}^n(q,r,s)\,\delta_h[\mathbf{x}-\mathbf{X}^n(q,r,s)]\,\Delta q\,\Delta r\,\Delta s. \tag{26}$$

Here $\sum_{q,r,s}$ denotes the sum over the values of q, r, s given by $(q,r,s)=(i\Delta q, j\Delta r, k\Delta s)$, where i, j and k are integers. The function δ_h is a smoothed approximation to the three-dimensional Dirac delta function. It will be constructed in the next section.

With $\mathbf{F}^n$ known, we are ready to update the fluid velocity by integrating the Navier–Stokes equations. This is done by solving the following linear system for $\mathbf{u}^{n+1}$, p^{n+1}:

$$\rho\left(\frac{\mathbf{u}^{n+1}-\mathbf{u}^n}{\Delta t}+\sum_{\alpha=1}^{3} u_\alpha^n D_\alpha^\pm \mathbf{u}^n\right) = -\mathbf{D}^0 p^{n+1} + \mu \sum_{\alpha=1}^{3} D_\alpha^+ D_\alpha^- \mathbf{u}^{n+1} + \mathbf{F}^n , \tag{27}$$

$$\mathbf{D}^0 \cdot \mathbf{u}^{n+1} = 0 . \tag{28}$$

In equation 27, the notation $u_\alpha^n D_\alpha^\pm$ allows for a choice between the forward and backward difference operators. This choice is to be made by upwind differencing. Thus:

$$u_\alpha^n D_\alpha^\pm = \begin{cases} u_\alpha^n D_\alpha^- & u_\alpha^n > 0 \\ u_\alpha^n D_\alpha^+ & u_\alpha^n < 0 . \end{cases} \tag{29}$$

Because of the upwind differencing, the scheme given by equations 27–28 is stable, provided that:

$$\sum_{\alpha=1}^{3} |u_\alpha^n| \, \Delta t \leqslant h \tag{30}$$

at all of the points of the fluid lattice.

Note that equations 27–28 are linear constant-coefficient difference equations in the unknowns $(\mathbf{u}^{n+1}, p^{n+1})$. They can therefore be solved by Fourier methods, and this can be made very efficient through the use of the Fast Fourier Transform (FFT) algorithm. It is a consequence of our use of a regular cubic lattice in the discretization of the fluid equations that we are able to exploit the FFT in this way. If the fluid grid had been made to conform to the geometry of the immersed elastic bodies. Fourier methods would not be applicable.

Once $\mathbf{u}^{n+1}$ has been determined, the next (and last) step is to move the fibers. This is done through a discretization of equation 11:

$$\mathbf{X}^{n+1}(q,r,s) = \mathbf{X}^n(q,r,s) + \Delta t \sum_{\mathbf{x}} \mathbf{u}^{n+1}(\mathbf{x})\, \delta_h[\mathbf{x} - \mathbf{X}^n(q,r,s)]\, h^3 , \tag{31}$$

where $\sum_{\mathbf{x}}$ denotes the sum over the cubic lattice of the fluid computation. This is the set of points $\mathbf{x}$ of the form $\mathbf{x}=\sum_{\alpha=1}^{3} h j_\alpha \mathbf{e}_\alpha$, where j_1, j_2 and j_3 are integers. As in equation 26, δ_h is a smoothed approximation to the Dirac delta function. The construction of δ_h is the subject of the next section. Since $\mathbf{u}$ and $\mathbf{X}$ have been updated, the time step is complete.

Construction of δ_h

Let

$$\delta_h(\mathbf{x}) = h^{-3}\phi\left(\frac{x_1}{h}\right)\phi\left(\frac{x_2}{h}\right)\phi\left(\frac{x_3}{h}\right), \tag{32}$$

where x_1, x_2 and x_3 are the components of $\mathbf{x}$, and where ϕ has the following properties: (i) ϕ is continuous; (ii) $\phi(r)=0$ for $|r|\geqslant 2$; (iii) $\sum_{i,\text{even}} \phi(r-i)=\sum_{i,\text{odd}} \phi(r-i)=\frac{1}{2}$, all r; (iv) $\sum_i (r-i)\,\phi(r-i)=0$, all r; (v) $\sum_i [\phi(r-i)]^2=C$, all r, where C is some constant independent of r. (It turns out that $C=3/8$. This can be shown by considering the special case $r=0$ and making use of all of the above-listed properties of ϕ.)

The motivation for imposing these requirements is as follows. Continuity of ϕ is needed to avoid sudden jumps in the fiber velocity or force as the fiber points move through the computational lattice of the fluid. Bounded support of ϕ is needed to keep down the computational cost of the algorithm: it would be very expensive to have each fiber point interact directly with all of the lattice points of the fluid. (The specific bound 2 which appears in property ii defines the smallest support that is consistent with the other criteria.)

Property iii has the immediate consequence that $\sum_i\phi(r-i)=1$ for all r. When δ_h is used for interpolation, this ensures that the interpolation of a constant is exactly correct. When δ_h is used for applying the fiber force to the fluid, this same property ensures that the correct total force is applied by each fiber point (conservation of momentum).

The stronger conditions of property iii concerning the separate sums over even and odd points are helpful because they prevent the appearance of a point-to-point oscillation that would otherwise be generated by the application of localized forces. This is related to the use of the central difference operator $\mathbf{D}^0$ in the discretization of the Navier–Stokes equations.

When combined with property iii, property iv guarantees that the interpolation of linear functions will be exact and that the correct total torque (with respect to any chosen origin) will be applied to the fluid by each fiber point (conservation of angular momentum).

Property v is the most interesting one. It is applied because it guarantees the following inequality:

$$\sum_i \phi(r_1-i)\,\phi(r_2-i)\leqslant C, \tag{33}$$

which holds for all (r_1, r_2) and which follows from property v by an application of the Schwarz inequality.

Expressions such as those on the left-hand side of this inequality arise if the function δ_h is used first to apply the fiber forces to the fluid lattice and then to interpolate the resulting force field back to the fiber points themselves. In this two-step process, one would like the interaction of a fiber point with itself to be constant, irrespective of where that point sits with respect to the fluid lattice, and this is precisely what property v asserts. Moreover, one would like the interaction of one fiber point with another to be bounded by the interaction of a fiber point with itself, which is precisely the content of the above inequality.

We leave it as an exercise for the reader to show that the five properties listed above uniquely determine the function ϕ, as follows:

$$\phi(r)=\begin{cases}\frac{1}{8}(3-2|r|+\sqrt{1+4|r|-4r^2}) & |r|\leqslant 1\\ \frac{1}{2}-\phi(2-|r|) & 1\leqslant |r|\leqslant 2\,.\\ 0 & 2\leqslant |r|\end{cases} \tag{34}$$

(Note that the second line defines ϕ on $1\leqslant|r|\leqslant2$ in terms of the values of ϕ on $|r|\leqslant1$. One could, of course, write out a formula for this, but it is more efficient to compute ϕ as indicated above, since the typical situation is that ϕ is simultaneously needed at four points of the form r–2, r–1, r and r+1, where $0\leqslant r\leqslant1$.)

Even though we have only postulated the continuity of ϕ itself and said nothing about its derivatives, it is a remarkable fact that the continuity of the first derivative of ϕ turns out to be implicit in the five properties proposed above. This can be checked by differentiating the above formulae for ϕ to obtain $\phi'(0)=0$, $\phi'(1^-)=\phi'(1^+)$ and $\phi'(2^-)=0$.

For readers who are familiar with our previous work, it should be noted that the ϕ function used here is different from the trigonometric function used previously:

$$\phi_{\text{old}}(r)=\begin{cases}\frac{1}{4}(1+\cos\frac{\pi r}{2}) & |r|\leqslant 2\\ 0 & |r|\geqslant 2\end{cases}\,. \tag{35}$$

One can check that ϕ_{old} satisfies four of the five properties that were used to define ϕ, the one exception being the first-moment or torque condition, property iv. Although the expressions for ϕ and ϕ_{old} may look very different, their numerical values are startlingly close: plot their graphs with a thick pen and you will have trouble distinguishing them. Thus, the change from ϕ_{old} to ϕ is not likely to have any practical effect on the computed results. We have gone ahead and made the change nonetheless, since it turns out that ϕ is slightly cheaper to compute than ϕ_{old}, and since it is satisfying to have δ_h uniquely determined by a reasonable list of axioms.

Example: a computer model of the heart and its valves

We have used the methodology described above to develop a three-dimensional computer model of the mammalian heart, including the heart valves and the nearby great vessels. The model is constructed as a collection of fibers immersed in a (periodic) box of fluid. These fibers are arranged in such a manner as to simulate the true fiber architecture of the heart, as described by Thomas (1957) and by Streeter *et al.* (1969, 1978). The general mode of construction that we use is to define surfaces within the heart wall on which the fibers are to run, and then to lay out the fibers as geodesics (curves of shortest length) on these surfaces. In the special case of the arterial valves, we have introduced a mathematical theory (Peskin and McQueen, 1994) that can be used to determine the fiber architecture of the valve leaflets from first principles, and we have used that theory to generate the arterial valves of the model heart. It is an open problem how to do the same for the atrioventricular valves, and indeed for the heart as a whole. [There is such a theory available for the left ventricle (Peskin, 1989), but it relies on axial symmetry and we have not used it here.]

The model that we have constructed is anatomically complete. It includes left and right atria; left and right ventricles; aortic, pulmonic, mitral and tricuspid valves; ascending aorta and main pulmonary artery; superior and inferior vena cavae; and four pulmonary veins. The model arteries and veins are equipped with sources and sinks which apply realistic pressure loads to the model heart. An external source/sink allows for the changes in volume of the heart that occur during the cardiac cycle. The fibers that comprise the model vessels and valve leaflets have fixed elastic parameters, but those of the atrial and ventricular walls have time-dependent stiffnesses and rest lengths so that they can contract and relax at appropriate times in the cardiac cycle. All fibers have nonlinear stress–strain relationships with increasing stiffness at greater loads.

All physical parameters of the model, with the exception of the blood viscosity, have been set appropriately for the human heart. The viscosity has been increased by a factor of 25, which means that the Reynolds number has been reduced by the same factor. Smaller viscosity requires a finer computational mesh, at least near the boundary. The present form of the immersed boundary method uses a uniform mesh, which is therefore expensive to refine, but future research may make it possible to perform local mesh refinement or indeed to use a grid-free method that automatically concentrates the computational effort in regions of high vorticity. Even with uniform meshes, future progress in computer hardware will gradually make it feasible to use finer and finer meshes and hence to reduce the viscosity of the simulated blood.

Figs 1–3 show the heart model in action. In all three of these figures, part A shows the model during ventricular diastole and part B during ventricular systole. The figures all show the heart in the same orientation, seen from the front, with the left atrial appendage in the foreground. Fig. 1 shows the external view of the model heart. In Fig. 2, the front of the heart has been cut away to reveal the blood flow inside. The sectioning plane passes through the mitral, aortic and pulmonic valves, and also cuts close to the apex of the left ventricle. Blood flow is depicted in terms of fluid markers which leave trails behind them so that their motion during the immediate past can be appreciated. Fig. 3 shows a somewhat transparent view of the entire heart model, with the blood flow seen through the fibers of the heart walls. Only a small subset of the model fibers is shown; otherwise the walls would appear solid and the blood flow could not be seen.

The model heart beats, but it is not yet a healthy heart. The most obvious pathology is mitral regurgitation, and aortic regurgitation is also present. Further work on the valves is needed, and other changes in the anatomy and physiology of the model heart may be required as well. It is not an easy task to imitate nature's design, but we are doing our best. Once the model has been perfected, it will be used as a test chamber for the computer-assisted design of prosthetic cardiac valves, in the simulation of disease processes affecting the mechanical function of the heart or its valves, and as a tool for achieving improved understanding of the normal physiology of the heart.

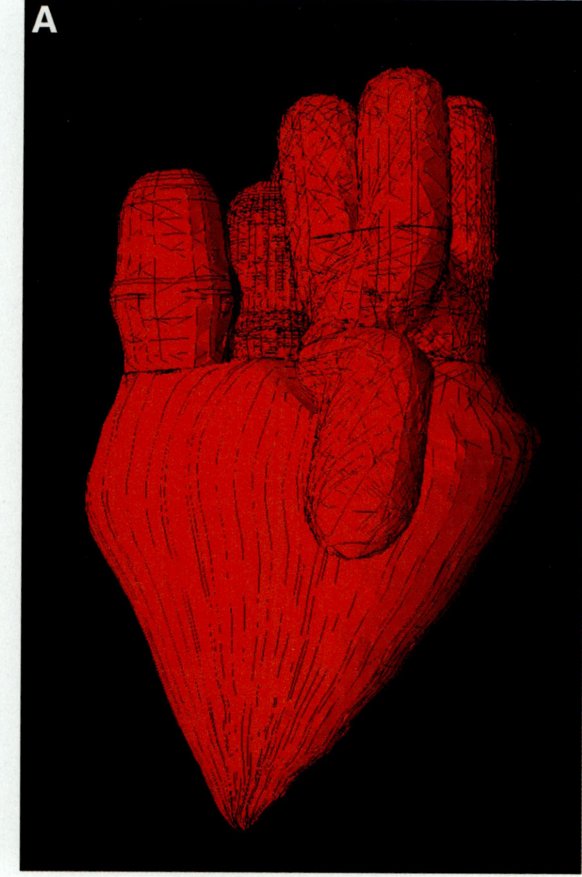

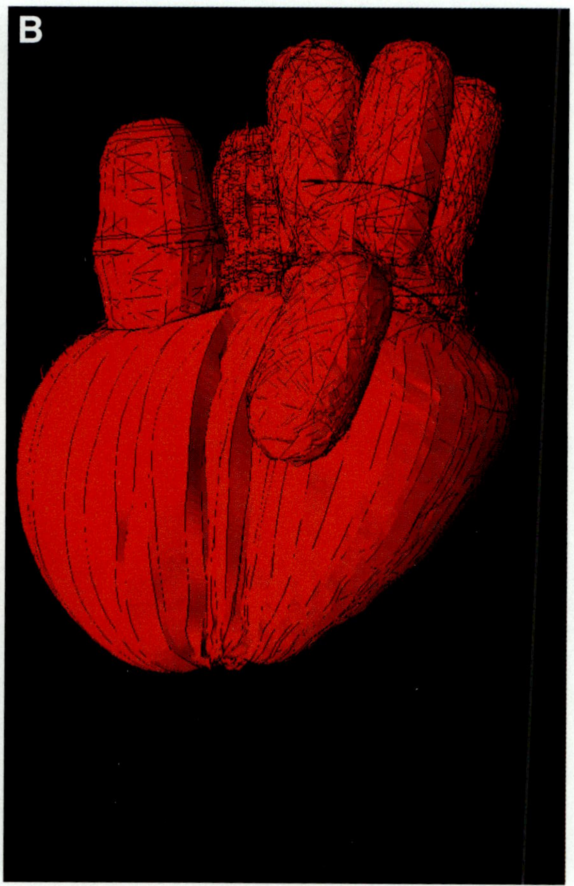

Fig. 1. External view of the model heart (A) during ventricular diastole and (B) during ventricular systole. The heart is shown from the front, so the left side of the heart is on the right side of the figure, with the left atrial appendage (auricle) in the foreground. Structures seen at the top of the figure are (from left to right in the figure) the main pulmonary artery, the ascending aorta and the left atrium with three of the four pulmonary veins visible. The right atrium and the vena cavae are at the back and cannot be seen. Thin black lines indicate some of the fiber trajectories on the surface of the model heart.

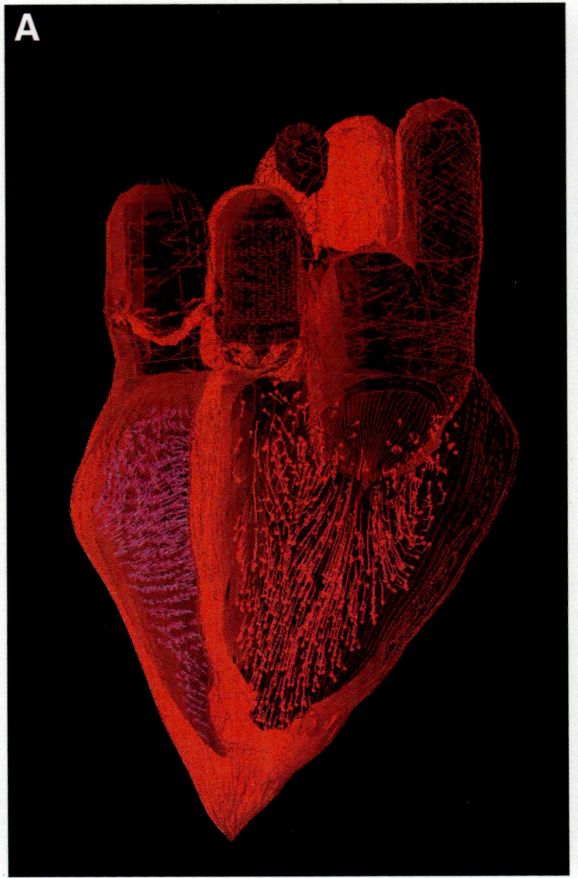

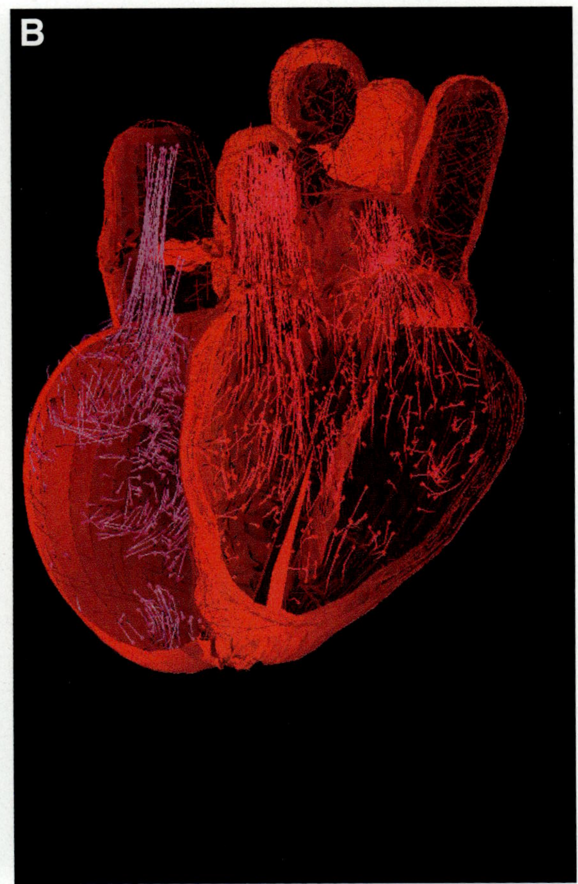

Fig. 2. Cut-away view of the model heart in the same orientation and at the same times in the cardiac cycle as in Fig. 1. Blood flow is depicted in terms of streak-lines. Mitral regurgitation is clearly visible during ventricular systole (B).

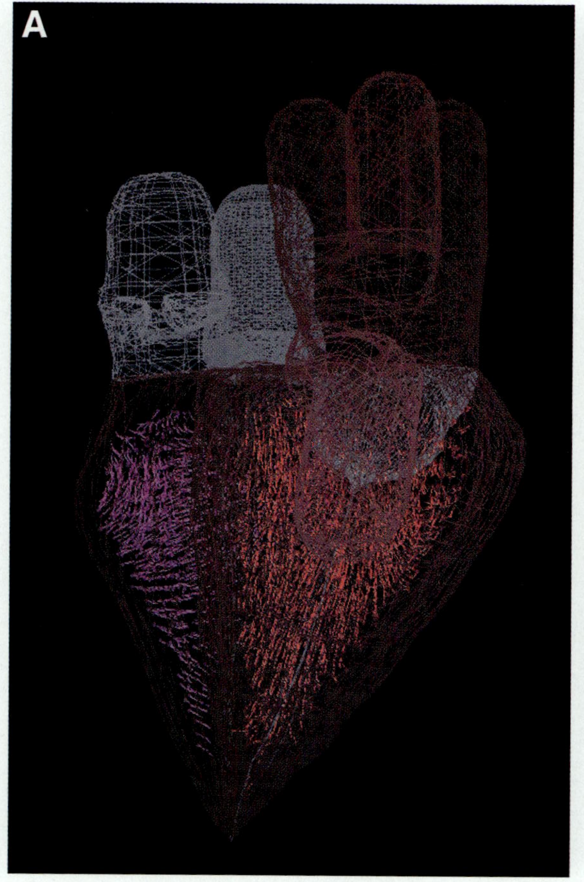

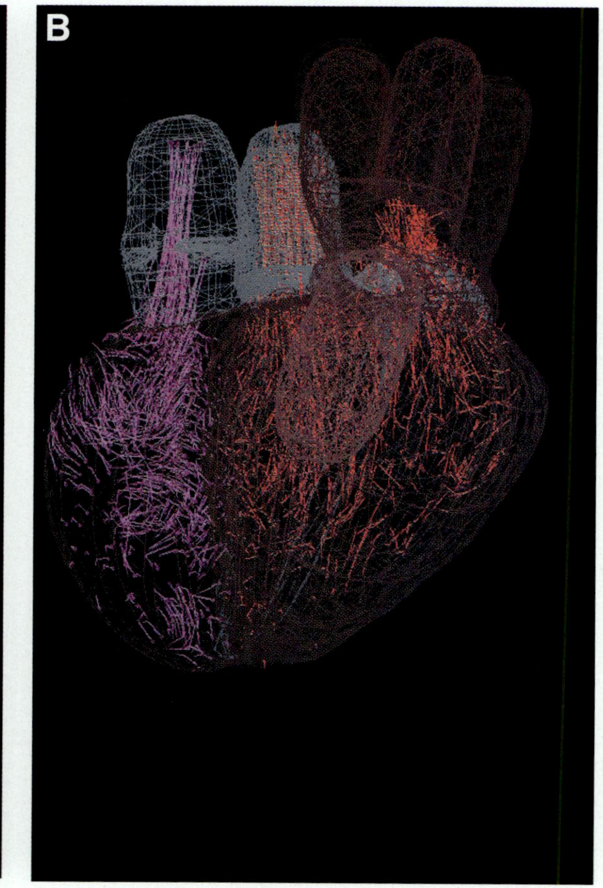

Fig. 3. Transparent view of the model heart showing selected fibers and the blood flow within the chambers. Frames shown correspond to those of Figs 1–2.

The work described in this paper is supported by the National Science Foundation (USA) under research grant BIR-9302545. Computation is performed at the Pittsburgh Supercomputing Center under a grant (MCA93S004P) of Cray C-90 computer time from the MetaCenter Allocation Committee (USA).

References

BEYER, R. P. (1992). A computational model of the cochlea using the immersed boundary method. *J. comput. Phys.* **98**, 145–162.

FAUCI, L. J. (1990). Interaction of oscillating filaments – a computational study. *J. comput. Phys.* **86**, 294–313.

FAUCI, L. J. AND FOGELSON, A. L. (1993). Truncated Newton methods and the modeling of complex immersed elastic structures. *Comm. Pure appl. Math.* **46**, 787–818.

FAUCI, L. J. AND PESKIN, C. S. (1988). A computational model of aquatic animal locomotion. *J. comput. Phys.* **77**, 85–108.

FOGELSON, A. L. (1984). A mathematical model and numerical method for studying platelet adhesion and aggregation during blood clotting. *J. comput. Phys.* **56**, 111–134.

FOGELSON, A. L. (1985). Mathematical and computational aspects of blood clotting. In *Proceedings of the 11th IMACS World Congress on System Simulation and Scientific Computation,* vol. 3 (ed. B. Wahlstrom), pp. 5–8. New York: North Holland.

FOGELSON, A. L. AND PESKIN, C. S. (1988). A fast numerical method for solving the three-dimensional Stokes' equations in the presence of suspended particles. *J. comput. Phys.* **79**, 50–69.

MCCRACKEN, M. F. AND PESKIN, C. S. (1980). A vortex method for blood flow through heart valves. *J. comput. Phys.* **35**, 183–205.

MCQUEEN, D. M. AND PESKIN, C. S. (1983). Computer-assisted design of pivoting-disc prosthetic mitral valves. *J. thorac. cardiovasc. Surg.* **86**, 126–135.

MCQUEEN, D. M. AND PESKIN, C. S. (1985). Computer-assisted design of butterfly bileaflet valves for the mitral position. *Scand. J. thorac. cardiovasc. Surg.* **19**, 139–148.

MCQUEEN, D. M. AND PESKIN, C. S. (1989). A three-dimensional computational method for blood flow in the heart. II. Contractile fibers. *J. comput. Phys.* **82**, 289–297.

MCQUEEN, D. M. AND PESKIN, C. S. (1990). A heart valve prosthesis. European Patent Publication Number EP 0 211 576 B1.

MCQUEEN, D. M. AND PESKIN, C. S. (1991). Curved butterfly bileaflet prosthetic cardiac valve. U.S. Patent Number 5026391.

MCQUEEN, D. M., PESKIN, C. S. AND YELLIN, E. L. (1982). Fluid dynamics of the mitral valve: physiological aspects of a mathematical model. *Am. J. Physiol.* **242**, H1095–H1110.

MEISNER, J. S., MCQUEEN, D. M., ISHIDA, Y., VETTER, H. O., BORTOLOTTI, U., STROM, J. A., FRATER, R. W. M., PESKIN, C. S. AND YELLIN, E. L. (1985). Effects of timing of atrial systole on LV filling and mitral valve closure: computer and dog studies. *Am. J. Physiol.* **249**, H604–H619.

PESKIN, C. S. (1972). Flow patterns around heart valves: a digital computer method for solving the equations of motion. PhD thesis, Physiology, Albert Einstein College of Medicine. University Microfilms no. 72–30, 378. 211pp.

PESKIN, C. S. (1977). Numerical analysis of blood flow in the heart. *J. comput. Phys.* **25**, 220–252.

PESKIN, C. S. (1980). Fluid dynamics of the heart and the ear. In *Computing Methods in Applied Sciences and Engineering* (ed. R. Glowinski and J. L. Lions), pp. 587–613. Amsterdam: North Holland.

PESKIN, C. S. (1989). Fiber architecture of the left ventricular wall: an asymptotic analysis. *Comm. Pure appl. Math.* **42**, 79–113.

PESKIN, C. S. (1992). Two examples of mathematics and computing in the biological sciences: blood flow in the heart and molecular dynamics. In *American Mathematical Society Centennial Publications*, vol. 2, pp. 395–416. Providence, RI: American Mathematical Society.

PESKIN, C. S. AND MCQUEEN, D. M. (1980). Modeling prosthetic heart valves for numerical analysis of blood flow in the heart. *J. comput. Phys.* **37**, 113–132.

PESKIN, C. S. AND MCQUEEN, D. M. (1989). A three-dimensional computational method for blood flow in the heart. I. Immersed elastic fibers in a viscous incompressible fluid. *J. comput. Phys.* **81**, 372–405.

PESKIN, C. S. AND MCQUEEN, D. M. (1992*a*). Computational biofluid dynamics. *Contemp. Math.* **141**, 161–186.

PESKIN, C. S. AND MCQUEEN, D. M. (1992*b*). Cardiac fluid dynamics. *Crit. Rev. Biomed. Eng.* **20**, 451–459.

PESKIN, C. S. AND MCQUEEN, D. M. (1994). Mechanical equilibrium determines the fractal fiber architecture of aortic heart valve leaflets. *Am. J. Physiol.* **266**, H319–H328.

PESKIN, C. S. AND PRINTZ, B. F. (1992). Improved volume conservation in the computation of flows with immersed elastic boundaries. *J. comput. Phys.* **105**, 33–46.

ROSAR, M. E. (1994). A three-dimensional computer model for fluid flow through a collapsible tube. PhD thesis, New York University.

STREETER, D. D., JR, POWERS, W. E., ROSS, M. A. AND TORRENT-GUASP, F. (1978). Three-dimensional fiber orientation in the mammalian left ventricular wall. In *Cardiovascular System Dynamics* (ed. J. Baan, A. Noordergraaf and J. Raines), pp. 73–84. Cambridge, MA: MIT Press.

STREETER, D. D., JR, SPOTNITZ, H. M., PATEL, D. P., ROSS, J., JR AND SONNENBLICK, E. H. (1969). Fiber orientation in the canine left ventricle during diastole and systole. *Circulation Res.* **24**, 339–347.

SULSKY, D. AND BRACKBILL, J. U. (1991). A numerical method for suspension flow. *J. comput. Phys.* **96**, 339–368.

THOMAS, C. E. (1957). The muscular architecture of the ventricles of hog and dog hearts. *Am. J. Anat.* **101**, 17–57.

SHEAR-AUGMENTED DISPERSION IN THE RESPIRATORY SYSTEM

ROGER D. KAMM

Fluid Mechanics Laboratory, Department of Mechanical Engineering, Massachusetts Institute of Technology, Cambridge, MA, USA

Summary

Biological systems contain numerous examples of shear-augmented dispersion in which gradients in the velocity profile act in concert with lateral mixing or molecular diffusion to cause materials to disperse at an enhanced rate. Some of the better known examples are found in the respiratory or cardiovascular systems, but other applications include the dispersal of pollutants discharged into a flowing stream, the mixing of contaminants in groundwater flows and the possibility of enhanced transport rates through tissues subjected to transient loads.

This review focuses on two examples in the respiratory system, bolus dispersion and high-frequency ventilation, that draw upon a broad range of fundamental studies in shear-augmented dispersion. Simple examples are considered which contain specific features of the considerably more complex real situations. These features include, for example, the effects of turbulence, secondary flows, absorption by the walls, aerosol deposition, complex geometries and oscillatory flow.

A scaling analysis is presented that yields the approximate dependence of effective diffusivities associated with shear-augmented dispersion when more detailed analyses are either not warranted or too complex to be tractable.

Introduction

Shear-augmented dispersion plays a critical role in many biological and physiological phenomena. As the name implies, it occurs when a velocity gradient or shear in the primary flow direction interacts with either molecular diffusion or convective mixing in the lateral or cross-stream direction to augment the rate of transport along the direction of the primary flow.

Examples of shear-augmented dispersion abound in nature. It contributes to the progressive spread of an injected bolus (e.g. drugs, tracers, dissolved gases) through the circulation (Bassingthwaighte and Goresky, 1984). In the mammalian respiratory system, a bolus of trace gas or aerosol particles introduced during inspiration and measured again at the mouth on the subsequent expiration broadens as a result of the effects of shear-augmented dispersion as influenced by the complexity of the geometry and flow conditions found in the lung (Ultman, 1981; Heyder *et al.* 1988). A clinical application of

Key words: Taylor diffusion, augmented dispersion, shear-augmented dispersion, bolus dispersion, high-frequency ventilation, gas transport, gas mixing, indicator dilution, respiratory system.

shear-augmented dispersion is found in the use of small-volume, high-frequency oscillations introduced *via* an endotracheal tube to ventilate patients suffering from diseases such as respiratory distress syndrome (Froese and Bryan, 1987). Since the oscillation volumes used are often smaller than the volume of the conducting airways (those in which no gas exchange takes place), some form of augmentation must clearly be involved. This method has the advantage of maintaining adequate gas exchange while minimizing the pressure and volume excursions that might otherwise cause damage to a diseased lung (Drazen *et al.* 1984).

Shear-augmented dispersion is also likely to play a role in other biological systems, although these other cases have been much less studied. Situations that might give rise to shear-augmented dispersion include (i) the dispersal of drugs in tissues, especially those in which there exist mean or oscillatory convective flows, such as the arterial wall, cartilage or muscle, (ii) ventilation in other species, either *via* primitive lungs or through the body surface, and (iii) the movement of micro-organisms in convective flow fields.

On a larger scale, shear-augmented dispersion is prominent in the mixing and dispersal of pollutants discharged into rivers and estuaries. An understanding of shear-augmented dispersion in this situation could help, for example, to determine the size of the region exposed to dangerously high levels of toxic materials. Similar issues arise in the spread of toxic waste or other solutes introduced to groundwater flows. Methods of analyzing shear-augmented dispersion in porous media have been developed for this purpose, some of which will be discussed briefly.

In this brief review, I have chosen to focus on applications of shear-augmented dispersion in respiratory physiology, with some emphasis on contributions from my own laboratory. For readers interested in presentations with a different focus or a broader view, I recommend one of the following. Fischer (1976) reviewed the field of shear-augmented dispersion as applied to rivers and estuaries. The review by Bassingthwaighte and Goresky (1984) provides an excellent reference to transport and mixing phenomena in the cardiovascular system. Topics related to the broader issues of gas mixing in the lung are addressed in the comprehensive reviews by Ultman (1985) and Grotberg (1994). For those interested in theoretical methods, I recommend a recent text by Brenner and Edwards (1993), who present a wide variety of situations in the context of macro-transport theory, a generalized theoretical approach to the analysis of shear-augmented dispersion.

Classical Taylor dispersion

G. I. Taylor (1953) laid the foundation for all subsequent work in shear-augmented dispersion when he investigated the rapid rate of axial mixing that occurs when a solute is injected into a long piping system containing steady flow. The observation was that the injected bolus spread in a roughly Gaussian distribution, nearly symmetrical up- and downstream, the half-width of which varied as the square root of time. This is the character that one would expect to see if the bolus were to spread solely by molecular diffusion, but the rate of spreading observed was many times larger than could be accounted for by molecular diffusion alone.

Taylor considered a fully developed laminar flow in a pipe of circular cross-section A

in which the rate at which solute is exchanged across a cross-sectional plane can be expressed as:

$$\text{Mass flux} = \dot{m} = \int \left(uC - D_{\mathrm{m}} \frac{\partial C}{\partial z} \right) \mathrm{d}A\,, \tag{1}$$

where u is the component of velocity in the z-direction, C is solute concentration and D_{m} is the molecular diffusivity. If we confine our attention to the case of axial dispersion of an injected tracer bolus, then it is useful to consider transport across a plane which is itself traveling at the mean speed of the fluid, V_{m}, in which case velocity u in the above expression should be replaced by $u - V_{\mathrm{m}}$, the speed relative to this moving plane. The integrated result (from equation 1) is a net transport of solute across this moving reference plane in the direction of flow.

The second term in equation 1, which is unchanged by this transformation to a moving reference frame, simply represents axial molecular diffusion. The first term, representing convective transport and encompassing the effect of shear-augmentation, can be seen to be non-zero in the moving frame only when both the axial velocity and the solute concentration are non-uniformly distributed over the cross-section. The velocity distribution in this frame is parabolic in shape with a zero mean, so that fluid is moving forward through the plane in the core region and moving back along the walls as indicated by the arrows in Fig. 1. Although it has not appeared explicitly, note that radial molecular diffusion of solute between the core and the wall is a major factor in determining the difference in concentration between these two streams. Ahead of the contaminant bolus in Fig. 1, the solute concentration is greater in the core than near the wall since the core fluid originates from a region of high relative concentration. Similarly, the concentration near

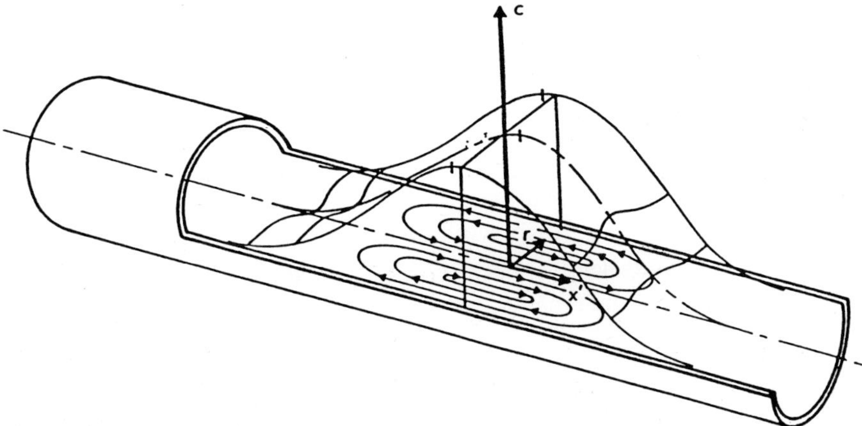

Fig. 1. Solute concentration distribution of an injected bolus in a reference frame translating with the mean fluid speed V_{m}. Arrows indicate the direction of solute transport giving rise to augmented transport. Note the local maximum in concentration along the tube centerline ahead of the peak of the axial distribution and the corresponding trough behind the axial peak. (After Probstein, 1994. Reprinted by permission of John Wiley and Sons, Inc.)

the wall is lower because it is convected from a region of *low* concentration. This sets up a radial concentration gradient that causes solute to diffuse from the core towards the wall. Convection is thus the *cause* of the radial concentration gradient which molecular diffusion acts to diminish. The rate of augmented transport [the integral of $(u-V_m)C$ in equation 1] is maximized for large radial differences in C and is therefore *reduced* by radial molecular diffusion. It also follows that the magnitude of the transport is dependent upon the magnitude and shape of the axial velocity profile, more 'peaked' profiles leading to greater augmentation.

The result of Taylor's analysis of this phenomenon is:

$$\frac{D_{\text{eff}}}{D_m} = 1 + \frac{1}{48}\left(\frac{V_m a}{D_m}\right)^2, \tag{2}$$

where a is the radius of the tube, D_{eff} is effective diffusivity and the parameter $V_m a/D_m$ is the Peclet number Pe. The second term on the right-hand side is Taylor's contribution (Taylor, 1953) and represents what is commonly referred to as Taylor diffusion; the first term, the existence of which was later demonstrated by Aris (1956) through a more rigorous analysis of the problem, represents the additive effect of axial molecular diffusion. Thus, in flow in which $Pe \gg 1$, axial dispersion occurs many times more rapidly through this interaction between axial shear and radial molecular diffusion than by molecular diffusion alone.

Although most of this paper is devoted to a discussion of behavior observed long after the injection of solute, it is essential to have an appreciation of the behavior for shorter times as well. This is especially true in networks such as the lung where, owing to axial variations in duct geometry and the continuing readjustment of the axial and secondary flow profiles, the dispersion is *never strictly* fully developed, even though it might sometimes be a reasonable approximation to treat it as such.

It is useful to consider axial transport in a tube of finite length L, when the mean residence time of a fluid particle is L/V_m. Dispersion in this instance is characterized by the two dimensionless parameters, a/L and Pe. On the basis of the foregoing discussion, in the limit of low Peclet number ($Pe \ll 1$) and short tubes (defined by the condition that the axial convection time L/V_m is small compared with the radial and axial diffusion times, a^2/D_m and L^2/D_m, respectively), molecular diffusion dominates over convection and axial transport is characterized by the molecular diffusivity. If the Peclet number is still small but the tube is long ($L^2/D_m \gg L/V_m$ or, equivalently, if $Pe \gg a/L$), the spread of the bolus remains dominated by molecular diffusivity but the center of the distribution is convected at a speed V_m. This is termed 'convective axial diffusion' and applies in the designated region of Fig. 2.

The situation can be analyzed in a similar manner when $Pe \gg 1$. In this case, if the solute bolus passes through the tube before it has an opportunity to diffuse over the tube cross section ($a^2/D_m \gg L/V_m$, or equivalently, $Pe \gg L/a$), then axial dispersion results predominantly from shear in the axial profile while the bolus is convected along the tube at a speed characterized by (but not necessarily equal to) V_m. Thus, axial transport is purely convective in nature. If the tube is long, so that $a^2/D_m \ll L/V_m$ ($Pe \ll L/a$), then Taylor dispersion (or, more precisely, Taylor/Aris dispersion) takes over (Fig. 2).

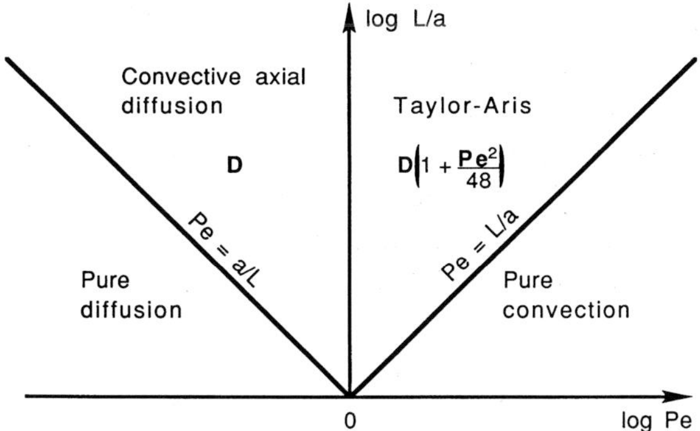

Fig. 2. A mapping in parameter-space of the different zones of solute dispersion in a tube of radius a and length L. Also shown are the applicable expressions for axial diffusivity in each zone. (After A. A. Sonin, M.I.T., personal communication.)

The different regimes exist in all the specific cases discussed below, although the complexity of the situation increases with the complexity of the flow. The main difference is that molecular diffusion can be accompanied by other forms of convective mixing, either by turbulence or by complex secondary flows. In qualitative terms, this has the effect of replacing D_m by some larger 'convective mixing coefficient'.

Scaling arguments

Because of the complexity of many biological applications of shear-augmented dispersion, it is often difficult to develop rigorous theories that are strictly applicable or even to perform realistic numerical experiments. Moreover, often what is needed is not a precise prediction, but rather simply an estimate of how the rate of shear-augmented dispersion depends on the various parameters of the problem. For both reasons, it is useful to establish a framework within which the general scaling laws for the effective axial diffusivity for a given situation can be obtained.

One general approach is based on the analysis of Taylor (1921), who determined that when the instantaneous axial velocity of a particle relative to the mean, $V_{rel}=u-V_m$, is a stationary random process, the effective axial diffusivity can be written as:

$$D_{eff} = \frac{1}{A}\int_A dA \int_0^{\infty} \langle V_{rel}(t)V_{rel}(t-t')\rangle dt', \tag{3}$$

where <> denotes a representative ensemble average over many fluid particles and A is the cross-sectional area of the tube or channel. The integrand initially has a magnitude $V_m{}^2$ and, owing to the nature of an ensemble average, vanishes to zero on a time scale that can be thought of as the time (t_c) for the instantaneous velocity (at time t') to become uncorrelated with its value at time t. This time can be seen to be of the same scale as the time for a particle randomly to sample all axial velocities. Keeping in mind that there are situations in which a significant fraction of the cross-sectional area may have a uniform axial velocity and hence not contribute to shear-augmented dispersion, the double integral in equation 3 can be approximated as (Pedley and Kamm, 1988):

$$D_{\text{eff}} \approx V_{\text{rel}}^2 t_c \boldsymbol{A}\,, \tag{4}$$

where $\boldsymbol{A}$ is the fraction of the total cross-sectional area containing axial velocity gradients in the lateral direction.

This approximate analysis can be applied to the case already discussed: laminar, fully developed flow. In that instance, $V_{\text{rel}} \approx V_m$, $t_c \approx a^2/D_m$ and $\boldsymbol{A}=1$, leading to the estimate, $D_{\text{eff}} \approx V_m^2 a^2/D_m$, the correct result, lacking only the numerical coefficient, 1/48.

Although much of the subsequent discussion is generally applicable to a wide variety of biologically relevant situations, it is useful to develop these general results in the context of specific examples. Here, I include two, both drawn from the field of respiration physiology.

Two examples from the respiratory system

Bolus dispersion

In a wide variety of biological phenomena, we often seek to gain knowledge of the distributed or local behavior of a complex system from measurements made at one site by means of a non-invasive or minimally invasive method. These methods often involve remote measurements that reflect the cumulative effects on the quantity measured of a range of differing conditions. One such example is found in the dispersion of a bolus of tracer injected into the inspiratory flowstream at the mouth and observed at a fixed point during both inspiration and expiration. In between, the bolus will have traversed many generations of the tracheobronchial tree and its appearance on expiration will reflect this complex history. This procedure has been performed both with boli of trace gases and with aerosol particles (see Fig. 3). If injected late in inspiration, the bolus penetrates only a short distance into the lung and passes the measurement site (typically at the mouth) early in expiration; the last gas entering the lung is the first to leave. The bolus has a greater variance than that observed on inspiration but is still relatively narrow. In a series of tests in which the tracer is injected progressively earlier in inspiration, and therefore penetrates further and further into the lung, the bolus is smeared over a progressively greater volume and the peak correspondingly falls (Fig. 3). Recent experiments with 1 μm diameter aerosol particles indicate that the half-width of the expired bolus increases approximately linearly with penetration volume over a wide range of penetration volumes up to 900 ml (Heyder *et al.* 1988). This behavior agrees with other measurements with gases (Ultman *et al.* 1978) for cases in which the bolus penetrates less than 200 ml into the lung. For larger penetration volumes, however, the two diverge with the gas dispersing much more rapidly, demonstrating the significant influence of molecular diffusion of gases in the lung periphery. In the case of a bolus of aerosol particles, the integrated volume of the bolus also falls as a result of deposition of some fraction of the aerosol particles on the airway walls.

Curves of concentration *versus* expired volume are characteristic of either a trace gas or an aerosol bolus, although the degree of dispersion, and possibly the mechanisms

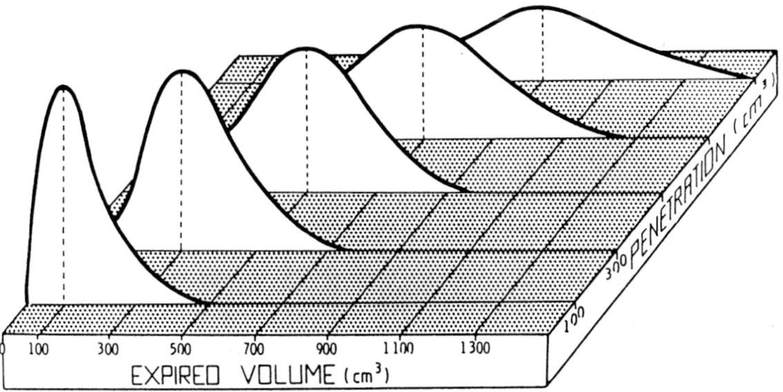

Fig. 3. A schematic representation depicting the increase in dispersion with increasing volumetric penetration of an inspired bolus of aerosol or tracer gas. Curves correspond to the concentration profiles seen on expiration following bolus injection at 100, 300, 500, 700 and 900 cm^3 before end inspiration. (After Heyder *et al.* 1988.)

producing dispersion, may differ somewhat. Studies of this type have been used to infer the nature of mixing in the lung as discussed extensively by Ultman (1985).

Gas exchange by high-frequency ventilation

Although bolus dispersion has caught the attention of many pulmonary physiologists and biomedical engineers because of the information it potentially contains about the mechanisms of gas mixing in the airways, the second example is one which has special clinical significance. Briscoe *et al.* (1954) observed that, contrary to the conventional view of gas exchange, some amount of gas reached the alveolar zone even when the inspired volume was less than the volume of the conducting airways. About 20 years ago, Lunkenheimer *et al.* (1972) rediscovered this result and extended it to make the observation that adequate gas exchange could be achieved by the use of low-volume but high-frequency oscillation imposed at the mouth or *via* an endotracheal tube. This realization led to a flurry of research activity primarily in the 1980s aimed at developing a fundamental understanding of the physical mechanisms responsible for this finding, and to the gradual adoption of high-frequency ventilation (HFV) for the ventilation of infants suffering from respiratory distress syndrome (see Drazen *et al.* 1984; Froese and Bryan, 1987; for further references).

Venegas *et al.* (1986) have demonstrated that adequate CO_2 elimination (eucapnia) can be achieved by HFV in a wide variety of species and that the conditions for eucapnia can be characterized by the following expression:

$$\frac{\dot{V}_{\mathrm{osc}}}{\dot{V}_{\mathrm{A}}} = \left(\frac{f}{0.19(\dot{V}_{\mathrm{A}}/V_{\mathrm{D}})} \right)^{0.54}, \tag{5}$$

for $f > 5(\dot{V}_A/V_D)$, where $\dot{V}_{osc}$ is the product of oscillation frequency f and tidal volume V_T, $\dot{V}_A$ is the required alveolar ventilation, and V_D is the dead space (conducting airway volume). These conditions are readily attainable in humans; for f=5 Hz, this corresponds to $\dot{V}_{osc}$ of about $0.7\,l\,s^{-1}$. This can be rearranged to demonstrate that alveolar ventilation (proportional to the rate of gas exchange) scales as $fV_T^{2.17}$.

In the context of these two examples, several studies will be described which are motivated by a need to elucidate the fundamental physics behind the results of bolus dispersion experiments and the enhanced gas exchange found with HFV. Typically, these studies focus on one or more specific mechanisms present in idealized models that mimic certain aspects of dispersion in the lung. For example, flow in the branching airway network has several features that can be examined separately, such as turbulence, secondary flows due to curvature of the airways, gas absorption or aerosol deposition, alveolar duct geometry in the periphery, and statistical variability in both geometry and flow distribution. Each of these is considered individually in the next sections.

Mechanisms of augmented dispersion

Turbulence

Flow conditions in the lung are such that turbulence is generally to be found, at least in the first several airways immediately below the trachea (Pedley and Kamm, 1991). This is especially true on inspiration, during which the constriction at the glottis produces a turbulent jet. The turbulent eddies promote lateral mixing and therefore reduce the time scale for lateral equilibration. On the basis of the scaling arguments discussed earlier, this causes t_c to fall and, according to equation 4, D_{eff} to decrease. The effect of turbulence can be understood as resulting from two phenomena. One is a blunting of the axial velocity profile due to the more efficient lateral exchange of momentum that reduces axial shear over much of the cross-sectional area, confining the steep gradients in axial velocity profile to the region near the wall and reducing D_{eff}. The other phenomenon is the turbulent mixing which can be viewed, in crude terms, as resulting in a change in the lateral diffusivity; molecular diffusion, characterized by D_m, is overwhelmed by the 'turbulent diffusivity', which scales approximately as the product of the length and velocity scales of the largest turbulent eddies. These scales are a and V_m, respectively, giving a turbulent diffusivity that scales as $V_m a$. When this is substituted for D_m in the expression for *laminar* flow, this results in an effective diffusivity that scales as (see equation 2):

$$D_{eff} \approx V_m^2 a^2/(V_m a) \approx V_m a\,. \tag{6}$$

Taylor (1954), using a more quantitatively accurate approach, obtained the result:

$$D_{eff} \approx \mathbf{f}(Re) V_m a\,, \tag{7}$$

where $\mathbf{f}(Re)$ is a weak function of Reynolds number ($Re = V_m a/\nu$, where ν is the gas kinematic viscosity), having a numerical value of about 0.6 for $Re = 10^4$.

Secondary flows

Flows in the plane perpendicular to the duct axis arise in the lung primarily because of the curvature found at bifurcations. A simple flow that exhibits similar secondary motion is fully developed flow in a curved tube of uniform curvature. If the curvature is not too great (that is, if $\delta \equiv a/R \ll 1$, where R is the radius of curvature of the tube) and the Dean number ($Dn = aV_m\delta^{1/2}/\nu$) is not too large ($Dn < 60$), then secondary flows develop but these have relatively little effect on the axial velocity profile which remains essentially parabolic. The generation of secondary flows has the effect of enhancing lateral mixing and thereby reducing t_c. Since the secondary flows in this instance, however, simply consist of two counter-rotating vortices, then mixing occurs only along the secondary flow streamlines and, for a particle to sample *all* cross-sectional locations, it must still rely on molecular diffusion to move *between* streamlines. Hence, although the secondary flows produce a reduction in D_{eff} (Fig. 4), the reduction is limited to that realized by complete and instantaneous mixing along the secondary flow streamlines; once this has been accomplished, further increases in mixing along these streamlines can have no further effect and D_{eff} asymptotes to a value roughly a factor of 5 lower than the straight tube result (Johnson and Kamm, 1986). The experimental data shown in the figure suggest some further reduction in D_{eff} which might be associated with distortions in the axial velocity profile or the influence of minor imperfections in the experimental tubes, which lead to low-order distortions in the secondary flow pattern and consequent mixing between streamlines.

Gas absorption by the wall

Many gases occasionally found in inspired air, especially some that pose potential health hazards, can be absorbed into the airway wall tissue. Aside from the obvious physiological and possible pathological consequences, this also influences the rate of axial dispersion of an injected bolus.

To understand the effect, consider a steady, fully developed laminar flow through a tube of circular cross-section with a layer of absorbing material of thickness b coating the

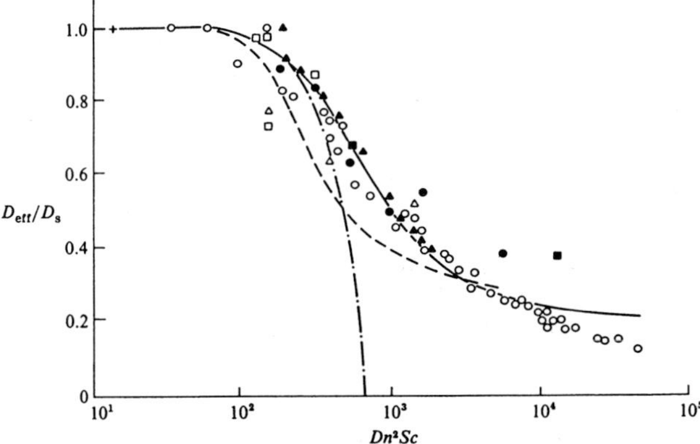

Fig. 4. The effective diffusivity of a curved tube, divided by the value for zero curvature D_S, as a function of Dn^2Sc. Experimental data from □, van Andel *et al.* (1964); ■, Trivedi and Vasudeva (1975); △, Nigam and Vasudeva (1976); ●, Shetty and Vasudeva (1977); ○, van den Berg and Deelder (1979); and ▲, Andersson and Berglin (1981). The solid line is the numerical prediction of Johnson and Kamm (1986); the dashed line a numerical solution from Janssen (1976); the dot-dash line a perturbation expansion solution from Erdogan and Chatwin (1967). (After Johnson and Kamm, 1986.)

wall. This layer must be considered to be part of the tube cross-section since the tracer can freely pass into and out of it. While in the wall, the tracer has essentially zero axial velocity. It is easy to imagine, therefore, that the effect of tracer being absorbed by the wall, residing there for some time, then escaping at quite another point along the propagating bolus is to increase D_{eff} dramatically. From the perspective of the scaling analysis presented earlier, it is clear that the time required to sample all cross-sectional locations is now much longer owing to reduced diffusivity in the wall material. The increase in t_c consequently increases D_{eff}. A second effect is that the bolus travels at a mean speed slower than the mean speed of gas flow in the tube. This can be explained by the fact that, as wall solubility increases, an increasing fraction of the tracer resides in the wall, where it moves at zero velocity.

This situation has been analyzed by Davidson and Schroter (1983), who expressed their results in the form:

$$\frac{D_{eff}}{D_m} = K_1(\tau) + Pe^2 K_2(\tau)\,, \tag{8}$$

where $\tau \equiv D_m t/a^2$, K_1 represents axial molecular diffusion (modified by wall solubility) and the second term represents the effect of shear-augmented dispersion. Because wall diffusivity is always smaller than diffusivity in the gas phase and since some fraction of the gas resides in the wall, K_1 is always less than unity. K_2 is a complex function, especially in the entrance region of the tube, up to a time of about a^2/D_m=100. Even the long-time behavior is somewhat complicated. For values typical of the lung (ratio of gas-to-wall diffusivities of 10^4, wall thickness-to-radius ratio of 0.1), K_2 at first increases, reaching a maximum value of about 1 as the solubility coefficient β_s (the ratio of wall concentration to gas concentration at equilibrium) approaches unity. When β_s increases further, D_{eff} begins to fall, attaining values even lower than the case without wall absorption for β_s>200. By way of explanation, note that in the limit of $\beta_s \to \infty$, all gas will reside in the wall. In that limit, dispersion will occur only as a result of axial diffusion in the wall, an *extremely* slow process.

Aerosol dispersion

The case of an inspired bolus of aerosol particles would seem to bear some similarity to the case just discussed with absorbing walls; the results, however, are quite different. To start with, the bolus travels *faster* on average than the mean speed of the gas. Unlike the previous example, we consider the speed only of the material that remains suspended in the gas since, once an aerosol particle strikes the wall, it can never return to the gas stream. Consequently, the region near the wall has a depressed concentration of particles, compared with the case of a gas with non-absorbing walls, producing a concentration profile skewed towards the high-velocity region near the tube axis. The mean aerosol velocity is found to be 56% higher than the mean gas velocity in this instance (Brenner and Edwards, 1993).

The effect on D_{eff} also differs from the previous case. The aerosol that remains suspended in the gas is dispersed by a process akin to normal Taylor dispersion and might be expected to behave according to equation 2. The skewing of the radial distribution of aerosol particles towards the tube axis, however, reduces D_{eff} by about a factor of 4 while retaining the same parametric dependence found in the classical Taylor result (Brenner and Edwards, 1993):

$$D_{\text{eff}} = Pe^2/200\,. \tag{9}$$

Note also that the effects of aerosol impaction and axial dispersion combine to cause the peak in concentration for an injected bolus of aerosol particles to fall off more rapidly than for a non-depleting bolus.

Complex geometries

Alveolated duct

There are many complexities of the tracheo-bronchial tree, but one in particular has been found to exert a strong influence on axial dispersion. In the lung periphery, the airways contain alveolar out-pouchings with increasing frequency as one approaches the alveolar duct. Earlier studies had suggested that, by the time gas reaches this region, the Peclet number is sufficiently small, falling to values of the order of 1 for normal breathing, for Taylor dispersion to have little or no influence on axial dispersion. What had not previously been appreciated, however, was that the alveoli themselves can augment the rate of axial dispersion in a manner not unlike that of the absorbing wall example above.

In a recent theoretical model (Federspiel and Fredberg, 1988), this situation was simulated by a central duct of circular cross-section with a periodic arrangement of axisymmetrical ‘alveoli’, each consisting of a torus with an opening to the central duct. As a bolus of tracer passes through such a duct, tracer molecules can diffuse into an alveolus, migrate around within the alveolus for some time as a result of molecular diffusion and the small convective currents present, and eventually rejoin the main gas stream in the central duct. As in the case of an absorbing wall, this increases the time required to sample all cross-sectional locations, and thereby increases t_c and consequently D_{eff}. The enhancement can be considerable, especially when the alveolar volume (V_a) is large compared with that of the central duct (V_d) or when the alveolar ‘mouth’ is particularly small. The results obtained in this situation are shown in Fig. 5. Note that A, the axial length of an alveolar mouth and L_c, the length of one unit cell, are both normalized to the diameter of the central duct.

Branching networks

Another mechanism for enhancing the rate of axial dispersion relates to the statistical nature of the branching airways in the sense that each pathway into the lung is unique, with its own distribution of pathlengths, airway diameters, branching angles, etc., that distinguish it from any other pathway. As a result of these complexities, if one were to follow the paths of a collection of fluid particles into the lung, all starting at an identical point in a major airway, they would each penetrate a different distance when observed at some later time during inspiration. If all these pathways were to rejoin *via* a convergent network with similar statistical variability, as occurs in the capillary bed of the circulatory system, the initial bolus would be spread over some axial distance depending on the degree of variability of the network, which would result in a distribution of transit times. Thus, even in the absence of all other mechanisms of shear-augmented dispersion

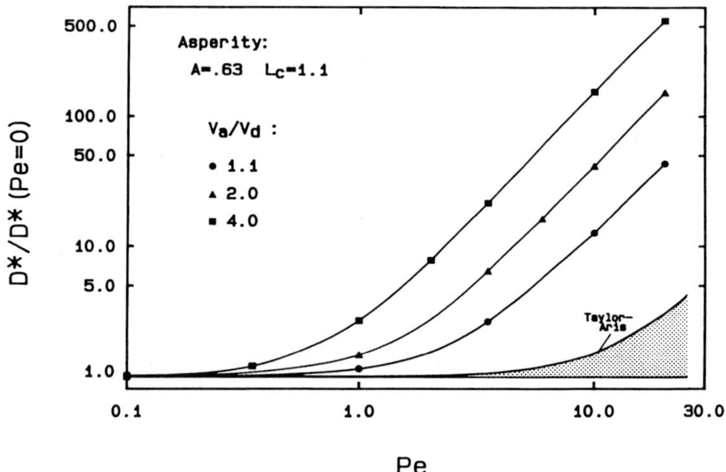

Fig. 5. The ratio of augmented axial diffusivity D^* to axial diffusivity with zero flow $D^*(Pe=0)$ as a function of Peclet number ($Pe=2V_{\mathrm{m}}a/D_{\mathrm{m}}$ in this figure only). The shaded region indicates the result for a tube without alveoli. Lines indicate the enhancement resulting from alveolar out-pouchings. Notation defined in text. (After Federspiel and Fredberg, 1988.)

discussed above, axial dispersion would result, as is readily observed in indicator dilution studies in the cardiovascular system (Zierler, 1962).

The situation in the lung is different since, if expiratory flow were the exact reverse of inspiration (and lacking other means of dispersion), all gas particles would return to precisely the same location at which they began their journey at precisely the same time. We know, however, that expiration is *not* the exact reverse of inspiration and the same dispersion process that is observed in the capillaries will occur, to some degree, in the lung.

The degree to which this occurs in the lung has been considered by Horsfield and Cumming (1968) and expressed in terms of an effective augmented diffusivity by Yu (1975). The situation is somewhat analogous to the dispersion process during flow though a random porous medium. In that case, dispersion occurs in both the axial and lateral directions, raising the important point that, in many situations of interest, the effective diffusivity is a tensorial rather than a scalar quantity, taking on different values depending upon the direction of interest. (For more on this, see Brenner and Edwards, 1993.) In such a porous medium, when the Peclet number (based on particle size L) is sufficiently large, mixing occurs predominantly by convective mixing, which is characterized by the product of a velocity scale (V_{m}) and a length scale (L), roughly analogous to the case of dispersion in turbulent pipe flow. As in the case discussed above, the role of D_{m} is taken over by a convective diffusivity that scales approximately as $V_{\mathrm{m}}L$. This leads to the prediction that D_{eff} scales as $V^2L^2/(VL)\approx VL$, again, as in the turbulent flow result. A much more thorough analysis of dispersion in porous media leads to the following predictions for the effective diffusivities parallel to the mean flow direction (Koch and Brady, 1985):

$$\frac{D_{\mathrm{eff}}}{D_{\mathrm{m}}} \approx 1+\frac{3}{4}\,Pe+\frac{1}{6}\,\pi^2\phi Pe\ln(Pe) \tag{10}$$

and perpendicular to it:

$$\frac{D_{\text{eff}}}{D_{\text{m}}} \approx 1 + \frac{63\sqrt{2}}{320}\,\phi^{1/2}Pe\,, \tag{11}$$

where ϕ represents the solids volume fraction of the material. Although additional terms appear in these equations (compared with the approximate result above) representing the effect of closed, stagnant pathways and boundary layers on the individual particles, the leading order behavior, dominant at low *Pe*, is that of the approximate expression. Finally, it is reassuring to note that these theoretical predictions agree well with experiments in random beds (Fried and Combarnous, 1971).

This scaling is entirely consistent with the predictions of Yu (1975) for dispersion in the lung due to a random distribution of branch lengths; $D_{\text{eff}}/D_{\text{m}}$ is found to vary as the first power of the Peclet number with a numerical coefficient of the order of 1.

Oscillatory flow in a straight tube

When the mechanisms of gas transport during HFV were first considered, one of the questions posed was how, in a purely oscillatory flow with zero mean, net transport could occur at a rate far in excess of what would be expected from molecular diffusivity alone. In view of the earlier work by Taylor and others summarized in the previous sections, it was obvious that shear-augmented dispersion could be responsible, at least in part. Following on this idea, investigators first focused on several previous theoretical studies of shear-augmented dispersion in oscillatory flow in a straight tube (Harris and Goren, 1967; Chatwin, 1975). These studies predicted that, at sufficiently low frequencies that the time for the lateral transport of both momentum and mass over the cross section (a^2/ν and a^2/D_{m}, respectively) were smaller than the cycle period, transport would follow the behavior predicted by steady Taylor diffusion (equation 2). For a gas, since the Schmidt number ($Sc \equiv D_{\text{m}}/\nu$) is typically of the order of 1, both conditions cease to be satisfied at approximately the same frequency, when the Womersley number $\alpha \equiv a\sqrt{(\omega/\nu)}$ [or $\beta \equiv a\sqrt{(\omega/D_{\text{m}})}$, where ω is the radian frequency] exceeds unity. When this condition is reached, a further increase in oscillation frequency, for a given velocity amplitude, produces a fall in D_{eff} relative to the steady prediction.

This result can be understood if we return to our scaling analysis summarized in equation 4. In steady flow, t_{c} is the time to sample all cross-sectional positions. To determine t_{c} in oscillatory flow, it is useful to examine the net displacement of a fluid particle after the completion of each oscillatory cycle. The net axial displacement of such a particle can be seen to depend upon whether the particle migrated in a direction of greater or lesser axial velocity during the course of the cycle. If it began near the wall where the axial velocity was small, then migrated as a result of molecular diffusion over the course of one cycle towards the axis where the velocity is high, it would first experience a small displacement in one direction (forward, say) then a greater displacement in reverse. The net displacement over that cycle would be in the reverse direction. On the next cycle, the same particle has an equal probability of migrating either towards the wall or towards the axis; therefore, its net displacement after the next cycle is essentially uncorrelated with its displacement on the previous cycle. The uncorrelation time (t_c) is therefore the cycle period, characterized by the inverse of the radian frequency, ω^{-1}.

Axial dispersion is clearly affected by the change in axial velocity profile as oscillation frequency increases. Velocity gradients come to be confined to a narrow region (the 'Stokes layer') close to the wall, the thickness of which scales with $\sqrt{(\nu/\omega)}$. Accordingly, α is seen to be the ratio of tube radius to the Stokes layer thickness. Still confining our attention to gases ($Sc \cong 1$), a decreasing fraction of the tube cross-section takes part in shear-augmented dispersion as frequency increases, characterized by the ratio of the Stokes layer area to the tube area, $2\pi a\sqrt{(\nu/\omega)}/(\pi a^2) \approx [a\sqrt{(\omega/\nu)}]^{-1}$, the inverse of the Womersley number, α^{-1}. The parameter $\boldsymbol{A}$ therefore falls, leading to further reductions in D_{eff}. The combination of effects, $t_c \approx \omega^{-1}$ and $\boldsymbol{A} \approx \alpha^{-1}$, leads to the following behavior [for $Sc \approx 1$ and $\alpha \rightarrow \infty$]:

$$\frac{D_{\mathrm{eff}}}{D_{\mathrm{m}}} \approx Pe^2 \alpha^{-3/2}, \tag{12}$$

as observed in the high-frequency limit of the theoretical solutions (Harris and Goren, 1967; Watson, 1983) and experimental results (Joshi *et al.* 1983; Gaver *et al.* 1992).

Oscillatory flow in a curved tube

As in steady flow, the straight tube result is altered in the presence of secondary flows such as those occurring in bends or bifurcations. In this case, however, secondary flows can either increase or decrease D_{eff} depending on the value of β. When $\beta \ll 1$, [and $Sc \approx 1$], both flow and transport are quasi-steady and the result is the same as for steady curved tube flow, where we saw that D_{eff} is reduced by the onset of the two-vortex secondary flow pattern. When $\beta > 1$, it was demonstrated in the absence of secondary flow that D_{eff} falls, partly because of a reduction in the portion of the tube $\boldsymbol{A}$ taking part in the transport process. Secondary flow, in that it transports both momentum and mass across the tube, opposes the confinement of velocity gradients to a narrow Stokes layer, making the axial velocity profile less blunt and distributing velocity gradients across the tube cross-section. Hence, $\boldsymbol{A}$ remains near unity and D_{eff} falls, primarily because of the fall in t_c. The net effect is a progressive reduction in D_{eff} with increasing frequency, but not as great a reduction as is found when the tube is straight (see Fig. 6).

One new phenomenon arises in this situation. When secondary flows are present, there are two characteristic times of importance: the oscillation period and the time required to traverse a secondary flow circuit, the latter being different for each secondary flow streamline. On those streamlines for which the oscillation period and secondary flow period coincide, or nearly do, a new phenomenon termed 'convective resonance' (Pedley and Kamm, 1988) comes into play. As a fluid particle makes its way around the secondary flow loop, it might reside in a region of high axial velocity during forward flow, then move into a region of low velocity on reverse flow. Such a fluid particle would tend to move consistently forward on each consecutive cycle, progressing in a rachet-like manner until either slight differences between the two time periods or diffusion to other, non-resonant streamlines breaks the pattern. For particles experiencing convective resonance, axial transport can be greatly enhanced. This is likely to account for the local

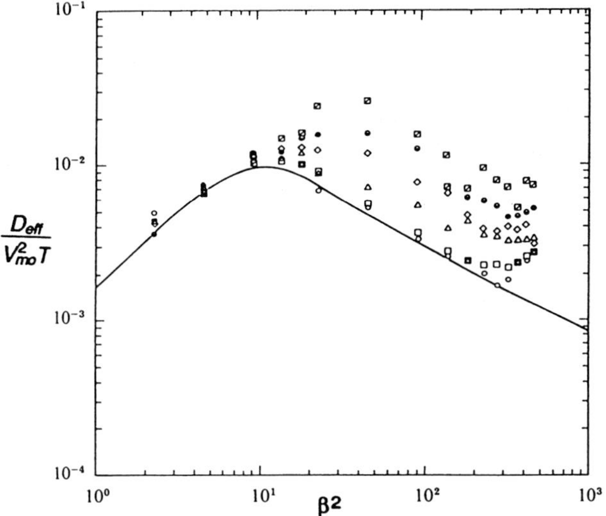

Fig. 6. Experimental results for normalized diffusivity $D_{eff}/(V_{mo}^2T)$ in a curved tube with oscillatory flow, where T is the cycle period and V_{mo} the area-averaged velocity amplitude, plotted against β^2, compared with the result for a straight tube with oscillatory flow (Watson, 1983). ○, Dn^2/α^4=0.658; □, 0.893; △, 1.30; ◇, 1.59; ⊖, 1.80; ◪, 2.37. (After Sharp *et al.* 1991.)

peaks in transport rate observed both experimentally and numerically by Sharp *et al.* (1991). Similar enhancement is observed when the curvature ratio a/R takes on values typical of those found in the lung, in which case the phase relationship between the axial velocity and concentration profiles comes into play as well (Eckman and Grotberg, 1988).

The effects of airway compliance

It has been observed that when oscillatory flow amplitude increases, it can produce large pressure excursions that cause the airway diameter to fluctuate as a result of wall compliance (Gavriely *et al.* 1985). The effect on shear-augmented dispersion has been studied in two ways. Dragon and Grotberg (1991) examined the effect on axial dispersion of a wave propagating along a compliant tube. They established that, in this case, transport is influenced by an additional dimensionless group, $\kappa \equiv Ea^2/(\rho_w \nu^2)$, where E is the elastic modulus and ρ_w the density of the tube wall material. Their findings indicated that wave propagation always reduced the rate of axial transport, but that D_{eff} attained a maximum when the phase angle between the wall motion and the axial flow approaches a minimum.

Hydon and Pedley (1993) considered the case in which flows were generated by an imposed oscillatory motion of the walls with the motion at every point being in phase. Steady streaming of the type discussed in the next section was observed and was able significantly to enhance transport rates in the larger airways. For conditions found in the more peripheral airways, flows generated by the axial pressure gradient were found to combine with those due to wall motion to enhance transport rates, but not in a purely additive fashion (Hydon, 1991).

Transport by convective streaming

To complete this discussion of axial transport in HFV, one further mechanism, termed 'convective streaming' by Scherer and Haselton (1982), must be considered. Through a series of experiments conducted in a single bifurcation, they demonstrated that, owing to directional asymmetries in the axial velocity profile, a net streaming motion could be produced in which gas travels into the lung over part of the cross-section and out of it over another cross-section when viewed over several consecutive cycles. Fig. 7 illustrates how this might occur in a simple duct with diverging walls. Since, even in quasi-steady flows, the profile of flow into a convergent duct is more blunted than into a divergent one, an asymmetry will exist, leading to a time-mean velocity profile as shown in Fig. 7C, in which flow streams towards the left near the walls and towards the right in the core.

A rigorous analysis of oscillatory flow in a tapered tube (Godleski and Grotberg, 1988) confirms the existence of a steady drift which, for frequencies that are not too large, is qualitatively of the type depicted in Fig. 7. For the range of conditions studied, however, the authors concluded that the rate of axial transport was not significantly enhanced by convective streaming and that D_{eff}, computed locally, was similar in magnitude to that for a straight tube with the same local diameter.

Other factors absent from these idealized scenarios but present in the lung, such as turbulence and the secondary flows associated with bifurcations, will tend to reduce further the importance of convective streaming, at least in the more central airways of the lung.

Combined effects in high-frequency ventilation

Among the influences of area taper, wall compliance and curvature, only the latter increases D_{eff} significantly above that for a straight tube (Grotberg, 1994). Since experimental results for dispersion in branching tube networks (Tarbell *et al.* 1982; Paloski *et al.* 1987) always show transport enhancement, this suggests that gas exchange in HFV may be largely attributable to the secondary flows generated in bifurcations. Further support for this conclusion can be found by noting the similarity of experimental results for D_{eff} obtained in a multiple-generation network (Fig. 8) to the results for a curved tube (Fig. 6). Both follow trends similar to those seen in oscillatory flow in a straight tube, but are uniformly higher, at least for $\beta>3$. In more recent experiments in a symmetrical branching network with more realistic curvatures in the the bifurcation region, C. Keramidas and R. D. Kamm (unpublished observations) obtained the result that gas transport rate varies as

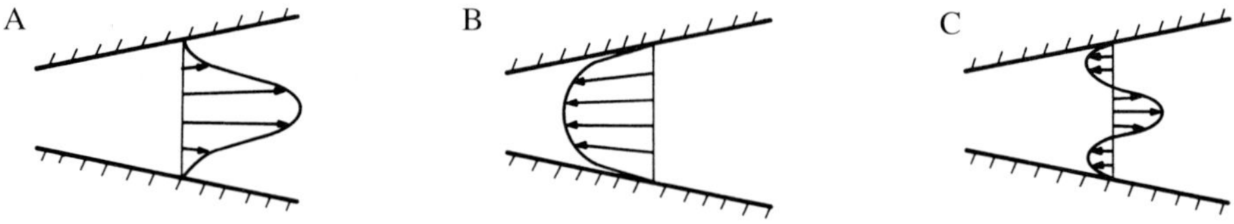

Fig. 7. A schematic representation of convective streaming. (A) Velocity profile towards divergent section; (B) velocity profile towards convergent section; (C) axial velocity when averaged over an integer number of cycles showing net transport to the right in the center and to the left along the walls.

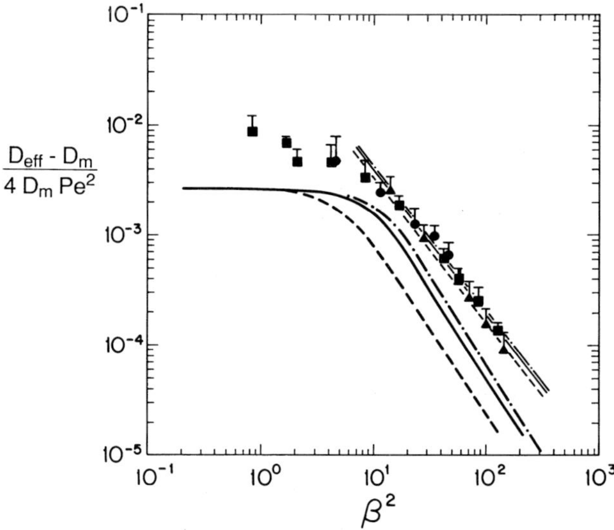

Fig. 8. Normalized effective axial diffusivity measured in a four-generation branching network using several different gas combinations and compared with the theoretical prediction for a straight tube (Watson, 1983). Squares and solid line, CH_4 in air; circles and dash-dot line, CH_4 in He; triangles and dashed line, CH_4 in SF_6. Regression results are shown as light lines. (After Paloski *et al.* 1987.)

$f^{0.86}V_T^{2.06}$, which compares favorably with the results of Venegas *et al.* (1986), discussed above, indicating a dependence as $fV_T^{2.17}$. These similarities, combined with the success of whole-lung models based on the empirical results of Fig. 8 in predicting gas exchange rates in other animal studies (Khoo *et al.* 1984), suggest that the dominant mechanisms have been identified and that shear-augmented dispersion is largely responsible for the gas exchange observed with HFV. That is not to say, however, that other mechanisms might not be important in devising alternative ventilation strategies or in developing schemes for enhancing the rate of gas exchange with HFV. This area is a continuing area of research and one that should certainly be pursued.

Conclusions

This review describes a collection of idealized model problems which help to elucidate the mechanisms of shear-augmented dispersion in the lung. Although much has been learned, our understanding of augmented transport in systems with more realistic complexity is still developing. Dispersion in other biological systems is at an even more primitive state since relatively few studies have been conducted.

Shear-augmented dispersion continues to be an active area of research. In just the past few years, new issues have been raised; for example, the potential role of chaotic mixing in shear-augmented dispersion (P. E. Hydon, personal communication). Also, though not discussed in this review, powerful new theoretical methods, such as those described in Brenner and Edwards (1993), have not been fully exploited, especially in their application to biological problems. These and other issues promise to make shear-augmented dispersion an important and exciting field of continued research.

The author would like to acknowledge the contributions to this work of many colleagues, but especially those of A. H. Shapiro, M. Johnson, T. J. Pedley and J. M. Drazen. The support for this work comes from the US National Institutes of Health (HL33009) and a grant from the Freeman Foundation.

References

ANDERSSON, B. AND BERGLIN, T. (1981). Dispersion in laminar flow through a circular tube. *Proc. R. Soc. Lond. A* **337**, 251–268.

ARIS, R. (1956). On the dispersion of a solute in a fluid flowing through a tube. *Proc. R. Soc. Lond. A* **235**, 67–77.

BASSINGTHWAIGHTE, J. B. AND GORESKY, C. A. (1984). Modeling in the analysis of solute and water exchange in the microvasculature. In *Handbook of Physiology*, section 2, *The Cardiovascular System*, vol. IV, *Microcirculation*, part 1 (ed. E. M. Renkin, C. C. Michel and S. R. Geiger), pp. 549–626. Bethesda, MA: American Physiological Society.

BRENNER, H. AND EDWARDS, D. A. (1993). *Macrotransport Processes*. Boston: Butterworth-Heinemann.

BRISCOE, W. A., FORSTER, R. E. AND COMROE, J. H. (1954). Alveolar ventilation at very low tidal volumes. *J. appl. Physiol.* **7**, 27–30.

CHATWIN, P. C. (1975). On the longitudinal dispersion of passive contaminant in oscillatory flows in tubes. *J. Fluid Mech.* **71**, 513–527.

DAVIDSON, M. R. AND SCHROTER, R. C. (1983). A theoretical model of absorption of gases by the bronchial wall. *J. Fluid Mech.* **129**, 313–335.

DRAGON, C. A. AND GROTBERG, J. B. (1991). Oscillatory flow and transport in a flexible tube. *J. Fluid Mech.* **231**, 135–155.

DRAZEN, J. M., KAMM, R. D. AND SLUTSKY, A. S. (1984). High frequency ventilation. *Physiol. Rev.* **64**, 505–543.

ECKMANN, D. M. AND GROTBERG, J. B. (1988). Oscillatory flow and mass transport in a curved tube. *J. Fluid Mech.* **188**, 509–527.

ERGODAN, M. E. AND CHATWIN, P. C. (1967). The effects of curvature and buoyancy on the laminar dispersion of solute in a horizontal tube. *J. Fluid Mech.* **29**, 465–484.

FEDERSPIEL, W. J. AND FREDBERG, J. (1988). Axial dispersion in respiratory bronchioles and alveolar ducts. *J. appl. Physiol.* **64**, 2614–2621.

FISCHER, H. B. (1976). Mixing and dispersion in estuaries. *A. Rev. Fluid Mech.* **8**, 107–133.

FRIED, J. J. AND COMBARNOUS, M. A. (1971). Dispersion in porous media. *Adv. Hydrosci.* **7**, 169–282.

FROESE, A. B. AND BRYAN, A. C. (1987). High-frequency ventilation. *Am. Rev. Respir. Dis.* **135**, 1363–1374.

GAVER, D. P., III, SOLWAY, J., PUNJABI, N., ELAD, D., GROTBERG, J. B. AND GAVRIELY, N. (1992). Gas dispersion in volume-cycled tube flow. II. Tracer-bolus experiments. *J. appl. Physiol.* **72**, 321–331.

GAVRIELY, N., SOLWAY, J., DRAZEN, J. M., SLUTSKY, A. S. AND BROWN, R. (1985). Radiographic visualization of airway wall movement during oscillatory flow in dogs. *J. appl. Physiol.* **58**, 645–652.

GODLESKI, D. A. AND GROTBERG, J. B. (1988). Convection–diffusion interaction for oscillatory flow in a tapered tube. *J. Biomech. Eng.* **110**, 283–291.

GROTBERG, J. B. (1994). Pulmonary flow and transport phenomena. *A. Rev. Fluid Mech.* **26**, 529–571.

HARRIS, H. G. AND GOREN, S. L. (1967). Axial diffusion in a cylinder with pulsed flow. *Chem. Eng. Sci.* **22**, 1571–1576.

HEYDER, J., BLANCHARD, J. D., FELDMAN, H. A. AND BRAIN, J. D. (1988). Convective mixing in human respiratory tract: estimates of aerosol boli. *J. appl. Physiol.* **64**, 1273–1278.

HORSFIELD, D. K. AND CUMMING, G. (1968). Functional consequences of airway morphology. *J. appl. Physiol.* **24**, 384–390.

HYDON, P. E. (1991). Modeling the pulmonary circulation and gas transport in the lung. PhD thesis, Cambridge University.

HYDON, P. E. AND PEDLEY, T. J. (1993). Axial disperison in a channel with oscillating walls. *J. Fluid Mech.* **249**, 535–556.

JANSSEN, L. A. M. (1976). Axial dispersion in laminar flow through coiled tubes. *Chem. Eng. Sci.* **31**, 215–218.

JOHNSON, M. AND KAMM, R. D. (1986). Numerical studies of steady flow dispersion at low Dean number in a gently curving tube. *J. Fluid Mech.* **172**, 327–345.

JOSHI, C. H., KAMM, R. D., DRAZEN, J. M. AND SLUTSKY, A. S. (1983). An experimental study of gas exchange in laminar oscillatory flow. *J. Fluid Mech.* **13**, 245–254.

KHOO, M. C. K., SLUTSKY, A. S., DRAZEN, J. M., SOLWAY, J., GAVRIELY, N. AND KAMM, R. D. (1984). Gas mixing during high-frequency ventilation: an improved model. *J. appl. Physiol.* **57**, R493–R506.

KOCH, D. L. AND BRADY, J. F. (1985). Dispersion in fixed beds. *J. Fluid Mech.* **154**, 399–427.

LUNKENHEIMER, P. P., FRANK, L., ISING, H., KELLER, H. AND DICKHUT, H. H. (1972). Intrapulmonaler Gasechsel unter simultierter Apnoe durch Transtrachealen, periodishen intrathorakealen Druckweechsel. *Anesthetist* **22**, 232–238.

NIGAM, K. D. P. AND VASUDEVA, K. (1976). Influence of curvature and pulsations on laminar dispersion. *Chem. Eng. Sci.* **31**, 835–837.

PALOSKI, W. H., SLOSBERG, R. B. AND KAMM, R. D. (1987). Effects of gas properties and waveform asymmetry on gas transport in a branching tube network. *J. appl. Physiol.* **62**, 892–901.

PEDLEY, T. J. AND KAMM, R. D. (1988). The effect of secondary motion on axial transport in oscillatory tube flow. *J. Fluid Mech.* **193**, 347–367.

PEDLEY, T. J. AND KAMM, R. D. (1991). Dynamics of gas flow and pressure–flow relationships. In *The Lung: Scientific Fouundations*, vol. 1 (ed. R. C. Crystal and J. B. West), pp. 995–1010. New York: Raven Press.

PROBSTEIN, R. F. (1994). *Physicochemical Hydrodynamics: An Introduction*. New York: John Wiley and Sons, Inc. pp. 82–103.

SCHERER, P. W. AND HASELTON, F. R. (1982). Convective exchange in oscillatory flow through bronchial-tree models. *J. appl. Physiol.* **53**, R1023–R1033.

SHARP, M. K., KAMM, R. D., SHAPIRO, A. H., KIMMEL, E. AND KARNIADAKIS, G. E. (1991). Dispersion in a curved tube during oscillatory flow. *J. Fluid Mech.* **223**, 537–563.

SHETTY, V. D. AND VASUDEVA, K. (1977). Effect of Schmidt number on laminar disperison in helical coils. *Chem. Eng. Sci.* **32**, 782–783.

TARBELL, J. M., ULTMAN, J. S. AND DURLOFSKY, L. (1982). Oscillatory dispersion in a branching tube network. *J. Biomech. Eng.* **104**, 338–342.

TAYLOR, G. I. (1921). Diffusion by continuous movements. *Proc. Lond. math. Soc. 2* **20**, 196–212.

TAYLOR, G. I. (1953). Dispersion of solute matter in solvent flowing through a tube. *Proc. R. Soc. Lond. A* **219**, 186–203.

TAYLOR, G. I. (1954). The dispersion of matter in turbulent flow through a pipe. *Proc. R. Soc. Lond. A* **225**, 473–477.

TRIVEDI, R. N. AND VASUDEVA, K. (1975). Axial dispersion in laminar flow in helocal coils. *Chem. Eng. Sci.* **30**, 317–325.

ULTMAN, J. S. (1981). Gas mixing in the pulmonary airways. *Ann. Biomed. Eng.* **9**, 513–527.

ULTMAN, J. S. (1985). Gas transport in the conducting airways. In *Gas Mixing and Distribution in the Lung* (ed. L. A. Engel and M. Paiva), pp. 63–136. New York: Marcel Dekker.

ULTMAN, J. S., DOLL, B. E., SPIEGEL, R. AND THOMAS, M. W. (1978). Longitudinal mixing in pulmonary airways – normal subjects respiring at a constant flow rate. *J. appl. Physiol.* **44**, 297–303.

VAN ANDEL, E., KRAMERS, H. AND VOOGD, A. (1964). The residence time distribution of laminar flow in curved tubes. *Chem. Eng. Sci.* **19**, 77–78.

VAN DEN BERG, J. H. M. AND DEELDER, R. S. (1979). Measurements of axial dispersion in laminar flow through coiled capillary tubes. *Chem. Eng. Sci.* **34**, 1345–1347.

VENEGAS, J. G., HALES, C. A. AND STRIEDER, D. J. (1986). A general dimensionless equation of gas transport by high-frequency ventilation. *J. appl. Physiol.* **60**, 1025–1030.

WATSON, E. J. (1983). Diffusion in oscillatory pipe flow. *J. Fluid Mech.* **133**, 233–244.

YU, C. P. (1975). On equation of gas transport in the lung. *Respir. Physiol.* **23**, 257–266.

ZIERLER, K. L. (1962). Circulation times and the theory of indicator-dilution methods for determining blood flow and volume. In *Handbook of Physiology*, section 2, *The Circulation*, vol. I (ed. W. F. Hamilton and P. Dow), pp. 585–616. Washington, DC: American Physiological Society.

PRESSURE *VERSUS* FLOW IN BIOLOGICAL PUMPS

STEVEN VOGEL

Department of Zoology, Box 90325, Duke University, Durham, NC 27708, USA

Summary

The pumps with which organisms move fluids span nearly a ten-million-fold pressure range. As in human technology, positive displacement pumps (osmotic, valve-and-chamber, peristaltic, etc.) are used for high-pressure applications and fluid dynamic pumps (using hydrofoils, cilia, aspirators, etc.) for low pressures. But while pressure capability or system resistance dichotomizes pumps by operative mechanism, the values of a dimensionless pressure–flow index prove more relevant to their biological roles; this index is a ratio of overall pressure drop in the system to pressure drop due to viscous resistance to flow.

Introduction

Whether moving air or water, whether lifting sap or suspension feeding, whether involved in propulsion or circulation, all living pumps generate fluid motion against some opposing pressure. But in practice this common function has been obscured by the diversity of sizes, mechanisms and applications of the pumps.

For any pump, power output is the product of pressure change across it and volume flow through it. Almost all biological pumps driving internal flows operate at Reynolds numbers sufficiently low that volume flow is proportional to pressure drop, as with current and voltage in ohmic electrical circuits. Thus, we can define resistance as pressure drop divided by volume flow:

$$P = Q\Delta p = Q^2R = (\Delta p)^2/R\,, \tag{1}$$

where P is power, Q is volume flow, Δp is pressure change and R is resistance. Were power output constant, a graph of pressure change *versus* volume flow would be hyperbolic.

In fact, as shown in Fig. 1, output is ordinarily quite sensitive to operating load – most pumps develop maximal pressure at zero flow, maximal flow at negligible opposing pressure, and maximal power output somewhere between these extremes. While an organism might use a pump anywhere within the area defined by its pressure–flow capability line, the resistance of the system in which it works ordinarily sets more restricted conditions. The best it can do is thus the intersection of the system resistance and the output lines. While this point ought perhaps to align vertically with the peak of its power output curve, organisms are commonly biased towards volume flows a little greater than those that maximize power output (Foster-Smith, 1978).

A fixed, linear, origin-based resistance line, though, is merely the simplest case and

Key words: pumps, flow, pressure, jet, heart, circulation, transpiration, suction feeding.

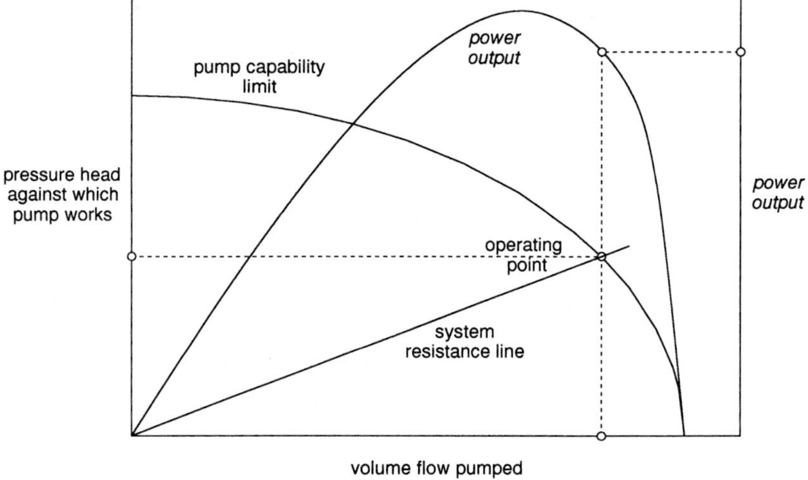

Fig. 1. The interrelationships among pressure, volume flow, power output and optimal operating point for a pump.

cannot be casually assumed to be applicable. Thus (i) turbulent flow will be characterized by an approximately parabolic curve – increasing flow takes a disproportionately increasing pressure. The value of the Reynolds number, 2000, commonly given for the onset of turbulent flow in a pipe is more of a best case scenario. The transition value will be lowered by such ordinary things as abrupt changes in diameter, bifurcations and flow through apertures. (ii) Some systems may have a fixed minimal pressure load whatever the flow, one to which fluid dynamic resistance then adds. For instance, in the evaporative sap-lifter of trees, gravity imposes a basic pressure drop of 101 kPa (1 atmosphere) for every 10 m of height. And (iii), biological conduits are not just passive plumbing. Thus, circulatory systems make major changes in their peripheral resistance in response to a host of factors, both normal and pathological.

Matching pumps and applications

If a pump produces a substantial flow with only a slight investment in pressure, it is best suited (as is evident from the Q^2R term in equation 1) for working in a system of conduits having a low resistance. If, by contrast, the pump generates a lot of pressure but only a limited flow, it is most suitable [from $(\Delta p)^2/R$] for systems of high resistance. Resistance, $\Delta p/Q$, is thus a measure of a pump's relative investment in pressure and flow.

In technological practice, the choice of pump depends strongly on the intended apportionment of output. Pumps are usually divided into two general categories – positive displacement (or hydrostatic) pumps and fluid dynamic (or hydrodynamic, rotodynamic or kinetic) pumps. (See, for instance, Karassik *et al.* 1976; Massey, 1989.) In positive displacement pumps, the fluid is introduced into a chamber whose volume is then reduced, and the fluid leaves through some pre-arranged opening; they are capable of generating high pressures and are thus most suitable for high-resistance applications.

Examples include piston pumps (manual tyre inflators, for instance), diaphragm pumps (many automotive fuel pumps), vane or gear pumps (many automotive oil pumps) and peristaltic pumps (analogous to biological ones).

Fluid dynamic pumps, by contrast, are most appropriate for low-resistance systems except when used in extensively serial arrangements, as in the axial compressors of jet engines. Even so, their performance spans a wide resistance range. Thus, pumps with centrifugal impellers (such as 'squirrel cage' fans) will work better against more resistive loads than do pumps with axial impellers (ordinary radial fan blades). Whether they fling fluid outwards or thrust it forwards, fluid dynamic pumps depend on the interactions of a moving fluid with solid surfaces or other fluids. A few do not depend on a rotating impeller – jet pumps use a fast flow through a nozzle to entrain another stream of fluid, and aspirators use a flow-induced pressure decrease to draw in another fluid.

This same dichotomization of both category and application proves applicable to the pumps used by organisms to move air and water through and around themselves. Table 1 lists a series of pumps used by organisms, divided into positive displacement and fluid dynamic devices and arranged in descending order of estimated system resistance.

Without a doubt, the evaporative pumps of tall plants exceed all others in the pressures they generate – values of up to 12 MPa (120 atmospheres) have been measured (Schlesinger *et al.* 1982). That these are negative pressures, drawing sap up from below the pump rather than pushing it higher, is no major matter here. Cellular osmotic pumps in parallel array can pump at substantial rates, as in generating root pressure in plants or in water transport *via* what Diamond and Bossert (1967) called 'standing gradient osmotic flow'. Valve-and-chamber devices may span the widest range of pressures of any kind of biological pump – from a mere 90 Pa in the burrow of the parchment worm *Chaetopterus variopedatus* (Riisgård, 1989) to over 30 kPa in the heart of a giraffe or the mantle cavity of a squid. Peristaltic pumps perform various tasks in digestive and circulatory systems as well as driving flow though the sand-occluded burrow of at least one annelid, *Arenicola*

Table 1. *Various kinds of pumps used in biological systems, arranged in descending order of estimated impedance during ordinary operation*

Pump type	Category	System resistance	Examples
Evaporative	Positive displacement	Highest	Evaporative sap lifter
Osmotic	Positive displacement	Very high	Root pressure sap pusher
Valve/chamber	Positive displacement	High	Heart, bird lungs, squid jet
Peristaltic	Positive displacement	High	Intestine, some worm hearts
Piston	Positive displacement	Medium	Some tubicolous worms
Vane or gear	Positive displacement	Medium	Other tubicolous worms
Valveless/chamber	Positive displacement	Medium	Jellyfish jet, mammalian lung
Drag-based paddles	Fluid dynamic	Medium	Crustaceans in burrows
Lift-based propellers	Fluid dynamic	Low	Hive-ventilating honeybees
Ciliary layer	Fluid dynamic	Low	Bivalve gills
Flagellar	Fluid dynamic	Low	Sponge choanocytes
Venturi aspirator	Fluid dynamic	Very low	Prairie dog burrow

marina, at about 1200 Pa (Foster-Smith, 1978). Burrow pumps using metachronal parapodia, in some other annelids, are closely analogous to vane or gear pumps. Bidirectional pumps, such as we use to ventilate our lungs, are essentially piston pumps without rectifying check-valves.

While the fluid dynamic pumps of organisms are more distant in appearance from their technological analogs than are the positive displacement pumps, both functional and applicational analogies are close. For such a pump, 90 Pa is a high pressure – a burrowing echinoderm, *Echinocardium cordatum*, manages it with a lengthy serial arrangement of cilia (Foster-Smith, 1978), the same solution as the jet engine's axial compressor. A burrowing amphipod crustacean, *Corophium volutator*, produces about 40 Pa by using its pleopods as paddles (Foster-Smith, 1978). 10–20 Pa is typical of the ciliary and flagellar pumps of suspension-feeding bivalve molluscs and sponges. And the various aspirators with which ambient flows are used to drive internal flows – as in sponges and prairie-dog burrows – operate at pressures below about 10 Pa (Vogel, 1978; Vogel *et al.* 1973).

If velocity were all that mattered, a circulatory system such as our own might be driven by ciliated capillaries, eliminating any need for a critical central pump. But resistance matters as much, a point missed by LaBarbera and Vogel (1982). Ciliary pumps, as fluid dynamic devices, are quite unsuitable for generating the pressures needed to force sufficient flow through the capillary beds of large, active animals.

A dimensionless index for pump performance

Matching pump type and system resistance may be as important for natural as for human technology, but resistance is a less useful quantitative variable for living systems. The principal difficulty lies in the dimensionality of system resistance and the wide size range of organisms. Whether using pressure or force, mass flow or volume flow, resistance involves some inverse power of length. If a pump capable of a given pressure difference is made smaller and its volumetric output decreases in proportion, the system resistance for which it is appropriate will rise. For example, for the hearts of mammals of small and moderate size, output flow is proportional to body mass to the power 0.81 (Schmidt-Nielsen, 1984) and output pressure is nearly constant. So a decrease in size from 10 kg to 10 g yields a 300-fold resistance increase. But the smaller mammal has a higher specific metabolic rate, a shorter length of circulatory circuit and a shorter circulation time – the higher resistance is misleading.

Is there a less size-contaminated variable? The essential element of resistance is the ratio of pressure needed to flow achieved. A dimensionless version of that ratio is used for expressing the distribution of pressure around bodies in flows – the pressure coefficient, C_p:

$$C_p = 2\Delta p/\rho U^2\,, \tag{2}$$

where ρ is fluid density and U is velocity.

But using the pressure coefficient entails two problems. First, it is most useful at high Reynolds numbers, where resistance is proportional to fluid density and the square of velocity. Second, the presence of velocity is awkward. Flow speeds in the internal fluid transport systems in organisms vary enormously from place to place without fully concomitant pressure changes, so the value of C_p will depend strongly on location in the system. Using the pump as a standard location is unsatisfactory, since pumps such as hearts are located where speeds are greatest while others such as ciliated gills are associated with minimal speeds.

One alternative is to replace the denominator, dynamic pressure, by a viscous resistance. The latter is, of course, proportional to flow speed and more appropriate for internal flows at low Reynolds numbers. An appropriate pressure–flow index I can be obtained by simplifying any operational definition of viscosity:

$$I = \Delta pt/\mu, \qquad (3)$$

where t is time and μ is dynamic viscosity.

The main uncertainty is now the interpretation of time. Its role is that of a rate or lengthless velocity in the denominator – the ratio is still one of pressure to flow, more specifically overall pressure drop in the system to pressure drop due to viscous resistance to flow. Thus, the most useful (if still somewhat arbitrary) interpretation is as the transit or residence time for a quantity of fluid as it passes through the parts of the system that contribute significantly to its resistance. For systems with well-distributed resistances, such as our circulatory system or the internal conduits of a sponge (LaBarbera, 1990), t is then the time needed for a pass through the entire system. For systems with locally concentrated resistance, such as the siphon in a jetting squid, t is the time needed to pass through that particular element.

Other pressure–flow indices can be easily contrived, but the variables of the present one seem to give the fewest problems of interpretation, of comparability in a diversity of systems and of being commonly or easily measured. For instance, since $\Delta p = RQ$, and the volume V of the system is, at least nominally, Qt, the index is equal to RV/μ. But consistent definition of system volume is not easily achieved.

Table 2 gives a selection of values of this pressure–flow index; some educated estimation was used in deriving transit times from anatomical information and total flow or speed, but few problems were associated with picking operating points for individual systems. Where the system resistance line (Fig. 1) is linear and origin-based, time will be inversely proportional to pressure, and the index will remain constant.

While scaling pumps by maximum pressure (Table 1) divided them by operative mechanism, scaling them with the pressure–flow index divides them more nearly by biological application. Values for all hearts are above 10^6 or, taking compound avian and mammalian hearts as single pumps, above 10^7. Values for pumps driving the main feeding activities of animals are below 10^6 and for those used for jet propulsion below 10^5. A few additional but equally preliminary generalizations follow; others may occur to readers of different background and perspective. While these points may be either self-evident or speculative, what matters here is that they emerge from consideration of a single parameter.

The index will be high for any system faced with a substantial gravitational load such as any large, terrestrial, liquid-pumping system that does not recirculate with siphoning – mainly sap ascent in tall plants and circulation in large mammals.

Table 2. *The pressure–flow index for a variety of biological pumps, arranged in descending order of the index*

Pump	Pressure (Pa)	Transit time (s)	Index	Reference
Liquid pumps				
Sap-lifter, red oak (*Quercus rubra*)	500 000	3 000	1.5×10^{12}	Zimmermann (1971)
Heart, pulmonate snail (*Helix pomatia*)	2 500	400	1.0×10^{9}	Jones (1983)
Heart, trout (*Salmo gairdneri*)	4 300	170	7.3×10^{8}	Jones and Randall (1978)
Heart, systemic (*Octopus vulgaris*)	2 500	120	3.0×10^{8}	Wells (1983)
Heart, systemic (Human)	13 000	50	1.9×10^{8}	Textbook values
Heart, crab (*Cancer magister*)	2 000	75	1.5×10^{8}	McMahon and Burnett (1990)
Heart, systemic (Chicken)	19 000	3.9	3.8×10^{7}	Jones and Johansen (1972)
Heart, pulmonary (Human)	2 500	5	3.6×10^{6}	Textbook values
Heart, pulmonary (Chicken)	3 600	0.6	1.1×10^{6}	Jones and Johansen (1972)
Nectar-feeding, butterfly (*Colias eurytheme*)	70 000	0.02	7.0×10^{5}	Kingsolver and Daniel (1979)
Urethral pump, (Human male)	4 000	0.10	5.6×10^{5}	Glemain *et al.* (1990)
Worm burrow piston pump (*Chaetopterus variopedatus*)	90	10	9.0×10^{5}	Riisgård (1989)
Pumped fish gills (*Micropterus salmoides*)	30	20	6.0×10^{5}	Lauder (1984)
Suction-feeding, sunfish (*Lepomis macrochirus*)	14 000	0.02	2.8×10^{5}	Lauder and Lanyon (1980)
Blood-sucking, louse (*Pediculus humanus*)	25 000	0.01	9.2×10^{4}	Daniel and Kingsolver (1983)
Ram-ventilated gills, tuna (*Katsuwonus pelamis*)	300	0.25	8.5×10^{4}	Stevens and Lightfoot (1986)
Jet, squid (*Loligo vulgaris*)	30 000	0.0025	7.5×10^{4}	Trueman and Packard (1968)
Suspension feeding, mussel (*Mytilus* sp.)	13	2.5	3.2×10^{4}	Meyhöfer (1985); Jørgensen (1989)
Suspension feeding, sponge (*Haliclona viridis*)	10	2.5	2.5×10^{4}	Vogel (1978)
Blood-sucking, bug (*Rhodnius prolixus*)	550 000	0.0004	2.2×10^{4}	Bennet-Clark (1963)
Jet, jellyfish (*Polyorchis penicillatus*)	30	0.5	1.5×10^{4}	Demont and Gosline (1988)
Air pumps				
Lung inflation (Human)	5 000	0.3	8.3×10^{7}	Textbook values
Lung inflation, lizard (*Gekko gekko*)	250	3.0	4.4×10^{7}	Milsom (1984)
Air-aspiration (Polypterid fishes)	680	0.3	1.1×10^{7}	Brainerd *et al.* (1989)
Burrow ventilation, prairie dog (*Cynomys ludovicianus*)	0.1	150	8.3×10^{5}	Vogel *et al.* (1973)

The hearts of birds and mammals operate at higher pressures than those of other animals. But, to move adequate volumes, their systemic hearts must operate at values of the pressure–flow index relatively low for valve-and-chamber hearts – their circulations must use short capillaries and arterioles, with many of each in parallel, for instance. Conversely, small or inactive animals that invest little in either construction or operation of a circulation can tolerate higher values. Thus, assuming linear resistances, reducing the transit time for trout to the value for mammals of the same size (around 3 s) just by raising pressure would require pressures of several atmospheres.

In fully serial circulations, the volume of blood contained in each circuit, pulmonary and systemic, must be proportional to the transit time. Thus, transit times in the pulmonary circuit must be kept low; but that is more safely done with low volumes than with high pressures. Consequently, pulmonary circuits must operate at lower values of the index.

The present index ought to vary inversely with Froude propulsion efficiency – in essence a measure of volume output *versus* velocity output (Vogel, 1994); and velocity will ordinarily vary with pressure. In short, if a jet-propelled animal has to be energetically competitive with ones using fins or flukes, it must maintain a low pressure–flow index.

Suspension feeding generally requires the movement of a lot of water to obtain a fairly small yield of food. That makes keeping the pressure–flow index low – investing in flow rather than pressure – especially urgent, by using filters of very large area and low resistance, even at some loss of filtration efficiency or ability to trap particles of diverse sizes.

The use of ambient flows as pumps (as in burrow ventilation of prairie dogs) or to augment active pumping (as in sponges) should be anticipated only in systems with intrinsically low pressure–flow indices. When inducing secondary flows, neither Bernoulli's principle nor viscous entrainment can generate very high pressures, although either is capable of moving substantial volumes of fluid (Vogel, 1994).

The striking similarity of the indices for respiratory air-pumping may be largely coincidental, but their elevation above those for gill ventilation probably reflects a real difference between the concentrations of oxygen in air and in water. Where the underlying resource is richer, higher values should be tolerable.

References

BENNET-CLARK, H. C. (1963). Negative pressures produced in the pharyngeal pump of the blood-sucking bug, *Rhodnius prolixus*. *J. exp. Biol.* **40**, 223–229.

BRAINERD, E. L., LIEM, K. F. AND SAMPER, C. T. (1989). Air ventilation by recoil aspiration in polypterid fishes. *Science* **246**, 1593–1595.

DANIEL, T. L. AND KINGSOLVER, J. G. (1983). Feeding strategy and the mechanics of blood sucking in insects. *J. theor. Biol.* **105**, 661–672.

DEMONT, M. E. AND GOSLINE, J. M. (1988). Mechanics of jet propulsion in the hydromedusan jellyfish, *Polyorchis penicillatus*. II. Energetics of the jet cycle. *J. exp. Biol.* **134**, 333–345.

DIAMOND, J. M. AND BOSSERT, W. H. (1967). Standing-gradient osmotic flow. *J. gen. Physiol.* **50**, 2061–2083.

FOSTER-SMITH, R. L. (1978). An analysis of water flow in tube-living animals. *J. exp. mar. Biol. Ecol.* **34**, 73–95.

GLEMAIN, P., CORDONNIER, J. P., LENORMAND, L. AND BUZELIN, J. M. (1990). Urodynamic consequences of urethral stenosis: hydrodynamic study with a theoretical model. *J. d'Urol.* **96**, 271–277.

JONES, D. R. AND JOHANSEN, K. (1972). The blood vascular system of birds. In *Avian Biology* (ed. D. S. Farner and J. R. King), pp. 158–265. New York: Academic Press.

JONES, D. R. AND RANDALL, D. J. (1978). The respiratory and circulatory systems during exercise. In *Fish Physiology*, vol. 7 (ed. W. S. Hoar and D. J. Randall), pp. 425–501. New York: Academic Press.

JONES, H. D. (1983). Circulatory systems of gastropods and bivalves. In *The Mollusca*, vol. 5 (ed. K. M. Wilbur), pp. 189–238. New York: Academic Press.

JØRGENSEN, C. B. (1989). Water processing in ciliary feeders with special reference to the bivalve filter pump. *Comp. Biochem. Physiol.* A **94**, 383–394.

KARASSIK, I. J., KRUTZSCH, W. C., FRAZER, W. H. AND MESSINA, J. P. (1976). *Pump Handbook.* New York: McGraw Hill.

KINGSOLVER, J. G. AND DANIEL, T. L. (1979). On the mechanics and energetics of nectar feeding in butterflies. *J. theor. Biol.* **76**, 167–179.

LABARBERA, M. (1990). Principles of design of fluid transport systems in zoology. *Science* **249**, 992–1000.

LABARBERA, M. AND VOGEL, S. (1982). The design of fluid transport systems in organisms. *Am. Sci.* **70**, 54–60.

LAUDER, G. V. (1984). Pressure and water flow patterns in the respiratory tract of the bass (*Micropterus salmoides*). *J. exp. Biol.* **113**, 151–164.

LAUDER, G. V. AND LANYON, L. E. (1980). Functional anatomy of feeding in the bluegill sunfish, *Lepomis macrochirus*: *in vivo* measurement of bone strain. *J. exp. Biol.* **84**, 33–55.

MASSEY, B. S. (1989). *Mechanics of Fluids*, sixth edn. London: Van Nostrand Reinhold.

MCMAHON, B. R. AND BURNETT, L. E. (1990). The crustacean open circulatory system: a reexamination. *Physiol. Zool.* **63**, 35–71.

MEYHÖFER, E. (1985). Comparative pumping rates in suspension-feeding bivalves. *Mar. Biol.* **85**, 137–142.

MILSOM, W. K. (1984). The interrelationship between pulmonary mechanics and the spontaneous breathing pattern in the Tokay lizard, *Gekko gekko*. *J. exp. Biol.* **113**, 203–214.

RIISGÅRD, H. U. (1989). Properties and energy cost of the muscular piston pump in the suspension feeding polychaete *Chaetopterus variopedatus*. *Mar. Ecol. Progr. Ser.* **56**, 157–168.

SCHLESINGER, W. H., GRAY, J. T., GILL, D. S. AND MAHALL, B. E. (1982). *Ceanothus megacarpus* chaparral: a synthesis of ecosystem processes during development and annual growth. *Bot. Rev.* **48**, 71–117.

SCHMIDT-NIELSEN, K. (1984). *Scaling: Why is Animal Size So Important?* Cambridge, UK: Cambridge University Press.

STEVENS, E. D. AND LIGHTFOOT, E. N. (1986). Hydrodynamics of water flow in front of and through the gills of skipjack tuna. *Comp. Biochem. Physiol.* A **83**, 255–259.

TRUEMAN, E. R. AND PACKARD, A. (1968). Motor performance of some cephalopods. *J. exp. Biol.* **49**, 495–507.

VOGEL, S. (1978). Evidence for one-way valves in the water-flow system of sponges. *J. exp. Biol.* **76**, 137–148.

VOGEL, S. (1994). *Life in Moving Fluids*, 2nd edn. Princeton: Princeton University Press.

VOGEL, S., ELLINGTON, C. P. AND KILGORE, D. C., JR (1973). Wind-induced ventilation of the burrow of the prairie dog, *Cynomys ludovicianus*. *J. comp. Physiol.* **85**, 1–14.

WELLS, M. J. (1983). Circulation in cephalopods. In *The Mollusca*, vol. 5 (ed. K. M. Wilbur), pp. 239–290. New York: Academic Press.

ZIMMERMANN, M. H. (1971). Transport in the xylem. In *Trees: Structure and Function* (ed. M. H. Zimmermann and C. L. Brown), pp. 169–220. New York: Springer-Verlag.

MECHANICS OF BLOOD FLOW IN THE MICROCIRCULATION

T. W. SECOMB

Department of Physiology, University of Arizona, Tucson, AZ 85724, USA

Summary

The microcirculation in most tissues consists of an intricate network of very narrow tubes. In analyses of blood flow through the microcirculation, inertial effects can be neglected, but continuum models for blood cannot be assumed, since blood is a concentrated suspension of cells with dimensions comparable to vessel diameters. These cells strongly influence blood flow. About 45 % of blood volume consists of red blood cells, whose key mechanical properties are known. A red cell has a fluid interior, surrounded by a flexible membrane, which strongly resists area changes, but bends and shears easily. White blood cells are comparable in size but much less numerous. They are less flexible than red cells and capable of active locomotion. Other suspended elements are much smaller than red cells.

This review focuses on the mechanics of red cell motion in the microcirculation. Experimental and theoretical studies of blood flow in uniform tubes, bifurcations and networks are discussed. Comparisons between predicted and observed flows in networks imply that resistance to blood flow in living microvessels is higher than that in uniform tubes with corresponding diameters. Living microvessels have non-uniform geometries, and red cells must deform continually to traverse them. Theoretical results are presented implying that these transient deformations contribute to increased flow resistance in the microcirculation.

Introduction

In most tissues, blood passes from the arterial side to the venous side of the circulatory system *via* an intricate network of microvessels, called the microcirculation. These vessels are responsible for exchange of materials between blood and surrounding tissues and cause most of the resistance to blood flow in the circulatory system. Therefore, the mechanics of blood flow in the microcirculation largely determines the workload of the heart and strongly influences material exchange in the circulatory system.

The microvessels can be classified into three main types: arterioles, capillaries and venules. Capillaries, with diameters in the range 3–10 μm, are the smallest. They are connected to the feeding arteries by arterioles and to the veins by venules. Arterioles and venules are larger than capillaries, with diameters up to about 100 μm.

The structure of the microcirculation varies from one tissue to another. In some tissues, the structure is not as described above. In the lungs and in the retina of the eye, capillaries form a dense mesh that is better described as a sheet than as a network (Fung, 1984).

Key words: microcirculation, blood flow, red blood cells, capillaries, flow resistance, blood rheology, lubrication theory, fluid mechanics.

Kidney and liver microcirculations have specialized anatomies reflecting their functions for exchange of materials. Nonetheless, the microcirculations of many tissues, including skeletal and cardiac muscles, brain and intestines, can be adequately described as networks of arterioles, capillaries and venules, and such structures are considered here.

The small diameters of microvessels imply small Reynolds numbers for blood flow, usually much less than 1. Therefore, inertial effects are negligible. Blood is not a homogeneous fluid, but a concentrated suspension of cells. In large blood vessels, a continuum description of the rheological properties of the blood is generally appropriate. However, microvessel diameters are comparable to blood cell dimensions. The resulting non-continuum behavior of blood in microvessels gives rise to a number of physiologically important phenomena and complicates the flow mechanics.

This review describes first the mechanics of blood constituents, then flow in microvessels, bifurcations and networks, and transient deformations of red cells in the microcirculation. Coverage of these topics is not comprehensive. In particular, the focus is on the mechanics of red blood cell motion, and the behavior of other blood cells is only briefly mentioned.

Mechanics of blood constituents

Blood is a suspension of cells in plasma. The plasma, a solution of proteins, electrolytes and other substances, is an incompressible, virtually Newtonian fluid. The cells are red blood cells (erythrocytes), white blood cells (leukocytes) of several different types and platelets. Normal human blood has a hematocrit (volume fraction of red cells) of about 45 %, and so red cells strongly influence the flow properties of blood.

The mechanical properties of human red blood cells have been studied extensively and are probably known better than those of any other cell type (see Skalak, 1976; Hochmuth and Waugh, 1987). A thin membrane surrounds the cytoplasm, which is essentially an incompressible Newtonian fluid. The membrane, consisting of a lipid bilayer and a cytoskeleton (network of protein molecules), exhibits viscoelastic properties. The elastic shear modulus (about $6\times10^{-6}\,\mathrm{N\,m^{-1}}$) is several orders of magnitude lower than the modulus of isotropic dilation (about $0.5\,\mathrm{N\,m^{-1}}$) and so the membrane shears readily but resists area changes. Also, bending resistance is small unless very small radii of curvature are involved; the bending modulus is about $1.8\times10^{-19}\,\mathrm{N\,m}$ (Evans, 1983). In transient deformations, the membrane exhibits a shear viscosity. A Kelvin solid model can be used to describe the viscoelastic behavior of the membrane, with the total stress represented as the sum of viscous and elastic contributions (Evans and Hochmuth, 1976).

In the absence of external stresses, a human red cell is a biconcave disk, approximately 8 μm in diameter and 2 μm thick. As a result of its fluid interior, and of the low resistance of its membrane to shear and bending deformations, it is highly deformable, as long as changes in surface area or volume are not required. This allows it to pass through capillaries with diameters much less than 8 μm. However, the incompressibility of the interior and the strong resistance of the membrane to area changes limit the deformations that a red cell can undergo. They imply a minimum diameter for tubes that will permit a red cell to pass through intact. For a typical human red cell, this diameter is about 2.8 μm (Canham and Burton, 1968; Halpern and Secomb, 1989).

In blood of humans and many other species, red cells spontaneously adhere to each other to form aggregates, unless flow forces are sufficient to keep them dispersed. Aggregation results from bridging of cells by plasma proteins or other macromolecules (Chien, 1975). Terminal segments of the macromolecules are adsorbed onto the surfaces of two adjacent cells, binding them together. The mechanics of aggregation may be analyzed in terms of the balance of energies involved in macromolecular bridging, electrostatic repulsion between cells, mechanical deformation of cells and external flow forces (Skalak *et al.* 1981).

Mechanical properties of red cells are modified in several diseases, including sickle cell anemia (Chien, 1977*b*), malaria (Nash *et al.* 1989), diabetes (Schmid-Schönbein and Volger, 1976) and sepsis (Hurd *et al.* 1988). Red cells' mechanical properties are also influenced by blood acidity (Chien, 1975) and oxygenation (Hakim and Macek, 1988). The aggregation tendency of red cells depends strongly on the composition of the plasma, especially its content of ions and proteins (Chien, 1975), and is modified in many diseases (Dintenfass, 1976). Viscometric testing shows that many of these changes in red cell properties significantly influence blood rheology. However, the consequences for blood flow in the microcirculation are not well understood, presenting an important challenge and motivation for studies in this field.

White blood cells are comparable in size to red blood cells but much less numerous. They are much stiffer than red cells and may contribute significantly to microvascular flow resistance (Schmid-Schönbein *et al.* 1981). The mechanical properties of white cells have been discussed by Yeung and Evans (1989) and Schmid-Schönbein (1990). Under normal physiological conditions, white cells frequently roll along the walls of venules. This motion is a consequence both of hydrodynamic effects and of specific molecular interactions between white cells and the endothelial cells lining the venules (Ley and Gaehtgens, 1991; Nazziola and House, 1992). In inflammatory reactions, white cells adhere to the endothelial cells and migrate between them by pseudopod formation and diapedesis, a form of active locomotion.

Platelets, which are essential to the blood's clotting process, are much smaller than red cells and do not contribute significantly to flow resistance. They are preferentially distributed near microvessel walls, probably as a result of hydrodynamic interactions with red cells (Tangelder *et al.* 1985).

Resistance to blood flow in microvessels

The resistance to blood flow through a vessel or a vascular bed is defined as the ratio of the driving pressure Δp to the volume flow rate Q. For steady laminar flow of a Newtonian fluid in a cylindrical tube, Q is related to Δp according to the relationship (known as Poiseuille's Law):

$$Q = \frac{\pi}{128} \frac{\Delta p D^4}{L\mu}, \tag{1}$$

where L is the tube length, D is the diameter and μ is the fluid viscosity. This may be used to estimate the flow resistance in blood vessels with diameters of about 500 μm or more, using values of μ obtained from bulk measurements. In microvessels, however, blood does not behave as a continuum, and μ is not a known constant. Instead, equation 1 is rearranged to define the *apparent viscosity*:

$$\mu_{\mathrm{app}} = \frac{\pi}{128} \frac{\Delta p D^4}{QL} . \tag{2}$$

The *relative apparent viscosity* is defined as $\mu_{\mathrm{rel}}=\mu_{\mathrm{app}}/\mu_{\mathrm{p}}$, where μ_{p} is the viscosity of the plasma or other suspending fluid. These parameters are useful for describing resistance to blood flow.

Starting with Martini *et al.* (1930) and Fåhraeus and Lindqvist (1931), numerous studies have been made of the apparent viscosity of blood in narrow glass tubes. As tube diameter decreases below about 500 μm, apparent viscosity declines to levels substantially lower than the bulk viscosity. This is known as the Fåhraeus–Lindqvist effect. Fig. 1 shows the empirical relationship between μ_{rel} and diameter for red cell suspensions with a hematocrit of 45 % in glass tubes (from Pries *et al.* 1992). For diameters of 5–10 μm, μ_{rel} is below 1.3, i.e. the apparent viscosity is less than 30 % greater than that of plasma. Below this diameter range, μ_{rel} increases rapidly as the minimum diameter for red cell passage is approached.

The reduced apparent viscosity of blood in narrow glass tubes results primarily from the tendency of red cells to migrate away from the tube wall in flow, creating a layer of zero or low hematocrit adjacent to the wall (Fung, 1981). This 'wall effect' reduces flow resistance because red cells interfere less with the flow if they are absent from the region near the wall, where the highest shear stresses occur. A further consequence is that the slowly moving fluid near the wall consists mainly of plasma, and so the mean red cell velocity exceeds the mean blood flow velocity. The mean transit time of red cells is

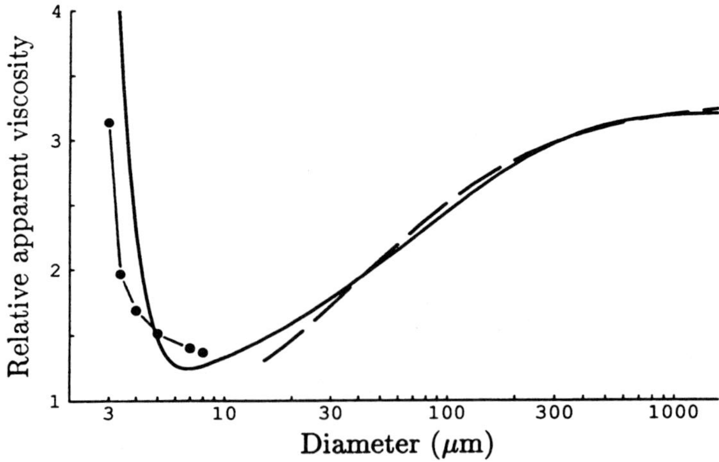

Fig. 1. Relative apparent viscosity of blood as a function of tube diameter for a discharge hematocrit of 45 %. Solid curve, empirical fit to experimental data for blood flow in glass tubes (Pries *et al.* 1992). Filled circles, theoretical predictions, cell velocity=1 mm s^{-1} (Secomb *et al.* 1986; Halpern and Secomb, 1989). Dashed curve, equation 4 with δ=1.8 μm.

therefore less than the overall mean transit time, implying that the concentration of red cells within the tube (tube hematocrit) is less than the concentration in the blood entering or leaving the tube (discharge hematocrit). This dynamic reduction of hematocrit in narrow tubes is called the Fåhraeus effect (Fåhraeus, 1928).

Direct measurements of apparent viscosity of blood in microvessels in living tissues are technically extremely difficult, requiring simultaneous pressure measurements at two points within a single microvessel. Lipowsky *et al.* (1978) performed such measurements in the cat mesentery and obtained estimates of apparent viscosity substantially higher than those observed in glass tubes with corresponding diameters. Further evidence for such a discrepancy between *in vitro* and *in vivo* apparent viscosities of blood was obtained by Pries *et al.* (1990) on the basis of observations and theoretical simulations of flow in microvascular networks of the rat mesentery. Possible explanations will be discussed later. First, the mechanics of blood flow in microvessels is discussed in more detail.

Mechanics of single-file flow

In capillaries, red cells often flow in single file, particularly if the diameter is 6 μm or less (Fig. 2). The stresses exerted on the cells by the surrounding plasma deform them into shapes that are narrower than the capillary, and the cells are surrounded by a sleeve of plasma. The effect of this plasma layer can be analyzed using the 'stacked-coins' (or 'axial-train') model for blood flow (Whitmore, 1968). Red cells are assumed to lie in a cylindrical core region of diameter λD co-axial with a tube of diameter D. This core is assumed to move as a rigid body. The velocity profile is a blunted parabola, and it is easily shown that:

$$\mu_{\text{rel}} = \frac{1}{1-\lambda^4}\,. \tag{3}$$

According to this model, even a narrow plasma layer leads to a relatively small value of

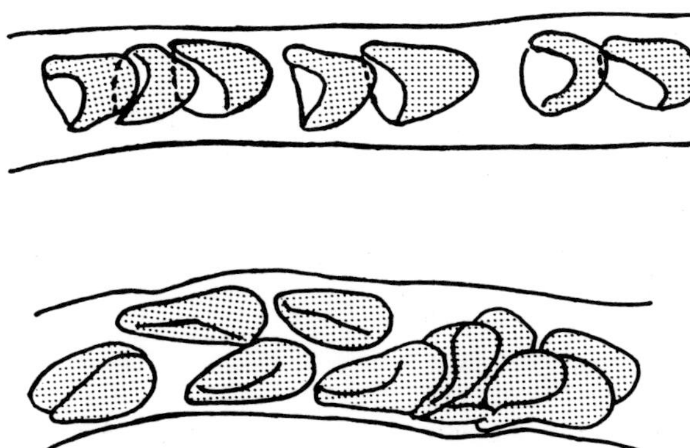

Fig. 2. Sketches of red blood cell shapes observed in capillaries *in vivo* (Secomb, 1991) based on photomicrographs by Skalak and Branemark (1969). Flow is from left to right. Upper diagram, single-file flow in a capillary approximately 7 μm in diameter. Lower diagram, flow in a capillary approximately 12 μm diameter. The five cells on the left have a 'zipper'-like arrangement.

μ_{rel}. For instance, if λ=0.8 then μ_{rel}=1.7, which is much less than the relative bulk viscosity of whole blood.

The shapes of the cells and the width of the plasma layer depend on the mechanics of cell deformation and plasma flow. Theoretical analyses were developed by Lighthill (1968) and Barnard *et al.* (1968), assuming axisymmetric shapes and using lubrication theory to describe the plasma flow in the gap between the cell and the wall. Further developments, with more realistic representations of red cell mechanics, were made by Zarda *et al.* (1977), Secomb *et al.* (1986) and Halpern and Secomb (1989) and are reviewed by Secomb (1991).

Examples of computed red cell shapes are shown in Fig. 3. The cell is deformed by flow forces into a cup- or bullet-like shape, convex at the front and concave at the rear. At the trailing edge, the membrane bulges slightly outwards. As the minimum diameter is approached, the cell becomes increasingly elongated. These features are also observed experimentally (Gaehtgens *et al.* 1980).

Fig. 1 includes predicted values of μ_{rel} for tube diameters ranging from 3 to 8 μm, derived from theoretical results of Secomb *et al.* (1986) and Halpern and Secomb (1989), assuming a discharge hematocrit of 45 % and taking into account the reduction in tube hematocrit by the Fåhraeus effect. Cell velocities of 1 mm s^{-1} are assumed, typical of the experimental data considered by Pries *et al.* (1992). The predictions agree well with the experimental data, considering the simplifications in the analyses.

Actual red cell shapes in capillaries are not axisymmetric, and so the question arises of whether non-symmetrical cell shapes would lead to appreciably different predictions of apparent viscosity. When the shape is not axisymmetric, continuous 'tank-treading' motion of the membrane relative to the cell occurs (Gaehtgens and Schmid-Schönbein, 1982). The mechanics of such membrane motions was considered by Secomb and Skalak (1982*a*). A two-dimensional analysis of single-file flow (Secomb and Skalak, 1982*b*) predicted a decrease in pressure required to drive motion of asymmetric cells, as a result

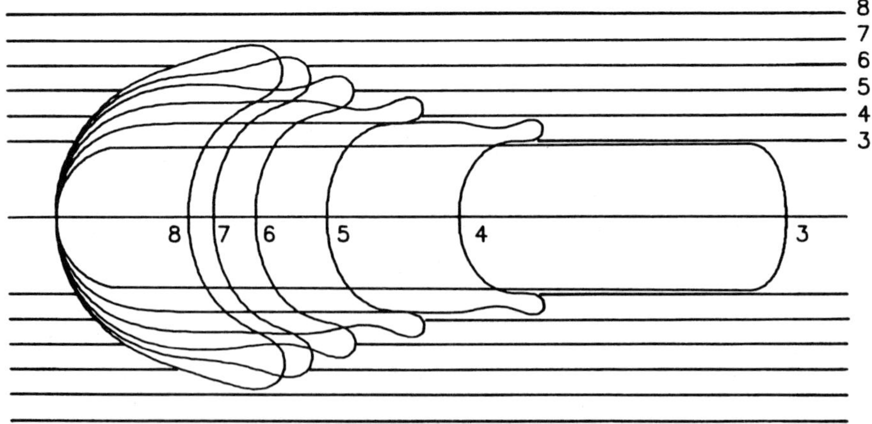

Fig. 3. Computed shapes of axisymmetric red blood cells in uniform tubes (Secomb, 1991). Cell velocity=0.1 mm s^{-1}; numerical values denote tube diameters in μm.

of cell asymmetry and tank-treading. However, Hsu and Secomb (1989) showed that the effects of asymmetry and tank-treading on apparent viscosity in a three-dimensional model were slight, consistent with the good agreement between axisymmetric model predictions and experimental findings.

Mechanics of multi-file flow

In larger microvessels, red cells flow in 'multi-file' rather than single file. Again, the cell-depleted wall layer is the major reason that μ_{rel} is lower than the bulk relative viscosity μ_{bulk}. Its effect can be shown by a modified axial train model, in which the core, instead of being rigid, is fluid with a relative viscosity μ_{bulk}, and the wall layer is cell-free. The velocity profile is a partially blunted parabola, and:

$$\mu_{\text{rel}} = \frac{1}{1 - \lambda^4(1 - 1/\mu_{\text{bulk}})} \tag{4}$$

(Vand, 1948). In this case, $\lambda = 1 - 2\delta/D$, where δ is the thickness of the wall layer. If δ is independent of the diameter D, a reasonable assumption if $\delta \ll D$, then μ_{rel} increases with increasing diameter, approaching μ_{bulk} for large diameters. Fig. 1 shows the variation of μ_{rel} with D if $\delta = 1.8\ \mu\text{m}$, demonstrating a close fit to the empirical curve for diameters from 30 to 1000 μm.

The above analysis has the limitation that the width of the cell-free layer is a fitted parameter. (In reality, the layer is generally cell-depleted rather than cell-free.) The physical exclusion of red cells by the wall is a major reason for the layer, and so its width should be comparable to cell size, as above. However, quantitative theories for the variation of hematocrit near the wall, taking into account the deformability and high concentration of red cells, are not available. For diameters below 30 μm, the further difficulty arises that representing the core as a continuum is unlikely to be a good approximation. Current theories of multi-file flow are either semi-empirical or qualitative with regard to their predictions for blood flow in microvessels. Theories for the wall effect in blood flow are reviewed by Goldsmith *et al.* (1989). The general subject of particle migration at low Reynolds numbers is reviewed by Leal (1980).

Fig. 2 shows an example of two-file flow, in which red cells often arrange themselves into a staggered 'zipper'-like arrangement. Sugihara-Seki *et al.* (1990) developed a two-dimensional model for such a flow, which can be used to predict the width of the plasma layer and the resistance to flow.

In multi-file flow, red cells frequently collide, making aggregation possible. At moderate or high flow rates, shear stresses are sufficient to break up aggregates, but at low flow rates, aggregates can persist. Aggregation markedly increases the bulk shear viscosity of blood at low shear rates (Chien, 1975). However, experimental studies using narrow vertical tubes (diameters 30–300 μm) show little change in apparent viscosity as flow rate is decreased to very low levels. Aggregation results in a wider cell-free or cell-depleted region at the tube wall, where shear stresses are highest. This largely compensates for the reduced relative motion of cells in the central part of the tube (Reinke *et al.* 1987; Cokelet and Goldsmith, 1991).

If the flow rate in a vertical tube is sufficiently low, virtually all the cells join a central aggregated core, co-axial with the tube. Flow resistance may then be estimated using the axial-train model. At higher flow rates, the core co-exists with a suspension of detached cells. A three-layer continuum model for such flow (Murata and Secomb, 1989) assumes a rigid core surrounded by a red cell suspension, with a cell-free layer of fixed width adjacent to the wall. The core width and the suspension hematocrit are dictated by a balance between red cell attachment and detachment at the core boundary. With increasing flow rate, the core progressively becomes disaggregated, increasing the hematocrit of the surrounding region and hence the apparent viscosity. This model accounts for the observed variation of apparent viscosity with flow rate (Reinke *et al.* 1987) in the range of velocities in which the transition from fully aggregated to dispersed flow occurs.

In narrow *horizontal* tubes, by contrast, a large increase in apparent viscosity is observed as flow rate decreases. This results from sedimentation of red cell aggregates, which reduces the width of the cell-depleted layer at the lower part of the tube wall (Reinke *et al.* 1987). In the experiments of Alonso *et al.* (1989), flow was suddenly reduced from a relatively high rate, at which cells were disaggregated, to a much lower rate. Soon after flow reduction, a core of aggregated cells formed, centered on the vessel axis. Contraction of this core resulted in the formation of an increased cell-free layer around the circumference of the tube, and flow resistance initially decreased slightly. Sedimentation of the core occurred over a period of minutes, with an increase in flow resistance. Secomb and El-Kareh (1994) analyzed the sedimentation of a cylindrical core within a horizontal tube and predicted rates of sedimentation consistent with experimental observations.

The significance of red cell aggregation and sedimentation in the microcirculation has long been discussed (Knisely, 1965) but remains unclear. Shear rates are lower in venules than in arterioles, so aggregation is most likely in venules. Under normal flow conditions, blood transit times in venules are probably 10 s or less (Secomb and El-Kareh, 1994), so sedimentation is probably slight. However, sedimentation may influence flow resistance substantially at low flow rates or for blood with an abnormally high aggregating tendency. The effects of aggregation and sedimentation in the microcirculation are complicated by the fact that microvessels have varying orientations and contain bifurcations and other geometric irregularities.

Flow in bifurcations

Bifurcations are the branch points of microvascular networks. At diverging bifurcations, flow from a parent vessel is divided between two daughter vessels. Flows recombine at converging bifurcations. The mechanics of blood flow in bifurcations is difficult to analyze because it involves the motion of deformable cells in geometrically complicated regions (Fig. 4). In a diverging bifurcation, both the plasma flow and the red cell flux are split between the two daughter vessels. Because of non-continuum behavior, the partition of red cells is generally not proportional to the overall flow partition, resulting in unequal hematocrits in the daughter vessels ('phase separation') and leading to wide variations of vessel hematocrit within networks.

The partition of red cells depends on the relative flow rates in the daughter vessels. The cell fraction (ϕ) entering one daughter vessel may be expressed as a function of the total flow fraction (ψ) entering that vessel (Schmid-Schönbein *et al.* 1980), as in Fig. 5 (Pries *et al.* 1989). Clearly, all such curves must pass through (0,0) and (1,1), since zero flow implies zero red cell flux. In relatively large microvessels, the ψ–ϕ relationship approaches a straight line through these two points, the continuum result. In smaller microvessels, however, the relationship is markedly nonlinear. If the flow rate in one daughter vessel is small, that vessel may draw only plasma from the parent vessel ('plasma skimming'), so that ϕ=0 for small values of ψ. At higher ψ, ϕ starts to rise. The relationship between ψ and ϕ depends on the distribution of red cells in the cross section of the parent vessel (Schmid-Schönbein *et al.* 1980). A uniform hematocrit profile results in nearly linear dependence, whereas a focused stream of oncoming cells gives nonlinear variation, with rapid dependence on ψ near ψ=0.5.

Several theoretical analyses for red cell partition have been developed, assuming that red cells follow streamlines of the plasma flow and taking into account the plasma layers in the parent vessel (Fenton *et al.* 1985*a*; Pries *et al.* 1989; Enden and Popel, 1992). The results are consistent with observations of blood flow both in model bifurcations and *in vivo*, particularly for vessels with diameters in the range 20–100 μm. However, such analyses do not realistically represent the mechanics of flow in smaller bifurcations, where the finite size of red cells must be considered. To examine this case, Audet and Olbricht (1987) used a two-dimensional model and represented red cells as rigid circular particles. Yan *et al.* (1991) considered the three-dimensional flow of fluid from a large tube into a small, perpendicular side branch, and the motion of a rigid spherical particle in this flow field. In these studies, the three-dimensional geometry of the bifurcation is not realistically represented. This is significant, since deviations of red cells from the streamlines of the plasma flow are probably the result of interactions between red cells and the curved dividing surface separating the daughter vessels. The interaction of a

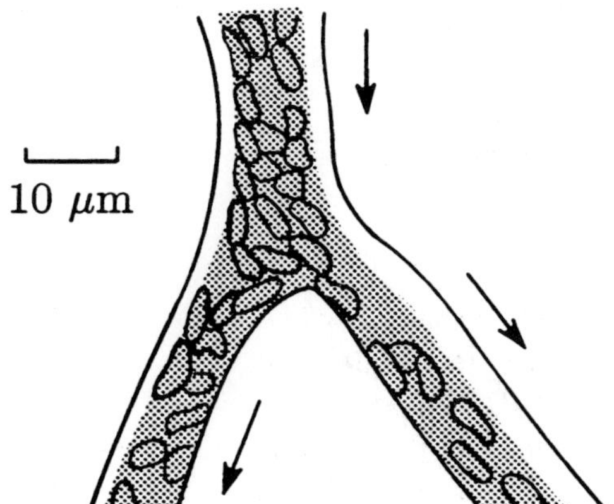

Fig. 4. Sketch of blood flow through a diverging capillary bifurcation, based on a photomicrograph by Schmid-Schönbein *et al.* (1980). Arrows show flow directions. Shaded area represents red-cell-containing regions; unshaded areas within vessels represent peripheral plasma layers.

particle with a flow impinging on a curved surface has been examined by El-Kareh and Secomb (1992).

In capillary bifurcations, red and white blood cells often undergo large deformations in order to enter narrow capillaries. White blood cells, being highly viscous, may take a relatively long time to deform and, during this period, they plug the capillary they are entering. This effect may contribute significantly to flow resistance (Fenton *et al.* 1985*b*). Red cells deform much more readily, but their viscous resistance to deformation contributes to flow resistance, as discussed below.

Flow in networks

A microvascular network consists of segments and bifurcations. The results described above provide a basis for simulating the distribution of blood flows and red cell fluxes in a network (Popel, 1987; Pries *et al.* 1990). Suppose first that the flow resistance of each segment is known. Then the flow in each segment can be expressed in terms of the pressures at the nodes (bifurcations), and the condition that the flows entering or leaving each node must add to zero gives a system of linear equations to be solved for the nodal pressures, subject to specified pressures or flows in vessels feeding or draining the network.

In reality, the resistance to flow in each segment depends on its red cell content, which itself depends on flow rates, because of phase separation at bifurcations. Two main approaches have been used to include this effect. One approach involves tracking the simulated motion of all red cells through the network (Schmid-Schönbein *et al.* 1980). This provides predictions about temporal fluctuations, but requires much computation. An alternative approach is to represent the red cell content of each segment by an average

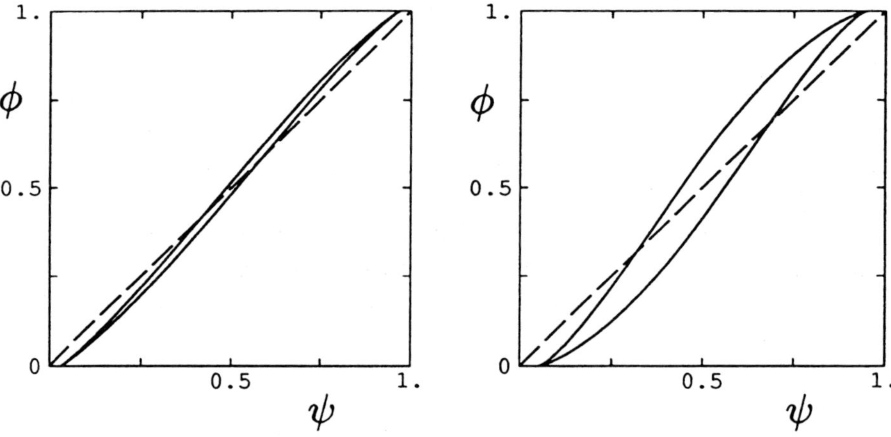

Fig. 5. Examples of empirical relationships (Pries *et al.* 1989) between red cell fraction (ϕ) and total flow fraction (ψ) entering a daughter vessel in a bifurcation. In each, the two solid curves show the relationships for the two daughter vessels. The dashed line shows the relationship in the absence of phase separation. Left-hand diagram, 20 μm feeding vessel, feed hematocrit 49 %. Right-hand digram, 7.5 μm feeding vessel, feed hematocrit 43 %.

hematocrit (Pries *et al.* 1990). Hematocrits in daughter branches are assigned as described in the previous section. This approach results in a nonlinear system of equations, which must be solved iteratively.

Microvascular networks are very heterogeneous in structure, both in topology (pattern of interconnections) and in geometry (lengths and diameters of segments). Simulations incorporating heterogeneous network structures predict large segment-to-segment variations in velocity and hematocrit (Dawant *et al.* 1986; Levin *et al.* 1986). Such heterogeneity is evident in experiments and must be taken into account in efforts to understand the transport functions of the microcirculation (Duling and Damon, 1987). Estimates of derived quantities based on averaged values of underlying parameters can be erroneous if these parameters are heterogeneous but correlated. For instance, hematocrit and flow velocity are correlated, as a result of unequal hematocrit partition at bifurcations. If mean values of velocity and hematocrit are used to estimate red cell flux through a network, flux is substantially underestimated (Pries *et al.* 1986).

The assumptions underlying network simulations may be tested by comparing predicted and observed values of hemodynamic parameters. If the topology and geometry of the network are established, and hemodynamic parameters are measured in each segment, comparisons can be made on a segment-by-segment basis. Such comparisons were made by Pries *et al.* (1990, 1994) in studies of microvessel hematocrits and velocities in networks of the rat mesentery, containing 383–913 segments. Flow resistance in each segment was initially estimated from *in vitro* data. Although overall *distributions* of predicted and measured parameters were in reasonable agreement, correlations between predicted and measured values in individual segments were poor. Part of the discrepancy was accounted for by known sources of error in measurement and in model assumptions. However, the remainder of the discrepancy could only be accounted for by assuming a different dependence of apparent viscosity on microvessel diameter. In particular, the results implied substantially higher apparent viscosities in the smallest vessels than are observed in glass tubes. Further support for this conclusion was obtained by direct measurements of flow resistance in similar networks.

The cause of this discrepancy between *in vivo* and *in vitro* resistance to blood flow in narrow tubes is not known. Possible mechanisms include (Pries *et al.* 1990) the effect of white cells, which are generally removed for glass-tube experiments; a layer of macromolecules lining the interior of microvessels, which might reduce the cross section available for flow (Desjardins and Duling, 1987); asymmetric radial distributions of red cells within microvessels *in vivo*; and irregularity of the internal cross sections of microvessels *in vivo*. These mechanisms are currently being investigated. Effects of capillary irregularity are discussed next.

Transient deformations of red cells

A red blood cell traversing the microcirculation encounters flow geometries that are not well represented by a uniform cylindrical tube. Capillaries have non-uniform cross sections, as indicated by systematic variations of red cell velocity along capillaries (Ellis *et al.* 1989). Endothelial nuclei project into the lumen, resulting in local narrowings. At diverging capillary bifurcations, red cells must adjust to the diameters of the daughter vessels. Driessen *et al.* (1984) suggested that 'the dynamic response of the red cell during transient deformations may limit the ability of the cell to negotiate the circulation'. In skeletal muscle, the number of flowing capillaries varies with total flow, in a phenomenon known as 'recruitment'. Secomb (1987) suggested that the inability of red cells to traverse irregularities at low driving pressures may contribute to this phenomenon. Transient deformations also occur in laboratory tests of blood cell deformability based on the rate of passage of cells through filters with cylindrical pores (Chien, 1977*a*).

During transient deformations of red cells, forces are generated in the membrane due to its shear viscosity, but previous analyses (e.g. Skalak and Özkaya, 1987) neglected this. A new model including the effects of membrane viscosity is outlined here. Axisymmetric cell shapes are assumed and lubrication theory is used. Shear and bending elastic resistance of the membrane are neglected, an approximation valid in the high-velocity limit, and predicted cell shapes have a cusp at the trailing edge. The concave rear of the cell is represented as part of a sphere. The governing equations are those of equilibrium of normal and tangential forces on the membrane, together with the lubrication equation. This approach was used in an earlier analysis of steady single-file red cell motion in uniform cylindrical tubes (Secomb and Gross, 1983), leading to estimates of apparent viscosity in good agreement with experimental findings in glass tubes.

When the viscous resistance of the membrane to shear deformation is included (Evans and Hochmuth, 1976), the axial (t_s) and circumferential (t_ϕ) components of membrane tension are:

$$t_s = t_0 - t_d \tag{5}$$

and

$$t_\phi = t_0 + t_d\,, \tag{6}$$

where:

$$t_d = \frac{2\pi_m}{r}\,\frac{\partial r}{\partial t}\,. \tag{7}$$

Here t_0 is the mean tension, r is the distance of the membrane from the axis, and the time derivative is evaluated following a fixed material point in the membrane. The membrane shear viscosity μ_m is $10^{-6}\,\mathrm{N\,s\,m^{-1}}$ (Hochmuth and Waugh, 1987). In transient deformations, gap widths are time-dependent. The leakback (flow rate in the gap) varies with position and time, and its spatial derivative is related to the time derivative of the gap width according to conservation of volume, leading to a time-dependent lubrication equation.

The resulting system consists of three coupled partial differential equations. The independent variables are s, a coordinate fixed in the membrane, and time t. The dependent variables are $r(s,t)$ as already defined, $p(s,t)$, the pressure difference across the membrane, and $t_s(s,t)$, the axial tension in the membrane. These equations are solved numerically by a finite difference method.

Fig. 6 shows an example in which a red cell in a 7 μm tube encounters a reduction in tube diameter to 4 μm. This could represent the entrance to a capillary at a diverging bifurcation. Since membrane elasticity is neglected, the flow resistance is proportional to the rate of viscous energy dissipation, which may be expressed as the sum of contributions from the membrane and from the lubrication layer. As the cell begins to squeeze through the constriction, the membrane is deformed and the width of the lubrication layer is reduced. Total resistance to flow increases to more than four times the

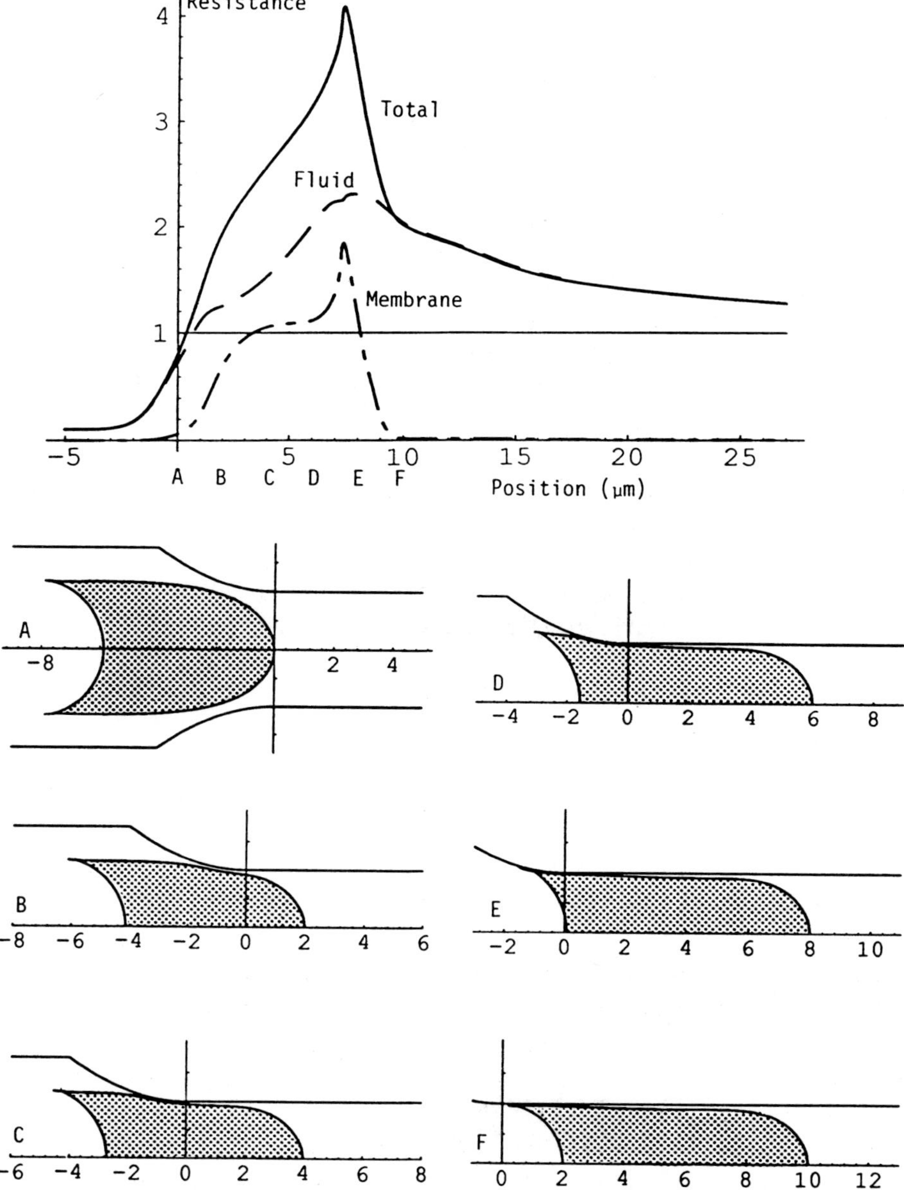

Fig. 6. Transient deformation of a red cell in a capillary narrowing from 7 to 4 μm. Upper diagram, flow resistance as a function of position, relative to flow resistance in a uniform 4 μm tube (horizontal line), showing contributions of fluid and membrane dissipation to total resistance. Lower diagram, cell shapes at several positions, denoted A–F. Horizontal scale in μm.

resistance that the cell would experience in a uniform 4 μm tube and remains elevated for a considerable distance as the red cell enters the narrow tube. This suggests that entrance effects could contribute significantly to overall pressure drop in a narrow capillary. Similar results are obtained for a red cell encountering other types of irregularity. These results imply that transient red cell deformations may contribute substantially to flow resistance in the microcirculation.

Conclusions

Much is known about the mechanical behavior of blood's constituents. In particular, the mechanical properties of red blood cells are well understood. This provides a basis for understanding and predicting the mechanics of blood flow in the normal microcirculation and for investigating the effects of modified blood cell properties.

Considerable effort has been devoted to the study of blood flow in uniform narrow cylindrical tubes. Experiments have shown that the apparent viscosity of blood in such tubes varies strongly with diameter, reaching low values for diameters of 5–10 μm. Theoretical studies have explained this finding on the basis of the motion and deformation of individual red cells. The behavior of blood in uniform microvessels larger than 10 μm is complex. At low flow rates, aggregation and sedimentation may occur. Theoretical analysis of flow in such vessels presents many challenges.

However, the microcirculation does not consist of uniform tubes, and the above findings do not adequately represent the mechanics of blood flow in the microcirculation. Microvessels are linked in networks, with bifurcations at nodal points. Flow behavior and red cell partition at diverging bifurcations strongly influence red cell distribution. Heterogeneous network structures lead to dispersion in hemodynamic variables, which in turn influences microvascular transport functions. Individual microvessel segments are not uniform in cross section. The transient deformations of red cells passing though microvessels may contribute significantly to flow resistance.

Therefore, future research into the mechanics of blood flow in the microcirculation should increasingly emphasize understanding blood flow in networks, bifurcations and irregular geometries. Such research has the potential to show more clearly how the mechanical properties of blood cells influence the functioning of the microcirculation.

The preparation of this review, and some of the studies described, were supported by NIH grants HL34555, HL17421 and HL07249. I thank my colleagues and collaborators who have contributed to many aspects of the work described, particularly R. Hsu and A. R. Pries.

References

ALONSO, C., PRIES, A. R. AND GAEHTGENS, P. (1989). Time-dependent rheological behavior of blood flow at low shear in narrow horizontal tubes. *Biorheology* **26**, 229–246.

AUDET, D. M. AND OLBRICHT, W. L. (1987). The motion of model cells at capillary bifurcations. *Microvasc. Res.* **33**, 377–396.

BARNARD, A. C. L., LOPEZ, L. AND HELLUMS, J. D. (1968). Basic theory of blood flow in capillaries. *Microvasc. Res.* **1**, 23–34.

CANHAM, P. B. AND BURTON, A. C. (1968). Distribution of size and shape in populations of normal human red blood cells. *Circulation Res.* **22**, 405–422.

CHIEN, S. (1975). Biophysical behavior of red cells in suspensions. In *The Red Blood Cell*, vol. II (ed. D. M. Surgenor), pp. 1031–1133. New York: Academic Press.

CHIEN, S. (1977*a*). Principles and techniques for assessing erythrocyte deformability. *Blood Cells* **3**, 71–99.

CHIEN, S. (1977*b*). Rheology of sickle cells and erythrocyte content. *Blood Cells* **3**, 283–303.

COKELET, G. R. AND GOLDSMITH, H. L. (1991). Decreased hydrodynamic resistance in the two-phase flow of blood through small vertical tubes at low flow rates. *Circulation Res.* **68**, 1–17.

DAWANT, B., LEVIN, M. AND POPEL, A. S. (1986). Effect of dispersion of vessel diameters and lengths in stochastic networks. I. Modeling of microcirculatory flow. *Microvasc. Res.* **31**, 203–222.

DESJARDINS, C. AND DULING, B. R. (1987). Microvessel hematocrit: measurement and implications for capillary oxygen transport. *Am. J. Physiol.* **252**, H494–H503.

DINTENFASS, L. (1976). *Rheology of Blood in Diagnostic and Preventative Medicine.* London: Butterworths.

DRIESSEN, G. K., FISCHER, T. M., HAEST, C. W. M., INHOFFEN, W. AND SCHMID-SCHÖNBEIN, H. (1984). Flow behaviour of rigid red blood cells in the microcirculation. *Int. J. Microcirc. Clin. Exp.* **3**, 197–210.

DULING, B. R. AND DAMON, D. H. (1987). An examination of the measurement of flow heterogeneity in striated muscle. *Circulation Res.* **60**, 1–13.

EL-KAREH, A. W. AND SECOMB, T. W. (1992). Particle trajectories near a dividing surface: Deviation from streamlines. *FASEB J.* **6**, A2073.

ELLIS, C. G., TYML, K. AND STRANG, B. K. (1989). Variation in axial velocity profile of red cells passing through a single capillary. In *Oxygen Transport to Tissue*, vol. X (ed. K. Rakusan, G. P. Biro, T. K. Goldstick and Z. Turek), pp. 543–550. New York: Plenum.

ENDEN, G. AND POPEL, A. S. (1992). A numerical study of the shape of the surface separating flow into branches in microvascular bifurcations. *J. Biomech. Eng.* **114**, 398–405.

EVANS, E. A. (1983). Bending elastic modulus of red blood cell membrane derived from buckling instability in micropipet aspiration tests. *Biophys. J.* **43**, 27–30.

EVANS, E. A. AND HOCHMUTH, R. M. (1976). Membrane viscoelasticity. *Biophys. J.* **16**, 1–11.

FÅHRAEUS, R. (1928). Die Strömungsverhältnisse und die Verteilung der Blutzellen im Gefässsystem. *Klin. Wschr.* **7**, 100–106.

FÅHRAEUS, R. AND LINDQVIST, T. (1931). The viscosity of the blood in narrow capillary tubes. *Am. J. Physiol.* **96**, 562–568.

FENTON, B. M., CARR, R. T. AND COKELET, G. R. (1985*a*). Nonuniform red cell distribution in 20–100 μm bifurcations. *Microvasc. Res.* **29**, 103–126.

FENTON, B. M., WILSON, D. W. AND COKELET, G. R. (1985*b*). Analysis of the effects of measured white blood cell entrance times on hemodynamics in a computer model of a microvascular bed. *Pflügers Arch.* **403**, 396–401.

FUNG, Y. C. (1981). *Biomechanics: Mechanical Properties of Living Tissues.* New York: Springer.

FUNG, Y. C. (1984). *Biodynamics: Circulation.* New York: Springer.

GAEHTGENS, P. AND SCHMID-SCHÖNBEIN, H. (1982). Mechanisms of dynamic flow adaptation of mammalian erythrocytes. *Naturwissenschaften* **69**, 294–296.

GAEHTGENS, P., DÜHRSSEN, C. AND ALBRECHT, K. H. (1980). Motion, deformation and interaction of blood cells and plasma during flow through narrow capillary tubes. *Blood Cells* **6**, 799–812.

GOLDSMITH, H. L., COKELET, G. R. AND GAEHTGENS, P. (1989). Robin Fåhraeus: evolution of his concepts in cardiovascular physiology. *Am. J. Physiol.* **257**, H1005–H1015.

HAKIM, T. S. AND MACEK, A. S. (1988). Effect of hypoxia on erythrocyte deformability in different species. *Biorheology* **25**, 857–868.

HALPERN, D. AND SECOMB, T. W. (1989). The squeezing of red blood cells through capillaries with near-minimal diameters. *J. Fluid Mech.* **203**, 381–400.

HOCHMUTH, R. M. AND WAUGH, R. E. (1987). Erythrocyte membrane elasticity and viscosity. *A. Rev. Physiol.* **49**, 209–219.

HSU, R. AND SECOMB, T. W. (1989). Motion of non-axisymmetric red blood cells in cylindrical capillaries. *J. Biomech. Eng.* **111**, 147–151.

HURD, T. C., DASMAHAPATRA, K. S., RUSH, B. F. AND MACHIEDO, G. W. (1988). Red blood cell deformability in human and experimental sepsis. *Arch. Surg.* **123**, 217–220.

KNISELY, M. H. (1965). Intravascular erythrocyte aggregation (blood sludge). In *Handbook of Physiology*, section 2, *Circulation*, vol. III (ed. W. F. Hamilton and P. Dow), pp. 2249–2292. Bethesda, MD: American Physiological Society.

LEAL, L. G. (1980). Particle motions in a viscous fluid. *A. Rev. Fluid Mech.* **12**, 435–476.

LEVIN, M., DAWANT, B. AND POPEL, A. S. (1986). Effect of dispersion of vessel diameters and lengths in stochastic networks. I. Modeling of microvascular hematocrit distribution. *Microvasc. Res.* **31**, 223–234.

LEY, K. AND GAEHTGENS, P. (1991). Endothelial, not hemodynamic, differences are responsible for preferential leukocyte rolling in rat mesenteric venules. *Circulation Res.* **69**, 1034–1041.

LIGHTHILL, M. J. (1968). Pressure-forcing of tightly fitting pellets along fluid-filled elastic tubes. *J. Fluid Mech.* **34**, 113–143.

LIPOWSKY, H. H., KOVALCHECK, S. AND ZWEIFACH, B. W. (1978). The distribution of blood rheological parameters in the microvasculature of cat mesentery. *Circulation Res.* **43**, 738–749.

MARTINI, P., PIERACH, A. AND SCHREYER, E. (1930). Die Strömung des Blutes in engen Gefässen. Eine Abweichung vom Poiseuille'schen Gesetz. *Dtsch. Arch. klin. Med.* **169**, 212–222.

MURATA, T. AND SECOMB, T. W. (1989). Effects of aggregation on flow properties of red blood cell suspensions in narrow vertical tubes. *Biorheology* **26**, 247–259.

NASH, G. B., O'BRIEN, E., GORDON-SMITH, E. C. AND DORMANDY, J. A. (1989). Abnormalities in the mechanical properties of red blood cells caused by *Plasmodium falciparum*. *Blood* **74**, 855–861.

NAZZIOLA, E. AND HOUSE, S. D. (1992). Effects of hydrodynamics and leukocyte–endothelium specificity on leukocyte–endothelium interactions. *Microvasc. Res.* **44**, 127–142.

POPEL, A. S. (1987). Network models of peripheral circulation. In *Handbook of Bioengineering* (ed. R. Skalak and S. Chien), pp. 20.1–20.24. New York: McGraw-Hill.

PRIES, A. R., LEY, K., CLAASEN, M. AND GAEHTGENS, P. (1989). Red cell distribution at microvascular bifurcations. *Microvasc. Res.* **38**, 81–101.

PRIES, A. R., LEY, K. AND GAEHTGENS, P. (1986). Generalization of the Fåhraeus principle for microvessel networks. *Am. J. Physiol.* **251**, H1324–H1332.

PRIES, A. R., NEUHAUS, D. AND GAEHTGENS, P. (1992). Blood viscosity in tube flow: dependence on diameter and hematocrit. *Am. J. Physiol.* **263**, H1770–H1778.

PRIES, A. R., SECOMB, T. W., GAEHTGENS, P. AND GROSS, J. F. (1990). Blood flow in microvascular networks – Experiments and simulation. *Circulation Res.* **67**, 826–834.

PRIES, A. R., SECOMB, T. W., GESSNER, T., SPERANDIO, M. B., GROSS, J. F. AND GAEHTGENS, P. (1994). Resistance to blood flow in microvessels *in vivo*. *Circulation Res.* **75**, 904–915.

REINKE, W., GAEHTGENS, P. AND JOHNSON, P. C. (1987). Blood viscosity in small tubes: effect of shear rate, aggregation and sedimentation. *Am. J. Physiol.* **253**, H540–H547.

SCHMID-SCHÖNBEIN, G. W. (1990). Leukocyte biophysics. *Cell Biophysics* **12**, 107–135.

SCHMID-SCHÖNBEIN, G. W., SKALAK, R., USAMI, S. AND CHIEN, S. (1980). Cell distribution in capillary networks. *Microvasc. Res.* **19**, 18–44.

SCHMID-SCHÖNBEIN, G. W., SUNG, K.-P., TÖZEREN, H., SKALAK, R. AND CHIEN, S. (1981). Passive mechanical properties of human leukocytes. *Biophys. J.* **36**, 243–256.

SCHMID-SCHÖNBEIN, H. AND VOLGER, E. (1976). Red-cell aggregation and red-cell deformability in diabetes. *Diabetes* **25**, 897–902.

SECOMB, T. W. (1987). Flow-dependent rheological properties of blood in capillaries. *Microvasc. Res.* **34**, 46–58.

SECOMB, T. W. (1991). Red blood cell mechanics and capillary blood rheology. *Cell Biophys.* **18**, 231–251.

SECOMB, T. W. AND GROSS, J. F. (1983). Flow of red blood cells in narrow capillaries: role of membrane tension. *Int. J. Microcirc. Clin. Exp.* **2**, 229–240.

SECOMB, T. W. AND EL-KAREH, A. (1994). A model for motion and sedimentation of cylindrical red-cell aggregates during slow blood flow in narrow horizontal tubes. *J. Biomech. Eng.* **116**, 243–249.

SECOMB, T. W. AND SKALAK, R. (1982*a*). Surface flow of viscoelastic membranes in viscous fluids. *Q. J. Mech. appl. Math.* **35**, 233–247.

SECOMB, T. W. AND SKALAK, R. (1982*b*). A two-dimensional model for capillary flow of an asymmetric cell. *Microvasc. Res.* **24**, 194–203.

SECOMB, T. W., SKALAK, R., ÖZKAYA, N. AND GROSS, J. F. (1986). Flow of axisymmetric red blood cells in narrow capillaries. *J. Fluid Mech.* **163**, 405–423.

SKALAK, R. (1976). Rheology of red blood cell membrane. In *Microcirculation*, vol. I (ed. J. Grayson and W. Zingg), pp. 53–70. New York: Plenum.

SKALAK, R. AND BRANEMARK, P.-I. (1969). Deformation of red blood cells in capillaries. *Science* **164**, 717–719.

SKALAK, R. AND ÖZKAYA, N. (1987). Models of erythrocyte and leukocyte flow in capillaries. In *Physiological Fluid Dynamics*, vol. II (ed. L. S. Srinath and M. Singh), pp. 1–10. New Delhi: Tata McGraw-Hill.

SKALAK, R., ZARDA, P. R., JAN, K. M. AND CHIEN, S. (1981). Mechanics of rouleau formation. *Biophys. J.* **35**, 771–781.

SUGIHARA-SEKI, M., SECOMB, T. W. AND SKALAK, R. (1990). Two-dimensional analysis of two-file flow of red cells along capillaries. *Microvasc. Res.* **40**, 379–393.

TANGELDER, G. J., TEIRLINCK, H. C., SLAAF, D. W. AND RENEMAN, R. S. (1985). Distribution of blood platelets flowing in arterioles. *Am J. Physiol.* **248**, H318–H323.

VAND, V. (1948). Viscosity of solutions and suspensions. I. Theory. *J. Phys. Colloid Chem.* **52**, 277–299.

WHITMORE, R. L. (1968). *Rheology of the Circulation.* Oxford: Pergamon.

YAN, Z.-Y., ACRIVOS, A. AND WEINBAUM, S. (1991). Fluid skimming and particle entrainment into a small circular side pore. *J. Fluid Mech.* **229**, 1–27.

YEUNG, A. AND EVANS, E. (1989). Cortical shell-liquid core model for passive flow of liquid-like spherical cells into micropipets. *Biophys. J.* **56**, 139–149.

ZARDA, P. R., CHIEN, S. AND SKALAK, R. (1977). Interaction of viscous incompressible fluid with an elastic body. In *Computational Methods for Fluid-Solid Interaction Problems* (ed. T. Belytschko and T. L. Geers), pp. 65–82. New York: American Society of Mechanical Engineers.

MODELLING THE STRUCTURAL PATHWAYS FOR TRANSCAPILLARY EXCHANGE

S. WEINBAUM[1] *and F. E. CURRY*[2]

[1]Department of Mechanical Engineering, The City College of CUNY, New York, NY 10031, USA *and* [2]Department of Human Physiology, School of Medicine, University of California at Davis, Davis, CA 95616, USA

Summary

The ultrastructural pathways and mechanisms whereby endothelial cells and the clefts between the cells modulate capillary permeability to water and solutes have been a central unresolved question in microvessel transport since the early 1950s. Freeze–fracture studies and ultrathin serial sections have demonstrated that endothelial cells are joined by an array of junctional strands which are interrupted at intervals, allowing for the passage of water and solutes, whereas cytochemical studies have indicated that the endothelial surface and portions of the wide part of the cleft contain matrix components. Neither constricted slit models based on the classic pore theory nor fiber matrix models are able to explain the large body of existing permeability measurements. In this review, we shall describe new three-dimensional modelling approaches which have resulted in a major revision of current ideas about the pathways for water and solutes through the junction strand and the structures that determine the molecular filter. For frog mesentery capillaries, these models predict (i) that the primary pathway for small ions is a previously unrecognized family of 2 nm small pores that are distributed along the length of the junction strand; (ii) that the primary pathway for water and intermediate-sized solutes (1–3.5 nm radius) is an infrequent 150 nm long orifice-like pore whose height is the same as that of the wide part of the cleft; (iii) that the sieving structure for these solutes is a fiber layer, typically 100 nm thick, which extends from the surface into the entrance region of the cleft and (iv) that the interpretation of low molecular weight tracer studies to define the permeability pathways depends on the time-dependent filling of the extravascular space.

Introduction

Vascular endothelium is the principal barrier to, and regulator of, material exchange between circulating blood and the body tissues. The ultrastrucural pathways and mechanisms whereby endothelial cells, their surface matrix and the junction and fiber structures in the clefts between the cells modulate microvessel permeability to water and solutes has been a central theme in capillary transport since Pappenheimer *et al.* (1951) proposed the first pore-slit theory more than 40 years ago. The relationship between the resistance to water and solute flows and the ultrastructure of the junctional strand and

Key words:capillary permeability, junctional pores, fiber matrix models, transcapillary exchange.

matrix components is still unresolved, but new three-dimensional modelling approaches, starting with the study by Tsay *et al.* (1989) and recent experiments in Charles Michel's laboratory and our own, have resulted in a major revision of long-standing ideas about the pathways for water and solutes through the junction strand and the structures that determine the molecular filter. In this review, we shall highlight these recent developments. Excellent reviews of earlier one-dimensional pore-slit models or fiber matrix models can be found in Crone and Levitt (1984), Curry (1984, 1986) and Michel (1984, 1988). These previous models and their various shortcomings are first briefly summarized below to establish the framework for the new three-dimensional models that are the primary focus of this paper.

One-dimensional pore-slit and fiber matrix models

In Fig. 1, taken from Weinbaum *et al.* (1992), two alternative hypotheses are illustrated for the size-selective structures that determine capillary permeability. These sketches form the basis for the earlier one-dimensional constricted slit and the fiber matrix models that were extensively used until the late 1980s. The model in Fig. 1A is based on published studies of the ultrastructure of the cleft between adjacent endothelial cells that were obtained from random thin section (40–50 nm) electron microscopic studies performed prior to 1980 using size-specific molecular probes (Karnovsky, 1967; Simionescu *et al.* 1973; Casely-Smith *et al.* 1975; Wissig, 1979). The molecular filter was assumed to be associated with slit-like openings of 6–8 nm gap height in an otherwise impermeable junctional barrier, where the opposing membranes appeared to be very close, but not fused. These constricted slits separated the wide portions of the cleft whose

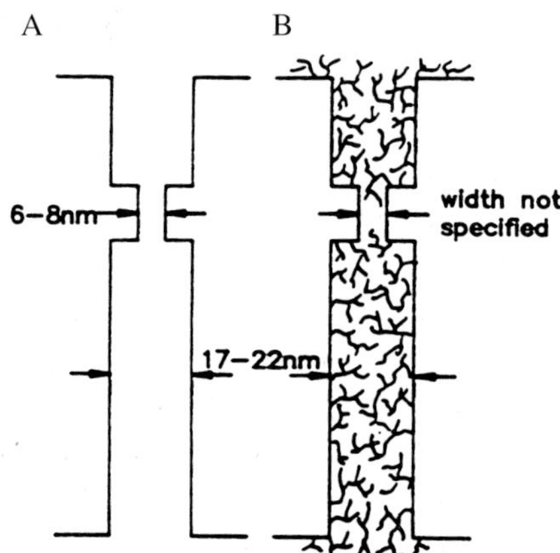

Fig. 1. (A) Constricted channel model. This model proposed that the junctional cleft is 17–22 nm wide except for one or more constrictions. The constriction is assumed to be the main molecular filter and its width, 6–8 nm, is chosen to fit reflection coefficient data. (B) Fiber matrix model. The fiber matrix is assumed to be contained in the wide part of the channel and acts as the molecular filter. Both models assume that the permeability is proportional to the fractional length of the tight junction, which is effectively open. From Weinbaum *et al.* (1992).

gap height is typically 17–22 nm. The size-selective slit-pore could also be formed by a tortuous pathway across a multi-strand array in which the slit-like openings could appear in different planes of section (Wissig, 1979). The dimensions of the constricted slit were deduced from the observation that the passage of horseradish peroxidase (HRP) (6 nm) appeared to be blocked by the constricted openings in most but not all planes of section. These dimensions also appeared to be roughly compatible with measurements of the reflection coefficient for different-sized solutes in different tissues (Curry, 1986). A reasonable fit for the reflection coefficient σ could be obtained for a parallel slit whose gap height was between 7 and 9 nm or a circular cylindrical pore of between 5 and 6 nm radius. Using one-dimensional models, Crone and Levitt (1984) estimated that the hydraulic conductivity L_p and diffusive permeability P of small solutes could be accounted for if 10 % of the junction barrier had these constricted slit openings in mammalian muscle capillaries and if 90 % of the junction length were open in frog mesentery capillaries.

All of the foregoing studies were performed using random transmission sections. The serial reconstructions in rat heart (Bundgaard, 1984) and frog mesentery capillaries (Adamson and Michel, 1993) have revealed several very important features that negate the above view. First, the serial section studies showed that the gap height at the interruptions in the junction strand are the same as that of the remaining wide part of the cleft (20 nm), suggesting that the strand itself is probably not the site of the primary molecular sieve. Second, the 40–80 nm breaks observed by Bundgaard (1984) and the 1500 nm breaks observed by Adamson and Michel (1993) were very infrequent and represented a fractional length of open junction that was small compared with the length predicted by the one-dimensional models for frog mesentery. Third, while multiple strands might be present in any given section, there was usually only a single strand that formed a nearly continuous circuit around the perimeter of the cell, and the remaining strands were short, at least in rat heart and frog mesentery capillaries. This suggested that the tortuous multi-strand pathway was not important in these tissues and that the appearance of tracer on the far side of a junction strand constriction did not necessarily reflect a slit opening in the plane of the random section, but could be due to lateral diffusion and convection in the wake of junction strand discontinuities.

Even prior to these more recent experimental observations, theoretical models based on a one-dimensional constricted slit concept were unable to predict a self-consistent set of values for the large body of experimental permeability measurements that had been performed on individually perfused frog mesentery microvessels using the modified Landis technique developed by Michel *et al.* (1973). In these experiments, the hydraulic conductivity L_p, the diffusive permeability P and reflection coefficient σ are determined by applying the Kedem–Katchalsky equations:

$$J_v = L_p(\Delta p - \sigma \boldsymbol{R} T \Delta C), \tag{1}$$

$$J_s = P \Delta C + (1 - \sigma) J_v C, \tag{2}$$

where Δp and ΔC are the transcapillary pressure and concentration difference, C is the concentration of the solute and $\boldsymbol{R}$ and T have their usual meaning, to measurements of the flux of water J_V and solute J_S across the microvessel wall. In general, the diffusive resistance of one-dimensional constricted slit models is too small by a factor of 5 to account for the measured resistance to intermediate-sized solutes and the width of the constriction, 6–8 nm, which satisfies the requirement for the molecular filter is too small to account for the measured L_P (Curry, 1986).

The inability to reconcile pore-slit theory with these experimental measurements led Curry and Michel (1980) to propose the fiber matrix model depicted in Fig. 1B. In this model, one assumes that a diffuse matrix of sulphated proteoglycan molecules at the endothelial surface and in the wide portion of the cleft provides the primary molecular filter. This fiber matrix could also strongly influence the filtration and permeability properties of the cleft. The existence of a surface glycocalyx was first observed by Luft (1966), and the most recent cytochemical studies by Adamson and Clough (1992) have demonstrated the existence of a continuous matrix both on the endothelial surface and in the entrance region of the clefts, provided that plasma proteins were present in the perfusate.

The principal drawbacks in the original formulation of the fiber matrix theory are that the expressions for L_P and P do not take into consideration the membrane boundaries of the interendothelial cleft or the hydrodynamic interaction of the solute molecules with the fibers. As we shall show later in this review, a more rigorous model which takes hydrodynamic and wall-fiber interactions into account shows that the fiber matrix model provides for too great a hydrodynamic resistance if the matrix occupies all of the wide portion of the cleft. Recent rapid freeze-etching techniques (Satcher, 1993) and goniometric tilting methods (Schulze and Firth, 1992) have revealed an ordered array of cleft-spanning fibers which are oriented perpendicular to the plasmalemma boundaries with a spacing of approximately 10 nm. This loose structure of cross-bridging fiber elements, where the space between fibers is of the order of half the channel height, does not meet the requirements of infinite medium theory.

These shortcomings of the simple one-dimensional models depicted in Fig. 1 have motivated a series of three-dimensional junction–pore–matrix models of increasing sophistication and accuracy which have the flexibility to examine in detail the permeability properties of a cleft with a bounded fiber array that is either ordered or random and a junction strand whose molecular structure can be varied to describe different junction protein arrangements. We shall first discuss the most likely possibilities for the pore structure in the junction strand.

Models for the junction protein strand

A central difficulty in determining the permeability pathways through breaks in the junction strand from random thin sections is that the frequency and length of such breaks cannot be determined. A further difficulty is that it is not possible directly to visualize small discrete pores that would allow the passage of small and intermediate-sized solutes using standard thin sections of 40–50 nm. These dimensions are much larger than the 5–6 nm radius circular pores suggested by the reflection coefficient data. Even if the pores were larger and visible they might be infrequent and thus hard to detect. The three-dimensional serial section reconstruction electron micrographs of rat heart capillaries by

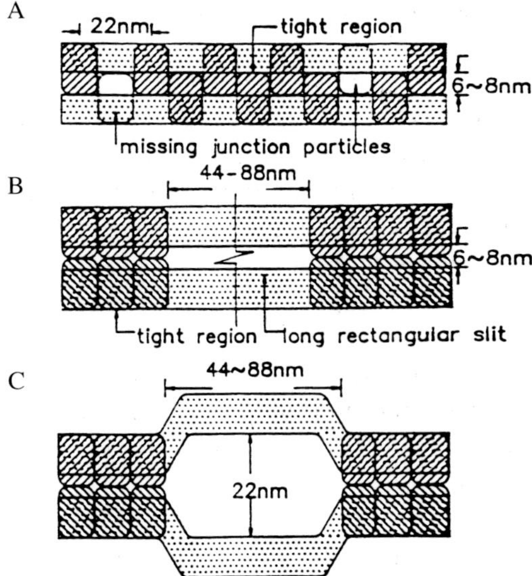

Fig. 2. Three schematic diagrams of junction protein arrangements. These protein arrangements correspond to (A) small gaps suggested by Bundgaard's (1984) ultrathin sections (the zigzag protein pattern was first proposed by Tsay *et al.* 1989), (B) long rectangular constricted slit pores, similar to those in the one-dimensional constricted channel model, and (C) large pores formed by discontinuities of 44–88 nm in the junctional strands with gap height the same as that of the wide part of the cleft. From Weinbaum *et al.* (1992).

Bundgaard (1984) provided the first ultrastructural insights into such questions. Bundgaard observed two possible pores. One was an infrequent large break typically of one or two standard section thicknesses whose frequency was approximately one per micrometer of junction strand length. The second was a more frequent small gap that was suggested by a small sample of ultrathin 12–15 nm sections, where slit-like pores as short as 12 nm were visible. The latter results were more speculative since they were at the borderline of the resolution of the electron micrographs.

The foregoing observations led Weinbaum *et al.* (1992) to propose three alternative structures for the arrangement of the proteins in the junction strands (Fig. 2). The molecular structure in Fig. 2A was first proposed by Tsay *et al.* (1989) as a way in which size-selective pores could be formed by individual missing proteins. The alternating arrangement of proteins between opposite membranes was motivated by the observation of Firth *et al.* (1983) that the average spacing between junctional proteins in each membrane of guinea pig placental capillaries in freeze cleavage electron micrographs of the junction strand arrays was 22 nm, just twice the diameter of the individual proteins, 11 nm. The length of the pore, one missing protein, was suggested by the ultrathin serial sections (12–15 nm) in Bundgaard (1984), mentioned previously, where there was evidence for small slit pores as short as 12 nm. A pore of these dimensions corresponds closely to a small circular hole of 5.5 nm radius, which, as noted previously, provides an excellent fit to reflection coefficient data for nearly all solutes up to the size of albumin (3.5 nm radius).

The second possibility shown in Fig. 2B is the constricted slit geometry that was the basis for the size-selective junction pore models in Fig. 1A. The slit height of 6–8 nm is selected so that the slit can function as the primary molecular filter and the length of the discontinuity, 4–8 missing junction proteins, is representative of the length of the larger breaks observed by Bundgaard (1984). Although the constricted slit can function as the molecular filter, the most recent serial section electron micrographs of Adamson and Michel (1993) of frog mesentery capillaries confirm the more tentative observations of Bundgaard (1984) that the gap height at the large junction strand discontinuities approaches that of the wide part of the cleft. Thus, the third and most realistic proposed junction structure for intermediate-sized solutes between 1 and 3.5 nm radius is the molecular configuration shown in Fig. 2C. The length of the large breaks shown in this figure, 44–88 nm, is for rat heart capillaries. This length varies with species, and the recent studies by Adamson and Michel (1993) show that this dimension for frog mesentery is approximately 150 nm. It is evident that the large breaks shown in Fig. 2C cannot function as the molecular sieve and that this model, unlike the models in Fig. 2A,B, requires the presence of matrix components to provide for the molecular filter.

Initial three-dimensional model

The initial three-dimensional model for a cleft with a junction strand and cross-

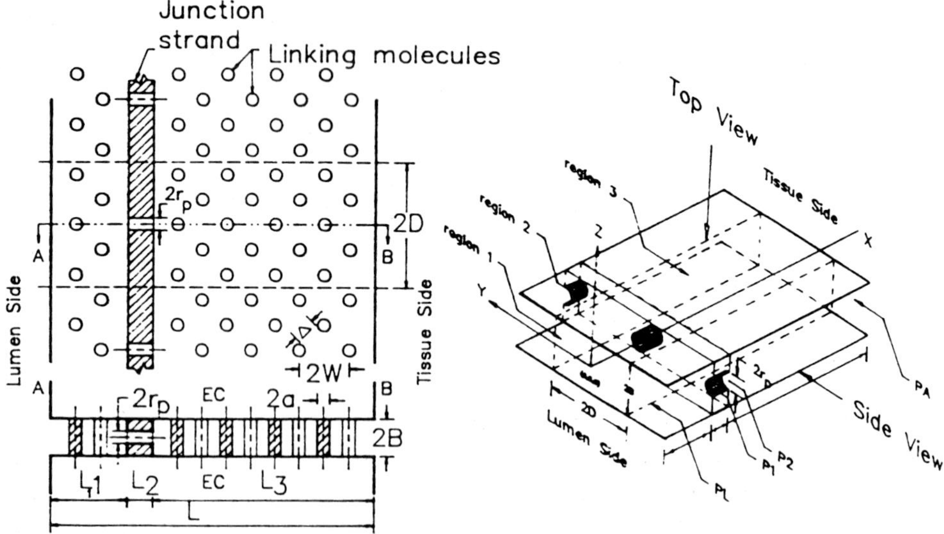

Fig. 3. Two diagrammatic views of the three-dimensional junction–pore–matrix model of the intercellular cleft. A junctional strand with periodic pores lies parallel to luminal front. L_2 is the depth of pores in the junctional strand and L_1 and L_3 are the depths between the junctional strand and the luminal and abluminal fronts. Within the wide portion of the cleft, cross-bridging fibers are represented by a periodic square array of transverse cylindrical fibers of radius a with an open gap spacing Δ. The distance between two adjacent pores in the junctional strand is $2D$. From Weinbaum *et al.* (1992).

bridging matrix fibers in its wide part was first proposed in Tsay *et al.* (1989) (see Fig. 3). Here, the junction strand is treated as an impermeable barrier with periodically distributed discrete circular pores of 5.5 nm radius representing the individual missing proteins corresponding to the molecular structure depicted in Fig. 2A. The matrix components in the wide part of the cleft are represented by an ordered square array of fibers of radius a aligned perpendicular to the plasmalemma boundaries with periodic spacing $2W$ and an open gap Δ between them. The fibers were assumed to fill the entire wide portion of the cleft, as was assumed in the original fiber matrix model of Curry and Michel (1980) sketched in Fig. 1B. The ordering of the fibers was based on Michel's hypothesis (1988) that the positive arginine groups at the ends of the albumin molecule ordered the negatively charged matrix. The recent ultrastructural studies of Schulze and Firth (1992) and Satcher (1993) have provided more direct evidence for both the regular ordering of the fibers in the wide part of the cleft and their perpendicular arrangement.

The initial model depicted in Fig. 3 was first solved to give L_p for the circular pore geometry by Tsay *et al.* (1989). A weak interaction theory for the fibers was also presented on the basis of Lee and Fung's (1969) two-term approximation for the flow past a cylindrical post in a channel. The results of this two-term approximation are not presented here since a more rigorous hydrodynamic theory for the fiber–boundary interaction was subsequently developed by Tsay and Weinbaum (1991). The latter theory was first applied by Weinbaum *et al.* (1992), who also developed a new approximate approach for calculating the permeability P of a solute molecule diffusing in a channel with matrix components. These three papers have set the stage for the more refined models of Fu *et al.* (1994, 1995). The key results from Tsay *et al.* (1989), Tsay and Weinbaum (1991) and Weinbaum *et al.* (1992) are presented in the next three sections.

Hydrodynamic pore interaction

The basic flow model in Fig. 3 involves two fundamental hydrodynamic interaction problems: (i) the three-dimensional interaction between the pores in the junction strand and (ii) the interaction between the fibers and the boundaries in the wide part of the cleft. Problem i is treated by Tsay *et al.* (1989). The expression for L_p for the entire cleft can be written in terms of three resistances in series:

$$L_p = (R_1 + R_2 + R_3)^{-1}, \tag{3}$$

where R_1 and R_3 describe the resistances of the wide parts of the channel and R_2 describes the resistance within the junction pore itself. Since the channel height $2B$ is much less than the pore spacing $2D$ or the cleft depth L, the pore interaction in regions 1 and 3 (see Fig. 3) is treated using Hele–Shaw flow theory. The flow within the circular pore of radius r_p is approximated by a Poiseuille flow; however, the flow through the wider breaks shown in Fig. 2B,C is more subtle and will be described later. The solution to the overall boundary value problem provides the expressions for R_1, R_2 and R_3, which are given for a circular pore by Tsay *et al.* (1989). These solutions show that L_p is insensitive to the location of the junction strand within the cleft and that a measured L_p for frog mesentery of $2 \times 10^{-7}\,\mathrm{cm\,s^{-1}\,cmH_2O^{-1}}$ can be achieved when roughly 1 in 25 proteins is missing from the junction strand if the resistance of the matrix components in the wide part of the cleft is neglected. The treatment of this matrix is discussed next.

Hydrodynamic interaction between fibers in the wide part of the cleft

Tsay and Weinbaum (1991) have developed a highly accurate solution for the additional flow resistance due to the fibers in the wide portion of the cleft. In this analysis, the actual viscosity μ is replaced by an effective viscosity μ_{eff} defined by $\mathrm{grad}\langle p\rangle=\mu_{\mathrm{eff}}\langle\bar{v}\rangle/B^2$, where $\langle p\rangle$ denotes an average over a region which is small compared with the depth of the cleft L. For the periodic fiber arrangement shown in Fig. 3, the averages of the pressure p and velocity $\bar{v}$ are taken over a periodic unit containing a single fiber. The effective increase in viscosity is given by a hydrodynamic interaction function f defined by $\mu_{\mathrm{eff}}=\mu f$, which depends only on the length ratios B/a and δ/B, where δ is the fiber interaction layer thickness. For our fiber-channel geometry, $2B\approx20$ nm and a=0.6 nm, if the fiber is a GAG sidechain on a typical proteoglycan, whereas a=2 nm if the fiber is the protein monomer of the proteoglycan. Thus, B/a lies in the range 5–18 and Δ/B is of the order of 1. For this range of values of B/a and Δ/B, fiber–fiber and fiber–boundary interactions are both important.

The boundary value problem for determining f and μ_{eff} requires that the no slip boundary conditions be satisfied on the surface of each fiber and on the channel walls. In Tsay and Weinbaum (1991) an exact infinite series solution to the full boundary value problem for the doubly periodic fiber array is constructed, using the fundamental singularities for a single circular post developed by Lee and Fung (1969) and a quasi-periodic function that is a linear combination of the Weierstrass zeta function and its derivatives, in order to describe the periodicity conditions for each fiber unit cell. This highly accurate theory is mathematically cumbersome and difficult to apply; however, it provides a benchmark for testing the accuracy of more simplified approaches, such as the effective medium theory of Brinkman (1947).

In Tsay and Weinbaum (1991) an expression for f is also derived using an effective medium approach based on the Darcy–Brinkman equation:

$$\mathrm{grad}p=-\frac{\mu}{K_{\mathrm{p}}}\bar{v}+\mu\Delta^2\bar{v}, \tag{4}$$

where $\bar{v}$ is the water velocity. In equation 4, K_{p} is a Darcy permeability coefficient which describes the flow through an infinite matrix that has the same fiber geometry as the interior of the bounded flow under consideration. In this case, this flow corresponds to the two-dimensional flow perpendicular to a doubly periodic array of infinitely long cylinders of radius a. It is shown in Tsay and Weinbaum (1991) that the following simple expression for K_{p} is accurate to within 10 % for all solid volume fractions $S<0.7$:

$$K_{\mathrm{p}}=0.0572a^2(\Delta/a)^{2.377}. \tag{5}$$

The final expression for f derived by Tsay and Weinbaum (1991) is given by:

$$f=-\frac{\beta^3}{3(\beta-\tanh\beta)}, \tag{6}$$

where $\beta=B/\sqrt{K_p}$ is a dimensionless length ratio whose denominator $\sqrt{K_p}$ is the fiber interaction layer thickness δ along the boundaries of the cleft. L_p for the matrix layer in the wide part of the cleft can be simply related to f as follows:

$$L_p = \frac{2B^3}{3\mu f}\left(\frac{L_{jt}}{L_m}\right), \tag{7}$$

where L_m is the depth of the channel with matrix components and L_{jt} is the total cleft length per unit endothelial surface area. A comparison of the exact infinite series solution for f with the Brinkman approximation (equation 6) reveals that the latter provides remarkably good agreement with the rigorous hydrodynamic solutions provided that the fiber aspect ratio $B/a>5$. Equation 7 can also be applied to random fiber geometries, if one uses a suitable approximation for the infinite medium value of K_p that appears in the expression for f in equation 6.

Diffusive permeability

A two-dimensional theory for calculating the permeability P of a solute of finite size diffusing through the cleft geometry in Fig. 3 is described by Weinbaum *et al.* (1992). Separate models are developed to predict (i) the diffusive resistance of the junction strand and (ii) the added resistance of the fiber matrix in the wide part of the cleft. An equivalent expression to equation 3 is written for P, where R_1, R_2 and R_3 are now diffusive resistances. Problem (i) is very similar to the boundary value problem already described for Hele–Shaw flow in regions 1 and 3, since the governing equations and boundary conditions for the pressure field are equivalent to the boundary value problem for pure diffusion of a solute through this same geometry. The solution of this boundary value problem leads to expressions for R_1 and R_3 (equation 19 in Weinbaum *et al.* 1992). The expression for R_2 in the junction strand breaks is given for both circular and rectangular pores by Curry (1984).

The foregoing expressions for R_1 and R_3 involve a new approximation for the diffusion coefficient for a solute in a channel with fiber matrix components. Instead of using the statistical theory of Ogston *et al.* (1973) for the diffusion of a solute molecule in an infinite matrix, the approximate expression derived by Weinbaum *et al.* (1992) attempts to describe the hydrodynamic interaction of the solute molecule with both the matrix and the walls of the cleft, boundary value problem ii above. To account for the hydrodynamic resistance of the fibers, one first solves the Brinkman equation (equation 4) for the motion of a sphere in an infinite medium. This leads to the following expression:

$$D_{im} = D_{iw}\left[1 + \frac{r_s}{\sqrt{K_p}} + \frac{1}{3}\frac{r_s^2}{K_p}\right]^{-1} \qquad (i=1,3) \tag{8}$$

for the diffusion coefficient D_{im}. The term in brackets describes the drag on a sphere of radius r_s in a matrix whose infinite medium Darcy permeability coefficient is K_p. To account for the cleft boundaries, the term in brackets is multiplied by D_{iw}, the restricted diffusion coefficient derived by Ganatos *et al.* (1980) which describes the Stokes solution for the drag on a spherical particle in a parallel-walled channel.

The above expression for D_{im} does not include the steric exclusion of the fibers and the spatial variation of the concentration in the available space of the matrix. To include these effects, Weinbaum *et al.* (1992) solved the diffusion equation for a periodic fiber array in which a zero flux boundary condition is applied at the exclusion radius $a+r_s$ of the fibers, where a is the fiber radius. The final result is an expression for $D_{iw,eff}/D_{im}$ which is a function of the effective fiber fraction $S_e=S(1+r_s/a)^2$ where S is the actual fiber fraction and S_e accounts for the exclusion radius. This function is plotted in Fig. 5 of Weinbaum *et al.* (1992). Having determined $D_{iw,eff}$, the permeability P is obtained from the expression:

$$P = \frac{2BL_{jt}}{L} D_{iw,eff}. \tag{9}$$

Predictions of the initial model for L_p *and* P

Results are presented in Weinbaum *et al.* (1992) for L_p and P for the three basic pore geometries sketched in Fig. 2, both with and without matrix components in the wide part of the cleft. For the basic junction pore model without matrix, one finds that the measured value of $L_p=5.9\times10^{-7}\,\mathrm{cm\,s^{-1}\,cmH_2O^{-1}}$ can be satisfied for the small 5.5 nm radius pore when $2D$=90 nm, for the 8 nm constricted slit when $2D$=370 nm, for the 22 nm×44 nm large break when $2D$=1.2 μm and for the 22 nm×88 nm large break when $2D$=1.65 μm. These predictions for $2D$ corresponding to the measured L_p are then used in equaton 9 to determine P. The key results are summarized in Fig. 4. The 5.5 nm radius pore and the 8 nm constricted slit, while they satisfied the measured data for NaCl and sucrose (first two data points), provide a very poor fit for the intermediate-sized solutes between 1.0 and 3.5 nm radius. In contrast, the larger 44 and 88 nm breaks suggest a better fit for the

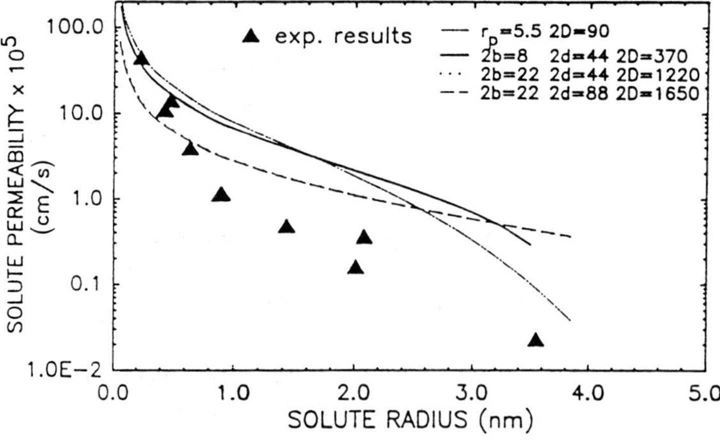

Fig. 4. Solutions for the diffusive permeability for clefts for the three basic pore geometries illustrated in Fig. 2. The spacing between pores ($2D$) is determined from the solutions for pore spacing $2D$ which satisfy $L_p=5.9\times10^{-7}\,\mathrm{cm\,s^{-1}\,cmH_2O^{-1}}$ (frog mesentery; Clough and Michel, 1988). The filled triangles are measured values for P taken from Curry (1986). From Weinbaum *et al.* (1992).

intermediate-sized solutes, but substantially underestimate P for the small solutes. No pore model provides a compatible prediction for both L_p and P regardless of the geometry of the junction strand pore.

In Weinbaum *et al.* (1992), the results for the basic junction strand model just summarized are supplemented by predictions for a cleft with just matrix components and a combined junction pore–fiber matrix model with both a junction strand and matrix components distributed throughout its wide part. The principal predictions of the combined junction pore–fiber matrix model are (i) that a matrix with a size-selective molecular filter for intermediate-sized solutes (Δ=7 nm) cannot fill the entire depth of the cleft since the additional hydraulic resistance is too large to satisfy the measured L_p; (ii) that large infrequent breaks provide a better fit for P for intermediate-sized solutes; however, matrix components must be present at the luminal surface and/or in the entrance region of the cleft to account for the molecular filter; (iii) that a fiber matrix offers little resistance to small ions, and the results shown in Fig. 4 for P for small solutes would not be significantly affected by a sieving matrix for intermediate-sized solutes.

The model predictions just summarized are based on four important assumptions: (i) that the flow in the junction pore has a velocity profile typical of a viscous flow in a duct with the same cross secion, (ii) that the matrix fills the entire depth of the wide part of the cleft (iii) that there is only a single family of pores in the junction strand and (iv) that the concentration at the cleft exit does not vary significantly with time and is close to zero because the tissue acts as an infinite reservoir. In the remainder of the paper, each of these assumptions will be examined in greater detail.

Flow profiles in junction pores

The flow in the vicinity of the junction strand pores when there are longer slit-like breaks of the type shown in Fig. 2B,C is a complicated hydrodynamic problem. In the limit where the break length $2d \gg 2B$, the channel height, the flow profiles in the plane of the junction strand in planes parallel to the channel walls should approach a potential flow solution with infinite velocities at the edges of the break and a minimum velocity along the pore axis according to the Hele–Shaw flow approximation. Thus, in contrast to the flow through the small circular pores shown in Fig. 2A, which is reasonably approximated by a parabolic velocity profile with a maximum on the pore axis, the flow through the large pores in Fig. 2B,C should deviate greatly from Poiseuille flow theory. Intuitively, one anticipates that the velocity profiles will change from potential flow to Poiseuille flow character, and the hydrodynamic resistance change accordingly, as the ratio d/B decreases. Only when d/B is of the order of 1 should the profiles resemble unidirectional Poiseuille flow in a rectangular pore.

To investigate the above behavior, Zeng and Weinbaum (1994) have developed a new exact three-dimensional solution to the Stokes equations for the flow through rectangular orifices in a channel. Such orifices are a realistic representation of the slit-like breaks in the junction strand illustrated in Fig. 2B,C. The characteristic velocity profiles in the midplane of the orifice for a 150 nm long pore typical of the large breaks observed by Adamson and Michel (1993) in the junction strand of frog mesentery microvessels are shown in Fig. 5. Also shown is the Hele–Shaw potential profile with the infinite edge

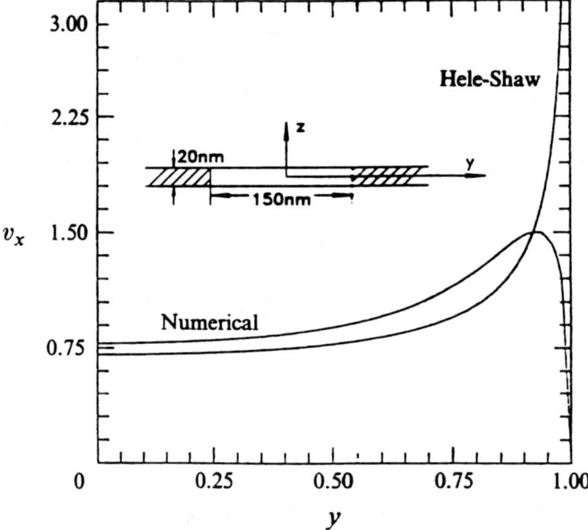

Fig. 5. Velocity profiles perpendicular to the y,z plane (v_x) at the orifice opening in the channel midplane z=0. A sketch of the corresponding cross section with barriers shaded is shown to scale in the inset. From Zeng and Weinbaum (1994).

velocities discussed above. One observes that the Hele–Shaw profile is a good approximation except in the localized region near the orifice edge, where a viscous flow must satisfy no-slip conditions.

Parker *et al.* (1993) in an Appendix to Adamson and Michel (1993) have used the Hele–Shaw approximation in Fig. 5 to obtain a potential solution for an isolated pore in a junction strand that is arbitrarily positioned within the cleft. They introduce a correction factor c to describe the increase in L_p compared with one-dimensional theory that results from the spreading of streamlines fore and aft of the junction strand break in the wide part of the cleft. The Hele–Shaw model predicts that for a 150 nm break in a 400 nm deep cleft, c=2.2 if the strand is positioned midway in the cleft and increases to 3.1 as the strand is moved to either the luminal or the tissue border of the cleft.

Junction–orifice–fiber entrance layer model

Experimental observations

Shortly after the theoretical calculations of Weinbaum *et al.* (1992) were completed, two experimental papers appeared which have had an important impact on the refinement of the initial model. In the first of these studies (Adamson and Clough, 1992), cytochemical studies were performed which provided the first accurate estimates of the thickness of the endothelial surface glycocalyx. They showed that the surface layer could extend up to 100 nm from the surface and that its structure was strongly dependent on the plasma proteins in the perfusate. Using cationized ferritin to visualize the outer border of the surface layer, these investigators observed that the average thickness of the surface fiber layer in plasma was 60 nm. In an earlier study, Adamson (1990) had shown that the enzymatic degradation of the surface matrix led to a 2.5-fold increase in L_p. These two experimental observations, the thickness of the surface glycocalyx and the increase in L_p after its removal, when combined, provided the first reliable experimental data for estimating the overall effective thickness of the matrix layer and its hydraulic resistance in our theoretical model.

In a more recent study, Adamson and Michel (1993) have obtained the first detailed measurements of the size and frequency of junction strand discontinuities in frog mesentery capillaries in which simultaneous measurements were also obtained for the cleft geometry and L_p. The frequency of the breaks was assessed using both conventional serial sections of 40–50 nm thickness and lanthanum-perfused microvessels in which the frequency and lateral spreading of the tracer wakes on the downstream side of the junction strand were quantified. Specifically, in vessels perfused without lanthanum, there were three interruptions with an average length of 150 nm in a total of 13.36 μm of junctional strand (mean distance between breaks was 4450 nm). In vessels perfused with lanthanum, 11 breaks were found in a total cleft length of 23.6 mm. The average length of the discontinuities for the lanthanum-perfused vessels was 160 nm, and the mean distance between the breaks was 2140 nm. In both experiments, the gap height of the breaks was the same size as the wide part of the cleft, confirming the pore model proposed in Fig. 2C. These data provided valuable realistic bounds on the model parameters describing the junction strand geometry for the quantitative evaluation of our three-dimensional mathematical models. The hydraulic conductivity of all vessels was measured and an average value for L_p of 2×10^{-7} cm s^{-1} cmH_2O^{-1} was obtained.

Hydraulic conductivity and the thickness of the fiber entrance

The experimental studies described above set the stage for a substantially refined model in which the other assumptions and predictions of Weinbaum *et al.* (1992) could be more accurately evaluated. In particular, one wished to examine the possibilities (i) that the sieving part of the fiber matrix was confined to a thin layer at the endothelial surface and the entrance region of the wide part of the cleft, (ii) that there were large infrequent junction strand discontinuities of typically 150 nm length in frog mesentery capillaries that occupied only a small percentage of the total cleft length and (iii) that a very small pore for small ions existed in parallel with the large pore breaks. A modified junction–orifice–fiber entrance layer model was proposed by Fu *et al.* (1994*b*) to test these hypotheses and is shown schematically in Fig. 6. The model contains three essential components: an entrance layer of sieving fibers of effective thickness L_f, orifice-like breaks in the junction strand of cross section $2d\times2B$ and spacing $2D$, and a family of narrow slits of approximately 2 nm height which will be discussed in the next section.

One would first like to determine the effective thickness L_f of a finite matrix layer that includes both the endothelial surface glyocalyx and some unknown thickness of matrix that penetrates the entrance region of the wide part of the cleft. The matrix layer that lies within the cleft is treated using the effective medium Brinkman theory described earlier. The matrix at the endothelial surface is well described by K_p in equation 5. The effective

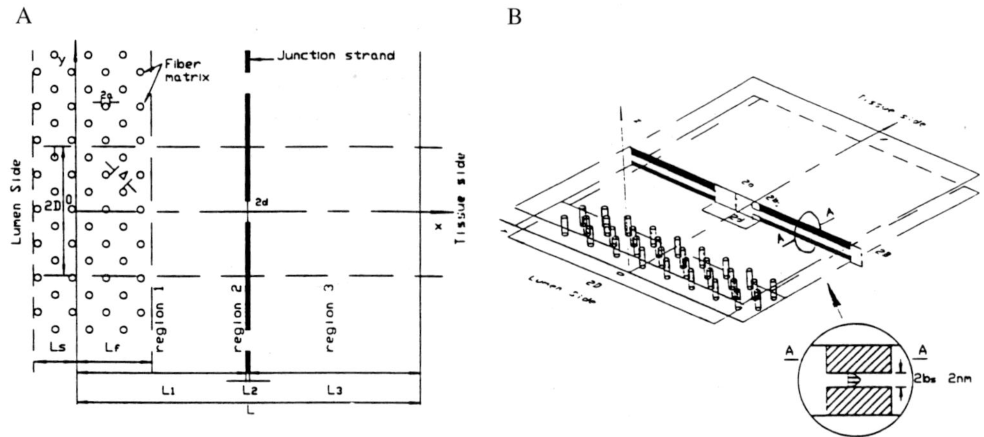

Fig. 6. (A) Plane view of the junction–orifice–matrix entrance layer model of the intercellular cleft. A junction strand with periodic openings lies parallel to the luminal front. The distance between two adjacent breaks in the junctional strand is $2D$. At the entrance of the cleft on the luminal side, fiber matrix is represented by an ordered square array of transverse cylindrical fibers whose spacing is $2a+\Delta$. (B) Three-dimensional sketch of a single periodic unit of width $2D$ showing the central orifice of height $2B$ and narrow slits of height $2b_s$. From Fu *et al.* (1994).

Darcy permeability in the wide part of the cleft, $K_{p,\mathrm{eff}}$, can be related to K_p using the function f defined in equation 6. Using the ratio of $K_{p,\mathrm{eff}}/K_p$, one can convert any thickness of surface layer L_s into an equivalent layer thickness of matrix in the wide part of the cleft and treat the matrix as a single layer of effective thickness L_f.

A mathematically rigorous treatment of the filtration boundary value problem for a finite entrance layer with $L_f<L_1$ requires that the pressure be treated as an unknown along the interface $x=L_f$ between the fiber-free and fiber-filled regions. A much simpler approach, with sufficient accuracy for the present purposes, is to assume an average effective viscosity in region 1, $\mu^{(1)}$, which is an average of μ_f in the fiber layer and μ in the fiber-free subregion and is proportional to the relative depth of each region. This simplification allows one to reduce the boundary value problem for the clefts to a two-region problem with different effective viscosities $\mu^{(1)}$ and $\mu^{(3)}$ in regions 1 and 3 whose x velocity component and pressure must match at the orifice opening.

In Fu *et al.* (1994) the simplified two-region problem is solved using the approximate Hele–Shaw velocity profile shown in Fig. 5 at the large pore breaks. Fig. 7 shows the solution for the decrease in hydraulic resistance as the ratio of the thickness of the sieving fiber layer to the cleft depth L_f/L is increased. Typical values for the total cleft depth (L) are 400 nm and all dimensions in the legend are in nanometers. $2D=2640$ nm is the average spacing of all 14 breaks (average break length $2d=150$ nm) observed in Adamson and Michel (1993) and the values $2D=2140$ nm and $2D=4450$ nm are the measured spacings with and without lanthanum tracer. One notes that the measured value of $L_p=2.0\,\mathrm{cm\,s^{-1}\,cmH_2O^{-1}}$ is achieved when $L_f/L=0.25$ or the fiber layer thickness is 100 nm if the frequency of the lanthanum wakes, $2D=2140$ nm, is used for the input data.

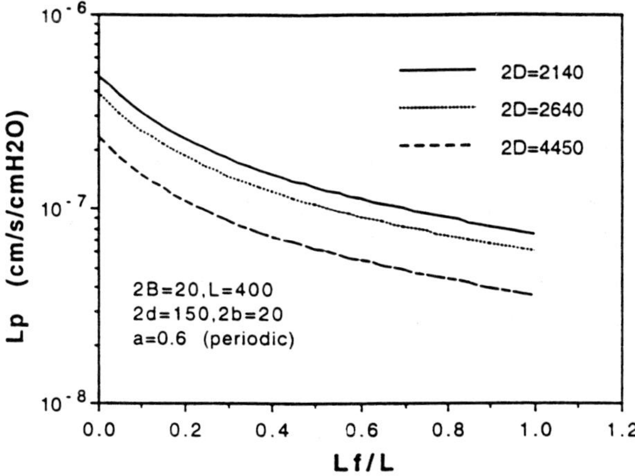

Fig. 7. L_p as a function of the dimensionless depth L_f/L of the fiber entrance layer for the minimum (2140 nm), maximum (4450 nm) and average (2640 nm) spacing $2D$ between adjacent breaks (Adamson and Michel, 1993). Solid fraction S_f=0.017 corresponds to a=0.6 nm and Δ=7 nm. All lengths are in nanometers. From Fu *et al.* (1994).

The $2D$=2640 nm curve in Fig. 7 almost exactly predicts the 2.5-fold increase in L_p to 4.9 cm s^{-1} cmH$_2$O^{-1} that was measured by Adamson (1990) when the surface glycocalyx was enzymatically removed, L_f/L=0. Using the ratio $K_{p,eff}/K_p$ described earlier, one finds that a surface glycocalyx of 60 nm is equivalent to a 45 nm thick fiber layer in the cleft. A predicted L_f of 100 nm would thus correspond to a matrix layer that penetrated to a depth of 55 nm in the entrance region of the cleft plus this surface layer.

Diffusive permeability: two-pore model

Equivalent results to those shown in Fig. 7 for L_p are presented in Fu *et al.* (1994) for P_l. One finds that the predicted curves for P_l, which satisfy the measured L_p of 2.0 cm s^{-1} cmH$_2$O^{-1}, underestimate small ion permeability by at least a factor of 3. However, the fit to the measured data for P_l for intermediate-sized solutes with a radius greater than 1 nm is far superior to the predictions in Fig. 4, where the model of Weinbaum *et al.* (1992) led to results for P that were larger than the measured P for these larger solutes by a factor of 3–5.

The foregoing predictions suggested that a heretofore unrecognized second pore system for the diffusion of small ions might exist in parallel with the large break discontinuities. A second pore of this nature would allow for a significant increase in P without significantly changing the results for L_p in Fig. 7, since the hydraulic resistance of the small pore would be much larger than its diffusive resistance. (L_p is proportional to the third power of the slit height $2b_s$, whereas P is proportional to the pore area). A narrow continuous slit is a particularly appealing choice for this second pore since Adamson and Michel (1993) have observed a narrow translucent region of roughly 2 nm gap height between outer membrane leaflets when thin sections with junctional occlusions were viewed after goniometric tilting.

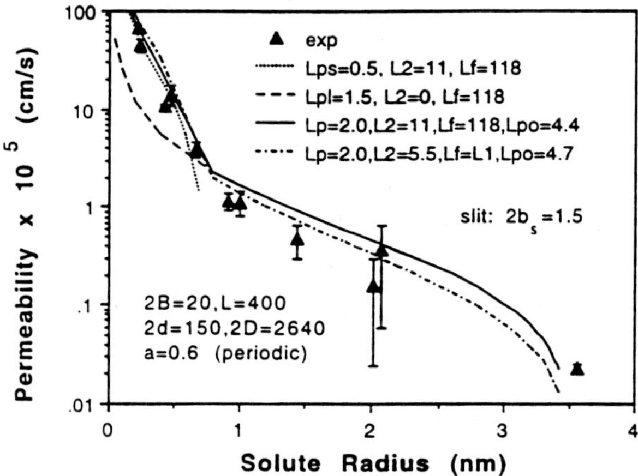

Fig. 8. Permeability P as a function of solute radius r_s for a two-pore model consisting of large 150 nm×20 nm orifice breaks and a continuous narrow slit of height 1.5 nm. L_{ps} is the contribution to L_p from small pores and L_{pl} is the contribution from large breaks. The total L_p is fixed at $2.0\times10^{-7}\,\mathrm{cm\,s^{-1}\,cmH_2O^{-1}}$. L_{po} is the value without matrix. All lengths are in nanometers and units of $L_p{=}\times10^{-7}\,\mathrm{cm\,s^{-1}\,cmH_2O^{-1}}$. S_f=0.017 periodic matrix, $L_1{=}L_3$ and $L_f{=}L_1$. From Fu *et al.* (1994*b*).

In Fu *et al.* (1994), two types of very small pores are explored, a narrow continuous slit of height $2b_s$, as shown in Fig. 6, and a small circular 1.5 nm radius pore whose spacing was set equal to the diameter of the intramembranous proteins in the junction strand, 11 nm. The latter pores could represent the interstices between abutting proteins (see Fig. 2B,C). In either case, the depth L_2 of these pores was assumed to lie between 5.5 and 11 nm, reasonable bounds for the thickness of the junction strands. The resistance of the narrow slit pore system is described by simple one-dimensional pore-slit theory and the small circular pores by the model shown in Fig. 3.

The predictions of the two-pore model (large breaks and very small pores) are illustrated in Fig. 8 for the case where the second pore is a narrow slit. In these calculations, the total hydraulic conductivity $L_p = L_{pl}$(large pore) + L_{ps}(small pore) and we require that $L_p{=}2.0\times10^{-7}\,\mathrm{cm\,s^{-1}\,cmH_2O^{-1}}$ remain unchanged. The predicted individual contributions of the large- and small-pore systems to L_p are shown in the figure, as is the predicted effective thickness L_f of the fiber entrance layer. The height $2b_s$ of the narrow slit was adjusted to provide an optimum fit of the data for small ion permeability, which for the narrow slit was achieved for a gap height of 1.5 nm. One observes that a very good fit to P can be obtained for solutes of all sizes for this two-pore system. The continuous dashed curve is the result that one obtains if only the large 150 nm orifice pores are present. It is clear that only the two-pore model is able to explain the intriguing change in slope of P at $r_s{\approx}1$ nm. Similar agreement to that shown in Fig. 8 can also be obtained for a small circular pore of 1.5 nm radius with spacing $2D{=}11$ nm. This combined model of large breaks, as the pathway for large solutes and much of the water, and very small pores or slits, as the primary pathway for small ions, is also able to account for the 2.5-fold increase in L_p that is observed when the surface glycocalyx is enzymatically removed (Adamson, 1990). The increase in hydraulic conductivity when the matrix is removed given by the L_{po} values in Fig. 8.

Junction strand wakes: time-dependent labelling studies

Very important additional evidence in support of the small pore hypothesis has been obtained from our latest time-dependent studies of the penetration of lanthanum into the cleft on the abluminal side of the junction strand, confocal microscopic measurements of the spread of sodium fluorescein in the tissue surrounding a perfused microvessel and a newly developed theoretical model for describing the time-dependent labelling behavior observed in these experiments. Both these low molecular weight tracers ($r_s \approx 0.4$ nm) should easily pass through the small pore system.

Experimental studies

As noted earlier, Adamson and Michel (1993) observed the penetration of lanthanum tracers beyond the junction strand approximately 15 s after tracer was introduced and concluded that about 6 % of the cleft length was labelled to the margins of the cleft exit. When these studies were repeated in our laboratory, a striking difference between the tracer distributions after short (10 s) and longer (60 s) perfusions was observed. At 10 s, the frequency of discontinuities in the junctional strand was similar to the earlier observations in Adamson and Michel. However, when serial sections of a frog mesenteric capillary were perfused for 60 s following the same procedure, lanthanum was observed to fill the cleft beyond the junctional constriction to the abluminal border in every section. Most significantly, all clefts from this vessel exhibited the same pattern of leakage.

These observations strongly suggest that clefts leak along their entire length but that the threshold for visibility of lanthanum at the cleft exit is exceeded only after sufficient diffusional filling of the surrounding tissue. Thus, the wakes from the large breaks are labelled at early times because their high flux density allows the local concentration at the cleft exit in the vicinity of these large pores to rise rapidly. However, the results of the two-pore model of Fu *et al.* (1994) predict that the total flux for small solutes through the infrequent large pores is less than one-third of the flux through the small-pore system (see Fig. 8) and that, after longer times, the latter flux will dominate and fill the entire tissue space surrounding the cleft exit. When this occurs, every cleft should be labelled on the abluminal side of the junction strand. The importance of the time-dependent labelling of the extravascular space had never previously been considered in the interpretation of electron microscopic labelled tracer studies. In fact, all previous permeability measurements have been based on the assumption that the tissue concentration was low and could be neglected in calculating endothelial permeability.

Strong evidence in support of this hypothesis has been provided by the first confocal microscopic images just obtained by Roger Adamson in our laboratory for the detailed time-varying distribution of a low molecular weight fluorescent tracer surrounding an individually perfused microvessel under well-controlled conditions *in situ*. The orientation of the vessels and the junction strands with their large breaks are shown schematically in cross-sectional and side views of the vessel in Fig. 9. Previous studies

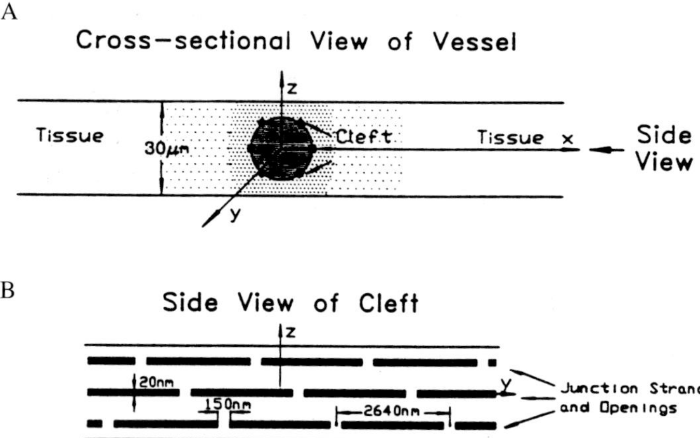

Fig. 9. Schematic of model for confocal microscopy. (A) Cross-sectional view of a frog mesenteric microvessel with several clefts distributed around the perimeter of the vessel wall. Shading indicates decreasing concentration of fluorescent probe as one proceeds into the tissue. (B) Side view looking into the cleft along the length of the junction strand. Three clefts are shown with periodically spaced large pore junction strand breaks.

have provided only two-dimensional integrated *en face* projections of the tracer distribution around the vessel, rather than the detailed distribution in a given plane. The new experimental technique provides critical information on the distribution of the tracer in a cross-sectional plane, the rate of tracer diffusion into the tissue and the concentration of the tracer at the capillary wall as it enters the tissue (cleft exit concentration). The laser can scan approximately 30 000 data points in a given plane in approximately 3 s. A typical profile in the plane $z=0$ is shown at different times from 0 to 58 s in Fig. 10. These time-dependent profiles show that the concentration at the cleft exit rose to about 50 % of the luminal concentration after 58 s of perfusion and suggest that the tracer wakes in our lanthanum studies become visible along the entire length of the junction strand when the cleft exit concentration is close to this value.

Time-dependent model for tracer wakes and tissue labelling

The intriguing results just summarized have motivated a much more sophisticated three-region model for analyzing the time-dependent labelling of the wakes on the abluminal side of the junction strand and the time-dependent, spatially varying labelling of a low molecular weight tracer in the tissue space surrounding the vessel. This more elaborate model is sketched in Fig. 11 and described in detail by Fu *et al.* (1995). As noted above, all previous models have tacitly assumed that in both tracer labelling and permeability studies the concentration $C(L,y,t)$ at the cleft exit vanishes because the tissue space is treated as an infinite reservoir. The model of Fu *et al.* (1995) attempts to predict not only the quasi-steady spatial variation of the cleft exit concentration but also how this concentration changes with time, since this will have a profound effect, as discussed above, on the time-dependent labelling of the lanthanum wakes that are observed downstream of the large breaks in the junction strand.

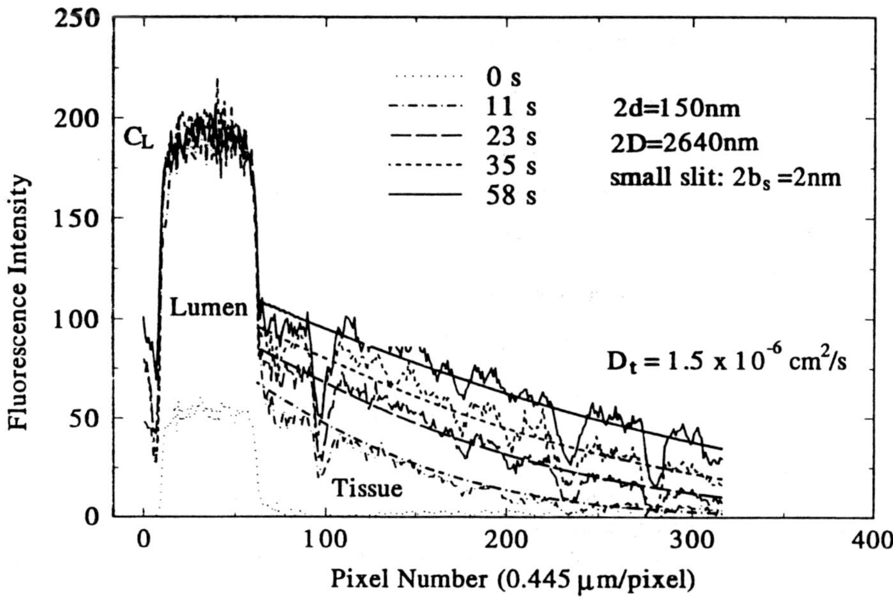

Fig. 10. Comparison of theory (continuous lines) and experimental results for the time-dependent concentration profiles in the tissue space surrounding a frog mesenteric microvessel in the midplane z=0 of the tissue specimen, see Fig. 9. Experimental data courtesy of R. Adamson. Theoretical curves courtesy of B. M. Fu.

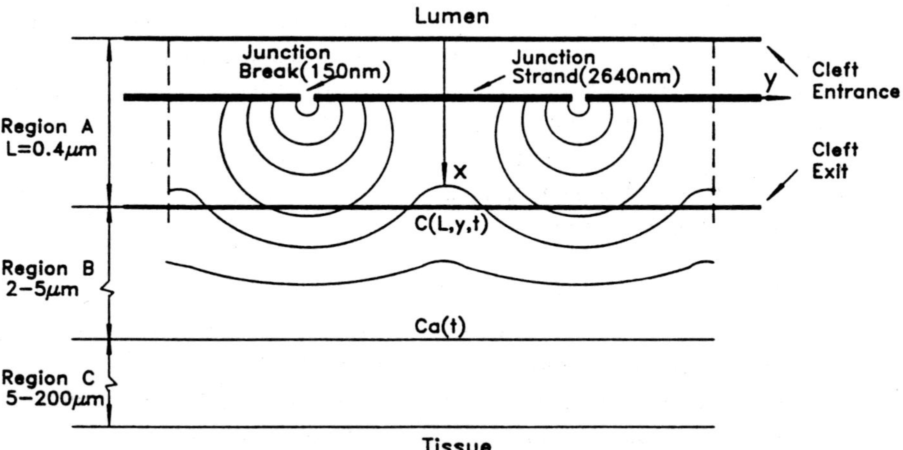

Fig. 11. Diagram of the mathematical model for predicting concentration profiles in the interendothelial cleft beyond the junction strand breaks and in the surrounding tissue space. The model is based on three regions with different characteristic length scales whose typical lengths are shown in the figure and are described in the text.

Fig. 11 is a sketch of the concentration profiles that one would observe at some time in the midplane of an idealized cleft and its continuation into the tissue space if one were to traverse the length of the cleft along the plane z=0 (see Fig. 9). The three regions depicted in Fig. 11 reveal that there is an inner length scale L (region A, 0.4 μm) which characterizes the development of the detailed concentration profiles on the abluminal side of junction strand in the cleft, an intermediate length scale (region B, 2–5 μm) which characterizes the mixing of the wakes from the large orifice discontinuities in the tissue space surrounding the cleft exit and a far field (region C, 200 μm) where these wakes have merged and the tissue transport satisfies one-dimensional, time-dependent diffusion from an integrated source whose strength varies with time.

Asymptotic analysis of the different length scales and characteristic times reveals that important simplifications can be introduced for each region. On the time scale in which the concentration is varying in the far field, the concentration in regions A and B can be treated as satisfying a quasi-steady diffusion equation. On the length scale of the intermediate region, the solute flux at the cleft exit can be treated as a time-varying line source whose strength varies along its length. The line integral of this source provides the unknown time-dependent source strength for the far field. On the length scale of the far field, the intermediate region B can be viewed as the origin x=0 of a lowest-order outer expansion in which the concentration $C_a(t)$ at large values of x in the intermediate region serves to define the flux entering the far field. The critical matching condition coupling the local continuity of flux leaving the cleft exit and entering the far field is given by:

$$\frac{\partial C}{\partial x} = \alpha(t)[C(L, y, t) - C_a(t)], \tag{10}$$

where $\alpha(t)$ is a time-varying function that is determined from the local solution for the line source at the cleft exit in the intermediate region and $\partial C/\partial x$ is the local gradient at the cleft exit. There are significant variations in α at early times (t<1 s), but it then approaches an asymptotic value that is a function of the gap height $2B$ and the diffusion coefficient ratio D_t/D_c for the diffusivity in the extravascular tissue compared with that in the cleft. Measurements of the tissue diffusivity indicate that this ratio is approximately 0.3. The integral of equation 10 along x=L, the cleft exit plane, provides the time-varying source strength for the far field. After a complicated matching procedure, one is able to reduce the overall boundary value problem to an integral equation for the unknown concentration $C_a(t)$, the far-field concentration as x approaches zero on the outer length scale. This is the effective average wall concentration that is measured in our confocal microscopic experiments.

Model predictions

Fu *et al.* (1995) present detailed results for the time-varying wake concentration profiles in the cleft in the vicinity of the junction strand discontinuities, the non-uniform time-varying concentration $C(L,y,t)$ along the cleft exit and the concentration profiles along the midplane z=0, where the confocal microscopic measurements shown in Fig. 10 were obtained. The solutions for the time variation of $C_a(t)$ are shown in Fig. 12 for both the large pore only and the two-pore model where the small pore is a narrow slit of 2 nm height. All the other input parameters are based on the morphometric measurements for the junction strand previously obtained in Adamson and Michel (1993). One observes

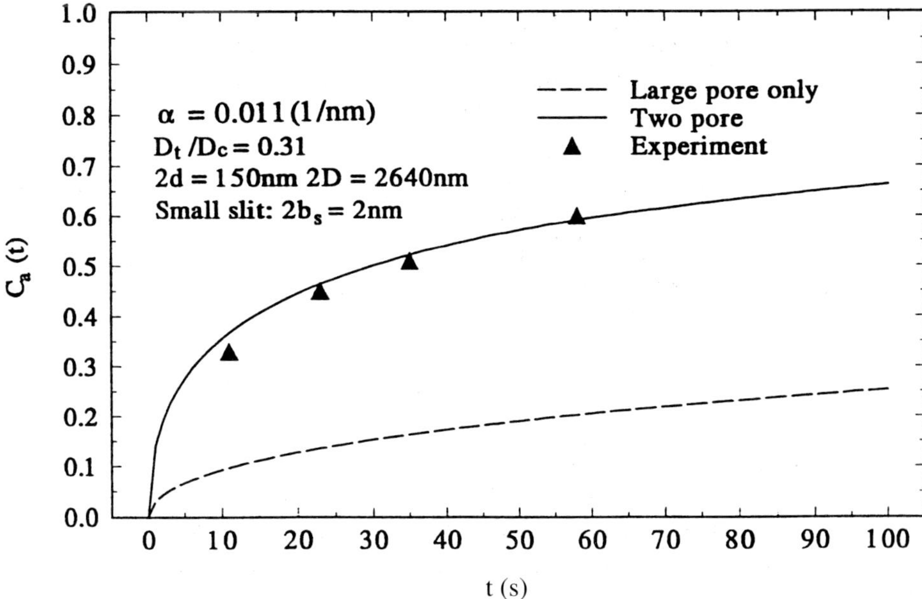

Fig. 12. The rise in average tissue concentration $C_a(t)$ at the wall of a microvessel as a function of time. Note that the two-pore model of large 150 nm breaks and a 2 nm slit in the region where the junction strand is continuous provides vastly improved agreement with confocal microscopic measurements of vessel wall concentration. Experimental data courtesy of R. Adamson. Theoretical curves courtesy of B. M. Fu.

that, as previously predicted in Fig. 8, the large pore provides only about one-third of the solute flux and that the solution of the integral equation for $C_a(t)$ provides remarkably good agreement with confocal microscopic measurements of the vessel wall concentration. The theoretically predicted profiles in the tissue (see Fig. 10) are also in excellent agreement with the measurements of the time-dependent mid-tissue profiles at z=0 obtained from the fluorescent intensity measurements using the confocal microscope. These combined results provide strong evidence in support of the hypothesis advanced by Fu *et al.* (1994) that there is a second very small pore that is the primary pathway for ions and small solutes.

In summary, a comparison of the predictions of Fu *et al.* (1995) and our electron and confocal microscopic experiments indicates the following. (i) Over the first 10 s of perfusion, there is little tracer detectable in the tissue. This is exactly the behavior that would be expected if the tracer crossing the wall were rapidly diluted as it spreads into the tissue volume. Tracer wakes distal to the junction strand are only detected in the region of the larger breaks, because the high local flux density creates a local elevation in cleft exit concentration that is not observed along most of the cleft length. (ii) Tracer is not detected on the abluminal side of a small pore pathway distributed along the length of junctional strand until the tissue concentration of the tracer increases sufficiently for the cleft exit concentration to be detectable. The data in Fig. 10 suggest that this threshold is close to 50 % of the perfusate concentration.

This research is supported by NIH grant HL-44485. The authors are indebted to Bing Mei Fu, Ruey Tsay and Roger Adamson for their many valuable contributions to this research.

References

ADAMSON, R. H. (1990). Permeability of frog mesenteric capillaries after partial pronase digestion of the endothelial glycocalyx. *J. Physiol., Lond.* **428**, 1–13.

ADAMSON, R. H. AND CLOUGH, G. F. (1992). Plasma proteins modify the endothelial cell glycocalyx of frog mesenteric microvessels. *J. Physiol., Lond.* **445**, 473–486.

ADAMSON, R. H. AND MICHEL, C. C. (1993). Pathways through the intercellular clefts of frog mesenteric capillaries. *J. Physiol., Lond.* **466**, 303–327.

BRINKMAN, H. C. (1947). A calculation of the viscous force exerted by a flowing fluid on a dense swarm of particles. *Appl. Sci. Res. Sect. A* **1**, 27–34.

BUNDGAARD, M. (1984). The three-dimensional organization of tight junctions in a capillary endothelium revealed by serial-section electron microscopy. *J. Ultrastruct. Res.* **88**, 1–17.

CASELY-SMITH, J. R., GREEN, J. L. AND WADEY, P. J. (1975). The quantitative morphology of skeletal muscle capillaries in relation to permeability. *Microvasc. Res.* **10**, 43–64.

CLOUGH, G. C. AND MICHEL, C. C. (1988). Quantitative comparisons of hydraulic permeability and endothelial intercellular cleft dimensions in single frog capillaries. *J. Physiol., Lond.* **405**, 563–576.

CRONE, C. AND LEVITT, D. (1984). Capillary permeability to small solutes. In *Handbook of Physiology*, section 2, vol. 4 (ed. E. M. Renkin and C. C. Michel), pp. 411–466. Bethesda, MD: American Physiological Society.

CURRY, F. E. (1984). Transcapillary exchange. In *Handbook of Physiology*, section 2, *The Cardiovascular System*, vol. 4, *The Microcirculation*, part 1 (ed. E. M. Renkin and C. C. Michel), pp. 309–374. Bethesda, MD: American Physiological Society.

CURRY, F. E. (1986). A fiber matrix model of capillary permeability. *Circulation Res.* **59**, 367–380.

CURRY, F. E. AND MICHEL, C. C. (1980). Determinants of capillary permeability: a review of mechanism based on single capillary studies. *Microvasc. Res.* **20**, 96–99.

FIRTH, J. A., BAUMAN, K. F. AND SIBLEY, C. P. (1983). The intercellular junctions of guinea-pig placental capillaries: A possible structural basis for endothelial solute permeability. *J. Ultrastruct. Res.* **85**, 45–57.

FU, B. M., ADAMSON, R. H., CURRY, F. E. AND WEINBAUM, S. (1995). A diffusion wake model for tracer ultrastructure permeability studies in microvessels. *Am. J. Physiol.* (in press).

FU, B. M., TSAY, R. Y., CURRY, F. E. AND WEINBAUM, S. (1994*b*). A junctional-orifice-fiber entrance layer model for capillary permeability: Application to frog mesenteric capillaries. *ASME J. Biomech. Eng.* **116**, 502–513.

GANATOS, P., WEINBAUM, S. AND PFEFFER, R. (1980). A strong interaction theory for the creeping motion of a sphere between plane parallel boundaries. II. Parallel motion. *J. Fluid Mech.* **99**, 755–783.

KARNOVSKY, M. J. (1967). The ultrastrucural basis of capillary permeability studies with peroxidase as a tracer. *J. Cell Biol.* **35**, 213–236.

LEE, J. S. AND FUNG, Y. C. (1969). Stokes flow around a circular cylindrical post confined between two parallel plates. *J. Fluid Mech.* **37**, 657–672.

LUFT, J. H. (1966). Fine structure of capillary and endo-capillary layer as revealed by ruthenium red. *Fedn Proc. Fedn Am. Socs exp. Biol.* **25**, 1773–1788.

MICHEL, C. C. (1984). Fluid movements through capillary walls. In *Handbook of Physiology*, section 2, vol. 4 (ed. E. M. Renkin and C. C. Michel), pp. 375–410. Bethesda, MD: American Physiological Society.

MICHEL, C. C. (1988). Capillary permeability and how it may change. *J. Physiol., Lond.* **404**, 1–29.

MICHEL, C. C., SNOW, G. R. AND TASKER, J. A. (1973). A method for measuring the permeability of individually perfused capillaries of the frog mesentery. *J. Physiol., Lond.* **234**, 25P–26P.

OGSTON, A. G., PRESTON, B. N. AND WELLS, J. D. (1973). On the transport of compact particles through solutions of chain polymers. *Proc. R. Soc. Lond. A* **333**, 297–316.

PAPPENHEIMER, J. R., RENKIN, E. M. AND BORRERO, L. M. (1951). Filtration, diffusion and molecular sieving through peripheral capillary membranes. A contribution to the pore theory of capillary permeability. *Am. J. Physiol.* **167**, 13–46.

SATCHER, R. L., JR. (1993). A mechanical model of vascular endothelial. PhD thesis, Department of Chemical Engineering, MIT.

SCHULZE, C. AND FIRTH, J. A. (1992). The interendothelial junction in myocardial capillaries: evidence for the existence of regularly spaced, cleft spanning structures. *J. Cell Sci.* **101**, 647–655.

SIMIONESCU, N., SIMIONESCU, M. AND PALADE, G. E. (1973). Permeability of muscle capillaries to exogenous myoglobin. *J. Cell Biol.* **57**, 424–452.

TSAY, R. AND WEINBAUM, S. (1991). Viscous flow in a channel with periodic cross-bridging fibers of arbitrary aspect ratio and spacing. *J. Fluid Mech.* **226**, 125–148.

TSAY, R., WEINBAUM, S. AND PFEFFER, R. (1989). A new model for capillary filtration based on recent electron microscopic studies of endothelial junctions. *Chem. Eng. Commun.* **82**, 67–102.

WEINBAUM, S., TSAY, R. AND CURRY, F. E. (1992). A three-dimensional junction–pore–matrix model for capillary permeability. *Microvasc. Res.* **44**, 85–111.

WISSIG, S. L. (1979). Identification of the small pore in muscle capillaries. *Acta physiol. scand.* (Suppl.) **463**, 33–44.

ZENG, Y. AND WEINBAUM, S. (1994). Stokes flow through periodic orifices in a channel. *J. Fluid Mech.* **263**, 207–226.

SEB SYMPOSIUM 'BIOLOGICAL FLUID DYNAMICS'
LEEDS, 4–9 JULY, 1994

Scientific Programme

Tuesday, 5 July, morning Session A: Swimming
Chairmen: D. Weihs & J.W.M. Osse

08.50–09.00 Welcome from the Chairman, Prof. T.J. Pedley

09.00–09.50 J.J. Videler (Groningen)
Body surface adaptations to boundary-layer dynamics.

09.50–10.10 T.L. Williams, J. Carling, G. Bowtell, K.A. Sigvardt & N.A. Curtin (London)
Interactions between muscle activation, body curvature and the water in the swimming lamprey.

10.10–10.30 J.Y. Cheng, T.J. Pedley & J.D. Altringham (Leeds)
Modelling swimming fish: hydrodynamics and fluid–solid interactive dynamics.

11.00–11.20 J. Glasheen & T.A. McMahon (Harvard)
A hydrodynamic model of basilisk lizards running on water.

11.20–11.40 E.V. Romanenko (Moscow)
Swimming of dolphins (experiments and modelling).

11.40–12.30 J. Lighthill (London)
The lateral line's role in active drag reduction by clupeoid fishes.

Tuesday, 5 July afternoon Session B: Flight
Chairmen: J. Lighthill and R.McN. Alexander

14.00–14.50 C.P. Ellington (Cambridge)
Unsteady aerodynamics of insect flight.

14.50–15.10 W. Nachtigall (Saarbrücken)
Hovering in syrphids.

15.10–15.30 M. Okamoto, K. Yasuda M. Okamoto & A. Azuma (Kawasaki)
Aerodynamic characteristics of wings and body of a dragonfly.

16.00–16.20 R. Bannasch (Berlin)
Penguin swimming.

16.20–16.40 K. Kawachi, S. Sunada and H. Liu (Tokyo)
Application of numerical methods to the aerodynamics of insect flight.

16.40–17.30 J.M.V. Rayner (Bristol)
Force generation mechanisms and wake structure for swimming or flying at high Reynolds number.

18.00 University Reception, University House, Dining Room 4/5.

Wednesday, 6 July, morning Session C: Large vessel blood flow.
Chairmen: T. Yamaguchi and C. Oddou

09.00–09.50 T.J. Pedley (Leeds)
High Reynolds number flow in tubes of complex geometry with application to arteries and airways.

09.50–10.10 B. Hillen (Utrecht)
'Form and flow': morphologic influence on the flow and *vice versa*.

10.10–10.30 P.G. Walker and others (Atlanta)
Magnetic resonance: a new tool to study cardiovascular fluid mechanics.

11.00–11.20 M. Sugawara, Y. Kondoh, K. Uchida, C.J.H. Jones (Tokyo)
Interactions between the heart and the arterial system.

11.20–11.40 R.E. Shadwick (La Jolla) & J.M. Gosline (Vancouver)
Windkessels in whales: an analysis of haemodynamics from arterial mechanics.

11.40–12.30 C.S. Peskin (New York)
A general method for the computer simulation of biological systems interacting with fluids.

Wednesday, 6 July, afternoon Session D: Microcirculation and Tissue Transport.
Chairmen: C.G. Caro and B. Hillen

14.00–14.50 T.W. Secomb (Arizona)
Mechanics of blood flow in the micro-circulation.

14.50–15.10 G. Schmid-Schonbein (La Jolla)
Perfusion of skeletal muscle.

15.10–15.30 T.M. Griffith & D.H. Edwards (Cardiff)
Mathematical, pharmacological and mechanical characterisation of chaotic resistance artery vaso motion.

16.00–16.20 P. Cerasi, P. Mills, J. Durussel, G. Guiffaut & J. Dufaux (Paris VII)
Study of instability amplification in a non-consolidated porous medium as applied to angiogenesis.

16.20–16.40 A. Roth (Tübingen)
Water transport in vascular plants – numerical simulations.

16.40–17.30 S. Weinbaum (New York) & F.E. Curry (Davis)
Modelling the structural pathways for transcapillary exchange.

20.00 Evening Poster and video session (with wine)

Thursday, 7 July, morning Session E: Micro-organisms, Filter feeding, etc.
Chairmen: M.A. Sleigh and M.A.R. Koehl

09.00–09.50 J.R. Blake (Birmingham)
Hydrodynamics of filter feeding.

09.50–10.10 M.J. Holwill (London)
Structure and function in flagellar avoidance responses.

10.10–10.30 C. van den Berg, J.W.M. Osse & T.J. Schaafsma (Wageningen)
An attempt to visualise the water flow in the head of a breathing carp using NMRI.

10.30–10.50 S. Vogel (Duke)
Who's Who among the fluid pumps of organisms.

11.15–11.55 J.O. Kessler (Arizona)
Paths and patterns: the biology and physics of swimming algal and bacterial populations.

11.55–12.45 H.C. Bennet-Clark (Oxford)
Insect sound production: transduction mechanisms and impedance matching.

Thursday, 7 July
Afternoon: free
Evening: conference dinner in the York Railway Museum.

Friday, 8 July, morning Session F: Invertebrates and intermediate Reynolds number
Chairmen: T.A. McMahon and S. Vogel

09.00–09.50 T.L. Daniel (Seattle)
Invertebrate swimming: integrating internal and external mechanics.

09.50–10.10 C. Jordan (Chicago)
A predictive model of undulatory locomotion: combining muscle and soft tissue mechanics with external fluid dynamics.

10.10–10.30 E.J. Stamhuis (Groningen).
Application of laser-sheet particle image velocimetry to quantify flow around aquatic animals.

11.00–11.20 J.W.M. Osse & J.G.M. van den Boogaart (Wageningen)
Resistive and reactive components in swimming of carp larvae.

11.20–11.40 C. Loudon (Berkeley)
The influence of airspeed on the rate of chemical signal interception by insect antennae.

11.40–12.30 M.A.R. Koehl (Berkeley)
The fluid dynamics of hairy appendages at low and intermediate Reynolds number.

Friday, 8 July, afternoon Session G: Respiration
Chairmen: D. Isabey and J.B. Grotberg

14.00–14.50 P. Scheid (Bochum)
Diffusion, convection and structure determine gas exchange in vertebrate gills and lungs.

14.50–15.10 C.D. Bertram (Sydney)
The dynamics of collapsible tubes.

15.10–15.30 L. Huang & J.E. Ffowcs Williams (Cambridge)
Two major mechanisms of human snoring.

16.00–16.50 R.D. Kamm (M.I.T.)
Shear-augmented dispersion in biological systems.

16.50–17.10 M. Nishida, Y. Inaba, H. Fujioka & K. Tanishita (Yokohama)
Gas dispersion in oscillatory flow in a model pulmonary bifurcation.

17.10–17.30 W. Limberg, R. Opitz & L. Lorang (Aachen)
Theoretical and experimental studies based on a new model of the mechanics of breathing.

17.30 Close of Symposium

Steering Committee
Chairman T.J. Pedley (Leeds)
Co-Chairman C.P. Ellington (Cambridge)
R.McN. Alexander (Leeds)
J.D. Altringham (Leeds)
C.R. Bridges (SEB)
N.A. Hill (Leeds)
J.M.V. Rayner (Bristol)

LIST OF PARTICIPANTS

Dr P Aerts
University of Anterp (U.I.A)
Biology Dept
Universiteitsplein
Wilrijk (Antwerpen) B-2610
Belgium

Mr A A Ahmed
University of Birmingham
Dept of Mathematics & Statistics
Edgbaston
Birmingham B15 2TT
UK

Dr G K Aldis
Australian Defence Force Academy
Dept of Mathematics
Canberra ACT 2600
Australia

Prof R McNeill Alexander
University of Leeds
Dept of Pure & Applied Biology
Leeds LS2 9JT
UK

Dr J D Altringham
University of Leeds
Dept of Pure & Applied Biology
Leeds LS2 9JT
UK

Prof A Azuma
University of Tokyo
37-3 Hiyako-Cho
Saiwai-Ku
Kawasak 210
Japan

Dr R Bannasch
Technische Universitat Berlin
Bionik und Evolutionstechnik
Ackerstrasse 71-76
Berlin D-13355
Germany

Dr H C Bennet-Clark
Oxford University
Dept of Zoology
South Parks Road
Oxford OX1 3PS
UK

Dr C D Bertram
University of New South Wales
Centre for Biomedical Engineering
Sydney 2052
Australia

Ms G Biehle
Albert-Ludwigs-Universitat Freiburg
Institut fur Biologie III
Abt. Prof. Dr. Spatz
Schanzlestr.1
Freiburg 79104
Germany

Prof J R Blake
University of Birmingham
School of Mathematics & Statistics
Edgbaston
Birmingham B15 2TT
UK

Dr R W Blake
University of British Columbia
Dept of Zoology
Vancouver, BC
Canada

Dr G Borger
Carl von Ossietzky Universitat
Fachbereich Physik
Postfach 2503
Oldenburg D-26111
Germany

Dr G Bowtell
The City University
Dept of Mathematics
Northampton Square
Islington
London EC1 0HB
UK

Dr M D Brown
Birmingham University
Dept of Physiology
Birmingham B15 2TJ
UK

Dr J C Carling
St George's Hospital Medical School
Dept of Physiology
Cranmer Terrace
Tooting
London SW17 0RE
UK

Prof Colin G Caro
Imperial College
Centre for Biological & Medical Systems
Exhibition Road
London SW7 2BX
UK

Mr Cerasi
Universite Paris 7
LBHP
2 etage, Tour 33-4, Case 7056
2 Place Jussieu
Paris 75251
France

Dr J-Y Cheng
St Francis Xavier University
Biology Dept
PO Box 5000
Antigonish, N.Scotia B2G 2W5
Canada

Dr A J Cooper
University of Cambridge
Zoology Dept
Downing Street
Cambridge CB2 3EJ
UK

Prof T L Daniel
University of Washington
Dept of Zoology
Seattle, WA 98195
USA

Dr M E De Mont
St Francis Xavier University
Biology Dept
Box 5000
Antigonish, N.Scotia B2G 2WS
Canada

Dr R H Dillon
Tullane University
Dept of Mathematics
New Orleans, LA 70118
USA

Dr P Domenici
Dunstaffnage Marine Laboratory
PO Box 3
Oban, Argyll
Scotland

Dr D J Doorly
Imperial College
Centre for Biological & Medical Systems
London SW7 2AZ
UK

Dr A I D'Yachenko
Institute of Biomedical Problems
Dept of Hyperbaric Physiology
Khotosheskoje Shosse, 76-A
Moscow 123007
Russia

Dr S Egginton
University of Birmingham
Dept of Physiology
Birmingham B15 2TJ
UK

Prof D Elad
Tel Aviv University
Dept of Biomedical Engineering
Faculty of Engineering
Tel Aviv 69978
Israel

Dr C P Ellington
University of Cambridge
Dept of Zoology
Downing Street
Cambridge CB2 3EJ
UK

Prof L J Fauci
Tulane University
Dept of Mathematics
New Orleans, Lousiana 70118
USA

Dr F Fish
West Chester University
Dept of Biology
West Chester, PA 19383
USA

Mr H Fujioka
Keio University
Bio-Med Engineering, Science & Technology
3-14-1, Hiyoshi
Kohoku-ku
Yokohama 223
Japan

Mr N Furuta
Tokai University, Dept Bio-Med Eng
School High Technology for Human Welfare
317 Nishino
Numazu
Shizuoka 410-03
Japan

Ms Gabet
Universite Paris 7
LBHP
2 etage, Tour 33-4, Case 7056
2 Place Jussieu
Paris 75251
France

Mr J W Glasheen
Harvard University
Organismal & Evolutionary Biology
Biomechanics Lab, ESL
40 Oxford Street
Cambridge, MA 02138
USA

Dr J Goodfellow
University of Wales College of Medicine
Cardiology Dept
Cardiff
UK

Dr T M Griffith
University of Wales
College of Medicine
Dept of Diagnostic Radiology
Heath Park, Cardiff CF4 4XN
UK

Prof J B Grotberg
Northwestern University
Biomedical Engineering Dept
2145 Sheridan Road
Evanston, IL 60208
USA

Mr A B Haines
Royal Aeronautical Society
3 Bromham Road
Biddenham
Bedford
UK

Ms B G Hamer
Massachusetts Inst of Technology
Dept of Mechanical Engineering
77 Massachusetts Ave 3-243
Cambridge, MA 02139
USA

Dr D G Harper
University of Cambridge
Dept of Zoology
Downing Street
Cambridge CB2 3EJ
UK

Dr N Hill
The University of Leeds
Dept of Applied Mathematical Studies
Leeds LS2 9JT
UK

Prof B Hillen
Utrecht University
Dept of Functional Anatomy
PO Box 80039
Utrecht 3508 TA
The Netherlands

Dr M E J Holwill
King's College London
Dept of Physics
Strand
London WC2R 2LS
UK

Dr L Huang
Peterhouse
Cambridge CB2 1RD
UK

Dr P E Hydon
University of Northumbria
Dept of Mathematics & Statistics
Ellison Building
Newcastle-upon-Tyne NE20 9UZ
UK

Ms H Igarishi
Tokai University, Dept Bio-Med Eng
School High Technology for Human Welfare
317 Nishino
Numazu
Shizuoka 410-03
Japan

Dr D Isabey
INSERM
U-296-Physiologie Respiratoire
Faculte de Medecine
8 rue General Sassail
Creteil 94010
France

Dr G Jayaraman
Indian Istitute of Technology
Centre for Atmospheric Sciences
New Delhi
India

Dr C J H Jones
University of Wales College of Medicine
Cardiology Dept
Cardiff
UK

Dr C E Jordan
University of Chicago
Dept of Organismal Biology & Anatomy
1025 E 57th Street
Chicago, IL 60637
USA

Ms M Junge
Universitat des Saarlandes
FB 13.4 Zoologie
Saarbrucken 66041
Germany

Prof R D Kamm
Massachusetts Inst of Technology
Dept of Mechanical Engineering, Rm 3-260
77 Massachusetts Ave
Cambridge, MA 02139
USA

Ms A Kamphuis
Universitat Bonn, Botanisches Institut
Abteilung Theoretische Biologie
Kirschallee 1
Bonn 53115
Germany

Prof K Kawachi
University of Tokyo
Research Centre for Adv. Science & Tech.
4-6-1 Komaba
Meguro-Ku
Tokyo 153
Japan

Ms A B Kesel
Universitat des Saarlandes
FB 13.4 Zoologie
Saarbrucken 66041
Germany

Prof J O Kessler
University of Arizona
Physics Dept
Tucson, AZ 85721
USA

Dr E Kimmel
Technion
Dept of Agricultural Engineering
Haifa 32000
Israel

Ms T Knower
University of California, San Diego
Scripps Institution of Oceanography
214 Scholander Hall
Mail Code 0204
La Jolla, CA 92093
USA

Prof M A R Koehl
University of California, Berkeley
Dept of Integrative Biology
Berkeley, CA 94720
USA

Dr J K B Krijger
Utrecht University
Dept of Functional Anatomy
PO Box 80039
Utrecht 3508 TA
The Netherlands

Sir James Lighthill
University College London
Dept of Mathematics
Gower Street
London WC1E 6BT
UK

Prof G M Lilley
University of Southampton
Dept of Aeronautics & Astronautics
Southampton S017 1BJ
UK

Mr Q Long
Imperial College, London
Centre for Biological & Medical Systems
Sir Leon Bagrit Centre
London SW7 2BX
UK

Mr L Lorang
RWTH Aachen
Aerodynamisches Institut Aachen
Wullnerstrasse ZW.5U.7
Aachen D-52062
Germany

Dr C Loudon
Kansas State University
Dept of Entomology
Waters Hall
Manhattan, Kansas
USA

Dr T W Lowe
University of Leeds
Dept of Applied Mathematical Studies
Leeds LS2 9JT
UK

Mr E Luiker
University of British Columbia
Dept of Zoology
6170 University Road
Canada

Dr X Y Luo
The University of Leeds
Dept of Applied Mathematical Studies
Leeds LS2 9JT
UK

Prof T A McMahon
Harvard University
Division of Applied Sciences
Pierce Hall 325
Cambridge, MA 02138
USA

Dr A J Mestel
Imperial College, London
Mathematics Dept
180 Queensgate
London SW7 2BZ
UK

Dr R N Miftakhov
United Arab Emirates University
Dept of Biophysics
PO Box 17666
Al Ain
UAE

Mr H Mitsutake
Tokai University, Dept Bio-Med Eng
School High Technology for Human Welfare
317 Nishino
Numazu
Shizuoka 410-03
Japan

Mrs A J Mokady
Imperial College, London
Centre for Biological & Medical Systems
Exhibition Road
London SW7 2BX
UK

Ms U K Muller
University of Groningen
Dept of Marine Biology
Biological Centre
PO Box 14
Haren 9750 AA
The Netherlands

Prof W Nachtigall
Universitat des Saarlandes
FB 13.4 Zoologie
Saarbrucken 66041
Germany

Mr M Nishida
Keio University
Bio-Med Engineering, Science & Technology
3-14-1, Hiyoshi
Kohoku-ku
Yokohama 223
Japan

Prof C O Oddou
Universite Paris XII Val du Marne
Laboratoire Mecanique Physique
61 Avenue du General de Gaulle
Creteil 94010
France

Prof K Ohba
Kansai University
Dept of Mechanical & Systems Engineering
Suita
Osaka 564
Japan

Prof J W M Osse
Agricultural University, Wageningen
Experimental Animal Morph. & Cell Biol.
PO Box 338
Wageningen 6700 AH
The Netherlands

Prof T J Pedley
University of Leeds
Dept of Applied Mathematics
Leeds LS2 9JT
UK

Dr G Pelle
Universite Paris XII Val du Marne
Laboratoire Mecanique Physique
61 Avenue du General de Gaulle
Creteil 94010
France

Prof C S Peskin
New York University
Courant Inst of Mathematical Sciences
251 Mercer Street
New York, NY 10012
USA

Dr J Ravensbergen
Utrecht University
Dept of Functional Anatomy
PO Box 80039
Utrecht 3508 TA
The Netherlands

Dr J M V Rayner
University of Bristol
School of Biological Sciences
Woodland Road
Bristol BS8 1UG
UK

Ms I Roche
Universite Paris 7
LBHP
2 etage, Tour 33-4, Case 7056
2 Place Jussieu
Paris 75251
France

Dr A Roth
Universitat Tubingen
Institut fur Geologie und Palaeontologie
Sigwarstr.10
Tubingen D-72076
Germany

Prof Dr P Scheid
Ruhr-Universitat Bochum
Institut fur Physiologie
Bochum 44780
Germany

Prof G W Schmid-Schoenbein
University of California, San Diego
Institute for Biomedical Engineering
La Jolla, CA-92093
USA

Dr R C Schroter
Imperial College
Centre for Biological & Medical Systems
London SW7 2AZ
UK

Dr P J Schulte
University of Nevada
Dept of Biological Sciences
Las Vegas, NV 89154
USA

Dr T W Secomb
University of Arizona
Dept of Physiology
Tucson, AZ 85724
USA

Dr N Shadrina
Pavlov Institute of Physiology
Fax 812 218 0501

Dr R Shadwick
University of California, San Diego
Scripps Institute of Oceanography
Dept of Marine Biology
La Jolla, CA 92093
USA

Mr K Shindo
Tokai University, Dept Bio-Med Eng
School High Technology for Human Welfare
317 Nishino
Numazu
Shizuoka 410-03
Japan

Dr Z Skalak
Institute of Hydrodynamics
Dept of Biomechanics
Podbabska 13
Prague 6
166 12
Czech Republic

Mr M J C Smith
Purdue University
School of Aeronautics & Astronautics
Grissom Hall
West Lafayette, IN 47907
USA

Dr S W Smye
St James's University Hospital
Dept of Medical Physics
Leeds

Mr E J Stamhuis
University of Groningen
Dept of Marine Biology
Biological Centre
PO Box 14
Haren 9750 AA
The Netherlands

Prof M Sugawara
Tokyo Women's Medical College
Dept of Cardiovascular Sciences
8-1 Kawada-cho
Shinjuku-ku
Tokyo 162
Japan

Mr G Tanaka
Keio University
Bio-Med Engineering, Science & Technology
3-14-1, Hiyoshi
Kohoku-ku
Yokohama 223
Japan

Dr J W Tang
University of Sheffield
Faculty of Medicine and Dentistry
Sheffield S10 2TN
UK

Prof K Tanishita
Keio University
Biomed Engineering, Science & Technology
3-14-1, Hiyoshi
Kohoku-ku
Yokohama 223
Japan

Dr M A Taylor
National Museums of Scotland
Dept of Geology
Chambers Street
Edinburgh EH1 1JF
UK

Prof Dr B E Ungerechts
Katholieke Universiteit Leuven
Fac Lichamelijke Opleidingenkin Aquatics
Tervaurvest 101
Heverlee B-3001
Belgium

Dr C van den Berg
University of Cambridge
Dept of Zoology
Downing Street
Cambridge CB2 3EJ
UK

Ms L A van Duren
University of Groningen
Dept of Marine Biology
Biological Centre
PO Box 14
Haren 9750 AA
The Netherlands

Mr P W J van Hengel
Rijksuniversiteit Groeningen
Vakgroep biofysica
Nijenborgh 4
Groningen 9747 AG
The Netherlands

Dr J Th P W van Maarseveen
Rijksuniversiteit Groningen
Dept Biofysica
Nijenborgh 4
Groningen NL-9747
The Netherlands

Dr S M van Netten
University of Groningen
Dept of Biophysics
Nijenborgh 4
Groningen 9747 AG
The Netherlands

Dr J J Videler
Groningen University
Dept of Marine Biology
PO Box 14
Haren 9750 AA
The Netherlands

Prof S Vogel
Duke University
Zoology Dept
Box 90325
Durham, NC 27708
USA

Mr J M Wakeling
University of Cambridge
Zoology Dept
Downing Street
Cambridge CB2 3EJ
UK

Dr P G Walker
Georgia Institute of Technology
School of Chemical Engineering
778 Atlantic Drive
Atlanta, GA 30332
USA

Dr C Walsh
University of Toronto
Institute of Biomedical Engineering
4 Taddle Creek Road, rm 407
Toronto M5S 1A4
Canada

Prof D Weihs
Technion
Dept of Aerospace Engineering
Haifa 32000
Israel

Prof S Weinbaum
City College of New York
Dept of Mechanical Engineering
137th St & Convent Avenue
New York, NY 10031
USA

Dr P J W Wensing
Utrecht University
Dept of Functional Anatomy
PO Box 80039
Utrecht 3508 TA
The Netherlands

Dr P J Wilkin
Purdue University North Central
Dept of Biology/Chemistry
Westville, IN 46391
USA

Dr T L Williams
University of London
St George's Hospital Medical School
Physiology Dept
Tooting
London SW17 0RE
UK

Mr A P Willmott
University of Cambridge
Dept of Zoology
Downing Street
Cambridge CB2 3EJ
UK

Dr R J Wootton
University of Exeter
Dept of Biological Sciences
Hatherley Laboratories
Prince of Wales Road
Exeter EX4 4PS
UK

Dr X Y Xu
City University
Dept of Mech Engineering & Aeronautics
Northampton Square
London EC1V 0HB
UK

Prof R Y Yamaguchi
Shibaura Institute of Technology
Dept of Mechanical Engineering
3-9-14 Shibaura
Minato-ku
Tokyo 108
Japan

Prof T Yamaguchi
Tokai University, Bio-Med Engineering
School High Technology for Human Welfare
317 Nishino
Numazu
Shizuoka 410-03
Japan

Dr K Yasuda
Nihon University
Dept of Aerospace Engineering
7-24-1, Narashinodai
Funabashi
Chiba 274
Japan

INDEX OF SUBJECTS